VIRAL GENE THERAPY

Edited by **Ke Xu**

Viral Gene Therapy
Edited by Ke Xu

Published by InTech
Janeza Trdine 9, 51000 Rijeka, Croatia

Publishing Process Manager Romina Krebel

Technical Editor Teodora Smiljanic

Cover Designer InTech Design Team

Additional hard copies can be obtained from orders@intechopen.com

Viral Gene Therapy, Edited by Ke Xu
p. cm.
ISBN 978-953-307-539-6

For EU product safety concerns:
IN TECH d.o.o., Prolaz Marije Krucifikse Kozulić 3, 51000 Rijeka, Croatia,
info@intechopen.com or visit our website at intechopen.com.

Meet the editor

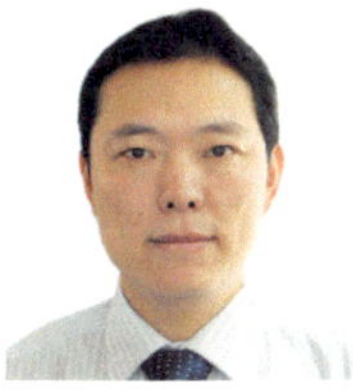

Dr. Ke Xu earned his first degree in Microbiology in 1989 from School of Life Sciences in Nankai University (China), and his Ph.D. in Cell and Molecular Biology in 2001 from University of Essex (UK). He completed his postdoctoral training at the Institute of Cancer Research (UK), studying on the induction of leukemia cell apoptosis and differentiation. Dr. Ke Xu carried out his research fellowship at Imperial College London (UK), investigating gene targeting and lung cancer. He joined the Tianjin Lung Cancer Institute of Tianjin Medical University General Hospital (China) in 2007 as a professor to establish an independent research group, studying the molecular mechanism of metastasis and chemoresistance of lung cancer. He also develops novel chemical compounds to interfere with key cancer promoting pathways. Dr. Ke Xu is an active member of American Association of Cancer Research, American Society for Cell Biology, Chinese Anti-Cancer Association and Chinese Pharmaceutical Association.

Contents

Preface

The general meaning of gene therapy is to correct defective genes that are responsible for disease development. The most common form of gene therapy involves the insertion, alteration or removal of genes within an individual's cells and biological tissues. Many of gene transfer vectors are modified viruses. The ability for the delivery of therapeutic genes made them desirable for engineering virus vector systems. Recently, the viral vectors in laboratory and clinical use have been based on RNA and DNA viruses processing very different genomic structures and host ranges. Various viral vectors have been developed and optimized, such as retrovirus, adenovirus, lentivirus and adeno-associated virus. This book provides broad coverage of the field of viral gene therapy.

In the first section of this book, 'Retroviral Vector', chapter one discusses the efficiency of retroviral DNA integration, the preferences of integration for certain regions, and advances on integration site selection and gene therapy. Chapter two reviews and discusses the current cell lines and bioreaction platforms used for production of retroviral and lentiviral vectors, focusing on the current bottlenecks and future directions with a particular emphasis in the metabolic constrains. Modification of the surface of these vectors is a key element for their successful research and clinical use. Chapter three discusses the methods to modify surfaces of retroviral vectors, and the applications for surface modification of retroviral vectors, such as targeting and immune modulation. Chapter four reviews the role of the nuclear glucocorticoid receptor in controlling retroviral infection and function, and highlights its potential importance in retroviral-based gene therapy applications.

Adenoviral vectors serve as an excellent gene delivery system for a variety of cell types or organs for gene therapy and immunization applications. In the second section 'Adenoviral Vector', chapter five introduces the history of adenovirus research, the advantage and disadvantage of adenoviral vector, the adenoviral vector induced innate immune response, the evolution of adenoviral vector system, the application of adenoviral vector in gene therapy, and adenoviral vaccine. Chapter six reviews the background of virotherapy and the approaches of conditionally replicating adenoviruses (CRAds) on cancer treatment. The author also points out the exiting problems and obstacles in this field. In chapter seven, Adams et al. discuss how adenoviral vectors interact with human immune cells, particularly how adenoviral vectors interact with professional antigen presenting cells, namely dendritic cells. Chapter eight reviews the properties of the immune response induced by adenoviral vaccines and the mechanisms which control the quality of T cell response generated during such vaccination. Holst et al. compare the adenovirus vectors with other vaccination tools in the immunological arsenal, and discuss potential future clinical application of adenovirus vectored vaccines.

The third section of this book is 'Adeno-associated-virus Vector'. Chapter nine by Sun et al. introduces the adeno-associated virus (AAV) mediated β-thalassemia gene therapy. Human hematopoietic stem cells (HSCs) were obtained from β-thalassemia patients, transfected with the recombinant AAV containing β-globin gene. The transfected cells were then transplanted into Nude/SCID mice, and the long term expression of β-globin *in vivo* was examined. In the tenth chapter, Korecka et al. compare AAV serotypes for gene delivery to dopaminergic neurons in the substantia nigra (SN). They found that AAV5 and 7-syn-GFP resulted in the highest percentage of nigral dopaminergic neurons transduction, where AAV7 showed the highest efficiency in transducing the nigrostriatal projection pathway. Accordingly, they conclude that AAV7-syn-GFP is the most suitable SN gene delivery vehicle in mice. In the eleventh chapter, Okada et al. developed a new method of producing AAV vectors. They applied these AAV vectors in muscle transduction for the treatment of Duchenne muscular dystrophy (DMD). In chapter twelve, Sunico et al. introduce their study on the function of 2 dysregulated proteins in pathological events occurring at the peripheral (nerve) and central (motoneuron) levels after the severe crushing of a motor nerve in adult rats, using AAV and lentiviral vector.

In the section on 'Lentiviral Vector', the generation of high-titre lentiviral vectors capable of efficiently expressing transgenes over long periods of time is governed by a number of vector design rules. Chapter thirteen highlights the guiding design principles and the technical of the successful lentiviral gene vector design. Chapter fourteen reviews current status of lentiviral vector development, especially the progress in the lentiviral vector systems allowing the controlling of gene expression. It also discusses the ability of future application of the gene regulatable lentiviral vectors to therapeutic approach for the treatment of HIV-1 infection and acquired immunodeficiency syndrome (AIDS). Chapter fifteen discusses the development of lentiviral vectors, their evaluation for *ex vivo* and *in vivo* gene delivery to dendritic cells, and the efforts made to improve the biosafety of the lentiviral vector system.

In the last section on 'Other Types of Viral Vector', chapter sixteen introduces the development of HIV vector pseudotyped with HIV envelope, and applications of these vectors for AIDS or adult T-cell leukemia. Chapter seventeen introduces the development of novel vector system for highly efficient retrograde gene transfer by pseudotyping the HIV-1 vector with fusion glycoprotein B type (FuG-B). Herpes simplex virus type 1 (HSV-1) is a human pathogen associated with keratitis and cold sores. Chapter eighteen reviews the biology of HSV-1, and clinical trails and challenges of oncolytic Herpesvirus. In chapter nineteen, Kaneda et al. develop a hemagglutinating virus of Japan envelope (HVJ-E) vector using inactivated Sendai virus, as a pseudovirion for gene and drug delivery. They evaluate the anti-tumor effects of HVJ-E itself on mouse and human melanoma in animal models, and also the enhancement of anti-tumor effects of HVJ-E containing IL-12 gene. The last chapter reviews the pharmacokinetic study of viral vectors for gene therapy, including pharmacokinetic characteristics of viral vectors, analysis methods used for pharmacokinetic evaluations of viral vectors, and challenges and prospects.

We hope that the reviews and research described here will provide a wide-ranging forum in the viral gene therapy field. It is clear from these chapters that much more progress is required for the improvement of viral gene therapy. It is believed that the next few decades will see the application of viral gene therapy in the treatment of diseases.

Ke Xu
Tianjin Lung Cancer Institute
Tianjin Medical University General Hospital
Tianjin, China

Part 1

Retroviral Vector

1

Retroviral Vectors in Gene Therapy: Mechanism of Integration, Successes in Gene Therapy Trials, Emerging Problems and Potential Solutions

Ahmed F. Salem, Johanna A. Smith, Michael P. Lisanti and René Daniel
[1]*Division of Infectious Diseases - Center for Human Virology, and Jefferson Center for Stem Cell Biology and Regenerative Medicine, Thomas Jefferson University, Philadelphia*
[2]*Department of Stem Cell Biology and Regenerative Medicine, Thomas Jefferson University, Philadelphia,*
U.S.A

1. Introduction

Retroviral vectors have gained an increasing value in gene therapy because they stably deliver therapeutic genes to the host cell genome. These therapeutic genes are supposed to rectify consequences of inherited and acquired mutated genes in the host cell genome, or alter host cell function to cure diseases. In the following section we will discuss the biology and life cycle of retroviruses which starts with viral entry into the host cell, reverse transcription of viral RNA, nuclear import of the provirus, and finally integration of viral DNA into the cell host genome (Flint, Racaniello et al. 2004). Integration involves viral and host cellular proteins. Their role is discussed in the third and fourth sections of this chapter. Recently, the process of integration site selection (which is where the viral DNA integrates with the host cell DNA) has been quite understood throughout many *in vitro* and *in vivo* studies. The human genome project has enabled us to identify integration site preferences for retroviral vectors in human trials. The results of these human trials are reviewed in the fifth section of the chapter. Finally, the last section of the chapter will demonstrate the latest gene therapy trials attempts to control integration sites by manipulation of retrovirus genes and proteins.

1.1 Retrovirus structure and life cycle

Viruses are obligate parasites which depend on living cells to multiply. Their ability to deliver stable RNA and DNA into cells has determined their use in gene therapy. In 1983 Mann et al. developed one of the first retroviral gene therapy vectors for delivery *in vitro* (Mann, Mulligan et al. 1983). This development was followed by many successfully gene therapy trials of retroviruses (Anderson, Blaese et al. 1990; Levine and Friedmann 1991; Blaese, Culver et al. 1993). Now, retrovirual vectors are implemented in nearly 22.2% of clinical trials (http://www.wiley.com//legacy/wileychi/genmed/clinical/[June 2010]).
Retroviruses belong to the *Retroviriade* family. The retroviral particle consists of 2 copies of positive-single strand (+ss) RNA and viral proteins (reverse trascriptase, integrase, and

protease) which are all contained by nucleocapsid. The nucleocapsid complex is surrounded by a protein shell called capsid to form the viral core. A layer of matrix protein, which is formed outside the capsid, interacts with the envelope (env) which consists of lipid envelope derived from the host cell and viral envelope glycoproteins. Viral glycoproteins are made of two units: a transmembrane portion, which attaches the protein into the lipid bilayer, and a surface portion, which binds to the cellular receptor.
The life cycle of the retrovirus consist of several steps. It begins with the binding of the viral envelope to cellular receptors, which enables fusion of the viral envelope with the cellular membrane. Consequently, the viral particle is uncoated, liberating the viral core into the cell cytoplasm. The viral DNA is reverse transcribed to DNA. Then, the viral DNA is transported to the nucleus where it is integrated into the host cell's genome. From there, viral DNA is transcribed to RNA, some of which is translated to proteins. The viral RNA is packed in a viral particle along with viral proteins. Then, virion is produced when viral particles bud from the hosting cells (Escors and Breckpot).

1.2 Integration

The retroviral enzyme integrase (IN) plays a vital role in integration. It exists as a tetramer (dimer-of-dimers) inside the virion or the preintegration complex. IN facilitate viral DNA integration *in vitro*, even in the absence of other viral or cellular proteins (Coffin, Hughes et al. 1997; Flint, Racaniello et al. 2004). Integration is classified into two distinct steps. The first step called processing, where the IN removes two nucleotides from the 3' ends of the viral DNA, the synthesis of which was produced by the viral enzyme reverse transcriptase (Coffin, Hughes et al. 1997; Flint, Racaniello et al. 2004). Then, when the viral preintegration complex is in the vicinity of targeted host DNA, IN catalyzes a coupled cleavage-joining reaction, where the 3' ends of viral DNA are joined to host cell DNA, in the joining step (Coffin, Hughes et al. 1997; Flint, Racaniello et al. 2004). The intermediate product of the integration process is flanked by short single-stranded gaps in host cell DNA. After the integration reaction, postintegration repair takes place, in which the 5' ends of viral DNA are trimmed, the gaps filled, and ligated to host cell DNA. Lastly, the appropriate chromatin structure is reconstituted at the integration site. Postintegration repair does not require viral proteins, but instead depends on host cell DNA repair proteins (Daniel, Katz et al. 1999; Lau, Swinbank et al. 2005).
In vitro experiments show that incubating IN with oligonucleotides as DNA substrate, and target DNA were sufficient to achieve integration of one end of the DNA substrate (Flint, Racaniello et al. 2004). However, *in vivo*, stable integration requires cellular proteins to be accomplished. These cellular proteins have invoked interest of their potential as cofactors of integration. Using a yeast two-hybrid screen, human immunodeficiency virus (HIV)-1 IN-binding protein termed integrase interactor 1 (INI1) was identified (Kalpana, Marmon et al. 1994). At the beginning, INI1 protein was found to boost integration efficiency when it was added to the integration reaction *in vitro* (Kalpana, Marmon et al. 1994). Also, small interfering RNA (siRNA) targeting INI1, demonstrated that knocking down INI1 was sufficient to significantly reduce HIV-1 replication (Ariumi, Serhan et al. 2006). However, another study showed that lacking INI1 protein did not affect integration reaction (Boese, Sommer et al. 2004). Now it is accepted that INI1 does not affect integration but it appears to be involved in other process of the retroviral life cycle (Ariumi, Serhan et al. 2006; Mahmoudi, Parra et al. 2006; Treand, du Chene et al. 2006). Another cellular non-histone chromatin protein called high-mobility group protein-1 (HMG-1) was found to enhance

integration *in vitro* (Aiyar, Hindmarsh et al. 1996). This enhancement was thought to be attributed to its DNA-bending ability (Aiyar, Hindmarsh et al. 1996; Flint, Racaniello et al. 2004). HMG-I(Y), another related protein in the HMG family, was found in HIV-1 preintegration complexes (Farnet and Bushman 1997). As with HMG-1, HMG-I(Y) and HMG-2 boost integration in in vitro (Aiyar, Hindmarsh et al. 1996; Farnet and Bushman 1997; Hindmarsh, Ridky et al. 1999). Unfortunately, studies using HMG-I(Y) deficient cells did not elucidate the role of this protein in the integration reaction (Beitzel and Bushman 2003). Thus the role of HMG proteins in integration remains unclear. Autointegration is the integration of the viral DNA into itself which will eventually abort the retroviral life cycle. An 89 amino acid protein, which was identified in murine leukemia virus (MLV) preintegration complexes, forbids autointegration of viral DNA, and was hence called the barrier-to-autointegration factor (BAF) (Lee and Craigie 1998). Also BAF was detected in HIV-1 preintegration complex to block autointegration (Lin and Engelman 2003). Finally, in 2003, a yeast two-hybrid system resulted in the isolation of a new HIV-1 IN-binding protein, a previously identified cellular protein termed LEDGF/p75 (lens epithelium-derived growth factor) (Cherepanov, Devroe et al. 2004). In knockout mice experiments, LEDGF/p75 was found not to be a lens growth factor, actually, the knockout mice of the mouse LEDGF/p75 homolog, PSIP1 (PC4 and SFRS1-interacting protein-1), had skeletal abnormalities, indicating that this protein is involved in bone development (Sutherland, Newton et al. 2006). Furthermore, many studies demonstrate that LEDGF/p75 targeting with siRNA or LEDGF/p75 null cells, from the LEDGF/p75 null transgenic animals, showed that integration of HIV-1-based vectors is reduced 89–96% in the absence of LEDGF/p75 (Llano, Saenz et al. 2006; Shun, Raghavendra et al. 2007). Therefore, LEDGF/p75 appears to be essential for efficient integration of HIV-1. Meanwhile, numerous studies displayed that LEDGF/p75 does not bind to MLV IN nor is it essential for MLV integration (Llano, Vanegas et al. 2004; Busschots, Vercammen et al. 2005; Shun, Raghavendra et al. 2007). In addition to the LEDGF/p75 role in enhancing integration in *in vitro*, it has the ability to target HIV-1 and HIV-1-based vector integration sites (Ciuffi, Llano et al. 2005; Llano, Vanegas et al. 2006; Shun, Raghavendra et al. 2007).

In summary, retroviral DNA integration is catalyzed by the viral protein integrase, but host cell proteins play a significant role in enhancing the efficiency of the reaction, and preventing autointegration.

2. Integration site preferences of retroviruses and retroviral vectors

While Integration of viral DNA can take place anywhere in the host cell genome and there is no strict host sequence for site selection, many studies showed that site selection is not a haphazard process (Schroder, Shinn et al. 2002; Wu, Li et al. 2003; Mitchell, Beitzel et al. 2004). In vitro studies demonstrated that some DNA-binding proteins can prevent contact of IN to target DNA and subsequently block the integration reaction at their binding sites (Pryciak and Varmus 1992; Bushman 1994). On the contrary, bending or distortion of DNA seems to enhance integration (Pryciak, Muller et al. 1992; Pryciak and Varmus 1992; Katz and Skalka 1994; Pruss, Bushman et al. 1994; Pruss, Reeves et al. 1994). Furthermore, studies showed that DNA wrapping around nucleosomes promotes distortion of DNA and thus promotes integration in the nucleosomes-bound DNA (Pryciak, Sil et al. 1992; Pryciak and Varmus 1992; Pruss, Bushman et al. 1994). All of the previous studies show that there are certain integration site preferences in DNA substrate in *in vitro* models. However, it should be considered that host DNA exists in a higher order chromatin structure, as the results of these in vitro studies may not translate to what really happens in the infected cell. To mimic the *in vivo* model, Taganov et al. used a 13-nucleosome extended array which includes binding sites for specific transcription factors and can be compacted into a higher-ordered structure using the histone H1 (Taganov, Cuesta et al. 2004). They noticed that chromatin structure impacts the integration site selection of HIV-1 and avian sarcoma virus (ASV) IN proteins differentially. In particular, HIV-1 IN-mediated integration was reduced after compaction of the target DNA/chromatin structure, whereas ASV IN-mediated integration was more efficient after compaction (Taganov, Cuesta et al. 2004). These results reveal that a higher order chromatin structure is involved in integration site selection and variant retroviruses may exhibit differential selectivity of their integration. According to the International Human Genome Sequencing Consortium (IHGSC), in 2004, 25,000 genes had been identified in the human genome. In 1990, two studies indicated that retroviruses have a preference to integrate in the vicinity of transcriptionally active regions (Mooslehner, Karls et al. 1990; Scherdin, Rhodes et al. 1990). These studies were challenged by the relatively low number of identified transcription sites (Bushman, Lewinski et al. 2005). Also, due to incomplete human genome sequencing, the percentage of the genome containing these "favored" integration sites was not clear. Thus, after the IHGSC announcement, researchers were able to define accurate statistical analysis of integration sites. Large-scale studies on HIV-1 integration in human T cell lines revealed that roughly 70% of integration events occurred in genes (Schroder, Shinn et al. 2002; Bushman, Lewinski et al. 2005). Furthermore, the 11q13 chromosomal region was found to be a "hotspot" of integration. Also, Schroder et al. showed similar results when using pseudotyped HIV-1-based vectors (Schroder, Shinn et al. 2002). Many studies have revealed that many retroviruses and retroviral vectors like simian immunodeficiency virus, an SIV-based vector, HIV-2, and feline immunodeficiency virus (FIV) integration preferences resemble HIV-1 integration preferences (Hematti, Hong et al. 2004; Crise, Li et al. 2005; Kang, Moressi et al. 2006; MacNeil, Sankale et al. 2006). On the contrary, MLV and MLV-based vectors demonstrated diverse integration preferences compared with HIV-1 (Wu, Li et al. 2003; Mitchell, Beitzel et al. 2004; Lewinski, Yamashita et al. 2006). 20% of MLV integration occasions occur in the vicinity of the 5′ ends of transcription (Wu, Li et al. 2003), approximately 17% of MLV integration events take place in the vicinity of CpG islands (Mitchell, Beitzel et al. 2004), 11% of the integration sites were detected in the vicinity of DNase I-hypersensitive sites (Lewinski, Yamashita et al. 2006), and the remaining integration sites are scattered in a random manner (Wu, Li et al. 2003).

Avian retroviruses and vectors show only a weak preference for integration around genes (about 40%) and no MLV-like preference for 5′ ends of transcription units (Mitchell, Beitzel et al. 2004; Narezkina, Taganov et al. 2004). Interestingly, high levels of transcription may even inhibit ASV integration in genes (Weidhaas, Angelichio et al. 2000; Maxfield, Fraize et al. 2005). These preferences are consistent with the above-described data from the in vitro system, which used nucleosomal arrays (Taganov, Cuesta et al. 2004). Interestingly, the human T-leukemia virus type 1 (HTLV-1) and mouse mammary tumor virus (MMTV), like avian retroviruses, do not specifically target genes and transcription start sites (Derse, Crise et al. 2007; Faschinger, Rouault et al. 2008).

Lastly, it appears that there is a symmetric base preferences surrounding integration sites for integration of HIV-1, SIV, MLV, and avian sarcoma-leukosis viruses (Crise, Li et al. 2005; Holman and Coffin 2005). These weak consensus sequences are virus specific and possibly

reflect the influence of IN on integration site selection (Holman and Coffin 2005). This proposal is supported by the symmetry of the target site sequence, because IN likely functions as a tetramer (Coffin et al., 1997; Flint et al., 2004; Wu et al., 2005; and see above).
In summary, the integration preferences described in this section are distinct for different group of retroviruses. The first group including HIV-1, HIV-2, SIV, and FIV, show a preferential integration into genes (Daniel and Smith 2008). While the second group, consisting of MLV and FV, integrate in 5' ends of transcription units and CpG islands. The last group consists of AVLS, HTLV-1, and MMTV (Daniel and Smith 2008). This group shows weak or even no preferences for gene or transcription start sites. Also, it appears that DNA sequence has a role in integration site selection. However, other factors (cellular cofactors and cellular structures) are likely to be the principal controllers of integration site selection.

3. Mechanism of integration site selection

As mentioned before, IN has a low specificity for binding to host cell DNA. So, it seems that host cell proteins participate in the integration process. Using the yeast two-hybrid system, Debyser and coworkers have identified a new HIV-1 IN-binding protein, termed LEDGF/p75 (Cherepanov, Maertens et al. 2003). LEDGF/p75 is required for efficient integration of HIV-1 DNA. Also, LEDGF/p75 is a transcription factor and has a C-terminal IN-binding domain and N-terminal chromatin-binding domain (Cherepanov, Maertens et al. 2003; Cherepanov, Devroe et al. 2004; Vanegas, Llano et al. 2005; Llano, Vanegas et al. 2006; Turlure, Maertens et al. 2006). Chromatin binding is mediated by PWWP and AT-hook motifs in the N-termianl domain of LEDGF/p75 (Llano, Vanegas et al. 2006; Turlure, Maertens et al. 2006). In addition, LEDGF/p75 was detected in association with preintegration complexes of HIV-1 and FIV in cultured cells (Llano, Vanegas et al. 2006). Moreover, LEDGF/p75 halts proteasomal degradation of ectopically expressed HIV-1 IN, therefore it might assist to the stability of preintegration complexes during infection (Maertens, Cherepanov et al. 2003; Llano, Vanegas et al. 2006). Also, LEDGF/p75 null cells showed that the residual integration sites in these cells no longer take place in active genes (Shun, Raghavendra et al. 2007). However, integration occurred preferentially near promoters and CpG islands (Shun, Raghavendra et al. 2007). The symmetric base preferences surrounding the integration site remained preserved (Holman and Coffin 2005). As a result, in the absence of LEDGF/p75, HIV-1 integration site preferences resemble those of MLV (Shun, Raghavendra et al. 2007). All these results strongly support the hypothesis that LEDGF/p75 targets HIV-1 (and other lentiviral) integration into active genes by tethering the IN protein to chromatin.
Although LEDGF/p75 appears to be a major HIV-1 IN-binding cellular protein, other factors are likely involved in integration site selection by HIV-1 and HIV-1-based vectors. Analysis of robust number of integration sites demonstrated that preferred integration sites are found in the vicinity of certain computer-predicted epigenetic marks, such as histone H3 K4 methylation, H4 acetylation, or H3 aceytlation (Kalpana, Marmon et al. 1994). These results may suggest that the chromatin structure, including the histone code, may also affect integration site selection. However the decisive evidence that these marks play a role in integration site selection has yet to be revealed. Moreover, other factors which affect integration site selection have been identified. Knockdown of the T-cell lineage-specific chromatin organizer, SATB1 (special AT-rich sequence-binding protein-1), reduces HIV-1

integration in the vicinity of SATB1-binding sites (Kumar, Mehta et al. 2007). Consequently, SATB1 seems to be implicated in integration site selection by an unknown mechanism. Lastly, it has been shown that the cellular protein Ku80, which is present in the preintegration complex, directs integration to chromatin domains prone to silencing (Li, Olvera et al. 2001; Masson, Bury-Mone et al. 2007). In contrast to HIV-1, integration of MLV-based and ASV-based vectors does not seem to be determined by LEDGF/p75 (Mitchell, Beitzel et al. 2004; Narezkina, Taganov et al. 2004). It is still unknown what controls ASV integration site selection. While in the case of MLV, a study using HIV chimeras with MLV genes demonstrated that MLV IN appears to be the major director for integration site selection (Lewinski, Yamashita et al. 2006). Furthermore, Gag-derived proteins play an auxiliary role in the integration selection process, as an HIV-1 chimera with MLV Gag demonstrated other site preferences different from both HIV and MLV (Lewinski, Yamashita et al. 2006). All the previous data support a different mechanism of integration site selection for MLV versus HIV.

In conclusion, current data has promoted our understating of the retroviral site selection process and demonstrates a major role of host cell proteins in the process. Yet, the process is not entirely understood, and there will likely be new determinate members involved in the retroviral integration site selection process revealed in the near future.

4. Integration site selection and gene therapy

MLV and HIV-1 vectors are the two most widely used vectors in gene therapy. It was hypothesized that even if a retroviral vector integrates in the "wrong spot", it may not necessarily lead to the development of a tumor (Hahn and Weinberg 2002; Baum, Kustikova et al. 2006). However, this hypothesis was challenged when serious adverse effects emerged in gene therapy trials involving children to treat X-linked severe combined immunodeficiency (SCID-X1) (Hacein-Bey-Abina, Von Kalle et al. 2003; Alexander, Ali et al. 2007; Bushman 2007; Deichmann, Hacein-Bey-Abina et al. 2007; Faschinger, Rouault et al. 2008). In one these trials, which used an MLV-based vector, 4 out of 11 patients developed T cell leukemia. Moreover, in another SCID-X1 gene therapy trial, it has been reported that a patient, of 10 patients enrolled, developed leukemia (Alexander, Ali et al. 2007; Schwarzwaelder, Howe et al. 2007; Thrasher and Gaspar 2008). Using sequencing analysis, T cells from two of the patients in the first trial who developed leukemia, showed an insertion of the vector near (and subsequent activation of) Lin-1, IsI-1, Mec-3 (LIM) domain only-2 (LMO2) protooncogene by the long terminal repeat (LTR) enhancer of the vector (Hacein-Bey-Abina, Von Kalle et al. 2003). Also, in the second trial, the vector insertion was in the vicinity of the LMO2 protooncogene (Thrasher and Gaspar 2008). These striking data demonstrate that vector integration at a dangerous spot of the human genome could lead to cancer development. It is also true that there could be other unknown factors that contributed to the leukemia development. Proposed factors that may have been involved are expression of the transgenes and chromosomal rearrangement (Hacein-Bey-Abina, Von Kalle et al. 2003; Pike-Overzet, de Ridder et al. 2006; Thrasher, Gaspar et al. 2006; Woods, Bottero et al. 2006). A follow-up analysis of the patients of these gene therapy trials exhibited a nonrandom distribution of integration sites *in vivo* (Deichmann, Hacein-Bey-Abina et al. 2007; Schwarzwaelder, Howe et al. 2007). Integration of vectors occurred preferentially near the 5' ends of genes and associated CpG islands, which is consistent with the data obtained with MLV in in vitro studies (Bushman 2007; Deichmann, Hacein-Bey-

Abina et al. 2007; Schwarzwaelder, Howe et al. 2007). Comparison of integration sites, in transduced-cells before and after infusion into patients, showed that vector integration manipulates cell growth, survival and proliferation *in vivo* (Deichmann, Hacein-Bey-Abina et al. 2007; Schwarzwaelder, Howe et al. 2007). Similarly, clonal evolution was noticed in a gene therapy trial using ADA-SCID. However, in this trial, no adverse effects were related with vector integration site (Aiuti, Cassani et al. 2007). In similar trials, vector insertion caused a deregulation of gene expression without any development of cancer (Ott, Schmidt et al. 2006; Recchia, Bonini et al. 2006). Likewise, animal gene therapy model results were similar to results obtained in human gene therapy trials (Li, Dullmann et al. 2002; Hematti, Hong et al. 2004; Modlich, Kustikova et al. 2005; Baum, Kustikova et al. 2006; Montini, Cesana et al. 2006). Moreover, Kaiser described in his article the first successful gene therapy for Beta-thalassemia disease using an HIV vector to correct β-globin coding gene (Kaiser 2009). The infused cells with corrected genes were highly proliferating due to overexpression of mutated HMGA2. The follow-up of the patient did not show any serious adverse effects, still the elevation of HMGA2 seems to be a caveat.

In conclusion, integration of a retroviral vector into the human genome contributed to the development of leukemia both in animal models and human patients. Nevertheless, these insertions may not be directly involved in cancer development, few patients of gene therapy trials developed malignancies (Hacein-Bey-Abina, Von Kalle et al. 2003; Dave, Jenkins et al. 2004). These cases emphasize the need for further improvements of retroviral vector designs to obtain vectors with low preferences for "wrong spots" to increase the safety margin in gene therapy applications.

5. Retargeting integration

The hypothetical need for integration targeting was realized even prior to the adverse events described above. Thus, attempts to target integration were made in the last decade of the 20th century. These attempts involved attaching a specific DNA binding domain (binding to a known DNA sequence) to the retroviral integrase protein. It had been shown that these fusion proteins target integration *in vitro* ("testube"), however, when these proteins were introduced into a vector particle, they either failed to perform integration or did not target it efficiently to predicted sites ((Goulaouic and Chow 1996)). Following the discovery of LEDGF/p75, it has been hypothesized that it is possible to retarget integration using a modified LEDGF/p75 protein. Thus, the Daniel laboratory created a fusion protein, in which the LEDGF/p75 chromatin binding domain was replaced by the chromatin binding domain of the heterochromatin protein 1a (HP-1a, (Silvers, Smith et al.)). HP-1a binds to the trimethylated lysine 9 of the histone H3, which is a hallmark of heterochromatin. It should be noted that cellular chromatin consists of euchromatin, containing most genes, and heterochromatin, which contains mainly repetitive sequences and relatively few genes. Thus, integration into heterochromatin should be "safer" than integration into euchromatin and genes. This fusion protein, when transfected into cells prior to infection with a HIV-1 vector, indeed reduced integration events occurring in genes. Other labs, following a similar strategy, demonstrated that further reduction in genes can be achieved by knocking down the endogenous LEDGF/p75 (Ferris, Wu et al. 2010; Gijsbers, Ronen et al. 2010). It should be noted that the knockdown did not result in reduced integration efficiency, because the novel fusion proteins efficiently replaced LEDGF/p75 function. These results thus pave the way to retargeting integration, and reducing the safety risk in gene therapy trials. However, caveats remain. One disadvantage of these methods is that targeting requires two vectors, one to deliver the fusion LEDGF/p75-based protein, and one to deliver the therapeutic genes. In addition, a significant percentage of integrations still occurred in genes. One possible approach to address the first weakness is to introduce the targeting protein directly into a vector particle. It is possible that the second disadvantage can be removed by using chromatin binding domains that show more specificity for heterochromatin than that of HP-1a. These approaches are currently being explored. We hope they ultimately result in self-targeting HIV-1 vectors that can carry negligible risk of adverse events in gene therapy trials.

6. References

Aiuti, A., B. Cassani, et al. (2007). "Multilineage hematopoietic reconstitution without clonal selection in ADA-SCID patients treated with stem cell gene therapy." J Clin Invest 117(8): 2233-40.

Aiyar, A., P. Hindmarsh, et al. (1996). "Concerted integration of linear retroviral DNA by the avian sarcoma virus integrase in vitro: dependence on both long terminal repeat termini." J Virol 70(6): 3571-80.

Alexander, B. L., R. R. Ali, et al. (2007). "Progress and prospects: gene therapy clinical trials (part 1)." Gene Ther 14(20): 1439-47.

Anderson, W. F., R. M. Blaese, et al. (1990). "The ADA human gene therapy clinical protocol: Points to Consider response with clinical protocol, July 6, 1990." Hum Gene Ther 1(3): 331-62.

Ariumi, Y., F. Serhan, et al. (2006). "The integrase interactor 1 (INI1) proteins facilitate Tat-mediated human immunodeficiency virus type 1 transcription." Retrovirology 3: 47.

Baum, C., O. Kustikova, et al. (2006). "Mutagenesis and oncogenesis by chromosomal insertion of gene transfer vectors." Hum Gene Ther 17(3): 253-63.

Beitzel, B. and F. Bushman (2003). "Construction and analysis of cells lacking the HMGA gene family." Nucleic Acids Res 31(17): 5025-32.

Blaese, R. M., K. W. Culver, et al. (1993). "Treatment of severe combined immunodeficiency disease (SCID) due to adenosine deaminase deficiency with CD34+ selected autologous peripheral blood cells transduced with a human ADA gene. Amendment to clinical research project, Project 90-C-195, January 10, 1992." Hum Gene Ther 4(4): 521-7.

Boese, A., P. Sommer, et al. (2004). "Ini1/hSNF5 is dispensable for retrovirus-induced cytoplasmic accumulation of PML and does not interfere with integration." FEBS Lett 578(3): 291-6.

Bushman, F., M. Lewinski, et al. (2005). "Genome-wide analysis of retroviral DNA integration." Nat Rev Microbiol 3(11): 848-58.

Bushman, F. D. (1994). "Tethering human immunodeficiency virus 1 integrase to a DNA site directs integration to nearby sequences." Proc Natl Acad Sci U S A 91(20): 9233-7.

Bushman, F. D. (2007). "Retroviral integration and human gene therapy." J Clin Invest 117(8): 2083-6.

Busschots, K., J. Vercammen, et al. (2005). "The interaction of LEDGF/p75 with integrase is lentivirus-specific and promotes DNA binding." J Biol Chem 280(18): 17841-7.

Cherepanov, P., E. Devroe, et al. (2004). "Identification of an evolutionarily conserved domain in human lens epithelium-derived growth factor/transcriptional co-activator p75 (LEDGF/p75) that binds HIV-1 integrase." J Biol Chem 279(47): 48883-92.

Cherepanov, P., G. Maertens, et al. (2003). "HIV-1 integrase forms stable tetramers and associates with LEDGF/p75 protein in human cells." J Biol Chem 278(1): 372-81.

Ciuffi, A., M. Llano, et al. (2005). "A role for LEDGF/p75 in targeting HIV DNA integration." Nat Med 11(12): 1287-9.

Coffin, J. M., S. H. Hughes, et al. (1997). Retroviruses. Plainview, NY, Cold Spring Harbor Laboratory Press.

Crise, B., Y. Li, et al. (2005). "Simian immunodeficiency virus integration preference is similar to that of human immunodeficiency virus type 1." J Virol 79(19): 12199-204.

Daniel, R., R. A. Katz, et al. (1999). "A role for DNA-PK in retroviral DNA integration." Science 284(5414): 644-7.

Daniel, R. and J. A. Smith (2008). "Integration site selection by retroviral vectors: molecular mechanism and clinical consequences." Hum Gene Ther 19(6): 557-68.

Dave, U. P., N. A. Jenkins, et al. (2004). "Gene therapy insertional mutagenesis insights." Science 303(5656): 333.

Deichmann, A., S. Hacein-Bey-Abina, et al. (2007). "Vector integration is nonrandom and clustered and influences the fate of lymphopoiesis in SCID-X1 gene therapy." J Clin Invest 117(8): 2225-32.

Derse, D., B. Crise, et al. (2007). "Human T-cell leukemia virus type 1 integration target sites in the human genome: comparison with those of other retroviruses." J Virol 81(12): 6731-41.

Escors, D. and K. Breckpot "Lentiviral vectors in gene therapy: their current status and future potential." Arch Immunol Ther Exp (Warsz) 58(2): 107-19.

Farnet, C. M. and F. D. Bushman (1997). "HIV-1 cDNA integration: requirement of HMG I(Y) protein for function of preintegration complexes in vitro." Cell 88(4): 483-92.

Faschinger, A., F. Rouault, et al. (2008). "Mouse mammary tumor virus integration site selection in human and mouse genomes." J Virol 82(3): 1360-7.

Ferris, A. L., X. Wu, et al. (2010). "Lens epithelium-derived growth factor fusion proteins redirect HIV-1 DNA integration." Proc Natl Acad Sci U S A 107(7): 3135-40.

Flint, S. E., V. R. Racaniello, et al. (2004). Principles of Virology. Washington, D.C., ASM Press.

Gijsbers, R., K. Ronen, et al. (2010). "LEDGF hybrids efficiently retarget lentiviral integration into heterochromatin." Mol Ther 18(3): 552-60.

Goulaouic, H. and S. A. Chow (1996). "Directed integration of viral DNA mediated by fusion proteins consisting of human immunodeficiency virus type 1 integrase and Escherichia coli LexA protein." J Virol 70(1): 37-46.

Hacein-Bey-Abina, S., C. Von Kalle, et al. (2003). "LMO2-associated clonal T cell proliferation in two patients after gene therapy for SCID-X1." Science 302(5644): 415-9.

Hahn, W. C. and R. A. Weinberg (2002). "Rules for making human tumor cells." N Engl J Med 347(20): 1593-603.

Hematti, P., B. K. Hong, et al. (2004). "Distinct genomic integration of MLV and SIV vectors in primate hematopoietic stem and progenitor cells." PLoS Biol 2(12): e423.

Hindmarsh, P., T. Ridky, et al. (1999). "HMG protein family members stimulate human immunodeficiency virus type 1 and avian sarcoma virus concerted DNA integration in vitro." J Virol 73(4): 2994-3003.

Holman, A. G. and J. M. Coffin (2005). "Symmetrical base preferences surrounding HIV-1, avian sarcoma/leukosis virus, and murine leukemia virus integration sites." Proc Natl Acad Sci U S A 102(17): 6103-7.

Kaiser, J. (2009). "Gene therapy. Beta-thalassemia treatment succeeds, with a caveat." Science 326(5959): 1468-9.

Kalpana, G. V., S. Marmon, et al. (1994). "Binding and stimulation of HIV-1 integrase by a human homolog of yeast transcription factor SNF5." Science 266(5193): 2002-6.

Kang, Y., C. J. Moressi, et al. (2006). "Integration site choice of a feline immunodeficiency virus vector." J Virol 80(17): 8820-3.

Katz, R. A. and A. M. Skalka (1994). "The retroviral enzymes." Annu Rev Biochem 63: 133-73.

Kumar, P. P., S. Mehta, et al. (2007). "SATB1-binding sequences and Alu-like motifs define a unique chromatin context in the vicinity of human immunodeficiency virus type 1 integration sites." J Virol 81(11): 5617-27.

Lau, A., K. M. Swinbank, et al. (2005). "Suppression of HIV-1 infection by a small molecule inhibitor of the ATM kinase." Nat Cell Biol 7(5): 493-500.

Lee, M. S. and R. Craigie (1998). "A previously unidentified host protein protects retroviral DNA from autointegration." Proc Natl Acad Sci U S A 95(4): 1528-33.

Levine, F. and T. Friedmann (1991). "Gene therapy techniques." Curr Opin Biotechnol 2(6): 840-4.

Lewinski, M. K., M. Yamashita, et al. (2006). "Retroviral DNA integration: viral and cellular determinants of target-site selection." PLoS Pathog 2(6): e60.

Li, L., J. M. Olvera, et al. (2001). "Role of the non-homologous DNA end joining pathway in the early steps of retroviral infection." Embo J 20(12): 3272-81.

Li, Z., J. Dullmann, et al. (2002). "Murine leukemia induced by retroviral gene marking." Science 296(5567): 497.

Lin, C. W. and A. Engelman (2003). "The barrier-to-autointegration factor is a component of functional human immunodeficiency virus type 1 preintegration complexes." J Virol 77(8): 5030-6.

Llano, M., D. T. Saenz, et al. (2006). "An essential role for LEDGF/p75 in HIV integration." Science 314(5798): 461-4.

Llano, M., M. Vanegas, et al. (2004). "LEDGF/p75 determines cellular trafficking of diverse lentiviral but not murine oncoretroviral integrase proteins and is a component of functional lentiviral preintegration complexes." J Virol 78(17): 9524-37.

Llano, M., M. Vanegas, et al. (2006). "Identification and characterization of the chromatin-binding domains of the HIV-1 integrase interactor LEDGF/p75." J Mol Biol 360(4): 760-73.

MacNeil, A., J. L. Sankale, et al. (2006). "Genomic sites of human immunodeficiency virus type 2 (HIV-2) integration: similarities to HIV-1 in vitro and possible differences in vivo." J Virol 80(15): 7316-21.

Maertens, G., P. Cherepanov, et al. (2003). "LEDGF/p75 is essential for nuclear and chromosomal targeting of HIV-1 integrase in human cells." J Biol Chem 278(35): 33528-39.

Mahmoudi, T., M. Parra, et al. (2006). "The SWI/SNF chromatin-remodeling complex is a cofactor for Tat transactivation of the HIV promoter." J Biol Chem 281(29): 19960-8.
Mann, R., R. C. Mulligan, et al. (1983). "Construction of a retrovirus packaging mutant and its use to produce helper-free defective retrovirus." Cell 33(1): 153-9.
Masson, C., S. Bury-Mone, et al. (2007). "Ku80 participates in the targeting of retroviral transgenes to the chromatin of CHO cells." J Virol 81(15): 7924-32.
Maxfield, L. F., C. D. Fraize, et al. (2005). "Relationship between retroviral DNA-integration-site selection and host cell transcription." Proc Natl Acad Sci U S A 102(5): 1436-41.
Mitchell, R. S., B. F. Beitzel, et al. (2004). "Retroviral DNA integration: ASLV, HIV, and MLV show distinct target site preferences." PLoS Biol 2(8): E234.
Modlich, U., O. S. Kustikova, et al. (2005). "Leukemias following retroviral transfer of multidrug resistance 1 (MDR1) are driven by combinatorial insertional mutagenesis." Blood 105(11): 4235-46.
Montini, E., D. Cesana, et al. (2006). "Hematopoietic stem cell gene transfer in a tumor-prone mouse model uncovers low genotoxicity of lentiviral vector integration." Nat Biotechnol 24(6): 687-96.
Mooslehner, K., U. Karls, et al. (1990). "Retroviral integration sites in transgenic Mov mice frequently map in the vicinity of transcribed DNA regions." J Virol 64(6): 3056-8.
Narezkina, A., K. D. Taganov, et al. (2004). "Genome-wide analyses of avian sarcoma virus integration sites." J Virol 78(21): 11656-63.
Ott, M. G., M. Schmidt, et al. (2006). "Correction of X-linked chronic granulomatous disease by gene therapy, augmented by insertional activation of MDS1-EVI1, PRDM16 or SETBP1." Nat Med 12(4): 401-9.
Pike-Overzet, K., D. de Ridder, et al. (2006). "Gene therapy: is IL2RG oncogenic in T-cell development?" Nature 443(7109): E5; discussion E6-7.
Pruss, D., F. D. Bushman, et al. (1994). "Human immunodeficiency virus integrase directs integration to sites of severe DNA distortion within the nucleosome core." Proc Natl Acad Sci U S A 91(13): 5913-7.
Pruss, D., R. Reeves, et al. (1994). "The influence of DNA and nucleosome structure on integration events directed by HIV integrase." J Biol Chem 269(40): 25031-41.
Pryciak, P. M., H. P. Muller, et al. (1992). "Simian virus 40 minichromosomes as targets for retroviral integration in vivo." Proc Natl Acad Sci U S A 89(19): 9237-41.
Pryciak, P. M., A. Sil, et al. (1992). "Retroviral integration into minichromosomes in vitro." EMBO J 11(1): 291-303.
Pryciak, P. M. and H. E. Varmus (1992). "Nucleosomes, DNA-binding proteins, and DNA sequence modulate retroviral integration target site selection." Cell 69(5): 769-80.
Recchia, A., C. Bonini, et al. (2006). "Retroviral vector integration deregulates gene expression but has no consequence on the biology and function of transplanted T cells." Proc Natl Acad Sci U S A 103(5): 1457-62.
Scherdin, U., K. Rhodes, et al. (1990). "Transcriptionally active genome regions are preferred targets for retrovirus integration." J Virol 64(2): 907-12.
Schroder, A. R., P. Shinn, et al. (2002). "HIV-1 integration in the human genome favors active genes and local hotspots." Cell 110(4): 521-9.
Schwarzwaelder, K., S. J. Howe, et al. (2007). "Gammaretrovirus-mediated correction of SCID-X1 is associated with skewed vector integration site distribution in vivo." J Clin Invest 117(8): 2241-9.

Shun, M. C., N. K. Raghavendra, et al. (2007). "LEDGF/p75 functions downstream from preintegration complex formation to effect gene-specific HIV-1 integration." Genes Dev 21(14): 1767-78.

Silvers, R. M., J. A. Smith, et al. "Modification of integration site preferences of an HIV-1-based vector by expression of a novel synthetic protein." Hum Gene Ther 21(3): 337-49.

Sutherland, H. G., K. Newton, et al. (2006). "Disruption of Ledgf/Psip1 results in perinatal mortality and homeotic skeletal transformations." Mol Cell Biol 26(19): 7201-10.

Taganov, K. D., I. Cuesta, et al. (2004). "Integrase-specific enhancement and suppression of retroviral DNA integration by compacted chromatin structure in vitro." J Virol 78(11): 5848-55.

Thrasher, A. J. and H. B. Gaspar (2008) "Severe adverse event in clinical trial of gene therapy for X-SCID." Volume, DOI:

Thrasher, A. J., H. B. Gaspar, et al. (2006). "Gene therapy: X-SCID transgene leukaemogenicity." Nature 443(7109): E5-6; discussion E6-7.

Treand, C., I. du Chene, et al. (2006). "Requirement for SWI/SNF chromatin-remodeling complex in Tat-mediated activation of the HIV-1 promoter." Embo J 25(8): 1690-9.

Turlure, F., G. Maertens, et al. (2006). "A tripartite DNA-binding element, comprised of the nuclear localization signal and two AT-hook motifs, mediates the association of LEDGF/p75 with chromatin in vivo." Nucleic Acids Res 34(5): 1653-65.

Vanegas, M., M. Llano, et al. (2005). "Identification of the LEDGF/p75 HIV-1 integrase-interaction domain and NLS reveals NLS-independent chromatin tethering." J Cell Sci 118(Pt 8): 1733-43.

Weidhaas, J. B., E. L. Angelichio, et al. (2000). "Relationship between retroviral DNA integration and gene expression." J Virol 74(18): 8382-9.

Woods, N. B., V. Bottero, et al. (2006). "Gene therapy: therapeutic gene causing lymphoma." Nature 440(7088): 1123.

Wu, X., Y. Li, et al. (2003). "Transcription start regions in the human genome are favored targets for MLV integration." Science 300(5626): 1749-51.

2

Production of Retroviral and Lentiviral Gene Therapy Vectors: Challenges in the Manufacturing of Lipid Enveloped Virus

Ana F. Rodrigues, Paula M. Alves and Ana S. Coroadinha
Instituto de Biologia Experimental e Tecnologia/ Instituto de Tecnologia Química e Biologica – Universidade Nova de Lisboa (IBET/ITQB-UNL)
Portugal

1. Introduction

Gamma-retroviral vectors, commonly designated retroviral vectors, were the first viral vector employed in Gene Therapy clinical trials in 1990 and are still one of the most used. More recently, the interest in lentiviral vectors, derived from complex retroviruses such as the human immunodeficiency virus (HIV), has been growing due to their ability to transduce non-dividing cells (Lewis et al. 1992; Naldini et al. 1996), an attribute that distinguishes them from other viral vectors, including their simple counterparts, gamma-retroviral vectors. Retroviral and lentiviral vectors most attractive features as gene transfer tools include the capacity for large genetic payload (up to 9 kb), minimal patient immune response, high transducing efficiency *in vivo* and *in vitro*, and the ability to permanently modify the genetic content of the target cell, sustaining a long-term expression of the delivered gene (Coroadinha et al. 2010; Schweizer and Merten 2010).

According to the most recent updates, retroviral and lentiviral vectors represent 23% of all the vector types and 33% of the viral vectors used in Gene Therapy clinical trials. Moreover, retroviral vectors are currently the blockbuster vectors for the treatment of monogenic and infectious diseases and gene marking clinical trials (Edelstein 2010).

Retroviruses are double stranded RNA enveloped viruses mainly characterized by the ability to "reverse-transcribe" their genome from RNA to DNA. Virions measure 100-120 nm in diameter and contain a dimeric genome of identical positive RNA strands complexed with the nucleocapsid (NC) proteins. The genome is enclosed in a proteic capsid (CA) that also contains enzymatic proteins, namely the reverse transcriptase (RT), the integrase (IN) and proteases (PR), required for viral infection. The matrix proteins (MA) form a layer outside the capsid core that interacts with the envelope, a lipid bilayer derived from the host cellular membrane, which surrounds the viral core particle (Coffin et al. 1997). Anchored on this bilayer, are the viral envelope glycoproteins (Env) responsible for recognizing specific receptors on the host cell and initiating the infection process. Envelope proteins are formed by two subunits, the transmembrane (TM) that anchors the protein into the lipid membrane and the surface (SU) which binds to the cellular receptors (Fig. 1).

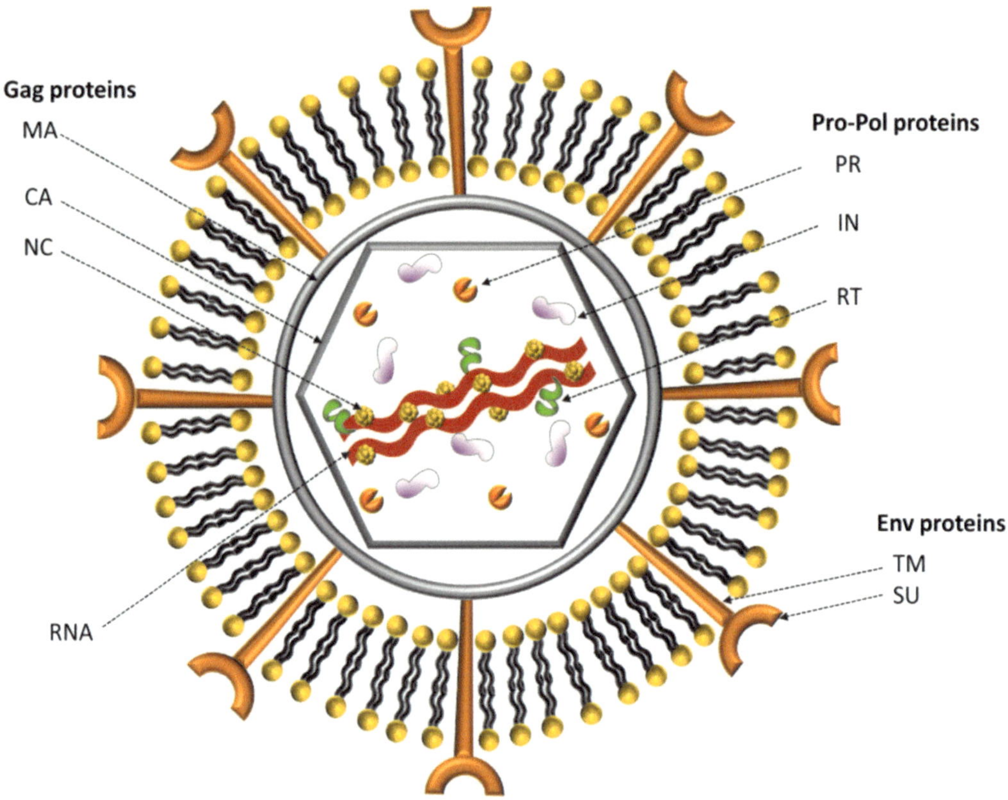

Fig. 1. Schematic representation of a retrovirus particle structure.

Based on the genome structure, retroviruses are classified into simple (e.g. MLV, murine leukemia virus) or complex retroviruses (e.g. HIV) (Coffin et al. 1997). Both encode four genes: *gag* (group specific antigen), *pro* (protease), *pol* (polymerase) and *env* (envelope) (Fig. 2). The *gag* sequence encodes the three main structural proteins: MA, CA, NC. The *pro* sequence, encodes proteases (PR) responsible for cleaving Gag and Gag-Pol during particles assembly, budding and maturation. The *pol* sequence encodes the enzymes RT and IN, the former catalyzing the reverse transcription of the viral genome from RNA to DNA during the infection process and the latter responsible for integrating the proviral DNA into the host cell genome. The *env* sequence encodes for both SU and TM subunits of the envelope glycoprotein. Additionally, retroviral genome presents non-coding *cis*-acting sequences such as, two LTRs (long terminal repeats), which contain elements required to drive gene expression, reverse transcription and integration into the host cell chromosome, a sequence named packaging signal (ψ) required for specific packaging of the viral RNA into newly forming virions, and a polypurine tract (PPT) that functions as the site for initiating the positive strand DNA synthesis during reverse transcription (Coffin et al. 1997).

Additionally to *gag*, *pro*, *pol* and *env*, complex retroviruses, such as lentiviruses, have accessory genes including *vif*, *vpr*, *vpu*, *nef*, *tat* and *rev* that regulate viral gene expression, assembly of infectious particles and modulate viral replication in infected cells (Fig 2B).

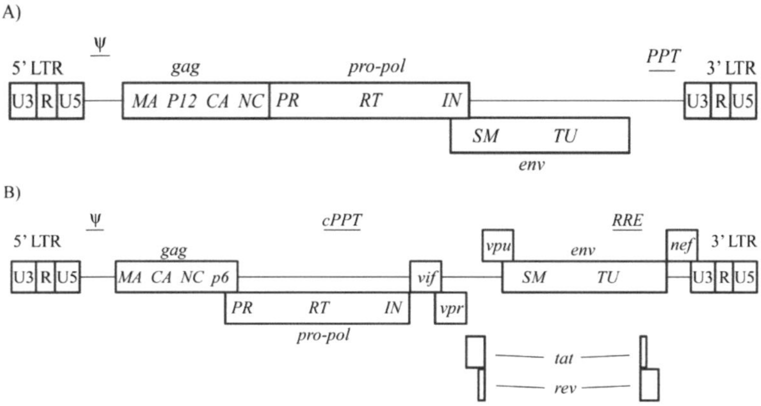

Fig. 2. Retroviral genomes. Schematic representation of (A) MLV and (B) HIV-1 wild-type genomes representing simple and complex retrovirus, respectively.

2. Cell line platforms for the production

The establishment of retroviral and lentiviral producer cells, named packaging cell lines, has been based on the physical separation of the viral genome into different transcriptional units to minimize the risk of generating replication-competent particles (RCPs) (Fig. 3). Some of

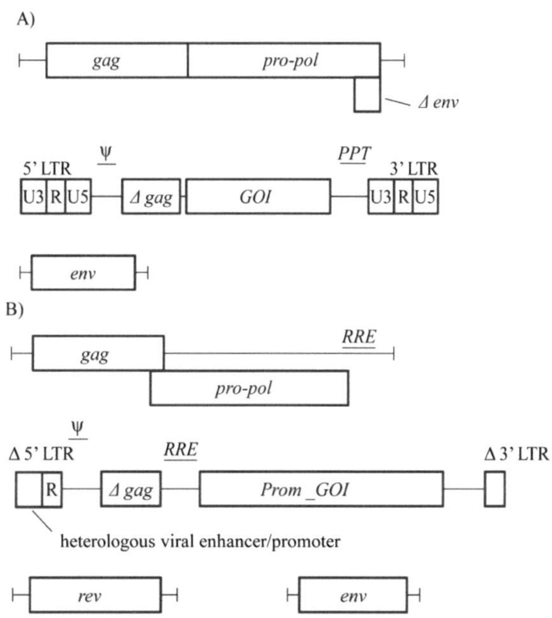

Fig. 3. Transcriptional units used for retroviral and lentiviral vector generation.
(A) Three construct system used for (simple) retroviral vector and (B) four construct system used for third generation lentiviral vector production. Only the most relevant parts of the constructs are show; for further details see (Blesch 2004; Sinn et al. 2005).
GOI: gene of interest; Prom_GOI: heterologous promoter and gene of interest.

these constructs are additionally engineered with heterologous sequences including: promoters (Dull et al. 1998) to support their independent expression or for improved safety, enhancers (Gruh et al. 2008) and stabilizing elements (Zufferey et al. 1999) to increase the overall levels of transcripts both in producer and target cells, hence increasing viral titers and transgene expression.

2.1 Retroviral vectors

For both retroviral and lentiviral vector production, different packaging systems, named generations, have been developed. Each new generation aimed at minimizing and reduce the risk of RCPs formation face to the previous one (Fig 3).

In the case of vectors based on MLV or other simple retrovirus, the non-cytotoxicity of the viral genes has allowed the establishment of cell lines stably and constitutively expressing viral vectors. Table 1 lists some of the available retroviral vector packaging cell lines.

The first packaging cells reported as so for simple retroviral vector production were established by providing the packaging functions (*gag-pro-pol*) with a retroviral genome where the packaging signal was deleted, thus preventing their incorporation into the viral particles (Cone and Mulligan 1984). However, a single event of homologous recombination was sufficient to restore replicative competence. This led to a second generation of retroviral packaging cells (Miller and Buttimore 1986), in which further modifications were introduced including the replacement of the 3'LTR and the second strand initiation site with the polyadenylation site of SV40. The third generation (Danos and Mulligan 1988) (Fig. 3A) further separates the construct that expresses *gag-pro-pol* from *env*, in a total of three independent transcriptional units. Although three homologous recombination events would be needed to restore replicative competence, which is very improbable, replicative competent viruses can still occur in third generation cell lines (Chong et al. 1998; Chong and Vile 1996). Therefore, additional improvements were made by means of decreasing the homology in the vector construct, using different LTR species to those used in the packaging functions (Cosset et al. 1995) or using heterologous promoters such CMV's (Rigg et al. 1996; Soneoka et al. 1995). The most recently developed retroviral vector packaging cell lines are based on this third generation optimized system. *Gag-pro-pol* genes are expressed from a single construct driven by a heterologous promoter. Vector construct contains a cassette for transgene expression typically driven by the 5'LTR promoter; it additionally contains the packaging signal (ψ) and the initial *gag* sequence known to provide enhanced packaging (Bender et al. 1987). The envelope expression is supplied by a third independent construct usually driven by a heterologous promoter. The separation of the envelope in an independent transcriptional unit offers great flexibility for envelope exchange - pseudotyping - and for the use of genetically or chemically engineered envelope proteins, thus allowing changing, restricting or broadening vector tropism (McTaggart and Al-Rubeai 2002; Yu and Schaffer 2005). For simple retroviruses several envelope glycoproteins have been used including MLV's amphotropic 4070A and 10A1 (Miller and Chen 1996), GaLV's (gibbon leukemia virus) (Miller et al. 1991), RD114 from cat endogenous virus (Takeuchi et al. 1994), HIV's gp120 (Schnierle et al. 1997) and the G protein from vesicular stomatitis virus (VSV-G) (Burns et al. 1993). Since the proteins encoded by these sequences are usually non-toxic, except for the last one, they can be constitutively expressed such that simple retroviral vector packaging cell lines are typically stable and continuously producing systems.

Retroviral producer cell lines	Cell origin	Envelope	Maximal Titers (I.P./mL)	Vector	Packaging generation	Reference
Ψ-AM	Murine NIH 3T3	Amphotropic	2.0×10^5	MLV based	1st	(Cone and Mulligan 1984)
PA317	Murine NIH 3T3	Amphotropic	3.0×10^6	MLV based	2nd	(Miller and Buttimore 1986)
Ψ-CRIP	Murine NIH 3T3	Amphotropic	6.0×10^6	MLV based	3rd	(Danos and Mulligan 1988)
PG13	Murine NIH 3T3	GaLV	5.0×10^6	MLV based		(Miller et al. 1991)
Gp + envAm12	Murine NIH 3T3	Amphotropic	1.0×10^6	MLV based		(Markowitz et al. 1988)
HAII	Human HT1080	Amphotropic	1.0×10^7	MLV based		(Sheridan et al. 2000)
FLY A4	Human HT1080	Amphotropic	1.0×10^7	MLV based		(Cosset et al. 1995)
FLY RD18	Human HT1080	RD114	1.2×10^5	MLV based		(Cosset et al. 1995)
Te Fly A	Human Te671	Amphotropic	1.0×10^7	MLV based		(Cosset et al. 1995)
Te Fly Ga 18	Human Te671	GaLV	1.0×10^6	MLV based		(Cosset et al. 1995)
CEM FLY	Human CEM	Amphotropic	1.0×10^7	MLV based		(Pizzato et al. 2001)
293-SPA	Human 293	Amphotropic	6.0×10^6	MLV based		(Davis et al. 1997)
293 *kat*	Human 293	Amphotropic Xenotropic 10A1	NR	MLV based		(Farson et al. 1999)
Phoenix	Human 293T	Amphotropic	1.0×10^5	MLV based		(Swift et al. 2001)
Flp293	Human 293	Amphotropic	2.0×10^7	MLV based	3rd with RMCE[1] technology	(Schucht et al. 2006)
293 FLEX	Human 293	GaLV	3.0×10^6	MLV based		(Coroadinha et al. 2006b)
PG368	Murine NIH 3T3	GaLV	1.0×10^6	MLV based		(Loew et al. 2009)

Table 1. Packaging cell lines for retroviral vector manufacture (1 – RMCE – Recombinase Mediated Cassette exchange; NR – Not reported: the titers reported for these packaging cells are expressed in terms of reverse transcriptase activity, which the correlation with infectious titers depends on the cell system.)

Retroviral vectors have been based on several viruses including avian, simian, feline and murine retroviruses, being the latter (MLV) the most used. As so, the majority of the retroviral vector packaging cell lines established were murine derived, being NIH/3T3 the most widely employed. However, it was rapidly found that the presence of galactosyl(α1-3)galactose carbohydrate moieties produced by murine cells in retroviral envelope lead to its rapid detection and inactivation by the human complement system (Takeuchi et al. 1994; Takeuchi et al. 1997; Takeuchi et al. 1996). Nowadays, murine cells are being replaced by human cell lines, to reduce the possibility of endogenous retroviral sequences packaging and also to improve vector half-life *in vivo* (Cosset et al. 1995).
Establishing a producer cell line involves at least three transfection and clonal selection steps, taking a time-frame of around one year which constitutes a major drawback in stable cell line development (see section 3.1). Yet, this process is undertaken for each new therapeutic gene and/or different envelope protein required (for changing vector tropism). On the other hand, high-titer packaging cells development has been based on an efficient method to facilitate the selection of a high producer cell clone in which a selectable marker gene is inserted in the vector construct downstream of the viral genes, so they are translated from the same transcript after ribosomal reinitiation (Cosset et al. 1995). This strategy, however, although very efficient for screening stable integration and/or high level long-term viral genome expression, raises considerable problems in therapeutic settings including immune response against the selection (foreign) gene product(s) (Liberatore et al. 1999). Therefore, a new generation of retrovirus packaging cell lines based on cassette exchange systems that allow for flexible switch of the transgene and/or envelope, as well as selectable marker(s) excision, were developed (Coroadinha et al. 2006b; Loew et al. 2004; Persons et al. 1998; Schucht et al. 2006; Wildner et al. 1998).
Schucht et al (2006) and Coroadinha et al (2006) established modular cell lines, based on targeted genome integration allowing to obtain rapidly high-titer retroviral producer cells (Figure 4).

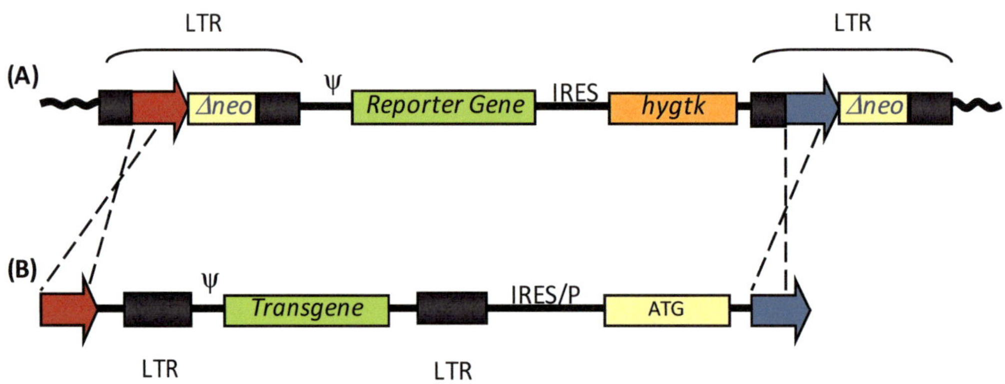

Fig. 4. Schematic representation of the modular cell lines based on the recombinase mediated cassette exchange (RMCE) technology. (A) Integrated retroviral transgene cassette harboring a marker gene and (B) targeting therapeutic transgene plasmid allowing a fast exchange and establishment of a new retroviral producer cell.

Two cell lines were created; Flp293A and 293 FLEX, both derived from 293 cells. The former pseudotyped with amphotropic and the latter with GaLV envelopes. Recently, a PG13-based murine producer cell line was also established using this strategy (Loew et al. 2009). A favorable chromosomal site for stable and high retroviral vector production is first identified and tagged. Due to the presence of two heterologous non-compatible FRT sites flanking the tagged retroviral genome, the subsequent re-use of this defined chromosomal site by means of RMCE is than performed to express a therapeutic gene. In order to select cell clones that underwent correct targeted integration reaction, the targeting viral vector contains a start codon that complements a transcriptionally inactive ATG-deficient selection marker after recombination.

The modular producer cell lines present several advantages: they are safer since integration of the vector within the packaging cell line was identified, the duration of the entire development process is much reduced as there is no need for screening and, in addition, production conditions are favorable due to the possibility of pre-adaptation of the master cell line to culture conditions and media. Thus, therapeutic virus production from bench to bedside becomes safer, faster, and cheaper (Coroadinha et al. 2010).

2.2 Lentiviral vectors

Similarly to retroviral vectors, the design of lentiviral vector packaging systems has evolved to minimize the risk of RCPs generation towards maximum safety. Currently, three generations of lentiviral vectors are considered. The first-generation (Naldini et al. 1996) closely resembles the three plasmid packaging system of simple retroviruses, except for the fact that the *gag-pol* expression is driven by a heterologous promoter instead of the viral LTR; additionally, the gp120 HIV-1's envelope was replaced by VSV-G's. However, this system contained all the necessary sequences for the generation of RCPs with three homologous recombination events which, although improbable, could not be accepted for a human and potentially lethal pathogen.

In the second generation (Zufferey et al. 1997), the three plasmid system was maintained but all the accessory genes were deleted including *vif, vpr, vpu,* and *nef*. The third generation (Fig. 3B) allowed for a *tat* independent lentiviral vector expression by engineering a chimeric 5′LTR with a heterologous viral promoter/enhancer, such as CMV's (cytomegalovirus) or RSV's (Rous sarcoma virus) (Dull et al. 1998); *rev* complementation was separately provided in *trans*, thus this system has a total of four constructs. A schematic representation of the third generation system is shown in Fig. 3B. *Gag-pro-pol* genes are expressed from a CMV promoter and none of the accessory or regulatory proteins is present in this construct. Only *rev* accessory gene is maintained but is provided by a nonoverlapping plasmid. Vector cassette for transgene expression is driven by a heterologous promoter, as virus LTRs were partially deleted. Similarly to simple retroviruses, the transgene vector construct additionally contains the packaging signal (ψ) and the initial sequence from *gag*. The envelope cassette encodes typically, but not necessarily, for VSV-G envelope glycoprotein.

The development of a fourth generation of lentiviral vectors, *rev* independent, has also been claimed by means of replacing RRE (*rev* responsive element) with heterologous viral sequences or by codon-optimization (Bray et al. 1994; Delenda 2004; Kotsopoulou et al. 2000; Pandya et al. 2001; Roberts and Boris-Lawrie 2000). However, its use is not widespread since, contrary to the other generations of lentiviral vectors, these packaging systems have not been made available for the research community; also the reported titers are typically one to two logs bellow the maximum titers obtained with the second or third generation systems.

In addition to HIV-derived, other lentiviral vectors have been developed and reported to retain identical features to those of HIV's based, including the ability to transduce non-dividing cells, high titers production, and the possibility to be pseudotyped with different envelope glycoproteins. These include lentiviral vectors based on SIV (simian immunodeficiency virus) (Pandya et al. 2001; Schnell et al. 2000), BIV (bovine immunodeficiency virus) (Matukonis et al. 2002; Molina et al. 2004), FIV (feline immunodeficiency virus) (Poeschla et al. 1998; Saenz and Poeschla 2004) and EAIV (equine infectious anaemia virus) (Balaggan et al. 2006; Mitrophanous et al. 1999; Stewart et al. 2009). Most of non-HIV derived lentiviral vectors have been reported to be *tat* and sometimes *rev* independent, thus falling in the 3rd or 4th generation of packaging systems. For clinical trials purposes, both second and third generation lentiviral vector systems were reported although only HIV-1 and EAIV derived vectors have been used (Schweizer and Merten 2010).

Contrarily to simple retroviral vectors, the cytotoxicity of some of the lentiviral proteins has hampered the establishment of stable cell lines constitutively expressing vector components. Therefore, the majority of the reported packaging cells for lentivirus manufacturing have been based on inducible systems that control the expression of the toxic proteins (for further details see section 3.1). Nevertheless, it is worth notice that transient production is still the main mean for lentiviral vector generation for both research and clinical purposes. Table 2 summarizes some of the available (stable) lentiviral vector packaging cell lines.

Except for the systems reported by and Ni et al. (2005), all the packaging cell lines for lentiviral vector production have been based on human 293 cells transformed with oncogenes such as the SV40 (simian vacuolating virus 40) large T antigen - 293T - or the Nuclear Antigen of Epstein-Barr Virus - 293EBNA.

For clinical application human 293 and 293T cells have been the exclusive cell substrates (Schweizer and Merten 2010). However, safety concerns arise from the fact that 90% of non-coding mobile sequences of the human genome are endogenous retrovirus and although most of them are defective, because of mutations accumulation, some are still active (Zwolinska 2006). Therefore, using human cell lines for the production of human retroviruses increases the chances of replicative-competent particles generation by homologous recombination (Pauwels et al. 2009). Also, the possibility of contamination with other human pathogens during the production process, poses additional hindrances to the use of human cells for biopharmaceuticals production, viral or not. In this context, the use of non-human cells would be strongly recommended, although the different glycosylation patterns of the envelope proteins could be an obstacle. For research purposes other human or monkey derived cells were tested (other 293 derived clones, HeLa, HT1080, TE671, COS-1, COS-7, CV-1), although most of them showed reduced vector production titers. Yet, COS-1 cells have shown to be capable of producing 3-4 times improved vector quality (expressed in infectious vector titer *per* ng of CA protein, p24), comparing with 293T cells (Smith and Shioda 2009).

Lentiviral packaging cell line	**Cell origin**	**Envelope**	**Maximal Titers (I.P./mL)**	**Vector**	**Packaging generation[1]**	**Observations**	**Reference**
SODk	Human 293T	VSV-G	1.0×10^7	HIV-1 based	2nd	Tet-off	(Cockrell et al. 2006; Kafri et al. 1999; Xu et al. 2001)
293G	Human 293T	VSV-G	-	HIV-1 based	2nd	Tet-off	(Farson et al. 2001)
STAR	Human 293T	Ampho GaLV RD114	1.2×10^7 1.6×10^6 8.5×10^6	HIV-1 based	2nd	Continuous system. Codon-optimized *gag-pol*	(Ikeda et al. 2003)
NR	Human 293	VSV-G	3.5×10^7	HIV-1 based	2nd	Tet-off. Three level cascade gene regulation system: TRE → tat+rev → VSV-G+Gag-Pol. Codon-optimized *gag-pol*	(Ni et al. 2005)
REr1.35	Human 293T	VSV-G	1.8×10^5	HIV-1 based	3rd	Ecdysone inducible system. Codon-optimized *gag-pol*	(Pacchia et al. 2001)
293SF-pacLV	Human 293 EBNA	VSV-G	3.4×10^7	HIV-1 based	3rd	Tet-on	(Broussau et al. 2008)
PC48	Human 293T	VSV-G	7.4×10^5	EIAV based	3rd	Tet-on	(Stewart et al. 2009)
SgpG109	Human 293T	VSV-G	1×10^5	SIV-based	3rd	Ponasterone inducible system. Codon-optimized *gag-pol*	(Kuate et al. 2002)
GPRG	Human 293T	VSV-G	5×10^7	SIV-based	3rd	Introduction of vector by concatemeric array transfection. Tet-off	(Throm et al. 2009)

Table 2. Packaging cell lines for lentiviral vector manufacture (1 – No lentiviral packaging cell line was developed based on the first generation lentiviral vector system.
Tet-on/ Tet-off – tetracycline inducible system; tet-on becomes active upon tetracycline (or an analogous molecule such as doxycycline) is added and tet-off is activated by tetracycline removal. NR: not reported)

3. Bioreaction platforms and production media

3.1 Stable vs. transient expression

Production platforms for lentiviral and retroviral vectors have been restrained to mammalian cells, typically murine or human derived, which are transfected with *gag-pol* the packaging functions, vector (transgene) and envelope constructions. This can be based on a short-term transfer of the viral constructs, known as transient production, into exponentially growing cells followed by 24-72 hours vector production and harvesting, or by their stable

integration and constitutive expression into the host cell genome, for continuous production (Fig. 5).
Transient production, makes use of transfection methods to introduce the viral constructions, commonly cationic agents that complex with the negatively charged DNA, thus allowing it to be up-taken by the cell *via* endocytosis (Al-Dosari and Gao 2009). From those, polyethylenimine (PEI) (Boussif et al. 1995) is probably the less expensive, one of the most efficient and the most widely used in the current protocols (Schweizer and Merten 2010; Segura et al. 2010; Toledo et al. 2009). Others methods such as calcium phosphate precipitation (Jordan and Wurm 2004; Mitta et al. 2005) and cationic lipids complexation including LipofectAMINE® and FuGENE®, have also been used, although at small-scale production or for research purposes only since, these are either difficult to scale-up or very expensive. Alternatively, viral infection has also been developed and validated namely for lentiviral vector production, using baculoviruses as transfection agents (Lesch et al. 2008). However, the additional downstream work to separate lentiviral vector and baculoviruses to achieve clinical-grade viral preparations standards, as well as the final titers reported (Lesch et al. 2011) reduced the competitiveness of lentiviral vector production using baculoviruses over plasmid DNA transfection methods.

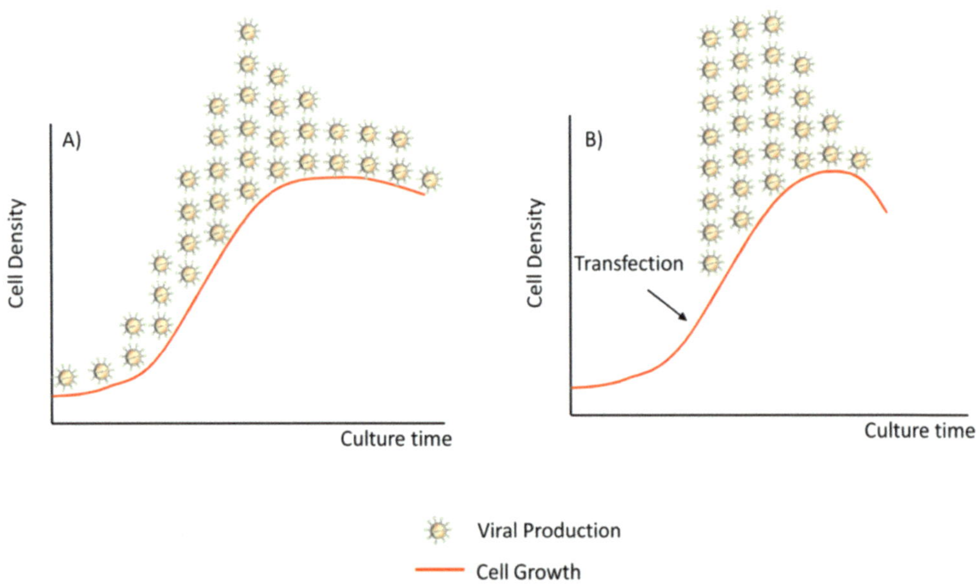

Fig. 5. Stable *vs.* transient viral vector production. (A) Stable and continuous production from cell lines constitutively expressing viral vector transgene, *gag-pro-pol* and *env*; vector titers are nearly dependent on cell density until the end of the exponential phase of cell growth. (B) Transient production after plasmid transfection of viral vector transgene, *gag-pro-pol* and *env*; high titers are obtained usually between 24 to 72 hours post-transfection, after which a pronounced decrease occurs, typically due to cell death.

Stable production relies on cell substrates in which the viral constructs where separately integrated into the cell genome, thus allowing their constitutive expression. Typically, the packaging functions are first inserted and after clonal selection of a high-level *gag-pol* expression, the envelope construction is then inserted and a second round of clonal selection is performed. At this point, a packaging cell line is established, in principal supporting the packaging of any viral vector (retroviral or lentiviral, depending on the *gag-pro-pol* functions). Finally, the transgene is introduced. If non-SIN vectors are used, this can be achieved directly by viral infection; otherwise, chemical transfection methods as those described above followed by stable integration and selection are required and equally suitable. Cosset and co-workers (1995) reported a very efficient method in which viral vector construct containing a (selectable) marker gene is firstly inserted in nude cells, facilitating the screening for stable integration and high-level long term expression (Cosset et al. 1995). This scheme was demonstrated to allow for the establishment of high-titer human derived retroviral vector packaging cell lines. Additionally, it permits high-titer retroviral vector production from single copy integration allowing for modular cell lines development, flexible platforms for transgene and/or envelope exchange (Coroadinha et al. 2006b; Schucht et al. 2006) (Fig. 4). Moreover, it allows optimization of the stoichiometry of the packaging constructs, maximizing viral titers and vector preparation quality, expressed by the ratio of infectious particles to total particles, which has a drastic impact on vector transduction efficiency a crucial parameter for clinical purposes (Carrondo et al. 2008).

Stable retroviral vector cell line development is a tedious and time consuming process which can take up to one year for a fully developed and characterized cell platform. However, it is compensated by obtaining continuously producing and highly consistent cell systems, prone to single-effort bioprocess and product characterization, a critical consideration for market approval.

Transient production is undoubtedly faster, when compared to the time frame necessary to develop a stable packaging cell line, presenting very competitive titers (up to 10^7 infectious vector *per* mL). Yet, for clinical purposes, continuous production by stable cell lines is highly desirable, since transient systems are difficult to scale-up, time and cost-ineffective at large scales and, more importantly, are unable to provide a fully characterized production platform with low batch-to-batch variability of the viral preparations. Therefore, transient production is unlikely to be of value after the transition from clinical to market. Retroviral vector manufacture, including those used in clinical trials, has been making use of stable and continuous cell lines for more than ten years (Cornetta et al. 2005; Eckert et al. 2000; Przybylowski et al. 2006; Wikstrom et al. 2004). However, the establishment of stable lentiviral vectors packaging cell lines has remained a challenge due to the inherent cytotoxicity of the lentiviral protease which has prohibited its constitutive expression (Schweizer and Merten 2010). It is well established that numerous HIV-1-encoded proteins are capable of causing cell death, including tat, nef, env, vpr and the protease (PR) (Gougeon 2003); from those, only the protease is still required in the current packaging systems. HIV protease mediates its toxicity *in vitro* and *in vivo*, by cleaving and activating procaspase 8, leading to mitochondrial release of cytochrome c, activation of the downstream caspases 9 and 3 and lastly, nuclear fragmentation (Nie et al. 2007; Nie et al. 2002). Ikeda and co-workers have reported the development of a 293T derived cell line, STAR, stable and continuously producing LV using an HIV-1 codon optimized *gag-pol* (Ikeda et al. 2003). However, significant titers could only be obtained by MLV-based vector transduction of the optimized *gag-pol*. This procedure raises biosafety issues, since it increases the chances of generating replicative-competent particles by homologous recombination and, posing further concerns of co-packaging (Pauwels et al. 2009).

At a laboratory scale, transient production by plasmid transfection has been the first choice to cope with the cytotoxic proteins. For larger-scale production purposes, conditional packaging systems have been developed in which the expression of those is under the control of inducible promoters (Broussau et al. 2008; Farson et al. 2001; Kuate et al. 2002; Pacchia et al. 2001; Stewart et al. 2009). However transient transfection systems are, as discussed above, difficult to scale-up and do not fulfill adequate batch-to-batch variability standards; and, although the clinical trials currently using lentiviral vectors have been provided exclusively with transiently produced batches (Schweizer and Merten 2010), it is unlikely that a transient based systems will be approved when going from clinical to market. Conditional systems, on the other hand, require the addition/removal of the induction agents cumbering the production and requiring further down-stream stringency in processing of the viral preparations.

3.2 Stirred bioreaction vs. adherent cultures

It is widely accepted that stirred bioreaction systems using suspension cultures offer more advantages from the bioprocess view-point when compared to those under static/adherent conditions. The most evident advantage is the higher volumetric productivity, since suspension cultures in stirred systems present increased ratios of cell number *per* volume of culture medium. Because of this, they are easier to scale-up with less space requirements; the agitation allows for homogeneous cells suspension preventing the formation of chemical (nutrient, waste products), physical (pH, oxygen, carbon dioxide) and thermal gradients, thus maximizing the productivity potential of the culture (Sadettin and Hu 2006).

The first suspension system reported for high-titer retroviral vector production was based on a T-lymphoblastoid cell line using a third generation packaging construct, producing MLV derived retroviral vectors pseudotyped with amphotropic envelope: CEMFLYA cells (Pizzato et al. 2001). These cells were able to produce in the range of 10^7 infectious units *per* mL and, the potential for scaled up vector production was demonstrated by continuous culture during 14 days in a 250 mL spinner flask. After CEMFLYA, other high-titer suspension cells were reported, namely suspension-adapted 293GPG cells producing MLV retrovirus vector pseudotyped with the vesicular stomatitis virus G (VSVG) envelope protein and expressing a TK-GFP fusion protein in a 3L acoustic filter-based perfusion bioreactor (Ghani et al. 2006). Another major landmark was achieved when the same group published for the first time retroviral vector production in suspension and under serum-free conditions (Ghani et al. 2007) (see section 3.4.1). Following retrovirus, lentiviral vector manufacture using suspension cultures has also been recently reported both for transfection-based transient production (Ansorge et al. 2009), as well as, for stable production using (inducible) packaging cell lines (Broussau et al. 2008).

Despite the advances in the development of suspension cultures for stirred tank bioreactors and its clear advantage from the bioprocess view-point, retroviral and lentiviral vector manufacture for clinical batches has mainly been based on adherent static and preferably disposable systems, including large T-flasks, cell factories and roller bottles (Fig. 6) (Eckert et al. 2000; Merten et al. 2011; Przybylowski et al. 2006; Wikstrom et al. 2004). A good example is retroviral vector production at the National Gene Vector Laboratory, Indiana University, (Indianapolis, IN), a US National Institutes of Health initiative that has as main mission provide clinical grade vectors for gene therapy trials (Cornetta et al. 2005). Also for clinical-grade lentiviral vector production, the bioreaction system of choice has been Cell Factory or equivalent multitray systems (Merten et al. 2011; Schweizer and Merten 2010). These systems allow for 10 to 40 L vector production under GMP conditions, meeting the needs for initial trials, where usually a reduced number of patients are involved. In the future, if lentiviral and retroviral vector Gene Therapy products reach the market, it is still not clear if such systems will continue to be used. In fact, several restrictions arise from the use of disposable systems and bioreactors including the increase in the costs of solid waste disposal and consumables, in addition to low scalability and the single-use philosophy itself (Eibl et al. 2010). However, the low infectivity stability of retro and lentiviral vectors has hampered the perspective of the "thousand-liter" production systems' for further storage. Nevertheless, significant efforts are being made to overcome this drawback including, at the bioprocess level, by developing storage formulations (Carmo et al. 2009a; Cruz et al. 2006) and at the viral vector design level, by developing mutant vectors with increased infectivity stability (Vu et al. 2008).

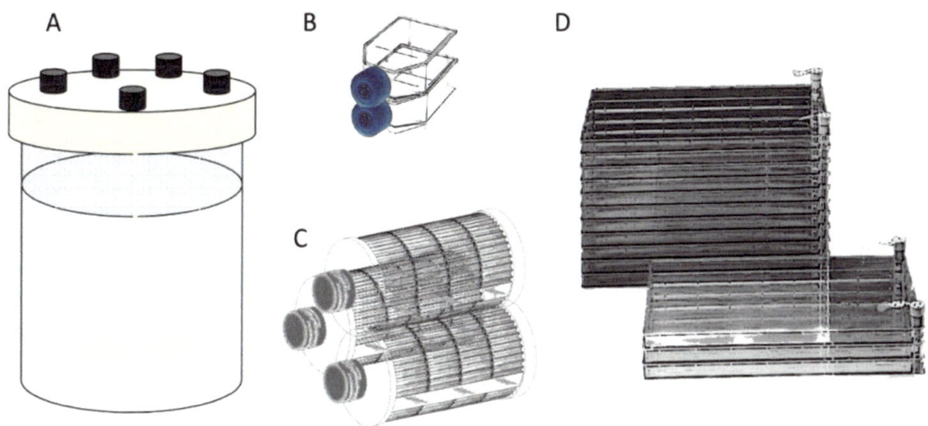

Fig. 6. Culture systems used for retroviral and lentiviral vector manufacture. Stirred tank bioreactor (A) vs. adherent disposable systems, T-flasks (B), roller bottles (C) and (D) cell factories.

3.3 Bioreaction physicochemical parameters

The cell culture parameters used in the bioreaction may have a profound effect on the virus titer by affecting the cellular productivities, vector stability or both. Several studies have been performed analyzing the impact of physicochemical parameters such as pH, temperature, osmolarity, O_2 and CO_2 concentrations. The optimal cell culture parameters have been shown to be producer cell line and viral vector dependent.

The optimal pH range for retroviral vector production was found to be between 6.8 and 7.2 for FLY RD18 and Te FLY A7; outside this range the cell specific productivities were considerable lower (McTaggart and Al-Rubeai 2000; Merten 2004), while the retroviral vector was observed to be stable between pH of 5.5 and 8.0 in ecotropic pseudotyped vectors (Ye et al. 2003). Both retroviral vectors (MLV derived) and lentiviral vectors (HIV-1 derived), VSV-G pseudotyped, were stable at pH 7. The half-lives of both viral vectors at pH 6.0 and pH 8.0 markedly decrease to less than 10 minutes (Higashikawa and Chang 2001). The viral half-life is also dependent on the temperature: at lower temperatures the vector decay kinetics are lower (Le Doux et al. 1999). Therefore one strategy explored in the production of retroviral vectors has been the reduction of the culture temperatures (28-32°C). Some authors reported increases in vector production at lower temperature (Kaptein et al. 1997; Kotani et al. 1994; Le Doux et al. 1999; Lee et al. 1996). The reduction of the

culture temperature from 37ºC to 32ºC extends vector stability allowing for the accumulation of more infectious virus and thus, increasing the volumetric titers. However, the increments are not always very significant as the temperature affects also the cell specific yields negatively. The improvement in the viral volumetric titer will be only observed if, the increase in the viral half-life is higher than the decrease in the cell specific production rate (Le Doux et al. 1999). Additionally, the viral vector inherent stability was also demonstrated to be lower when the viral vector was produced at 32ºC instead of 37ºC (Beer et al. 2003; Cruz et al. 2005). It was shown that the culture temperature affected the lipid viral membrane composition namely, the cholesterol content. The increase in cholesterol content was demonstrated to be inversely proportional to retroviral stability (Beer et al. 2003; Coroadinha et al. 2006c). Since enveloped virus, such as retrovirus and lentivirus, bud out of the host cells, they take part of the host cell lipidic membrane. Thus, the origin of the producer cell will have a pronounced effect on the viral particle stability and explain the discrepant results obtained for virus produced in different cells and at different temperatures. For PA317 cells, decreasing the production temperature from 37ºC to 32ºC resulted in an increase of 5-15 fold in the vector titers (Kaptein et al. 1997) while for PG13 lower titers were obtained (Reeves et al. 2000). The viral vector envelope glycoproteins also affect the viral particle inherent stability increasing the complexity and diversity of factors involved in the viral stability. Comparing lentiviral and retroviral vectors it was generally observed that HIV-1 derived vectors are more stable at 37ºC and at higher temperatures than MLV derived vectors (Higashikawa and Chang 2001).
Augmenting the media osmolarity was also shown to be a valid strategy to increase retroviral vector titers in Te FLY A7 (Coroadinha et al. 2006c). This increment was correlated with higher cell specific productivities and higher inherent viral stability. The high osmotic pressure altered the cellular and viral envelope lipid membrane composition. High osmotic media were tested showing to induce a decrease in the cholesterol to phospholipids ratio in the viral membrane and thus conferring higher stability to the viral vectors produced (Coroadinha et al. 2006c). These results, together with the studies of production at lower culture temperatures, strengthen the importance of lipid metabolism in the production of enveloped virus.
CO_2 gas concentration in the cultures did not affect virus production in packaging cell lines (Kotani et al. 1994; McTaggart and Al-Rubeai 2000). The dissolved oxygen levels used are between 20-80% and within this range do not affect viral production unless they became limiting to cell growth (Merten 2004).

3.4 Media composition and cell metabolic bottlenecks

Retroviral and lentiviral vector titers obtained in the production prior to purification are in the range of 10^6 to 10^7 infectious particles *per* mL of culture medium. Considering the average amount needed to treat a patient in a clinical trial, in the order of 10^{10} infectious vectors (Aiuti et al. 2009; Cavazzana-Calvo et al. 2000; Ott et al. 2006), around 10-100 L of culture volume can be previewed for each patient. Also, viral preparations are typically characterized by low ratios of infectious particles to total particles (around 1:100) which further reduce the therapeutic efficiency of the infectious ones (Carrondo et al. 2008). Additionally, these vectors are extremely sensitive losing their infectivity relatively fast, the reported half-lives are between 8-12 hours in cell culture supernatant at 37ºC (Carmo et al. 2009b; Carmo et al. 2008; Higashikawa and Chang 2001; Merten 2004; Rodrigues et al. 2009). Thus, the productivity performance of retroviral and lentiviral vector producing systems is below the therapeutic needs.

The problems of low titers, short half-life and low ratios of infectious particles to total particles have been subject of intensive bioprocess research. However, the infection with wild type retroviruses, in particular HIV-1, is typically chronically and characterized by persistent but low titers of the infectious agents in the blood stream, with high amounts of non-infectious particles contaminants and with equivalently low half-lives (Perelson et al. 1996; Rusert et al. 2004). Therefore, retrovirus and lentiviral manufacture starts in disadvantage - when compared to other viral vectors - in what concerns to such parameters. Several strategies have been attempted to circumvent these "natural" drawbacks in packaging cell lines, including engineering mutant vectors with improved resistance features and understanding and optimizing the metabolic pathways leading to improved productivities. Studying the metabolic features driving to high titer performances has been one important work lines of research. Therefore, this section will mainly focus on the metabolic bottlenecks of viral vector production.

3.4.1 Serum supplemented vs. serum-free media

The supplementation of mammalian cell culture media with animal sera has been common practice in biomedical and biotechnological research, since it provides critical nutrients and factors that support cell growth and proliferation. However, the ill-defined composition and high batch-to-batch variability of serum together with its potential source of contaminations, hinders safety and standardization of cell cultures, making it a highly undesirable supplement in the production of biopharmaceuticals (Falkner et al. 2006). Also, in the case of retroviral and lentiviral vectors, serum needs to be removed from the medium and/or viral preparations to prevent immunological responses in the patients.

Retroviral and lentiviral vector manufacture has been reported to rely on considerable amounts (5-10% (v/v)) of animal sera in the culture medium; although some authors reported improved titers in short-term serum-free productions (Gerin et al. 1999a; McTaggart and Al-Rubeai 2000), the issue of serum dependence for retroviral and lentiviral vector production will be next discussed in the perspective of long-term cultures. The majority of the latest generation of packaging cell lines, specially the HEK293 (human embryonic kidney) derived ones, seem to require high concentrations of serum in the culture medium to support elevated viral productivities for long term culture (Chan et al. 2001; Gerin et al. 1999a; Gerin et al. 1999b; Pizzato et al. 2001; Rodrigues et al. 2009).

The need of serum for retroviral and lentiviral vector production has been mainly associated with the lipidic needs of packaging cell lines. Unless other supplements are added, serum is the only lipid source of the culture medium and, although cells should be able to sense lipid absence in the culture medium and activate biosynthetic pathways to stand up to lipid deprivation, the activation of lipid *de novo* synthesis may take hours or days, depending on the cell type (Alberts et al. 1974; Spector et al. 1980). In some cases, cells can no longer synthesize certain lipids (Seth et al. 2005). Membrane lipids are active players in the complex process of retroviral assembling, and pseudotyping that takes place at the host cell membrane, in which interactions of membrane lipid rafts select both envelope and core proteins, recruiting later the other viral components by cooperative interaction. The production of infectious particles is known to rely on the efficiency of this process, which is dependent upon a delicate equilibrium of lipid type and amounts, easily disturbed by lipid deprivation (Briggs et al. 2003). Therefore, changes in serum concentration that disturb cell membrane lipid composition will ultimately affect viral particle membrane properties (Rawat et al. 2003) possibly resulting in a higher production of non-infectious particles. In fact, it has been not only demonstrated that lipids are one of the main serum components correlated with high retroviral infectious vector titers but also, that the reduction of serum in the culture medium affects infectious titers only, i.e. the total number of particles produced remained unaltered (Rodrigues et al. 2009). Indeed, high-titer production of retroviral and lentiviral vectors under serum-free conditions has only been achieved in the presence of lipid supplements, lipid carriers and lipoproteins addition (Broussau et al. 2008; Ghani et al. 2007).

The work done so far, addressing the issue of serum supplementation and infectious vector production, has mainly been focused on retroviral vectors, less attention has been paid to serum/lipid requirements in lentiviral vector production. Of notice is the work developed by B. Mitta et al (2005) in which optimal lentiviral production parameters were established, resulting in up to 132-fold improved productivities, and quality. The later is defined as the viral infectious titer (reflecting the number of transduction-competent lentiviral particles) relative to the number of total physical lentiviral particles produced (analysed by the levels of p24). A reduced-serum formulation was used and supplemented. Among others, lipid supplementation, included cholesterol, lecithin and chemically defined lipid concentrates. The lipid supplements were identified as the main responsibles for the improved viral productivities obtained.

In the case of lentiviral vectors, the short-term production periods associated with either the transient or conditional productions have not elucidated the extent of serum dependence in the production of high-infectious vector titers. Yet, the large majority of the current protocols for the production of lentiviral vectors still make use of 5 to 10% (v/v) of serum in the culture medium and up to now, only two publications have reported the production of lentiviral vectors under serum-free conditions (Ansorge et al. 2009; Broussau et al. 2008), both of them requiring lipid supplementation.

More recently, studies on the effects of adapting retroviral vector packaging cell lines to serum deprivation conditions and how it impacts infectious vector production have been performed. These studies identified differences in cell lipid metabolism as a requirement needed by the packaging cells to be able to adapt to serum deprivation: cells capable of activating *de novo* lipid biosynthesis under serum withdrawal, particularly cholesterol, are able to be adapted to serum deprivation without significant loss of infectious vector titer production. On the other hand, cells facing serum removal from the culture medium that are unable to activate lipid biosynthesis - HEK293 - lose infectious titer productivity after a few passages (Rodrigues et al., 2011). In this context, it should be noticed that long term serum-free production of retro and lentiviral vectors reported so far has been based not only in lipid supplemented media but also on oncogene transformed 293 cells, namely 293T, transformed with SV40 large T antigen (T-Ag) and 293 EBNA, transformed with Nuclear Antigen of Epstein-Barr Virus. These cells exhibit very different physiological features when compared to their non-transformed counterparts, 293, potentially facilitating serum-independence for vector production. For instance, SV40 transformed cells were shown to require minimal serum amounts or no serum at all, in the culture medium in order to proliferate. T-Ag expression is known to allow to overcome growth arrest mediated by contact inhibition and provide to the transformed cells an anchorage independent phenotype (Ahuja et al. 2005). Additionally, T-Ag expression drives even quiescent cells to the S-Phase (Ahuja et al. 2005), potentially providing raw material for viral replication. Besides those changes mentioned above, not much is known about the long-term physiological modifications induced by T-Ag and EBNA transformation. However, it is possible that some of those changes target lipid biosynthetic pathways, given that oncogenic neoplastic transformation is typically characterized by an increase in lipid biosynthesis and turnover (Barger and Plas 2010; Swinnen et al. 2006). In conclusion, the major metabolic hinge between serum and high titers has been demonstrated to be the lipids and cellular lipid metabolism.

3.4.2 Sugar carbon source

Glucose has been the traditional sugar source employed in animal cell culture media and thus, the most used in the production of retroviral and lentiviral vectors. Together with glutamine, glucose is the major energy and carbon source in the culture medium. It is also the universal carbohydrate in animal cell culture, since glucose cellular transporters are present in the majority of the mammalian cell types. However, glucose is rapidly consumed and inefficiently metabolized to lactate which, *per se,* is toxic to the cell. Concentrations of lactate above 5 mM can inhibit cell growth of Te Fly Ga18 cells and retroviral production (Merten et al. 2001).

The use of alternative sugar sources to glucose is a possible strategy to decrease lactate production. Indeed, the use of fructose and galactose was shown to improve the retroviral production in Te FLY A7, Te FLY Ga18, PG13 and Tel CeB cell lines (Coroadinha et al. 2006a; Merten 2004). The lactate production decreased 2 to 6 fold in galactose and fructose media and the vector titers increased up to 8 fold. Both galactose and fructose consumption rates were lower than glucose in Te Fly A7, possible due to lower specificity of the sugar transporters expressed in these cells. The best results in terms of vector titers were obtained at high concentrations of fructose (15-25 g/L) (Coroadinha et al., 2006, Merten, 2004). Additionally to the metabolic shift induced by an alternative carbon source, an effect of high osmotic pressure can also be of relevance in the improvement of viral titers (see section 3.3). The increment of infectious titers observed at high sugar concentrations in Te Fly A7 was confirmed to be the result of higher cell specific productivities, higher vector stability and lower production of defective non-infective particles (Coroadinha et al., 2006a and 2006b) (Table 3).

Medium	Osmolality (mOsm/kg)	Cell Productivity (I.P. cells^{-1}.h^{-1})	Virus Half-Life (h)	Cholesterol/Phospholipid molar ratio in viral particles
Glucose 25 mM	335	0.18 ± 0.01	8 ± 0.7	0.53±0.03
Glucose 25 mM + sorbitol	450	0.80± 0.09	14± 1	0.33±0.01
Fructose 140 mM	450	1.0± 0.1	14±2	0.30±0.01

Table 3. Effect of alternative sugar sources and media osmolality in retroviral vector production. Te Fly A7 producer cells were used in this study. Sorbitol is a non-ionic osmotic agent, non-metabolized by the cells.

Further metabolic studies were performed using ^{13}C-NMR spectroscopy indicating changes in the lipid metabolism, namely higher synthesis of phospholipids (Coroadinha et al., 2006 and Amaral et al., 2008). These results show that packaging cell line metabolism deeply influences the productivity performances, in particular lipid biosynthesis, thus suggesting it to be an important target for further improve retroviral and possibly lentiviral vector titers.

No studies with alternative sugar sources have been reported with lentiviral vectors. Nevertheless, the above studies were performed with, Te671 and NIH 3T3 cells and most lentiviral vectors are produced in 293 derived cells.

4. Conclusions and outlook

Murine leukemia virus (MLV) derived vectors were the first viral vectors used in clinical trials and remain among the preferentially used vehicles for gene therapy applications due to their advantages relatively to other vectors. Lentiviral vectors have been developed more recently. From the therapeutic perspective they present the additional advantage of transducing non-dividing cells. From the manufacturing perspective lentiviral vectors present however, an additional difficulty as they contain cytotoxic proteins, requiring either the use of transient transfection or inducible systems. Both lentiviral and retroviral vectors are derived from virus belonging to the *retroviridae* family sharing many characteristics in terms of genome, biochemistry, structure and viral cycle. Thus many of the metabolic constraints in their production are common and reviewed herein.

The success of the application of retroviral vectors in phase I and II clinical trials is now moving the prospects to phase III trials. This will create momentum to increase the efforts in research related with retroviral vectors development and production due to the large amounts of vectors needed, and the stringent demands by the regulatory agencies. Lentiviral vectors in particular possess many of the characteristics of MLV retroviral vectors, and as mentioned present the additional advantages of being able to transduce quiescent cells. The diversity of human gene therapy as well as the possibility of patients being treated more than once with viral vectors, which are recognized by the adaptive immune system, leaves space to both alternative vector technologies. MLV present a large safety record in clinical application that cannot be discarded. Since MLV retroviral vectors are not derived from human viruses they also show reduced vector genome mobilization and recombination in the host-cell and pre-existing immune response against the retroviral vector particle. Additionally, they are simple to develop in terms of plasmid cloning, transfection and cell culture; and from the clinical perspective they can be easily produced at large scale from stable packaging cell lines with satisfactory yields. From the manufacturing point of view, HIV-1 derived vector still requires further optimization, particularly in what concerns cell line development. There is still less clinical experience with this vector and the results on the ongoing clinical trials will be certainly important for their improvement.

Thus the recent manufacturing strategies together with future innovations will certainly be important to increase productivity, stability, quality and safety of retroviral and lentiviral vectors for clinical applications.

5. Acknowledgements

The authors acknowledge the financial support received from the European Commission (CLINIGENE -LSHB-CT2006-018933) and the Fundação para a Ciência e a Tecnologia-Portugal (PTDC/EBB-BIO/100491/2008). Ana F. Rodrigues acknowledges FCT for her PhD grant (SFRH/BD/48393/2008).

6. References

Ahuja D, Saenz-Robles MT, Pipas JM. 2005. SV40 large T antigen targets multiple cellular pathways to elicit cellular transformation. Oncogene 24(52):7729-45.

Aiuti A, Cattaneo F, Galimberti S, Benninghoff U, Cassani B, Callegaro L, Scaramuzza S, Andolfi G, Mirolo M, Brigida I and others. 2009. Gene therapy for immunodeficiency due to adenosine deaminase deficiency. N Engl J Med 360(5):447-58.

Al-Dosari MS, Gao X. 2009. Nonviral gene delivery: principle, limitations, and recent progress. Aaps J 11(4):671-81.

Alberts AW, Ferguson K, Hennessy S, Vagelos PR. 1974. Regulation of lipid synthesis in cultured animal cells. J Biol Chem 249(16):5241-9.

Ansorge S, Lanthier S, Transfiguracion J, Durocher Y, Henry O, Kamen A. 2009. Development of a scalable process for high-yield lentiviral vector production by transient transfection of HEK293 suspension cultures. J Gene Med 11(10):868-76.

Balaggan KS, Binley K, Esapa M, Iqball S, Askham Z, Kan O, Tschernutter M, Bainbridge JW, Naylor S, Ali RR. 2006. Stable and efficient intraocular gene transfer using pseudotyped EIAV lentiviral vectors. J Gene Med 8(3):275-85.

Barger JF, Plas DR. 2010. Balancing biosynthesis and bioenergetics: metabolic programs in oncogenesis. Endocr Relat Cancer 17(4):R287-304.

Beer C, Meyer A, Muller K, Wirth M. 2003. The temperature stability of mouse retroviruses depends on the cholesterol levels of viral lipid shell and cellular plasma membrane. Virology 308(1):137-46.

Bender MA, Palmer TD, Gelinas RE, Miller AD. 1987. Evidence that the packaging signal of Moloney murine leukemia virus extends into the gag region. J Virol 61(5):1639-46.

Blesch A. 2004. Lentiviral and MLV based retroviral vectors for ex vivo and in vivo gene transfer. Methods 33(2):164-72.

Boussif O, Lezoualc'h F, Zanta MA, Mergny MD, Scherman D, Demeneix B, Behr JP. 1995. A versatile vector for gene and oligonucleotide transfer into cells in culture and in vivo: polyethylenimine. Proc Natl Acad Sci U S A 92(16):7297-301.

Bray M, Prasad S, Dubay JW, Hunter E, Jeang KT, Rekosh D, Hammarskjold ML. 1994. A small element from the Mason-Pfizer monkey virus genome makes human immunodeficiency virus type 1 expression and replication Rev-independent. Proc Natl Acad Sci U S A 91(4):1256-60.

Briggs JA, Wilk T, Fuller SD. 2003. Do lipid rafts mediate virus assembly and pseudotyping? J Gen Virol 84(Pt 4):757-68.

Broussau S, Jabbour N, Lachapelle G, Durocher Y, Tom R, Transfiguracion J, Gilbert R, Massie B. 2008. Inducible packaging cells for large-scale production of lentiviral vectors in serum-free suspension culture. Mol Ther 16(3):500-7.

Burns JC, Friedmann T, Driever W, Burrascano M, Yee JK. 1993. Vesicular stomatitis virus G glycoprotein pseudotyped retroviral vectors: concentration to very high titer and efficient gene transfer into mammalian and nonmammalian cells. Proc Natl Acad Sci U S A 90(17):8033-7.

Carmo M, Alves A, Rodrigues AF, Coroadinha AS, Carrondo MJ, Alves PM, Cruz PE. 2009a. Stabilization of gammaretroviral and lentiviral vectors: from production to gene transfer. J Gene Med 11(8):670-8.

Carmo M, Dias JD, Panet A, Coroadinha AS, Carrondo MJ, Alves PM, Cruz PE. 2009b. Thermosensitivity of the reverse transcription process as an inactivation mechanism of lentiviral vectors. Hum Gene Ther 20(10):1168-76.

Carmo M, Panet A, Carrondo MJ, Alves PM, Cruz PE. 2008. From retroviral vector production to gene transfer: spontaneous inactivation is caused by loss of reverse transcription capacity. J Gene Med 10(4):383-91.
Carrondo MJT, Merten OW, Haury M, Alves PM, Coroadinha AS. 2008. Impact of retroviral vector components stoichiometry on packaging cell lines: Effects on productivity and vector quality. Human Gene Therapy 19(2):199-210.
Cavazzana-Calvo M, Hacein-Bey S, de Saint Basile G, Gross F, Yvon E, Nusbaum P, Selz F, Hue C, Certain S, Casanova JL and others. 2000. Gene therapy of human severe combined immunodeficiency (SCID)-X1 disease. Science 288(5466):669-72.
Chan LM, Coutelle C, Themis M. 2001. A novel human suspension culture packaging cell line for production of high-titre retroviral vectors. Gene Ther 8(9):697-703.
Chong H, Starkey W, Vile RG. 1998. A replication-competent retrovirus arising from a split-function packaging cell line was generated by recombination events between the vector, one of the packaging constructs, and endogenous retroviral sequences. J Virol 72(4):2663-70.
Chong H, Vile RG. 1996. Replication-competent retrovirus produced by a 'split-function' third generation amphotropic packaging cell line. Gene Ther 3(7):624-9.
Cockrell AS, Ma H, Fu K, McCown TJ, Kafri T. 2006. A trans-lentiviral packaging cell line for high-titer conditional self-inactivating HIV-1 vectors. Mol Ther 14(2):276-84.
Coffin JM, Hughes SH, Varmus H. 1997. Retroviruses: Cold Spring Harbor.
Cone RD, Mulligan RC. 1984. High-efficiency gene transfer into mammalian cells: generation of helper-free recombinant retrovirus with broad mammalian host range. Proc Natl Acad Sci U S A 81(20):6349-53.
Cornetta K, Matheson L, Ballas C. 2005. Retroviral vector production in the National Gene Vector Laboratory at Indiana University. Gene Ther 12 Suppl 1:S28-35.
Coroadinha AS, Gama-Norton L, Amaral AI, Hauser H, Alves PM, Cruz PE. 2010. Production of retroviral vectors: review. Curr Gene Ther 10(6):456-73.
Coroadinha AS, Ribeiro J, Roldao A, Cruz PE, Alves PM, Merten OW, Carrondo MJ. 2006a. Effect of medium sugar source on the production of retroviral vectors for gene therapy. Biotechnol Bioeng 94(1):24-36.
Coroadinha AS, Schucht R, Gama-Norton L, Wirth D, Hauser H, Carrondo MJ. 2006b. The use of recombinase mediated cassette exchange in retroviral vector producer cell lines: predictability and efficiency by transgene exchange. J Biotechnol 124(2):457-68.
Coroadinha AS, Silva AC, Pires E, Coelho A, Alves PM, Carrondo MJ. 2006c. Effect of osmotic pressure on the production of retroviral vectors: Enhancement in vector stability. Biotechnol Bioeng 94(2):322-9.
Cosset FL, Takeuchi Y, Battini JL, Weiss RA, Collins MK. 1995. High-titer packaging cells producing recombinant retroviruses resistant to human serum. J Virol 69(12):7430-6.
Cruz PE, Carmo M, Coroadinha AS, Bengala A, Gonçalves D, Teixeira M, Merten O-W, Genny-Fiamma C, Carrondo MJT. Retroviral Vector Stability: Inactivation Kinetics and Membrane Properties. In: Gòdia F, Fussenegger M, editors. Animal Cell Technology meets Genomics; 2005. Springer. p 303-308.

Cruz PE, Silva AC, Roldao A, Carmo M, Carrondo MJ, Alves PM. 2006. Screening of novel excipients for improving the stability of retroviral and adenoviral vectors. Biotechnol Prog 22(2):568-76.

Danos O, Mulligan RC. 1988. Safe and efficient generation of recombinant retroviruses with amphotropic and ecotropic host ranges. Proc Natl Acad Sci U S A 85(17):6460-4.

Davis JL, Witt RM, Gross PR, Hokanson CA, Jungles S, Cohen LK, Danos O, Spratt SK. 1997. Retroviral particles produced from a stable human-derived packaging cell line transduce target cells with very high efficiencies. Hum Gene Ther 8(12):1459-67.

Delenda C. 2004. Lentiviral vectors: optimization of packaging, transduction and gene expression. J Gene Med 6 Suppl 1:S125-38.

Dull T, Zufferey R, Kelly M, Mandel RJ, Nguyen M, Trono D, Naldini L. 1998. A third-generation lentivirus vector with a conditional packaging system. J Virol 72(11):8463-71.

Eckert HG, Kuhlcke K, Schilz AJ, Lindemann C, Basara N, Fauser AA, Baum C. 2000. Clinical scale production of an improved retroviral vector expressing the human multidrug resistance 1 gene (MDR1). Bone Marrow Transplant 25 Suppl 2:S114-7.

Edelstein M. 2010. Gene Therapy Clinical Trials Worldwide - http://www.wiley.com//legacy/wileychi/genmed/clinical/. Wiley InterScience.

Eibl R, Kaiser S, Lombriser R, Eibl D. 2010. Disposable bioreactors: the current state-of-the-art and recommended applications in biotechnology. Appl Microbiol Biotechnol 86(1):41-9.

Falkner E, Appl H, Eder C, Losert UM, Schoffl H, Pfaller W. 2006. Serum free cell culture: the free access online database. Toxicol In Vitro 20(3):395-400.

Farson D, McGuinness R, Dull T, Limoli K, Lazar R, Jalali S, Reddy S, Pennathur-Das R, Broad D, Finer M. 1999. Large-scale manufacturing of safe and efficient retrovirus packaging lines for use in immunotherapy protocols. J Gene Med 1(3):195-209.

Farson D, Witt R, McGuinness R, Dull T, Kelly M, Song J, Radeke R, Bukovsky A, Consiglio A, Naldini L. 2001. A new-generation stable inducible packaging cell line for lentiviral vectors. Hum Gene Ther 12(8):981-97.

Gerin PA, Gilligan MG, Searle PF, Al-Rubeai M. 1999a. Improved titers of retroviral vectors from the human FLYRD18 packaging cell line in serum- and protein-free medium. Hum Gene Ther 10(12):1965-74.

Gerin PA, Searle PF, Al-Rubeai M. 1999b. Production of retroviral vectors for gene therapy with the human packaging cell line FLYRD18. Biotechnol Prog 15(5):941-8.

Ghani K, Cottin S, Kamen A, Caruso M. 2007. Generation of a high-titer packaging cell line for the production of retroviral vectors in suspension and serum-free media. Gene Ther 14(24):1705-11.

Ghani K, Garnier A, Coelho H, Transfiguracion J, Trudel P, Kamen A. 2006. Retroviral vector production using suspension-adapted 293GPG cells in a 3L acoustic filter-based perfusion bioreactor. Biotechnol Bioeng 95(4):653-60.

Gougeon ML. 2003. Apoptosis as an HIV strategy to escape immune attack. Nat Rev Immunol 3(5):392-404.

Gruh I, Wunderlich S, Winkler M, Schwanke K, Heinke J, Blomer U, Ruhparwar A, Rohde B, Li RK, Haverich A and others. 2008. Human CMV immediate-early enhancer: a useful tool to enhance cell-type-specific expression from lentiviral vectors. J Gene Med 10(1):21-32.

Higashikawa F, Chang L. 2001. Kinetic analyses of stability of simple and complex retroviral vectors. Virology 280(1):124-31.

Ikeda Y, Takeuchi Y, Martin F, Cosset FL, Mitrophanous K, Collins M. 2003. Continuous high-titer HIV-1 vector production. Nat Biotechnol 21(5):569-72.

Jordan M, Wurm F. 2004. Transfection of adherent and suspended cells by calcium phosphate. Methods 33(2):136-43.

Kafri T, van Praag H, Ouyang L, Gage FH, Verma IM. 1999. A packaging cell line for lentivirus vectors. J Virol 73(1):576-84.

Kaptein LC, Greijer AE, Valerio D, van Beusechem VW. 1997. Optimized conditions for the production of recombinant amphotropic retroviral vector preparations. Gene Ther 4(2):172-6.

Kotani H, Newton PB, 3rd, Zhang S, Chiang YL, Otto E, Weaver L, Blaese RM, Anderson WF, McGarrity GJ. 1994. Improved methods of retroviral vector transduction and production for gene therapy. Hum Gene Ther 5(1):19-28.

Kotsopoulou E, Kim VN, Kingsman AJ, Kingsman SM, Mitrophanous KA. 2000. A Rev-independent human immunodeficiency virus type 1 (HIV-1)-based vector that exploits a codon-optimized HIV-1 gag-pol gene. J Virol 74(10):4839-52.

Kuate S, Wagner R, Uberla K. 2002. Development and characterization of a minimal inducible packaging cell line for simian immunodeficiency virus-based lentiviral vectors. J Gene Med 4(4):347-55.

Le Doux JM, Davis HE, Morgan JR, Yarmush ML. 1999. Kinetics of retrovirus production and decay. Biotechnol Bioeng 63(6):654-62.

Lee SG, Kim S, Robbins PD, Kim BG. 1996. Optimization of environmental factors for the production and handling of recombinant retrovirus. Appl Microbiol Biotechnol 45(4):477-483.

Lesch HP, Laitinen A, Peixoto C, Vicente T, Makkonen KE, Laitinen L, Pikkarainen JT, Samaranayake H, Alves PM, Carrondo MJ and others. 2011. Production and purification of lentiviral vectors generated in 293T suspension cells with baculoviral vectors. Gene Ther.

Lesch HP, Turpeinen S, Niskanen EA, Mahonen AJ, Airenne KJ, Yla-Herttuala S. 2008. Generation of lentivirus vectors using recombinant baculoviruses. Gene Ther 15(18):1280-6.

Lewis P, Hensel M, Emerman M. 1992. Human immunodeficiency virus infection of cells arrested in the cell cycle. Embo J 11(8):3053-8.

Liberatore C, Capanni M, Albi N, Volpi I, Urbani E, Ruggeri L, Mencarelli A, Grignani F, Velardi A. 1999. Natural killer cell-mediated lysis of autologous cells modified by gene therapy. J Exp Med 189(12):1855-62.

Loew R, Meyer Y, Kuehlcke K, Gama-Norton L, Wirth D, Hauser H, Stein S, Grez M, Thornhill S, Thrasher A and others. 2009. A new PG13-based packaging cell line for stable production of clinical-grade self-inactivating gamma-retroviral vectors using targeted integration. Gene Ther 17(2):272-80.

Loew R, Selevsek N, Fehse B, von Laer D, Baum C, Fauser A, Kuehlcke K. 2004. Simplified generation of high-titer retrovirus producer cells for clinically relevant retroviral vectors by reversible inclusion of a lox-P-flanked marker gene. Mol Ther 9(5): 738-46.

Markowitz D, Goff S, Bank A. 1988. Construction of a safe and efficient retrovirus packaging cell line. Adv Exp Med Biol 241:35-40.

Matukonis M, Li M, Molina RP, Paszkiet B, Kaleko M, Luo T. 2002. Development of second- and third-generation bovine immunodeficiency virus-based gene transfer systems. Hum Gene Ther 13(11):1293-303.

McTaggart S, Al-Rubeai M. 2000. Effects of culture parameters on the production of retroviral vectors by a human packaging cell line. Biotechnol Prog 16(5):859-65.

McTaggart S, Al-Rubeai M. 2002. Retroviral vectors for human gene delivery. Biotechnol Adv 20(1):1-31.

Merten O, Landric L, Danos O. 2001. Influence of the metabolic status of packaging cells on retroviral vector production. Recombinant Protein Production with Prokaryotic and Eukaryotic Cells. Dordrecht: Kluwer Academic Publishers.

Merten OW. 2004. State-of-the-art of the production of retroviral vectors. J Gene Med 6 Suppl 1:S105-24.

Merten OW, Charrier S, Laroudie N, Fauchille S, Dugue C, Jenny C, Audit M, Zanta-Boussif MA, Chautard H, Radrizzani M and others. 2011. Large scale manufacture and characterisation of a lentiviral vector produced for clinical ex vivo gene therapy application. Hum Gene Ther.

Miller AD, Buttimore C. 1986. Redesign of retrovirus packaging cell lines to avoid recombination leading to helper virus production. Mol Cell Biol 6(8):2895-902.

Miller AD, Chen F. 1996. Retrovirus packaging cells based on 10A1 murine leukemia virus for production of vectors that use multiple receptors for cell entry. J Virol 70(8):5564-71.

Miller AD, Garcia JV, von Suhr N, Lynch CM, Wilson C, Eiden MV. 1991. Construction and properties of retrovirus packaging cells based on gibbon ape leukemia virus. J Virol 65(5):2220-4.

Mitrophanous K, Yoon S, Rohll J, Patil D, Wilkes F, Kim V, Kingsman S, Kingsman A, Mazarakis N. 1999. Stable gene transfer to the nervous system using a non-primate lentiviral vector. Gene Ther 6(11):1808-18.

Mitta B, Rimann M, Fussenegger M. 2005. Detailed design and comparative analysis of protocols for optimized production of high-performance HIV-1-derived lentiviral particles. Metab Eng 7(5-6):426-36.

Molina RP, Ye HQ, Brady J, Zhang J, Zimmerman H, Kaleko M, Luo T. 2004. A synthetic Rev-independent bovine immunodeficiency virus-based packaging construct. Hum Gene Ther 15(9):865-77.

Naldini L, Blomer U, Gallay P, Ory D, Mulligan R, Gage FH, Verma IM, Trono D. 1996. In vivo gene delivery and stable transduction of nondividing cells by a lentiviral vector. Science 272(5259):263-7.

Ni Y, Sun S, Oparaocha I, Humeau L, Davis B, Cohen R, Binder G, Chang YN, Slepushkin V, Dropulic B. 2005. Generation of a packaging cell line for prolonged large-scale production of high-titer HIV-1-based lentiviral vector. J Gene Med 7(6):818-34.

Nie Z, Bren GD, Vlahakis SR, Schimnich AA, Brenchley JM, Trushin SA, Warren S, Schnepple DJ, Kovacs CM, Loutfy MR and others. 2007. Human immunodeficiency virus type 1 protease cleaves procaspase 8 in vivo. J Virol 81(13):6947-56.

Nie Z, Phenix BN, Lum JJ, Alam A, Lynch DH, Beckett B, Krammer PH, Sekaly RP, Badley AD. 2002. HIV-1 protease processes procaspase 8 to cause mitochondrial release of cytochrome c, caspase cleavage and nuclear fragmentation. Cell Death Differ 9(11):1172-84.

Ott MG, Schmidt M, Schwarzwaelder K, Stein S, Siler U, Koehl U, Glimm H, Kuhlcke K, Schilz A, Kunkel H and others. 2006. Correction of X-linked chronic granulomatous disease by gene therapy, augmented by insertional activation of MDS1-EVI1, PRDM16 or SETBP1. Nat Med 12(4):401-9.

Pacchia AL, Adelson ME, Kaul M, Ron Y, Dougherty JP. 2001. An inducible packaging cell system for safe, efficient lentiviral vector production in the absence of HIV-1 accessory proteins. Virology 282(1):77-86.

Pandya S, Boris-Lawrie K, Leung NJ, Akkina R, Planelles V. 2001. Development of an Rev-independent, minimal simian immunodeficiency virus-derived vector system. Hum Gene Ther 12(7):847-57.

Pauwels K, Gijsbers R, Toelen J, Schambach A, Willard-Gallo K, Verheust C, Debyser Z, Herman P. 2009. State-of-the-art lentiviral vectors for research use: risk assessment and biosafety recommendations. Curr Gene Ther 9(6):459-74.

Perelson AS, Neumann AU, Markowitz M, Leonard JM, Ho DD. 1996. HIV-1 dynamics in vivo: virion clearance rate, infected cell life-span, and viral generation time. Science 271(5255):1582-6.

Persons DA, Mehaffey MG, Kaleko M, Nienhuis AW, Vanin EF. 1998. An improved method for generating retroviral producer clones for vectors lacking a selectable marker gene. Blood Cells Mol Dis 24(2):167-82.

Pizzato M, Merten OW, Blair ED, Takeuchi Y. 2001. Development of a suspension packaging cell line for production of high titre, serum-resistant murine leukemia virus vectors. Gene Ther 8(10):737-45.

Poeschla EM, Wong-Staal F, Looney DJ. 1998. Efficient transduction of nondividing human cells by feline immunodeficiency virus lentiviral vectors. Nat Med 4(3):354-7.

Przybylowski M, Hakakha A, Stefanski J, Hodges J, Sadelain M, Riviere I. 2006. Production scale-up and validation of packaging cell clearance of clinical-grade retroviral vector stocks produced in cell factories. Gene Ther 13(1):95-100.

Rawat SS, Viard M, Gallo SA, Rein A, Blumenthal R, Puri A. 2003. Modulation of entry of enveloped viruses by cholesterol and sphingolipids (Review). Mol Membr Biol 20(3):243-54.

Reeves L, Smucker P, Cornetta K. 2000. Packaging cell line characteristics and optimizing retroviral vector titer: the National Gene Vector Laboratory experience. Hum Gene Ther 11(15):2093-103.

Rigg RJ, Chen J, Dando JS, Forestell SP, Plavec I, Bohnlein E. 1996. A novel human amphotropic packaging cell line: high titer, complement resistance, and improved safety. Virology 218(1):290-5.

Roberts TM, Boris-Lawrie K. 2000. The 5' RNA terminus of spleen necrosis virus stimulates translation of nonviral mRNA. J Virol 74(17):8111-8.

Rodrigues AF, Carmo M, Alves PM, Coroadinha AS. 2009. Retroviral vector production under serum deprivation: The role of lipids. Biotechnol Bioeng 104(6):1171-81.

Rodrigues AF, Amaral AI, Veríssimo V, Alves PA, Coroadinha AS 2011. Adaptation to serum deprivation: implications in lipid biosynthesis and vector production (submitted)

Rusert P, Fischer M, Joos B, Leemann C, Kuster H, Flepp M, Bonhoeffer S, Gunthard HF, Trkola A. 2004. Quantification of infectious HIV-1 plasma viral load using a boosted in vitro infection protocol. Virology 326(1):113-29.

Sadettin SO, Hu W. 2006. Cell culture technology for pharmaceutical and cell-based therapies. Sadettin SO, Hu W, editors. Boca Raton, FL, USA: CRC Press Taylor & Francis Group

Saenz DT, Poeschla EM. 2004. FIV: from lentivirus to lentivector. J Gene Med 6 Suppl 1:S95-104.

Schnell T, Foley P, Wirth M, Munch J, Uberla K. 2000. Development of a self-inactivating, minimal lentivirus vector based on simian immunodeficiency virus. Hum Gene Ther 11(3):439-47.

Schnierle BS, Stitz J, Bosch V, Nocken F, Merget-Millitzer H, Engelstadter M, Kurth R, Groner B, Cichutek K. 1997. Pseudotyping of murine leukemia virus with the envelope glycoproteins of HIV generates a retroviral vector with specificity of infection for CD4-expressing cells. Proc Natl Acad Sci U S A 94(16):8640-5.

Schucht R, Coroadinha AS, Zanta-Boussif MA, Verhoeyen E, Carrondo MJ, Hauser H, Wirth D. 2006. A new generation of retroviral producer cells: predictable and stable virus production by Flp-mediated site-specific integration of retroviral vectors. Mol Ther 14(2):285-92.

Schweizer M, Merten OW. 2010. Large-scale production means for the manufacturing of lentiviral vectors. Curr Gene Ther 10(6):474-86.

Segura MM, Garnier A, Durocher Y, Ansorge S, Kamen A. 2010. New protocol for lentiviral vector mass production. Methods Mol Biol 614:39-52.

Seth G, Philp RJ, Denoya CD, McGrath K, Stutzman-Engwall KJ, Yap M, Hu WS. 2005. Large-scale gene expression analysis of cholesterol dependence in NS0 cells. Biotechnol Bioeng 90(5):552-67.

Sheridan PL, Bodner M, Lynn A, Phuong TK, DePolo NJ, de la Vega DJ, Jr., O'Dea J, Nguyen K, McCormack JE, Driver DA and others. 2000. Generation of retroviral packaging and producer cell lines for large-scale vector production and clinical application: improved safety and high titer. Mol Ther 2(3):262-75.

Sinn PL, Sauter SL, McCray PB, Jr. 2005. Gene therapy progress and prospects: development of improved lentiviral and retroviral vectors--design, biosafety, and production. Gene Ther 12(14):1089-98.

Smith SL, Shioda T. 2009. Advantages of COS-1 monkey kidney epithelial cells as packaging host for small-volume production of high-quality recombinant lentiviruses. J Virol Methods 157(1):47-54.

Soneoka Y, Cannon PM, Ramsdale EE, Griffiths JC, Romano G, Kingsman SM, Kingsman AJ. 1995. A transient three-plasmid expression system for the production of high titer retroviral vectors. Nucleic Acids Res 23(4):628-33.

Spector AA, Mathur SN, Kaduce TL, Hyman BT. 1980. Lipid nutrition and metabolism of cultured mammalian cells. Prog Lipid Res 19(3-4):155-86.

Stewart HJ, Leroux-Carlucci MA, Sion CJ, Mitrophanous KA, Radcliffe PA. 2009. Development of inducible EIAV-based lentiviral vector packaging and producer cell lines. Gene Ther 16(6):805-14.

Swift S, Lorens J, Achacoso P, Nolan GP. 2001. Rapid production of retroviruses for efficient gene delivery to mammalian cells using 293T cell-based systems. Curr Protoc Immunol Chapter 10:Unit 10 17C.
Swinnen JV, Brusselmans K, Verhoeven G. 2006. Increased lipogenesis in cancer cells: new players, novel targets. Curr Opin Clin Nutr Metab Care 9(4):358-65.
Takeuchi Y, Cosset FL, Lachmann PJ, Okada H, Weiss RA, Collins MK. 1994. Type C retrovirus inactivation by human complement is determined by both the viral genome and the producer cell. J Virol 68(12):8001-7.
Takeuchi Y, Liong SH, Bieniasz PD, Jager U, Porter CD, Friedman T, McClure MO, Weiss RA. 1997. Sensitization of rhabdo-, lenti-, and spumaviruses to human serum by galactosyl(alpha1-3)galactosylation. J Virol 71(8):6174-8.
Takeuchi Y, Porter CD, Strahan KM, Preece AF, Gustafsson K, Cosset FL, Weiss RA, Collins MK. 1996. Sensitization of cells and retroviruses to human serum by (alpha 1-3) galactosyltransferase. Nature 379(6560):85-8.
Throm RE, Ouma AA, Zhou S, Chandrasekaran A, Lockey T, Greene M, De Ravin SS, Moayeri M, Malech HL, Sorrentino BP and others. 2009. Efficient construction of producer cell lines for a SIN lentiviral vector for SCID-X1 gene therapy by concatemeric array transfection. Blood 113(21):5104-10.
Toledo JR, Prieto Y, Oramas N, Sanchez O. 2009. Polyethylenimine-based transfection method as a simple and effective way to produce recombinant lentiviral vectors. Appl Biochem Biotechnol 157(3):538-44.
Vu HN, Ramsey JD, Pack DW. 2008. Engineering of a stable retroviral gene delivery vector by directed evolution. Mol Ther 16(2):308-14.
Wikstrom K, Blomberg P, Islam KB. 2004. Clinical grade vector production: analysis of yield, stability, and storage of gmp-produced retroviral vectors for gene therapy. Biotechnol Prog 20(4):1198-203.
Wildner O, Candotti F, Krecko EG, Xanthopoulos KG, Ramsey WJ, Blaese RM. 1998. Generation of a conditionally neo(r)-containing retroviral producer cell line: effects of neo(r) on retroviral titer and transgene expression. Gene Ther 5(5):684-91.
Xu K, Ma H, McCown TJ, Verma IM, Kafri T. 2001. Generation of a stable cell line producing high-titer self-inactivating lentiviral vectors. Mol Ther 3(1):97-104.
Ye K, Dhiman HK, Suhan J, Schultz JS. 2003. Effect of pH on infectivity and morphology of ecotropic moloney murine leukemia virus. Biotechnol Prog 19(2):538-543.
Yu JH, Schaffer DV. 2005. Advanced targeting strategies for murine retroviral and adeno-associated viral vectors. Adv Biochem Eng Biotechnol 99:147-67.
Zufferey R, Donello JE, Trono D, Hope TJ. 1999. Woodchuck hepatitis virus posttranscriptional regulatory element enhances expression of transgenes delivered by retroviral vectors. J Virol 73(4):2886-92.
Zufferey R, Nagy D, Mandel RJ, Naldini L, Trono D. 1997. Multiply attenuated lentiviral vector achieves efficient gene delivery in vivo. Nat Biotechnol 15(9):871-5.
Zwolinska K. 2006. Retroviruses-derived sequences in the human genome. Human endogenous retroviruses (HERVs). Postepy Hig Med Dosw (Online) 60:637-52.

3

Surface Modification of Retroviral Vectors for Gene Therapy

Christoph Metzner and John A. Dangerfield
University of Veterinary Medicine Vienna
Austria

1. Introduction

If biomedicine is considered to be the use of biological or botanical agents in medicine then it is certainly the oldest kind of therapy. Since drugs, however, it is no longer the most prolifically used, at least in the developed world. Will this change, and if so will it be in the near or more distant future? It has been discussed amongst experts in the industry for some time that, despite ever-increasing funding and new high-tech methods of discovery and screening, amounts of new drugs and drug leads are declining. In part, this has opened the way for biologics. The frontrunner is of course antibody technologies, mainly monoclonals, the use of which has exploded over the last 5 years to the point where most of the major pharma players are involved or are getting involved in what has now become a multi-billion dollar industry. Antibodies have reached the point of being a well trusted and accepted form of medical product across the industry and communities from bench to bedside.

Many believe the next similar success story will be for cell therapy, probably some differentiated form of stem cells. Although it has been happening for 20 years, it is only in the past 5 years that the amount of patients being treated with cells, as a therapy, has increased into the thousands per year. The vast majority of these are autologous cell treatments, undertaken by hospitals and private clinics on a patient to patient basis using the patients' own cells to treat a wide variety of diseases and conditions. These are not officially approved medical products. However, there are several non-pharmaceutical giant companies now in clinical trials, notable amongst these are Geron in the USA, Mesoblast in Australia and ReNeuron in the UK, although there are some interesting endeavors in Southeast Asia too, e.g. Medipost in Korea. All of these are undergoing various stages and sizes of clinical trials for diverse indications, some of which are showing already very encouraging results. It is predicted that within the next few years one or more of these potential products will reach the market as an approved medical product. Having said this, other than showing ongoing safety and efficacy in the trials, some hurdles do remain in the industry as whole, such as up-scaling for mass production of the cells which is considered necessary for generating an off-the-shelf product.

If this trend continues, it is only reasonable to assume that gene therapy will follow, most probably some years after cell therapy has been more widely accepted, but possibly in parallel to some extent, as there are also a number of human gene therapy trials already in progress. So, how significant will retroviral (RV) and lentiviral (LV) vectors be in this future gene therapy industry? One approach to answer this is to look at how popular they have been up to now, both in terms of previous and ongoing trials as well as the interest that the research community has in them compared to other forms of gene therapy tools.

In order to asses this one must firstly consider all forms of gene delivery tools, as this is a pre-requisite for gene therapy. In general, gene delivery can be achieved either by viral or non-viral means. Mostly, when non-viral gene delivery is discussed, it involves the use of plasmid DNA, although there is much interest in other forms of nucleic acids such as bacterial artificial chromosomes (BACs) (for recent review on BACs see Tunster et al. 2011). Nucleic acids can be transduced into the patients' cells by physical or chemical mechanisms. Physical methods include obvious ways like direct injection, or aerosolisation/inhalation but also more ingenious techniques like the gene gun or using sound waves, such as ultrasound (Passineau et al. 2011) or by electroshock, which can intriguingly even work *in vivo* (De Vry et al. 2010; Kaneda 2010). Such non-viral means have classically been considered to be safer because viral vectors may cause insertional mutagenesis, revert to wild-type via recombinations during preparation or *in vivo* with other viruses (infections or endogenous viruses). But, at the same time, non-viral means are also considered to be far less effective, as once the nucleic acid is inside the cell it is only by chance that it will enter the nucleus and be expressed. Both of these views are changing somewhat though. From a safety perspective, as techniques for producing and detecting virus vectors are advancing and people's understandings of viral vector safety is improving, and, from an efficiency perspective, as chemical and nanomaterial technologies improve.

It boils down to a risk/benefit calculation and viral based methods are still generally considered to be far more efficient tools, and as such, outweighing the risks. Mammalian cells could be transformed with virus-based methods as early as the 1960's, yet virus related vectorology, with respect to gene delivery, only started to strongly emerge in the early 1980's (Figure 1), showing that this is somewhat a matter of definition. In any case, adenoviruses (AdV) have always been and still are the most popularly researched and used vectors. One would expect that over the years, the number of different types of viruses and new viruses being researched as vectors would increase, and this is indeed the case (Fig. 1, see "others" from 1 in 1985 to over 400 in 2010). However, one trend that was not as expected is that the amount of studies on herpes simplex (HSV) as a vector has not increased. In other words, in 1980 the first talk of using viruses in connection with gene delivery was concerning HSV (Anderson et al. 1980), by 1985 a few publications related to RV, but the most were still HSV related, and surprisingly this number has almost not changed up to 2010 where still only approximately 20 publications related to using HSV as a vector for gene therapy or delivery. Is it fair to conclude from this that they may simply be unsuitable for the job? Further investigation would be required to make such a claim but it may be reasonable to suggest that if more successful steps had been made, then increasing popularity would be inevitable. Most surprising, however, is that over the last 10 years, publications of research and use of viruses as vectors seems to have reached a plateau, and in the last four years, have begun to decrease (see Figure 1, All). This may be a sign that that some technologies are being absorbed by industrial processes, e.g. patent before publication, trade secrets. Such translational activities, although more practical, are less academically novel and may reduce the number of research papers.

Most relevant perhaps for this chapter on surface modifications of enveloped viruses and their application, is the changing relationship of interest between RV and LV vectors in the research community over the last ten years (Figure 1, compare RV and LV).

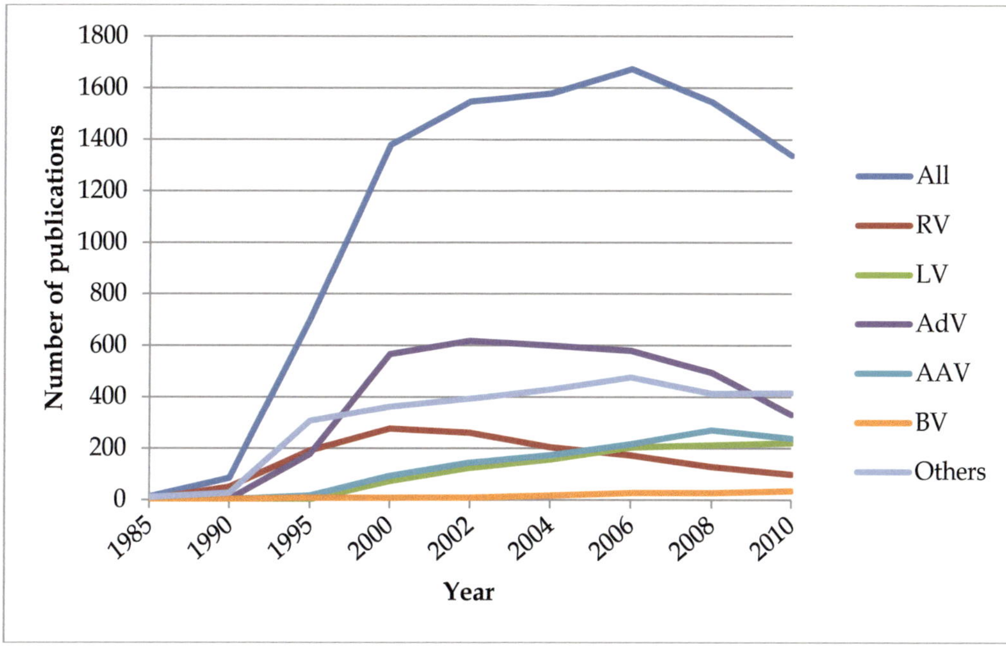

Fig. 1. The trend of scientific publications in the area of viral vectors for gene delivery over the last 25 years. A study was undertaken using the scientific reference collating programme, Endnote. The method used was to search and cross-reference various terms. For example, both "retrovirus" and "retroviral" were searched together with either "gene delivery" or "gene therapy" and "vector" and each were cross-referenced with each other, which allowed not only to be sure that the topic in question was relating to gene delivery/therapy with viral vectors, and that nothing was missed, but it also gave an idea of publications which were using both types of system, i.e. that these were not counted twice. The same was done for lentivirus, adenovirus and adeno-associated virus vectors.
Key: All = total number of all viral vectors for gene delivery and includes the following: RV = retroviral vectors; LV = lentiviral vectors; AdV = adenovirus vectors; AAV = adeno-associated virus vectors; BV = baculoviral vectors; Others = vectors based on the following viruses: alphaviruses (e.g. Sindbis, Semliki Forest, Ross River, Venezuelan equine encephalitis), vaccinia viruses, poxviruses, infectious bursal disease, herpes simplex, Sendai/hemagglutinating virus of Japan, measles, transmissible gastroenteritis virus, human and avian influenza, oncolytic vesicular stomatitis, papilloma viruses, lymphocytic choriomeningitis, rabies, hepatitis B/C, combinations of viruses (e.g. RV-LV, AdV-RV) as well as replicons, amplicons, retroelements and virally related transposons.

Although the actual numbers are not huge, there is clearly a significant shift in the focus of interest from RV vectors to LV vectors. When RV vectors are discussed, this means mainly the two forms of murine leukemia virus (MLV), the Friend and Moloney strains, although, studies also include vector work with mouse mammary tumour virus (MMTV) and Rous sarcoma virus (RSV) (Gunzburg 2003). When LV vectors are discussed, this means mainly human immunodeficiency virus type-1 (HIV-1), although again, studies also include vector work with simian and feline immunodeficiency viruses (SIV and FIV). There may be many reasons for this shift in interest in the scientific community. One is certainly that LV vectors, in contrast to RV vectors, offer the ability to transduce non-dividing cells (Sakoda et al. 2007). This is generally seen as an advantage, however, it may not be desirable in all gene delivery cases, as it may be useful to target only dividing cells (e.g. in cancer therapy). Another reason is likely to be the sheer amount of interest in HIV as its affliction on humans continues to globally expand, i.e. relatively large amounts of finance available and research undertaken to understand the virus for human medicine not only leads to drug targets but also to ingenious ways of using the virus as a vector for gene delivery or therapy, e.g. self-inactivating vectors to increase safety (Liehl et al. 2007).

Other than RV, LV, AdV and AAV, there are many types of viruses being developed as gene delivery vectors, all with limited impact, but it seems in more recent years that the numbers of these studies are no longer increasing (see Figure 1, Others). One explanation may be that this correlates with the amount of new viruses being discovered. Either man has discovered most viral entities already or a future technological breakthrough will allow discovery of viral or viral related entities of a new dimension. It may also be surprising to some to see how many "nasty" viruses are being used to make vectors. For example, HSV BACs were developed around 2000 mainly for studying viral genetics, but more recently they are being explored for gene therapy (Warden et al. 2011). Other ongoing examples include measles, influenza and papilloma viruses, the latter of which cause cancer. When considering this, however, one just has to remember what has happened with HIV over the last 15 years. First suggestions of using HIV vectors for human medicine were met with serious concern in the general media, and even scientists were skeptical, but now they are well accepted and even approved for use in human clinical trials (Sheridan 2011, also see below).

Some publications relate to expression of viral genes within other more common types of vector system, e.g. the thymidine kinase gene of the HSV (HSV-TK) expressed using a RV or AdV vector, so it is somewhat a matter of definition as to whether they are included as virus based gene delivery systems. For this study, such cases were not included. In some cases there were also hits for viral components such as the envelope proteins of vesicular stomatitis virus (VSV), lymphocytic choriomeningitis virus (LCMV) and amphotropic MLV (see also Table 2), but this is relating to pseudotyping, and, although there are a few genuine cases of scientists developing true gene delivery vectors from these viruses, the pseudotyping cases were not counted in this study. Pseudotyping as a method for viral surface modification is discussed later in this chapter.

Finally, how has all the viral vector research culminated into gene therapy trials in the clinic? The majority of trials that have been undertaken and are currently ongoing (around 14 human trials) are using AdV and AAV (for a recent review see Sheridan 2011). More relating to the topic of this chapter, however, are past and ongoing successes for enveloped viral vector gene therapies, i.e. RV and LV vectors. Most worthy of mention are the studies, human trials and treatments made by Alain Fischer, Marina Cavazzana-Calvo and Salima Hacein-Bey-Abina. Children who were suffering from severe combined immunodeficiency (SCID-X1) had their T-cells treated *ex vivo* with a RV vector (Moloney MLV based) to replace a defective part of the gene for the interleukin-2 receptor (Cavazzana-Calvo et al. 2000; Hacein-Bey-Abina et al. 2008). Although four of the twenty patients treated developed leukemia (caused by insertional mutagenesis and activation of a proto-oncogene), they were able to be treated for this secondary issue, and seventeen from twenty have had their immunodeficiency corrected over the follow-up period of almost 10 years now (Cavazzana-Calvo et al. 2010). This is a great success in which the benefit clearly outweighed the risk, as without alternative treatment (the only one being a bone marrow transplant with only 25%

chance of success), the outcome would have been fatal within a few years at best. Other ongoing studies in the area of primary immunodeficiency are being undertaken by San Raffaele in Italy, also using a Moloney MLV vector (Aiuti et al. 2002), although it is unclear if more human trials are planned at present. Two USA companies have ongoing RV vector treatments in trials, namely Neurologix for Parkinson's disease (Kaplitt et al. 2007; Lewitt et al. 2011) and Tocagen for a form of brain cancer, glioblastoma multiforme. The Tocagen trial is of particular interest as it is the first study in humans using a replication competent RV. All RV and LV vectors previously used in trials (even the vast majority used in research) are non-replicating or self-inactivating, which means after one round of infection/gene delivery that the virus is "dead" and cannot replicate further. It has been classically developed this way for safety reasons, unfortunately, as it turns out, the *in vivo* infection efficiency of such vectors may never be good enough for many applications. The MLV based replication competent vector developed by Tocagen and its research associates (Anliker et al. 2010) has the therapeutic gene, cytosine deaminase (CD), inserted into the viral genome in a stable position where the virus cannot easily reject it, even after multiple rounds of infection (Logg et al. 2001; Paar et al. 2007). As the RV vector is limited to replicating in dividing cells, and only very few cells in the brain are dividing at a speed comparable to the tumour, it is the ideal setting. Also, the prodrug used for the treatment, 5-FC, can only pass the blood-brain barrier in its non-activated form, i.e. once activated to 5-FU by the CD gene product at the cancer location, it cannot pass back into the rest of the body, where there are faster dividing cells which could be affected. Once the infected tumour is destroyed, so in turn are the replicating viruses in this so called suicide-gene therapy system. This trial is being followed by many and with great interest.

Concerning clinical trials with LV, three companies are worth mentioning. Bluebird Bio (formerly Genetix Pharmaceuticals) in the USA, recently completed 2 trials with three patients in total who underwent *ex vivo* treatment of their own hematopoietic stem cells with a LV vector delivering corrective genes for either cerebral adrenoleukodystrophy (Cartier et al. 2009) or beta-thalassaemia (Cavazzana-Calvo et al. 2010). Although both showed positive results, no public announcement on further trials has been announced as yet. Lentigen, also in USA, are currently undertaking a pilot study through the University of Pennsylvania for several kinds of leukemia and lymphoma, whereby, once again, the patients T-cells will be modified *ex vivo*, but in this case the modification should turn-on the T-cells enabling them to attack and trigger the destruction of the cancerous B cells once re-implanted (ClinicalTrials.gov Identifier No. NCT00891215). Oxford BioMedica are currently undertaking Phase I/II trial for Parkinson's disease by injecting their LV vector technology via stereotactic injection directly into the striatum of patients' brains. Three genes which are necessary for dopamine production should be delivered/expressed and the results are predicted to be published soon (EudraCT No. 2007-001109).

2. Methods to modify surfaces of RV/LV vectors

2.1 Introduction - proteins of retroviral surfaces

When retroviral or lentiviral (RV/LV) particles exit infected cells, they are surrounded by a lipid membrane, termed the envelope, derived from the infected cells. The envelope contains both virus-derived and cellular proteins (VP and CP, respectively), which may perform distinct functions for the virus. Since proteins displayed on the envelope are the first to make contact with neighboring molecules, they are often involved in virus-cell and virus-medium interactions. In order to complete their life cycle, viruses are depending on this communication with their surroundings, specifically the soluble factors (i.e. antibodies or proteins of the complement system) contained in the liquid environment and elements displayed on the surface of potential host cells (i.e. the receptors found on the cell surface required for binding and entry of the virus).

This is maybe best demonstrated by the VPs found in the lipid membrane of the RV/LV particle, termed envelope or Env proteins. The function of these proteins is to initiate cell entry (for more details see chapter 3.5.). The RV/LV envelope proteins may be replaced by surface glycoproteins of different virus species in a process termed pseudotyping (Bischof and Cornetta 2010; Cronin et al. 2005). The resulting viral pseudotypes can be of interest for gene therapy applications (see section 2.2. for details). Apart from the virus encoded Env proteins, CP are also incorporated into the viral envelopes. Theoretically, this may happen as a consequence of three processes: (i) interaction of host proteins with viral proteins (type 1 incorporation), (ii) incorporation due to directed colocalisation (type 2 incorporation) and (iii) random incorporation (type 3 incorporation). The incorporation of the cytoplasmic protein cyclophilin A to HIV-1 particles is an example of a type 1 incorporation. The protein associates with the viral Gag proteins and is subsequently incorporated with a similar efficiency (Hammarstedt and Garoff 2004). A similar situation was shown for the tumor susceptibility gene 101 (Tsg-101) product, which presumably has a role in RV/LV particle release (Garrus et al. 2001; Pornillos et al. 2003). Additionally, in 1995 the incorporation of complement regulatory factors such as CD55 (decay accelerating factor) and CD59 (protectin) into viral envelopes was described (Breun et al. 1999; Saifuddin et al. 1994; Saifuddin et al. 1995; Saifuddin et al. 1997). The levels of these proteins are high enough to ensure protection from the human complement system, a part of the innate immune system (Breun et al. 1999; Saifuddin et al. 1997). Both the glycosylphosphatidylinositol-anchored CD55 and CD59 molecules are enriched in membrane microdomains, often termed lipid rafts. Interestingly, it has been demonstrated that a range of viral species including retroviruses and lentiviruses may use lipid rafts as sites of viral assembly (Metzner et al. 2008a). Thus co-localisation of these molecules at the site of viral budding would lead to their incorporation into viral envelopes. Thus, this may constitute a type 2 incorporation. The co-localisation of molecules at membrane microdomains may also form the framework for pseudotyping events (Briggs et al. 2003; Metzner et al. 2008a; Pickl et al. 2001) (see section 2.2.). Discriminating between type 2 and type 3 incorporation events may be difficult, since directed co-localisation is not easy to demonstrate and the concept of membrane microdomains is controversial (Shaw 2006). However, there is reason to believe that most incorporation events happen passively (Hammarstedt and Garoff 2004), i.e. concentration of proteins is not increased compared to normal membrane composition. To maintain a proteome not altogether dissimilar from the cellular membrane may generally be beneficial for the virus, since this would contribute to immune-camouflage, i.e. "hiding" the virus from the host's immune system.

A special case is the exclusion of host proteins from the viral particles. Several cases have been described including proteins such as CD45 (Esser et al. 2001), CD4 and the HIV co-receptors CXCR4 and CCR5 (Lallos et al. 1999). Excluding receptors and co-receptors from budding viral particles can be beneficial for the virus, since premature receptor engagement and induction of fusion can be avoided. The mechanisms responsible for exclusion of proteins from viral envelopes may be that the formation of a network of viral Gag proteins inhibits access of proteins with large cytoplasmic domains (such as CD45) or multiple transmembrane passes (such as the HIV co-receptors). Alternatively, involvement of excluded proteins in larger complexes may prevent them from being incorporated (such as CD4-p56lck). Recently, proteomics approaches have been used to identify host proteins found in viral envelopes to get an overview of incorporation (see Table 1) and to date, a long list of proteins have been identified in viral particle envelopes (Chertova et al. 2006; Segura et al. 2008b) including a range of molecules involved in cellular adhesion. Viruses may profit from these molecules, as they can provide additional or indeed, initial anchoring before specific interactions between Env and the cognate cell-membrane viral receptors.

Protein	Virus	Function	Comment	Reference
Tsg-101	HIV-1	MVB sorting; HIV budding	Interaction with Gag	Hammarstedt and Garoff, 2004; Pornillos et al.; 2002
CD55	HIV-1, MLV	Complement regulation	GPI-anchored	Saifuddin et al., 1995; Plewa et al., 2005
CD59	HIV-1, MLV	Complement regulation	GPI-anchored	Saifuddin et al., 1995; Plewa et al., 2005
CD14	HIV-1	Lipopolysaccharide receptor	GPI-anchored	Chertova et al., 2006
CD29 (Integrin ß1)	HIV-1, MLV	Adhesion	Random?	Chertova et al., 2006; Segura et al., 2008
CD44	HIV-1	Adhesion	Random?	Chertova et al., 2006
CD54 (ICAM 1)	HIV-1	Adhesion	Random?	Chertova et al., 2006
CD48	HIV-1	Signaling	Random?	Chertova et al., 2006
CD45	HIV-1	Signaling	Excluded	Esser et al., 2001
CD4	HIV-1	HIV receptor	Excluded	Lallos et al., 1999
CXCR4	HIV-1	HIV co-receptor	Excluded	Lallos et al., 1999
CCR5	HIV-1	HIV co-receptor	Excluded	Lallos et al., 1999

Table 1. Examples for cellular proteins incorporated to RV/LV envelopes. Tsg tumor suppressor gene 101; MVB multivesicular bodies; ICAM intercellular adhesion molecule.

Surface modification of RV/LV particles can be broadly separated into five categories (see Figure 2): (i) pseudotyping, (ii) generation of fusion proteins, (iii) post translational modification of proteins with lipophilic residues, most notably glycosylphosphatidylinositol (GPI) anchors, (iv) utilization of adaptor molecules, or (v) direct chemical modifications. These types of modification will be discussed in sections 2.2. to 2.6., while the purpose of such modifications and possible applications will be discussed in section 3. Special attention will be given to the "non-classical" methods for modification of viral surfaces discussed in section 2.4. to 2.6.

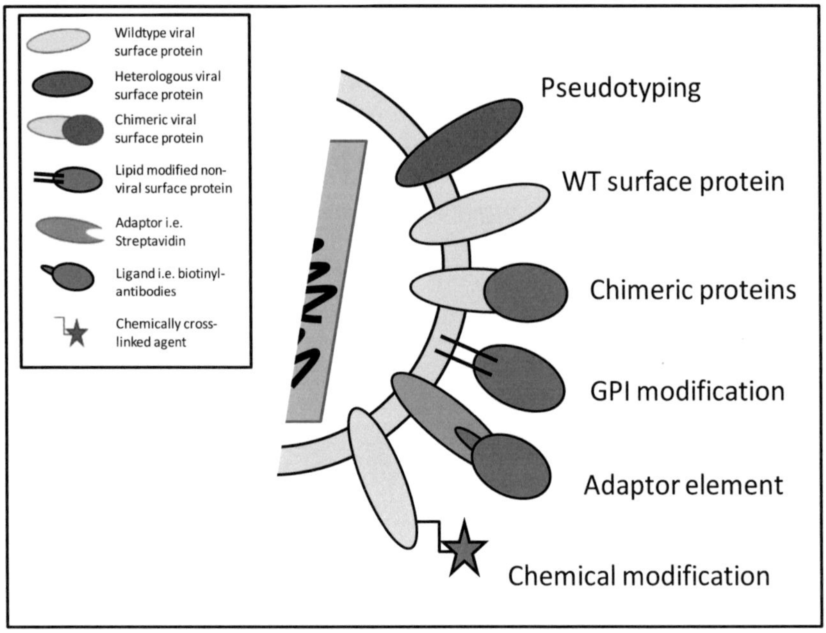

Fig. 2. Overview of strategies for modification of RV/LV vector surfaces.

2.2 Pseudotyping

The phenomenon that surface (glyco-)proteins of one virus species can be displayed on the surface of another retrovirus, or indeed other viral species has been termed "pseudotyping". It was first described more that 55 years ago, after the observation that cells infected with two different viruses, can give rise to phenotypically mixed particles (Granoff and Hirst 1954; Zavada 1982). Interestingly, surface glycoproteins from different families of viruses can be exchanged or mixed in such a manner (see Table 2), indicating some degree of similarity between these molecules or the mechanisms by which they are incorporated into the virions. Because of this compatibility, a limited set of modifications can be introduced to retroviral particles by displaying surface molecules of other viral species. Since the primary function of viral surface glycoproteins is to mediate binding and entry to host cells, the replacement of retroviral Env molecules in most cases changes the infectious range (the tropism) of the vector, because different receptors are engaged. This phenomenon can be exploited for gene therapy approaches, as it allows for example, the broadening or re-direction of the virus' host range (see Table 2). For example, HIV-1 based LV vectors, naturally having a very limited, highly specific tropism, infecting only CD4-expressing cells, can be redirected from these cells by replacing the Env proteins of HIV-1 with those of the vesicular stomatitis virus (VSV), thus generating a vector with a more diverse tropism (Bischof and Cornetta 2010). VSV-G, the surface glycoprotein of VSV, is probably the most often used molecule for pseudotyping applications. In addition to changing tropism, VSV-G also enhances virion stability (Burns et al. 1993) but is toxic to cells if expressed constitutively making it challenging to generate stable packaging cell lines. To overcome this, tetracycline-inducible promoters are frequently used to generate stable virus-producing cell lines (Ory et al. 1996). Additionally VSV-G pseudotypes are highly susceptible to inactivation by human serum complement (DePolo et al. 2000) and require additional treatment e.g. by polyethylene glycol (PEG) modification or PEGylation (Croyle et al. 2004). Other examples for pseudotyping are described in table 2. It is not in all cases that pseudotyping is used to transfer new cell binding properties to the RV/LV vector. Recent approaches employ pseudotyping to transfer fusion properties of surface glycoproteins from Sindbis (Morizono et al. 2009a; H. Yang et al. 2008a), Influenza (Lin et al. 2001; H. Yang et al. 2008a) or measles virus (Anliker et al. 2010; Frecha et al. 2011). In these molecules, fusion activity is not strictly dependent on receptor binding. In such cases the original binding activity may be abrogated and replaced with a binding function of choice. This constitutes a "mixed" modification, since both, pseudotyping and generation of chimeric proteins are employed to generate vector particles (see also sections 2.3 and 3.5.).

Viral Surface Protein	Virus Family	Vector Background	Targeting Preference	References
MLV amphotropic	Retroviridae	HIV-1, SIV	broad, fibroblasts	Strang et al., 2004
GALV	Retroviridae	HIV-1	hematopoietic, cancer	Diaz et al., 2000; Sandrin et al., 2002
RD114	Retroviridae	HIV-1, SIV	hematopoietic	Sandrin et al., 2002; Zhang et al., 2004
LCMV	Arenaviridae	HIV-1, EIAV, SIV	CNS, glioma, pancreas	Miletic et al., 2004; Kobinger et al., 2004
Sindbis	Togaviridae	HIV-1	broad	Morizono et al. 2009
Ross River	Togaviridae	HIV-1, FIV	Liver (non-hepatocyte)	Kang et al. 2002
VSG-G	Rhabdoviridae	HIV-1, HIV-2, SIV, FIV, EIAV	CNS, Liver, retina	Watson et al. 2002; Park et al. 2003; Auricchio et al. 2001
Ebola	Filoviridae	HIV-1, FIV	Lung, muscle	Kobinger et al. 2004; MacKenzie et al. 2002
Rabies	Rhabdoviridae	HIV-1, EIAV	CNS	Stein et al. 2005
Influenza A	Orthomyxoviridae	HIV-1, EIAV, SIV	Lung	McKay et al. 2006
Measles	Paramyxoviridae	HIV-1	broad (Edmonston strain)	Anliker et al. 2010
Sendai	Paramyxoviridae	HIV-1, SIV	Liver, Lung	Kowolik et al. 2002; Sinn et al. 2005
Hepatitis C	Flaviviridae	HIV-1	Liver	Hsu et al. 2003

Table 2. Examples for the use of pseudotyping events for gene therapy approaches. MLV murine leukemia virus; SIV simian immunodeficiency virus; GALV gibbon ape leukemia virus; LCMV lymphocytic choriomeningitis virus; EIAV equine infectious anemia virus; FIV feline immunodefiency virus; VSV-G vesicular stomatitis virus glycoprotein.

The mechanisms behind pseudotyping are believed to be related to the presence of membrane subdomains in cellular membranes which function as sites for viral assembly and/or budding of a range of different viral species (Briggs et al. 2003; Metzner et al. 2008a; Pickl et al. 2001). Since viruses from quite different taxonomical origins are assembled at such sites, incorporation of proteins from different virus backgrounds can occur. Consequently, pseudotyping can be viewed as a form of type 2 incorporation. Another pre-requisite for pseudotyping, is that wild-type RV/LV Env proteins are not required for functional assembly of virions, inferring that the absence of the native glycoproteins does not interfere with particle production. Alternatively, direct or indirect (via a cellular intermediate) protein interaction may be responsible for pseudotyping. Recently, an indirect interaction model has been proposed using a scanning electron microscopy approach (Jorgenson et al. 2009) thus supporting involvement of type 1 incorporation events. To date, a large number of combinations have been tried and have been assessed in terms of their targeting potential in gene therapy approaches (see Table 2). Recent reviews provide a more extensive overview of pseudotyping of RV/LV vectors (Bischof and Cornetta 2010; Cronin et al. 2005).

2.3 Fusion proteins

Hybrid proteins consisting of amino acid sequence elements derived from more than one original polypeptide are termed fusion or chimeric proteins. To avoid confusion with proteins such as viral surface glycoproteins exhibiting membrane fusion activity, the latter term will be used. The technique of fusing protein parts by manipulation on the DNA level has been widely used to study the spatial distribution or kinetics of expression by utilizing fluorescent marker proteins such as green fluorescent protein (GFP). Fusing retroviral envelope proteins with molecules of interest allows for a more widespread modification of viral surfaces, since it is not limited by the availability of naturally occurring viral glycoproteins. In the case of chimeric proteins, the residual RV/LV Env molecule part is used as a sorting signal, directing the chimeric molecule to sites of budding. The advantage of this method is that theoretically no limit is placed on the type of amino acid sequence introduced and that incorporation to the viral particle is in most cases efficient (Ryu, 2008). The fused parts may be complete ligands (Kasahara et al. 1994), peptides (Gollan and Green 2002; Morizono et al. 2009a) or single-chain antibodies (Anliker et al. 2010; Somia et al. 1995). However, limits have been shown to apply to this technique, as structural or functional elements are typically disturbed by their introduction, leading to loss of infectivity, since cellular uptake is inhibited at the level of envelope-cell membrane fusion (Galanis et al. 2001; Ryu et al. 2008; Zhao et al. 1999). When a chimeric Env molecule, containing a CD33 specific single-chain antibody, was generated to target CD33 positive cells, the collected data indicated, that the chimeric protein could not initiate fusion of the virus and cell membranes during infection (Zhao et al. 1999). The most widely accepted explanation for this is that the chimeric proteins are unable to undergo a mandatory conformational change which activates the fusion activity (see also section 3.5.). Thus, the use of such modifications for targeting applications, i.e. the induction of cellular uptake upon engagement of the chimeric protein with a cognate receptor, is limited. Inclusion of wild-type RV Env proteins to targeted vectors can help to increase infectivity (Tai et al. 2003). This, however, may come at a cost for specificity of targeting. Studies conducted on chimeric Moloney murine leukemia virus (MoMLV) Env proteins suggest, that addition of as little as two point mutations might rescue targeted infection (Zavorotinskaya and Albritton 2001). More recent data suggests

that such mutations may need to be determined depending on the characteristics of the insert as well as the insertion site (Ryu, 2008).
However, for purposes other than targeting, such as labeling of viral particles or tagging for enrichment purposes, this technique still holds appeal. A GFP-Env chimeric protein, containing the sequence of enhanced GFP fused to the N-terminus of the amphotropic 4070A Env of MLV has been generated and in this case viral particles retained their natural infection range (Spitzer et al. 2003). The construct was used to stain viral receptor-carrying cells and may be used for monitoring the dynamics of virus-cell interactions (Spitzer et al., 2003). An interesting aspect is, that the "virion-targeting functions" of chimeric proteins may not necessarily have to be provided by RV/LV Env proteins, but could also be provided by the use of cellular proteins present or enriched in viral membranes such as Tsg-101 (see Table 2). Alternatively, virion-targeting function may be provided by GPI-anchoring (see section 2.4.) or indeed, by making use of mixed modifications using fusion proteins of non-RV/LV glycoproteins, such as Sindbis virus (Morizono et al. 2009b; Pariente et al. 2007) influenza (Lin et al. 2001; L. Yang et al. 2006b) or measles virus (Anliker et al. 2010; Frecha et al. 2008) with engineered novel binding properties. In these cases the wild-type binding specificity was destroyed and replaced with molecules conferring specific targeting to molecules such as integrin (Morizono et al. 2009a) or the B lymphocyte marker CD20 (Anliker et al. 2010). In these cases, membrane fusion activity is inhibited to a lesser degree by the change in binding properties. For Sindbis and influenza, virus fusion is triggered by a decrease in pH. First *in vivo* experiments indicated that such vectors can be used for targeting applications (Anliker et al. 2010; L. Yang et al. 2006b) (see also section 3.5.)

2.4 Glycosylphosphatidylinositol (GPI) modification

GPI anchoring is a type of post-translational modification occurring in eukaryotic cells and probably constitutes the most complex and metabolically challenging way of attaching proteins to lipid membranes. Proteins targeted for GPI anchoring contain a GPI signaling sequence (GSS) at the C-terminal end. The GSS is recognized in the endoplasmatic reticulum by the transamidase enzyme complex where it is cleaved at the omega site, the point at which the preformed GPI anchor is attached. The biochemical pathway for synthesis of the GPI anchors is complex and chemical structures of GPI anchors vary to a great degree (Ikezawa 2002) however a common backbone structure is observed: Linkage of the GPI anchor to the C-terminal end of the protein is achieved by an amide bond to phosphoethanolamine. The following central three mannose residues are linked via a non-acetylated glucosamine to the phosphoinositol part, which in turn is associated to the lipid residues, usually acyl or aryl fatty acid chains or sphingolipids e.g. ceramide (Ikezawa 2002). GPI anchored proteins have a variety of different functions. In addition to the mentioned complement regulatory activity of CD55 and CD59, GPI-linked proteins serve as hydrolytic enzymes like acetylcholinesterase and placental alkaline phosphatase (Ikezawa, 2002) or are involved in signal transduction like Thy1 (Haeryfar and Hoskin 2004). They share several unique properties: GPI-linked (or "glypiated") proteins are targeted to the outer surface of the cell membrane (Ferguson 1999; Nosjean et al. 1997) and are frequently associated with dynamic membrane microdomains also known as lipid rafts (Legler et al. 2005). As mentioned previously, they have been suggested as the site of viral assembly for certain enveloped viruses e.g. HIV-1 (Briggs et al. 2003; D. H. Nguyen and Hildreth 2000). GPI proteins can also be found in serum and other body fluids both with intact or absent GPI anchors (Landi et al. 2003). Processes that release GPI-linked proteins into the medium with intact GPI anchors are reversible and it has been shown in a variety of *in vitro* and *in vivo* systems that GPI-linked proteins can be re-inserted into cell membranes (Dunn et al. 1996; Kooyman et al. 1995; Rifkin and Landsberger 1990; Rooney et al. 1993; Rooney et al. 1996; Vakeva et al. 1994). Transfer has been demonstrated for CD59 from erythrocytes to endothelial cells (Kooyman et al. 1995) as well as for trypanosomal variant surface glycoprotein (VSG) to erythrocytes of infected patients (Rifkin and Landsberger 1990). Therefore GPI-anchored proteins can be considered to be "hypermobile". This hypermobility allows for the re-integration of purified GPI-anchored proteins to lipid membranes of cells (Legler et al. 2005; Medof et al. 1996) and viruses (Metzner et al. 2008b). This process has been termed cellular or viral painting, respectively.

Technically, introducing a GPI anchor to a protein is achieved in the same way fusion proteins are made: Following genetic engineering, the recombinant protein is translated and the amino acid sequence describing the GSS is included to the nascent polypeptide, thus artificially GPI-anchored proteins are produced. A range of recombinant GPI-anchored proteins have been produced including glypiated GFP and CD4 (for a review see Metzner et al. 2008a). GPI-anchored proteins can be employed for the modification of RV/LV vectors by two distinct pathways: (i) after transfection of virus producing cells, facilitated by the co-localisation of glypiated proteins at the site of viral budding and (ii) by viral painting, re-introducing purified GPI-anchored proteins to mature viral particles as a result of the GPI-anchored protein hypermobility.

Co-transfection of plasmid vectors carrying genes for the production of retroviral vectors with constructs expressing the GPI-anchored proteins or super-transfection of pre-existing virus producing cell lines, leads to the formation of viral particles displaying GPI-anchored molecules on their envelopes. These particles acquire novel properties as a consequence of the incorporation of the GPI-anchored protein e.g. super-transfection of the murine retroviral producer cell line PALSG/S with the human GPI-anchored protein CD59, yields viral particles that are resistant to the activity of complement in human serum (Breun et al. 1999). These results suggested for the first time that incorporation of recombinantly expressed GPI-anchored proteins into the envelopes of viral vectors is possible and that these modifications can be useful for gene therapy approaches. In two more recent studies, co-transfection approaches successfully produced virus-like particles (VLPs) containing glypiated proteins from mammalian (Kueng et al. 2007) or insect cells (Skountzou et al. 2007). In both cases, recombinant GPI-anchored different cytokine species were generated i.e. interleukin-2 (IL-2) and granuolocyte-macrophage colony stimulating factor (GM-CSF). In the first study, it was demonstrated that the GPI-anchored cytokines are functional and elicit cellular responses such as differentiation and proliferation with similar efficiency as their soluble counterparts when co-cultured with the appropriate target cells (Kueng et al. 2007); and in the second it was described that GPI-anchored cytokines engineered onto VLPs based on simian immunodeficiency virus (SIV) can enhance immunogenicity of the VLPs. In both cases a modulation of the immune responses was achieved by displaying GPI-anchored cytokine (Kueng et al. 2007; Skountzou et al. 2007). The major advantage of this approach is that stable transfection of RV/LV producer cell lines co- or super-transfected with GPI-anchored proteins can provide a reproducible long-term source of modified viral particles. In addition, no post-exit steps that may reduce infectivity of the vectors are required.

The second method to modify RV/LV vectors is by using GPI-anchored proteins that have been extracted and purified from cells and can be re-inserted after incubation with enveloped viruses. This was first described for the GPI-linked model protein CD59his which associates to viral vectors based on MLV and HIV-1 (Metzner et al. 2008b). The association is specific and painted virus particles remain infectious after insertion of the GPI-linked protein, albeit at reduced efficiencies caused by the duration of the painting process, rather than the actual introduction of GPI-anchored molecules into the viral outer shell (Metzner et al. 2008b). Estimates of the number of GPI-anchored proteins painted onto retroviral particles were in the range of the numbers observed for Env molecules per virion and are thus similar to that achieved after incorporation of hybrid proteins produced in co-transfection experiments (Skountzou et al. 2007). The main advantage of this approach is flexibility. Different GPI-anchored proteins can be attached to a range of enveloped viral particles without repeated genetic manipulations of the virus-producing cells. This also means a considerable gain of time, compared to transfection-based methods. Additionally, the amounts of protein deposited at the viral surface are controllable and only a limited amount of information about the genetic requirements of the virus is necessary for modification. Viral painting may be the method of choice for modification of enveloped viral particles in all situations where a degree of flexibility is favourable, e.g. in response to genetic heterogeneity in gene therapy approaches or in response to high antigen variability for vaccination. Also when genetic modification of virus producing cell lines is difficult, e.g. when applying toxic proteins or when genetically or biochemically poorly defined virus species are the targets of modification. Viral painting is an example of post-exit surface modification, since fully formed viral particles are the target for modification. While increasing the flexibility of such approaches, the time invested in modification after exit from cells most likely will result in loss of titer (Metzner et al. 2008b) depending on the duration of the modification steps. Thus, keeping post-exit incubation times as short as possible is vital.

2.5 Using adaptors structures

Another strategy to modify viral particles is to introduce adaptor molecule onto the particles which in turn can mediate association of other molecules. These adaptors can either be soluble, non-covalently attached molecules or membrane bound factors. Soluble adaptors have been used to enable targeting strategies in gene therapy. In these cases bispecific molecules or assemblies were used, contacting specifically a molecule present on the virus and another on the cells about to become infected. These bispecific adaptors or bridge complexes can take different forms. For example, two different antibodies, modified with biotin, can be linked via avidin or streptavidin (Roux et al. 1989) thus providing specificity for viral surface proteins and the target molecule on the cell. Such a system has been proposed as early as 1989, showing directed infection of MHC class I and II expressing cells with murine retroviruses (Roux et al. 1989). This system is highly flexible and versatile, since a wide range of antibodies which can be biotinylated are available. Pre-treatment of the viral vector with the anti-viral antibody would effectively neutralize the viral particle, thus increasing the safety of the application. Alternatively, a receptor/ligand chimeric protein, in which the binding partner for the viral attachment protein is coupled to a ligand, binding to the target molecule on the cell surface may be used. Vectors pseudotyped with Avian sarcoma and leukosis virus (ASLV) have been used for implementing such strategies. The chimeric bridge protein consisted of the extracellular domains of the cellular receptor for ASLV, fused to ligands such as epidermal growth factor (EGF), vascular endothelial growth factor (VEGF) or heregulin, thus targeting cells expressing the respective receptors (Snitkovsky et al. 2000; Snitkovsky et al. 2001; Snitkovsky and Young 2002). Since these receptors are commonly overexpressed on tumor cells, the approach is already of some medical relevance. Instead of the ligands, also single-chain antibodies may be used. An approach which has been used for targeting cells expressing a tumor-specific form of the EGF receptor (Snitkovsky et al. 2000).

When using membrane associated adaptors, in most cases, avidin or streptavidin engineered to contain a trans-membrane domain are utilised, due to their extraordinarily strong affinity to biotin and the comparative ease with which biotin can be attached to a wide range of compounds from DNA to antibodies. Avidin and streptavidin molecules are available in a wide range of modifications, tailor-made for different applications (Laitinen et al. 2007). Again, mixed modifications may be used, by generating fusion proteins of avidin/streptavidin with viral surface proteins (M.U. Kaikkonen et al. 2008; M. U. Kaikkonen et al. 2009) or even GPI-anchors (Pinaud et al. 2009). The main advantage of this system is its flexibility, since factors attached to avidin or streptavidin can be exchanged. However, similar to viral painting, post-exit modification steps may be necessary, which could potentially reduce infectivity of RV/LV vectors. Such a system has been implemented by fusing avidin and streptavidin with the transmembrane domain of VSV-G (M. U. Kaikkonen et al. 2009). The binding of biotin to such vectors was demonstrated and they could be used for dual imaging and for targeting application (see sections 3.2. and 3.5.). Other approaches lead to the biotinylation of the lentiviral vector. This can be achieved by direct chemical modification (G. Yang et al. 2006a) (see also section 2.6.) or after addition of a biotin-adaptor peptide (BAP), a site for specific enzymatic biotin ligation (G. D. Chen et al. 2010a; Nesbeth et al. 2006) (see also section 2.6.). The bacterial enzyme, biotin ligase, has to be provided as a form of metabolic engineering to allow the modification of the BAP-containing protein. Both a cellular protein, low-affinity nerve growth factor (Nesbeth et al. 2006) and a viral protein, Sindbis virus glycoprotein (Morizono et al. 2009b), have been modified in such a way to generate novel LV vectors. The latter in fact constitutes pseudotyping of an LV vector with a chimeric envelope molecule, containing an adaptor element, added by enzyme-mediated covalent chemical modification, thus mixing four different strategies to modify viral RV/LV vectors. Alternatively, membrane proteins binding antibodies may be used to modify viral surfaces. Insertion of immunoglobulin G-binding domains (the ZZ domain of staphylococcal protein A) into the Env protein of MLV vectors allowed for the binding of specific antibodies directed against the EGF receptor HER2. However, infectivity was significantly reduced, as can be expected (Tai et al., 2003). A similar approach utilizes a fusion of the same antibody binding domain with Sindbis envelope glycoproteins (L. Yang et al. 2006b). The main disadvantage of adaptor systems is that an additional, separate element is necessary for the system to work, thus introducing a new level of complexity. Additionally, adaptors may dissociate from one or the other binding partner, especially if antibody binding domains are used. Competition from serum antibodies *in vivo* may significantly enhance dissociation (Morizono et al. 2009b). Pre-treatment of viral vectors with the adaptor at least allows administering the virus/adaptor complex as a single entity (Boerger et al. 1999). However, adaptor association in most cases requires post-exit procedures, which can again contribute to loss of infectivity.

2.6 Direct chemical modification

Another option would be the direct chemical linkage of substrates to viral surfaces. While successful modification of polymers and polypeptides to adenovirues and adeno-associated viruses has been achieved (Croyle et al. 2000; Croyle et al. 2002) it has been difficult to carry out such modifications on RV/LV particles and attempts have been rare. A successful example is the attachment of monomethoxy-poly(ethylene)glycol (PEG) to VSV-G pseudotyped LV vectors (Croyle et al. 2004). In this case an activated form of PEG is covalently attached to lysine residues on proteins displayed on the virus. PEGylation reduces the susceptibility of these vectors for the human and murine complement system, while maintaining transduction efficiencies (Croyle et al. 2004), thus manipulating the host immune system (see also section 3.4.). In another, early attempt, MoMLV was modified by chemical addition of carbohydrate (galactose) moieties in order to change viral tropism (Neda et al. 1991). Introduction of these residues was supposed to specifically infect hepatocytes expressing asialoglycoprotein receptors recognizing the carbohydrate moieties on the viral vectors. However, the modification resulted in severely reduced infectivity of RV/LV particles. Direct chemical biotinylation of retroviral vectors has also been demonstrated, using sulfo-N-hydroxysuccinimide-biotin MoMLV derived vectors (G. Yang et al. 2006). For this approach neutravidin was covalently linked to poly-lysine. The resulting compound was then associated to the biotinylated vector. The aim of the study was to allow transduction of human cells with ecotropic MLV vectors, which normally cannot infect human cells. In this case, progeny of modified viruses would lack the modification, hence infection of neighboring cells, even if replication competent vectors were generated, would not be possible. This could contribute to safety of gene therapy approaches. Another strategy to biotinylate viral surfaces includes the potential for chemical display of biotin using a metabolic engineering approach as was described in section 2.5, i.e. that the introduction of biotin-adaptor peptides to viral surface glycoproteins allows for the specific biotinylation of these proteins by a secreted biotin ligase, conferring the possibility for avidin, streptavidin or neutravidin linkage. These adaptors can in turn be used for attachment of secondary biotinylated compounds (Morizono et al. 2009b). Alternatively, desthiobiotin can be metabolically introduced to RV/LV vectors (R. Chen et al. 2010b). In this case, the binding to avidin and its derivates will be easier to reverse, owing to lower affinity. More recently, developments in bioorthogonal chemistry could bring new impetus to the field. Bioorthogonal chemistry describes the possibility to allow controlled, specific chemical reactions amidst the background of a biological system i.e. in cell culture. Specifically, cell surfaces can be modified by oxidation of sialic acids present on glycosylated surface proteins by periodate, generating reactive aldehyde groups, which in turn can be modified by conjugation of aminooxy-functionalised compounds (Zeng et al. 2009). When this technique was applied to cells producing VSV-G pseudotyped MoMLV, resulting viral particles carried the modification (S. Wong and Kwon 2011). They used this to introduce aminooxy-biotin and could subsequently associate magnetic particles to the virus, facilitating purification and concentration of virus preparations (Wong and Kwon 2011; see also section 3.3.). This approach may also be applied to viral particles post-exit. Direct chemical modification of herpesvirus particles with radioactive labels has also been demonstrated and was used for biodistribution studies (Schellingerhout and Bogdanov 2002). Biological chemistry, by developing bioorthogonal methods, appears to have great potential for novel types of modification.

3. Applications for surface modification of RV

3.1 General aspects

The purpose of modifying the surface of RV/LV vectors is to facilitate more efficient delivery of the gene of interest to desired sites of expression (see Figure 3). Changes to the viral surface can facilitate this in a number of ways, such as helping to produce more efficient vector stocks by enabling purification and concentration of viral vector stocks (thereby helping to increase transduction efficiencies) (see section 3.3.), by ensuring optimal interactions with the host organism, especially the host's immune system (see 3.4.), or by limiting viral entry to a subset of host cells (see 3.5.). In its simplest form, physical vector surface modification leads to a more efficient way of detecting the viral particles, due to the association of labeling molecules, thus allowing for a controlled administration and delivery regime (see 3.2.). All of these aspects will also help to increase safety of gene therapy approaches, by eliminating potentially toxic or immunogenic contaminants and reducing adverse and off-target effects. Suitability of modification types for each application will be discussed in the following sections. Another important aspect of course is that multifunctional modifications can - and should - be applied to allow implementation of different applications such as easy detection by labeling and purification/concentration in one modification step.

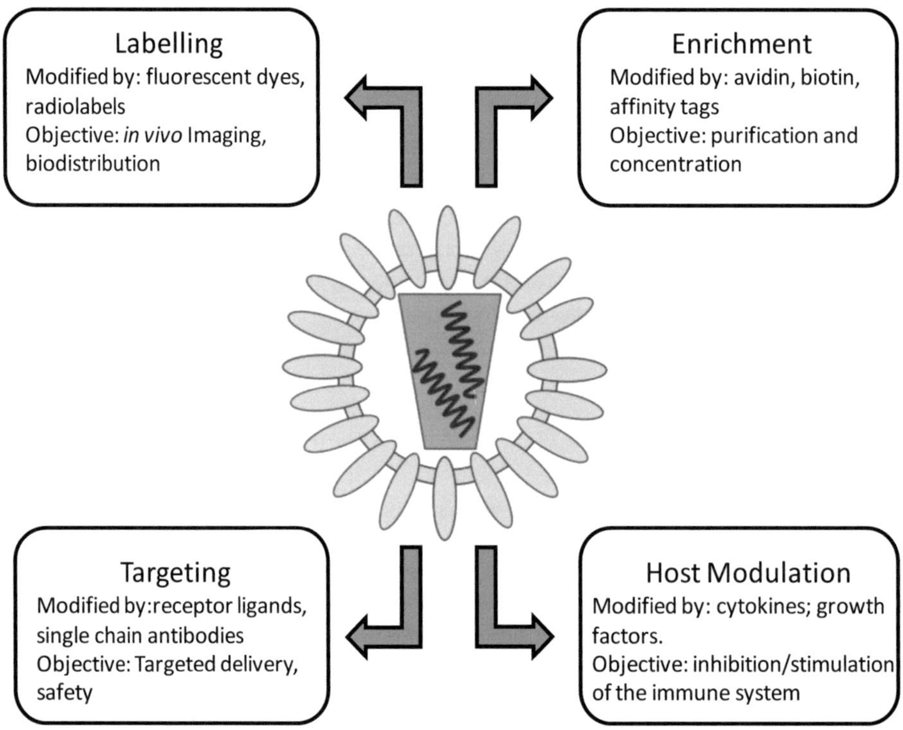

Fig. 3. Overview of applications for surface modifications of RV/LV vectors in gene therapy.

3.2 Imaging/biodistribution

Efficiency of gene therapy will be depending on administration regime and the subsequent distribution of vectors in the patient. Therefore, these events need to be controlled, already at the pre-clinical stages to assess vector performance i.e. in animal experiments. *In vivo* transgene expression analysis, as was used for the detection of specific targeting of LV vectors (Pariente et al. 2007) is not ideal, since the information yielded by measurement of transduction efficiency or, more generally, transgene expression is different from data describing physical particle distribution. Vector particles may be trapped or degraded long before transduction, subsequently not contributing to transgene expression. Thus detection of the physical vector particles is required (in addition to and in parallel to transgene expression analysis) and may need to be facilitated by labeling of the RV/LV vector particle. Generally, labeling approaches should have only minimal to no influence on the performance of the RV/LV vector and on the host or target organism (low toxicity and low immunogenicity). Another requirement is the stability of label attachment. Loss of label from viral particles would not only lead to decrease of signal, but also to an increase of background noise. Finally, detection of the label should be easy and easily achievable *in vivo*. Small, chemically inert substances, giving a strong and localized signal, enabling non-invasive detection methods will be the ideal tags. For practical reasons, a "one size fits all" approach to labeling may be preferred. Flexible and versatile procedures which can be applied to a broad range of RV/LV vectors are called for. All mentioned aspects will obviously influence choice of technique for labeling and subsequently, location and type of label.

RV/LV particles can be labeled at the level of the capsid, i.e. using chimeric proteins of capsid proteins and fluorescent proteins (Lampe et al. 2007; Lehmann et al. 2005). While loss of label will be less of a concern in such circumstances, changing the geometry of the capsid might very well have an influence on capsid and/or viral assembly. Modification can also be carried out at the level of viral surfaces, where they are much more susceptible to dissociation or degradation. So far viral particles are mainly labeled by incorporation of chimeric proteins of viral structural proteins and (fluorescent) marker proteins (Lampe et al. 2007; Lehmann et al. 2005), owing to a high degree of stability of association caused by the covalent association. However, fluorescent proteins are comparatively big, increasing the chance for steric hindrance and thus influence on vector performance. Detection of fluorescence signal may allow for a limited depth of penetration only. Standard immunohistochemistry methods use non-protein fluorophore-labelled secondary antibody, and while acceptable for *in vitro* purposes, it cannot provide the stability of a covalent bond and therefore may not be suitable for *in vivo* applications. For the same reason, most adaptor-based systems will also not be suitable for labeling, with the possible exception of systems using membrane-bound avidin/biotin (M. U. Kaikkonen et al. 2009), due to the extraordinarily strong association, which is comparable to covalent interactions. The use of GPI-anchored marker proteins provides an alternative, as the modification pathway does not interfere with viral structural components, i.e. the envelope surface protein required for target cell binding and infection. Infection efficiency is not disturbed by painting (Metzner et al. 2008b). The use of viral painting technology can provide the additional advantage of flexibility. Incorporation of label is mostly independent of viral producer cell lines and can be performed relatively quickly (Metzner et al. 2008b; Metzner et al. 2008a). However, still comparatively large polypeptide molecules are attached to the viruses and the degree of stability of interaction still needs to be determined. Direct chemical attachment seems to have good prospects in this area, since small molecules can be attached to virus particles covalently, in a relatively small amount of time (R. Chen et al. 2010b; S. Wong and Kwon 2011). However, such methods still need to be assessed in terms of their *in vivo* applications.

So far fluorescent molecules were considered as primary detection labels. While fluorescence detection, together with luminescence has been used for pre clinical *in vivo* detection approaches, it will not be suitable for application in human patients due to low penetration depth (Shah et al. 2004). Alternatively, detection based on magnetic resonance imaging (MRI) and two radiological methods, positron emission tomography (PET) and single photon emission computer tomography (SPECT), may be used (for a review on molecular imaging techniques in gene therapy see Shah et al. 2004; Raty et al. 2007). While MRI has been recently utilized for *in vivo* transgene expression, using ferritin as the reporter gene (Hasegawa et al. 2010; M. U. Kaikkonen et al. 2009), SPECT shows promising qualities, combining high sensitivity with comparatively low cost equipment and reagents, in analyzing physical particle distribution. Such an approach has been utilized to study biodistribution of herpes- (Schellingerhout and Bogdanov 2002) and baculovirus (Raty et al. 2007) *in vivo*. In these cases the radiolabels were attached to the virus either by direct chemical modification (Schellingerhout and Bogdanov 2007) or by adding a biotinylated radiolabel to streptavidin modified viral particles (Raty et al. 2007). Dual *in vivo* imaging of rats was demonstrated for LVvectors coding for transferring and displaying streptavidin adaptors (M. U. Kaikkonen et al. 2009). In this case, enrichment of iron in cells upon transferrin expression was used to enable MRI, while radiolabels were attached to the displayed streptavidin molecules to allow for SPECT detection. For this study, deposition of adaptor molecules on viral particles was additionally used for targeting applications, demonstrating the versatile nature of adaptor systems. However, also approaches using fluorescent labeling molecules may additionally have a function in enrichment or concentration prior to transduction i.e. viral particles modified with proteins containing 6xhis-tagged proteins can be enriched by using established immobilized metal ion affinity chromatography (IMAC) (Gaberc-Porekar and Menart 2001; Magnusdottir et al. 2009) or magnetic purification techniques (Franzreb et al. 2006) (see also section 3.3.).

3.3 Purification/concentration

Another important issue in gene therapy is generation of suitable vector preparations in terms of viral titer, purity, speed and costs. Cheap methods which allow for quick concentration and purification of RV/LV vectors after harvesting from producing cell lines are of great importance. Contaminants from producing cell cultures may inhibit transduction of target cells (Rodrigues et al. 2007). Additionally, with clinical use of vectors as a mid- to long-term aim, vector preparations need to be compliant with regulators' standards. In nearly all cases, purification and concentration of viruses starts with a micro-filtration step, using 0.45 µm filters to remove cells and cellular debris from culture supernatants. When large amounts of dead cells are present in the supernatant, centrifugation may be preferred for removal of micro-level contaminants. Subsequently, RV/LV particles are still concentrated and purified in most cases by ultra-centrifugation, often utilizing sucrose gradients to prevent mechanical damage to viruses. These methods are time-consuming and require the use of expensive equipment, i.e. high velocity centrifuges. Additionally, not all RV/LV vectors tolerate ultra-centrifugation well. Sucrose may need to be removed from preparations afterwards, adding another preparatory step. Additionally, high sucrose content can harm virus by change in osmotic pressure. Taken together these aspects lead to often quite significant reductions of infectivity (Rodrigues et al. 2007). Using VSV-G pseudotypes as well as ultra-centrifugation-resistant virus strains can improve yield after ultra-centrifugation (Burns et al. 1993). While acceptable for laboratory scale preparation, ultra-centrifugation is unsatisfactory for larger scale preparations. Alternatively viruses may be concentrated and purified by ultra-filtration or dialysis protocols, separating virus and contaminants according to size using semi-permeable membranes. Conventional column based methods lead to problems regarding large-scale preparations, but use of tangential flow devices can circumvent this aspect (Geraerts et al. 2005; Kuiper et al. 2002).

What these methods have in common is that they do not rely on any modification of the virus. This is partially also true for purification strategies involving chromatography applications e.g. size exclusion or ion exchange approaches, both of which have been used for purification and concentration purposes (Rodrigues et al. 2007). Affinity chromatography is a very powerful tool for removal of contaminants. Using naturally occurring affinity tags for purification and concentration such as heparin can work well (Segura et al. 2008a; Segura et al. 2010). In such an application the tag should interfere minimally with the virus activity, be easily accessible for the purification matrix and, in most cases, a transient interaction would be preferred, allowing for removal of virus under mild conditions. An additional advantage would be, if the same strategy would be applicable for a broad spectrum of vectors. After all, the key property of a purification label would be its affinity and specificity for the purification matrices used. Approaches utilising either biotin-streptavidin interactions or IMAC have been reported (Williams et al. 2005a; Williams et al. 2005b; Ye et al. 2004). In the latter strategy, the affinity of complexed nickel or cobalt ions to stretches of histidine aminoacids is exploited. Viruses may be modified for application of the streptavidin/biotin system in numerous ways, as described in sections 2.5 and 2.6. Direct chemical modification was chosen to biotinylate retroviral vectors prior to purification using a streptavidin coated stationary phase (Chan et al. 2005; Williams et al. 2005a; Williams et al. 2005b). As a result of the strong interaction of biotin and avidin/streptavidin, removal of viral particles from the purification matrix can require harsh conditions, which will reduce yield and infectivity of viral preparations. While IMAC was used successfully on viral vectors containing histidine tags in the Env protein (Ye et al., 2004), immediate dialysis of resulting samples is necessary to remove the chemicals necessary for desorption (imidazole, EDTA). These compounds would also need to be removed prior to any clinical application, as well as metal ions potentially leaking from the purification matrix, since both may lead to adverse side effects in patients (Rodrigues et al. 2007). In addition to chromatography based methods, attachment of magnetic particles to the viral vectors may enable purification and concentration. Recently, attempts have been made to attach micro- or nanoparticles with magnetic properties to modified viral surfaces (R. Chen et al. 2010b; M. U. Kaikkonen et al. 2009; Nesbeth et al. 2006; S. Wong and Kwon 2011). Again, avidin-biotin interactions were exploited to attach the magnetic particles. Such approaches are interesting due to their potential for up-scaling. Ideally, magnetic nanoparticles could be designed in such a way, that they may not have to be removed from viruses, but may serve additional function as contrast agents in detection via MRI. Generally, adaptor approaches can be considered most useful for labeling purposes, if only due to their versatility. Indeed, when an adaptor is present on a viral vector, it may as well be used for purification purposes in addition to the primary aim of modification, i.e. transduction targeting. Alternatively, quick post-exit approaches, such as viral painting with GPI-anchored proteins may be used, giving a great degree of flexibility, as they can be applied to a wide range of viral preparations, and again more than one objective may be achieved by a single modification i.e. by the use of a histidine-tagged, GPI-anchored immunomodulatory protein.

3.4 Modulation of host functions

Depending on the administration protocol planned, RV/LV vectors used in gene therapy may have to find their way to the target cells. During this journey, they will share contacts with both soluble and cell bound components of the host. Elements performing functions in the host's immune system will be of special interest, since in most patients, gene therapy vectors, including RV/LV vectors, will encounter an intact immune system. Navigating the immune system will be vital to any successful gene therapy approach. Interaction of virus particles with host molecules including immunological reactions are often mediated by molecules located in the envelope, thus modifying the envelope with immunologically competent molecules, e.g. cytokines or growth factors, allows for the manipulation of surrounding immune responses. This specifically includes protection of viral vectors from unwanted immune reactions such as complement activity. Immunoprotection can help to ensure efficient delivery to target cells by eliminating premature inactivation of vectors in gene therapy approaches. One example is the pegylation of VSV-G pseudotyped vectors (Croyle et al. 2004), as discussed in section 2.6. Other approaches to protect from complement activity include the introduction of complement regulatory factors such as CD55 or CD59 (Breun et al. 1999), if they are not already part of the envelope protein contents. In this case the presence of naturally occurring GPI-anchored proteins was exploited.

Protection from the complement or neutralizing antibodies is only one aspect of immune-modulation. Stimulation of immune responses may be a desired effect to augment therapeutic effect i.e. in cancer gene therapy or vaccine strategies. For example, presentation of antigen on the surface of virus-like particles (VLPs) is possible via the use of GPI-anchored molecules. GPI-anchored cytokines engineered onto simian immunodeficiency virus (SIV) can enhance immunogenicity of the VLPs (Skountzou et al. 2007). VLPs can be used to modulate the immune system in several ways (Kueng et al. 2011). These aspects may be of more importance in the development of vaccines or specific adjuvants enhancing vaccine efficacy, but variations may also prove useful for gene therapy approaches. For example, early acting cytokines such as interleukin 6, stem cell factor or thrombopoietin, have been shown to enhance gene transfer using RV/LV vectors to haematopoietic stem cells (Santoni de Sio et al. 2006; Zielske and Gerson 2003). Attachment of such factors to viral surfaces as discussed above can help to achieve stronger local effects. This may be considered also in the context of "targeting by activation", whereby efficient transduction is dependent on activation of the target cell by the ligand/receptor interaction (Verhoyen and Cosset 2004; see also section 3.5.).

A further aspect of modulation of host cell function is inducing differentiation e.g. for tissue engineering purposes. Proof of principle was shown through differentiation of monocytes to dendritic cells (Kueng et al. 2007). Again, the GPI-anchored cytokines used were functional and elicited cellular responses such as differentiation and proliferation with similar efficiency as their soluble counterparts when co-cultured with the appropriate target cells. The major advantage of this approach is that stable transfection of RV/LV producer cell lines co- or super-transfected with GPI-anchored proteins can provide a long-term source of modified viral particles reproducibly. In addition, no post-exit steps that may reduce infectivity of viral vectors are required. Alternatively, viral painting may be used in cases where flexibility is required. Immunomodulation appears to be an area of great possibilities, allowing potentially for the "fine tuning" of gene therapy approaches, by enhancing distribution or transgene expression and providing additional beneficial side effects such as increased tumor cell killing.

3.5 Infection targeting

A key element of successful and efficient gene therapy is the ability to target only a certain subset of cells for treatment after systemic administration. This constitutes both, a measure to ensure safety, since (ideally) no non-target cells should become genetically modified, and enhance efficacy, since (again, ideally) all vector particles present should recognize and infect target cells. Targeted infection is an especially important feature when using replication-competent vectors. Such vectors can replicate in infected cells and produce progeny virus which in turn can infect new target cells. Whilst highly efficient, i.e. in the case of tumor gene therapy, safety of course is an important issue, as a form of viremia is part of the delivery strategy, which needs to be tightly controlled. Additionally, infection targeting is equally important for all *in vivo* gene therapy approaches (as opposed to *ex vivo* approaches, were infection can be limited by other means), especially upon systemic administration. Here, viral vectors are introduced to the patient and non-specific infection is a definitive risk, especially considering integration of viral DNA into the host genome and the associated potential for insertional mutagenesis.

In the case of RV/LV vectors, the viral glycoproteins located in the envelope function as recognition and entry devices to allow access to the target cells. The so called Env proteins consist of two subunits, the surface (SU) and transmembrane (TM), both with distinct functions. The Env protein complex is a hexamer consisting of 3 copies of each of the TM and SU subunits. SU mediates the first contact to the host cells by engaging the viral receptor and, eventually co-receptors. The binding specificity of the SU subunit therefore determines the host cell range of the virus. Upon this first contact, TM activates fusogenic properties, which allow viral and cellular membranes to fuse, resulting in viral entry. The interaction of SU and TM is highly sensitive to changes in SU and already small changes can disturb the activation of the TM activity (Zhao et al. 1999). Subsequently, modifications introduced to the Env proteins are tolerated badly, quite often leading to severe reduction in infectivity. Nevertheless, modification of these properties is crucial to achieve infection or transduction targeting - one of the most important goals of viral gene therapy. The choice of method being used for targeting applications may also be influenced by the specific target molecule, cell or tissue and the target's distribution in the organism, since access to the targets will add additional obstacles to delivery/targeting, for example regarding the stability of the interaction between viral vector, targeting molecule and target. In targeting approaches, specificity is the most important parameter.

A range of different strategies have been tested to change the infection tropism including the use of glycoproteins from heterologous viral species (pseudotyping) or chimeric envelope glycoproteins (Env fusion proteins) as well as bridging molecules (adaptors) (Waehler et al. 2007). The application of pseudotyping for transduction targeting (Croyle et al. 2004; Engelstadter et al. 2001; Miller et al. 1991) is limited by the range of available glycoproteins with useful infection tropisms. A more versatile strategy is the use of chimeric envelope proteins in which parts of the protein responsible for receptor binding are replaced with peptides (Gollan and Green 2002), ligands (Cosset et al. 1995; Kasahara et al. 1994) or single-chain antibodies (Anliker et al. 2010; Somia et al. 1995) conferring binding to the desired receptors for viral entry. Additionally, adaptors, which are capable of associating with both the viral glycoprotein and the cellular receptor, can be used to mediate between virus and target cell (Boerger et al. 1999; Snitkovsky et al. 2001).

Another concept is targeting by activation. Retroviral vectors displaying the amphotropic MLV Env containing the original receptor binding domain and elements coding for IL2 (Maurice et al. 1999) or hepatocyte growth factor (HGF) (T. H. Nguyen et al. 1998) were generated. These vectors would allow binding of and entry to a broad range of cells. However, only upon cell activation due to binding of IL2 or HGF to their cognate receptor would lead to

significant transduction, as introducing proliferation enabled the progress of MLV provirus to the nucleus and subsequent integration and transgene expression (Maurice et al. 1999). Although lentiviral vector can infect non-dividing cells, blocks to transduction occur, for example in monocytes (Kootstra et al. 2000; Neil et al. 2001) and resting T cells (Dardalhon et al. 2001). Activation targeting can help to overcome such blocks. Problems encountered in such approaches include differentiation of stimulated cells or background infection in rapidly dividing cells (Verhoeyen and Cosset 2004). What these approaches have in common is that they often lead to significantly reduced infection rates (Galanis et al. 2001).
Progress in transduction targeting has been made by separating binding and fusion properties (Lin et al. 2001; L. Yang et al. 2006b). This is possible as in several viral species, binding and fusion properties are independent features and fusion activity is triggered by different stimuli, i.e. low pH after endocytosis (L. Yang et al. 2006b). Most promising candidates for the use as heterologous fusogenic proteins in RV are genetically engineered variants of the Sindbis virus (SIN) glycoprotein (Morizono et al. 2005; L. Yang et al. 2006b; L. Yang et al. 2008b; H. Yang et al. 2008a; Ziegler et al. 2008), the influenza virus hemagglutinin (Lin et al. 2001; L. Yang et al. 2006b) and measles virus surface glycoproteins (Anliker et al. 2010). In such a case, the use of adaptor systems may help to construct flexible targeting systems, as well as deposition of specific binding factors by using GPI-anchored proteins, especially in cases where binding and entry of viral particles are mediated by independent proteins, i.e. *in trans* (Lin et al. 2001; L. Yang et al. 2006b). The same basic viral particle can be modified with a range of binding properties to suit the specific needs of the applications. Antibody molecules, for example, in the form of single-chain antibody molecules, engineered to contain a GPI anchor, can provide a vast range of binding specificities. Summing up, the use of non RV/LV viral surface glycoproteins capable of inducing virus/cell fusion independent of specific binding taken together with a flexible such as an adaptor system or viral painting seems currently the most promising candidates for targeting applications.

4. Outlook and discussion

Due to their average size of 100 nm, RV and LV particles can be considered as bionanotechnological devices. Modification thus becomes the - in the field of nanotechnology - more commonly used term "functionalisation". Multiple modifications could lead to using viral vectors as multifunctional platforms for biomedicine combined with other nanotechnological elements. For example, magnetic micro- and nanoparticles are already commercially available to allow the purification of proteins containing tags such as the histidine tag or Flag tag. GPI-anchored proteins used for painting of enveloped viral vectors have also been engineered to contain histidine tags, allowing the particles to be coated with GPI-anchored protein and attached to the viral vectors by means of the GPI-anchor. Or, alternatively, biolinker proteins such as streptavidin can potentially be modified at the genetic level to contain a GPI signal sequences, and as such, after production in a suitable expression system, can be purified as reactive reagents to link up with biotinylated nanoparticles. In both cases the recombinant GPI-anchored protein acts as a linker or interface between the organic viral particles and inorganic nanomaterials, either magnetic or fluorescent capabilities (or both). With such a system in place to functionalise the surface of viral vectors without affecting the viral infectivity pathway, one can imagine many biomedical applications such as targeting of gene therapy vectors *in vivo* to tumours using magnetic force and tracking via bioimaging techniques based on magnetic field, i.e. MRI or high-sensitivity camera *in vivo* fluorescence imaging. However, with all of this in mind one must not forget the safety issues as the effects of such materials cannot always be predicted in biological systems, an issue that has already emerged for carbon nanotubes which would not have been expected to be as toxic as has proven to be the case in many instances (Patlolla et al. 2010; van der Zande et al. 2011). Sometimes the speed of development can lead to rashness when translating into the clinic, a fate that already befell gene therapy in some regards (Sheridan 2011), so the same mistakes should be avoided when mixing together such new technologies with clinically used viral vectors (Subbiah et al. 2010).

5. Conclusions / summary

RV/LV vectors are already proving to be useful delivery vehicles for gene therapy applications but in order to establish more efficient vectors for *in vivo* delivery, the viral surface can potentially be modified to provide better means of preparation, purification, concentration, detection, tracking, imaging, and targeting in order to not only successfully manufacture the product but also to navigate interactions within the patient and infect pre-defined target cells selectively. To achieve this aim several techniques may be employed for surface engineering or RV/LV vectors. Table 3 provides a concise overview of these techniques and the applications for which they have been used and may conceivably be used in the future. Pseudotyping has been used for targeting applications, however, can only make use of a limited amount of targeting options. Chimeric proteins have been used for labeling and targeting applications, and can be useful for immunomodulation approaches. Enrichment may be achieved as a secondary objective. Modifications employing GPI-anchored proteins may prove to be versatile and efficient; however, further research will be necessary. A similar assessment can be made for the use of membrane-bound adaptor systems and direct chemical modifications. Finally, combining different strategies will allow broadening possibilities for the surface modification of viral vectors considerably.

Modification		Comment	Labelling	Enrichment	Modulation	Targeting
Pseudotyping		limited possibilities				X
Chimeric Protein		versatile, decreased infectivity	X	(x)	(x)	X
GPI Modifications	via budding	versatile, time-consuming		(x)	X	(x)
	via painting	flexible, quick, post-exit	(x)	(x)	(x)	(x)
Adaptors	soluble	additional component, post-exit	(x)	(x)		X
	membraneous	flexible, versatile	X	X	(x)	X
Chemical Modification		flexible, quick, maybe post-exit	X	X	X	X

Table 3. Methods for engineering RV/LV vector surfaces and potential applications.
X applications mentioned in the text; (x) potential for future applications.

6. References

Aiuti, A., et al. (2002), 'Immune reconstitution in ADA-SCID after PBL gene therapy and discontinuation of enzyme replacement', *Nat Med,* 8 (5), 423-5.

Anderson, W. F., et al. (1980), 'Replication and expression of thymidine kinase and human globin genes microinjected into mouse fibroblasts', *Proc Natl Acad Sci U S A,* 77 (9), 5399-403.

Anliker, B., et al. (2010), 'Specific gene transfer to neurons, endothelial cells and hematopoietic progenitors with lentiviral vectors', *Nat Methods,* 7 (11), 929-35.

Auricchio, A., et al. (2001), 'Exchange of surface proteins impacts on viral vector cellular specificity and transduction characteristics: the retina as a model', *Hum Mol Genet,* 10 (26), 3075-81.

Azzouz, M., et al. (2004), 'Lentivector-mediated SMN replacement in a mouse model of spinal muscular atrophy', *J Clin Invest,* 114 (12), 1726-31.

Bischof, D. and Cornetta, K. (2010), 'Flexibility in cell targeting by pseudotyping lentiviral vectors', *Methods Mol Biol,* 614, 53-68.

Boerger, A. L., Snitkovsky, S., and Young, J. A. (1999), 'Retroviral vectors preloaded with a viral receptor-ligand bridge protein are targeted to specific cell types', *Proc Natl Acad Sci U S A,* 96 (17), 9867-72.

Breun, S., et al. (1999), 'Protection of MLV vector particles from human complement', *Biochem Biophys Res Commun,* 264 (1), 1-5.

Briggs, J. A., Wilk, T., and Fuller, S. D. (2003), 'Do lipid rafts mediate virus assembly and pseudotyping?', *J Gen Virol,* 84 (Pt 4), 757-68.

Burns, J. C., et al. (1993), 'Vesicular stomatitis virus G glycoprotein pseudotyped retroviral vectors: concentration to very high titer and efficient gene transfer into mammalian and nonmammalian cells', *Proc Natl Acad Sci U S A,* 90 (17), 8033-7.

Cartier, N., et al. (2009), 'Hematopoietic stem cell gene therapy with a lentiviral vector in X-linked adrenoleukodystrophy', *Science,* 326 (5954), 818-23.

Cavazzana-Calvo, M., et al. (2000), 'Gene therapy of human severe combined immunodeficiency (SCID)-X1 disease', *Science,* 288 (5466), 669-72.

--- (2010), 'Transfusion independence and HMGA2 activation after gene therapy of human beta-thalassaemia', *Nature,* 467 (7313), 318-22.

Chan, L., et al. (2005), 'Conjugation of lentivirus to paramagnetic particles via nonviral proteins allows efficient concentration and infection of primary acute myeloid leukemia cells', *J Virol,* 79 (20), 13190-4.

Chen, G. D., et al. (2010a), 'Concentration and purification of human immunodeficiency virus type 1 virions by microfluidic separation of superparamagnetic nanoparticles', *Anal Chem,* 82 (2), 723-8.

Chen, R., et al. (2010b), 'Affinity recovery of lentivirus by diaminopelargonic acid mediated desthiobiotin labelling', *J Chromatogr B Analyt Technol Biomed Life Sci,* 878 (22), 1939-45.

Chertova, E., et al. (2006), 'Proteomic and biochemical analysis of purified human immunodeficiency virus type 1 produced from infected monocyte-derived macrophages', *J Virol,* 80 (18), 9039-52.

Cosset, F. L., et al. (1995), 'Retroviral retargeting by envelopes expressing an N-terminal binding domain', *J Virol,* 69 (10), 6314-22.

Cronin, J., Zhang, X. Y., and Reiser, J. (2005), 'Altering the tropism of lentiviral vectors through pseudotyping', *Curr Gene Ther,* 5 (4), 387-98.
Croyle, M. A., Yu, Q. C., and Wilson, J. M. (2000), 'Development of a rapid method for the PEGylation of adenoviruses with enhanced transduction and improved stability under harsh storage conditions', *Hum Gene Ther,* 11 (12), 1713-22.
Croyle, M. A., et al. (2002), 'PEGylation of E1-deleted adenovirus vectors allows significant gene expression on readministration to liver', *Hum Gene Ther,* 13 (15), 1887-900.
--- (2004), 'PEGylation of a vesicular stomatitis virus G pseudotyped lentivirus vector prevents inactivation in serum', *J Virol,* 78 (2), 912-21.
Dardalhon, V., et al. (2001), 'Lentivirus-mediated gene transfer in primary T cells is enhanced by a central DNA flap', *Gene Ther,* 8 (3), 190-8.
De Vry, J., et al. (2010), 'In vivo electroporation of the central nervous system: a non-viral approach for targeted gene delivery', *Prog Neurobiol,* 92 (3), 227-44.
DePolo, N. J., et al. (2000), 'VSV-G pseudotyped lentiviral vector particles produced in human cells are inactivated by human serum', *Mol Ther,* 2 (3), 218-22.
Diaz, R. M., et al. (2000), 'A lentiviral vector expressing a fusogenic glycoprotein for cancer gene therapy', *Gene Ther,* 7 (19), 1656-63.
Dunn, D. E., et al. (1996), 'A knock-out model of paroxysmal nocturnal hemoglobinuria: Pig-a(-) hematopoiesis is reconstituted following intercellular transfer of GPI-anchored proteins', *Proc Natl Acad Sci U S A,* 93 (15), 7938-43.
Engelstadter, M., et al. (2001), 'Targeted gene transfer to lymphocytes using murine leukaemia virus vectors pseudotyped with spleen necrosis virus envelope proteins', *Gene Ther,* 8 (15), 1202-6.
Esser, M. T., et al. (2001), 'Differential incorporation of CD45, CD80 (B7-1), CD86 (B7-2), and major histocompatibility complex class I and II molecules into human immunodeficiency virus type 1 virions and microvesicles: implications for viral pathogenesis and immune regulation', *J Virol,* 75 (13), 6173-82.
Ferguson, M. A. (1999), 'The structure, biosynthesis and functions of glycosylphosphatidylinositol anchors, and the contributions of trypanosome research', *J Cell Sci,* 112 (Pt 17), 2799-809.
Franzreb, M., et al. (2006), 'Protein purification using magnetic adsorbent particles', *Appl Microbiol Biotechnol,* 70 (5), 505-16.
Frecha, C., et al. (2008), 'Stable transduction of quiescent T cells without induction of cycle progression by a novel lentiviral vector pseudotyped with measles virus glycoproteins', *Blood,* 112 (13), 4843-52.
--- (2011), 'Measles virus glycoprotein-pseudotyped lentiviral vector-mediated gene transfer into quiescent lymphocytes requires binding to both SLAM and CD46 entry receptors', *J Virol.*
Gaberc-Porekar, V. and Menart, V. (2001), 'Perspectives of immobilized-metal affinity chromatography', *J Biochem Biophys Methods,* 49 (1-3), 335-60.
Galanis, E., Vile, R., and Russell, S. J. (2001), 'Delivery systems intended for in vivo gene therapy of cancer: targeting and replication competent viral vectors', *Crit Rev Oncol Hematol,* 38 (3), 177-92.
Garrus, J. E., et al. (2001), 'Tsg101 and the vacuolar protein sorting pathway are essential for HIV-1 budding', *Cell,* 107 (1), 55-65.

Geraerts, M., et al. (2005), 'Upscaling of lentiviral vector production by tangential flow filtration', *J Gene Med,* 7 (10), 1299-310.

Gollan, T. J. and Green, M. R. (2002), 'Redirecting retroviral tropism by insertion of short, nondisruptive peptide ligands into envelope', *J Virol,* 76 (7), 3558-63.

Granoff, A. and Hirst, G. K. (1954), 'Experimental production of combination forms of virus. IV. Mixed influenza A-Newcastle disease virus infections', *Proc Soc Exp Biol Med,* 86 (1), 84-8.

Gunzburg, W. H. (2003), 'Retroviral gene therapy--where now?', *Trends Mol Med,* 9 (7), 277-8.

Hacein-Bey-Abina, S., et al. (2008), 'Insertional oncogenesis in 4 patients after retrovirus-mediated gene therapy of SCID-X1', *J Clin Invest,* 118 (9), 3132-42.

Haeryfar, S. M. and Hoskin, D. W. (2004), 'Thy-1: more than a mouse pan-T cell marker', *J Immunol,* 173 (6), 3581-8.

Hammarstedt, M. and Garoff, H. (2004), 'Passive and active inclusion of host proteins in human immunodeficiency virus type 1 gag particles during budding at the plasma membrane', *J Virol,* 78 (11), 5686-97.

Hasegawa, S., Furukawa, T., and Saga, T. (2010), 'Molecular MR imaging of cancer gene therapy: ferritin transgene reporter takes the stage', *Magn Reson Med Sci,* 9 (2), 37-47.

Hsu, M., et al. (2003), 'Hepatitis C virus glycoproteins mediate pH-dependent cell entry of pseudotyped retroviral particles', *Proc Natl Acad Sci U S A,* 100 (12), 7271-6.

Ikezawa, H. (2002), 'Glycosylphosphatidylinositol (GPI)-anchored proteins', *Biol Pharm Bull,* 25 (4), 409-17.

Jorgenson, R. L., Vogt, V. M., and Johnson, M. C. (2009), 'Foreign glycoproteins can be actively recruited to virus assembly sites during pseudotyping', *J Virol,* 83 (9), 4060-7.

Kaikkonen, M. U., et al. (2009), '(Strept)avidin-displaying lentiviruses as versatile tools for targeting and dual imaging of gene delivery', *Gene Ther,* 16 (7), 894-904.

Kaikkonen, M.U., et al. (2008), 'Avidin-displaying lentiviruses as versatile tools for targeting and dual-imaging of gene delivery', : *Consert Lab Course Lentiviral Vectors* (Evry, France).

Kaneda, Y. (2010), 'Update on non-viral delivery methods for cancer therapy: possibilities of a drug delivery system with anticancer activities beyond delivery as a new therapeutic tool', *Expert Opin Drug Deliv,* 7 (9), 1079-93.

Kang, Y., et al. (2002), 'In vivo gene transfer using a nonprimate lentiviral vector pseudotyped with Ross River Virus glycoproteins', *J Virol,* 76 (18), 9378-88.

Kaplitt, M. G., et al. (2007), 'Safety and tolerability of gene therapy with an adeno-associated virus (AAV) borne GAD gene for Parkinson's disease: an open label, phase I trial', *Lancet,* 369 (9579), 2097-105.

Kasahara, N., Dozy, A. M., and Kan, Y. W. (1994), 'Tissue-specific targeting of retroviral vectors through ligand-receptor interactions', *Science,* 266 (5189), 1373-6.

Kobinger, G. P., et al. (2004), 'Transduction of human islets with pseudotyped lentiviral vectors', *Hum Gene Ther,* 15 (2), 211-9.

Kootstra, N. A., Zwart, B. M., and Schuitemaker, H. (2000), 'Diminished human immunodeficiency virus type 1 reverse transcription and nuclear transport in primary macrophages arrested in early G(1) phase of the cell cycle', *J Virol,* 74 (4), 1712-7.

Kooyman, D. L., et al. (1995), 'In vivo transfer of GPI-linked complement restriction factors from erythrocytes to the endothelium', *Science,* 269 (5220), 89-92.
Kowolik, C. M. and Yee, J. K. (2002), 'Preferential transduction of human hepatocytes with lentiviral vectors pseudotyped by Sendai virus F protein', *Mol Ther,* 5 (6), 762-9.
Kueng, H. J., Schmetterer, K. G., and Pickl, W. F. (2011), 'Lipid rafts, pseudotyping, and virus-like particles: relevance of a novel, configurable, and modular antigen-presenting platform', *Int Arch Allergy Immunol,* 154 (2), 89-110.
Kueng, H. J., et al. (2007), 'General strategy for decoration of enveloped viruses with functionally active lipid-modified cytokines', *J Virol,* 81 (16), 8666-76.
Kuiper, M., et al. (2002), 'Purification of a functional gene therapy vector derived from Moloney murine leukaemia virus using membrane filtration and ceramic hydroxyapatite chromatography', *Biotechnol Bioeng,* 80 (4), 445-53.
Laitinen, O. H., et al. (2007), 'Brave new (strept)avidins in biotechnology', *Trends Biotechnol,* 25 (6), 269-77.
Lallos, L. B., et al. (1999), 'Exclusion of HIV coreceptors CXCR4, CCR5, and CCR3 from the HIV envelope', *AIDS Res Hum Retroviruses,* 15 (10), 895-7.
Lampe, M., et al. (2007), 'Double-labelled HIV-1 particles for study of virus-cell interaction', *Virology,* 360 (1), 92-104.
Landi, A. P., et al. (2003), 'Determination of CD59 protein in normal human serum by enzyme immunoassay, using octyl-glucoside detergent to release glycosyl-phosphatidylinositol-CD59 from lipid complex', *Immunol Lett,* 90 (2-3), 209-13.
Legler, D. F., et al. (2005), 'Differential insertion of GPI-anchored GFPs into lipid rafts of live cells', *Faseb J,* 19 (1), 73-5.
Lehmann, M. J., et al. (2005), 'Actin- and myosin-driven movement of viruses along filopodia precedes their entry into cells', *J Cell Biol,* 170 (2), 317-25.
Lewitt, P. A., et al. (2011), 'AAV2-GAD gene therapy for advanced Parkinson's disease: a double-blind, sham-surgery controlled, randomised trial', *Lancet Neurol,* 10 (4), 309-19.
Liehl, B., et al. (2007), 'Simian immunodeficiency virus vector pseudotypes differ in transduction efficiency and target cell specificity in brain', *Gene Ther,* 14 (18), 1330-43.
Lin, A. H., et al. (2001), 'Receptor-specific targeting mediated by the coexpression of a targeted murine leukemia virus envelope protein and a binding-defective influenza hemagglutinin protein', *Hum Gene Ther,* 12 (4), 323-32.
Logg, C. R., et al. (2001), 'A uniquely stable replication-competent retrovirus vector achieves efficient gene delivery in vitro and in solid tumors', *Hum Gene Ther,* 12 (8), 921-32.
Magnusdottir, A., et al. (2009), 'Enabling IMAC purification of low abundance recombinant proteins from E. coli lysates', *Nat Methods,* 6 (7), 477-8.
Maurice, M., et al. (1999), 'Efficient gene delivery to quiescent interleukin-2 (IL-2)-dependent cells by murine leukemia virus-derived vectors harboring IL-2 chimeric envelope glycoproteins', *Blood,* 94 (2), 401-10.
McKay, T., et al. (2006), 'Influenza M2 envelope protein augments avian influenza hemagglutinin pseudotyping of lentiviral vectors', *Gene Ther,* 13 (8), 715-24.
Medof, M. E., Nagarajan, S., and Tykocinski, M. L. (1996), 'Cell-surface engineering with GPI-anchored proteins', *Faseb J,* 10 (5), 574-86.

Metzner, C., et al. (2008a), 'Rafts, anchors and viruses - A role for glycosylphosphatidylinositol anchored proteins in the modification of enveloped viruses and viral vectors', *Virology.*

--- (2008b), 'Association of glycosylphosphatidylinositol-anchored protein with retroviral particles', *Faseb J,* 22 (8), 2734-9.

Miletic, H., et al. (2004), 'Selective transduction of malignant glioma by lentiviral vectors pseudotyped with lymphocytic choriomeningitis virus glycoproteins', *Hum Gene Ther,* 15 (11), 1091-100.

Miller, A. D., et al. (1991), 'Construction and properties of retrovirus packaging cells based on gibbon ape leukemia virus', *J Virol,* 65 (5), 2220-4.

Morizono, K., et al. (2009a), 'Redirecting lentiviral vectors by insertion of integrin-tageting peptides into envelope proteins', *J Gene Med,* 11 (7), 549-58.

--- (2009b), 'A versatile targeting system with lentiviral vectors bearing the biotin-adaptor peptide', *J Gene Med,* 11 (8), 655-63.

--- (2005), 'Lentiviral vector retargeting to P-glycoprotein on metastatic melanoma through intravenous injection', *Nat Med,* 11 (3), 346-52.

Neda, H., Wu, C. H., and Wu, G. Y. (1991), 'Chemical modification of an ecotropic murine leukemia virus results in redirection of its target cell specificity', *J Biol Chem,* 266 (22), 14143-6.

Neil, S., et al. (2001), 'Postentry restriction to human immunodeficiency virus-based vector transduction in human monocytes', *J Virol,* 75 (12), 5448-56.

Nesbeth, D., et al. (2006), 'Metabolic biotinylation of lentiviral pseudotypes for scalable paramagnetic microparticle-dependent manipulation', *Mol Ther,* 13 (4), 814-22.

Nguyen, D. H. and Hildreth, J. E. (2000), 'Evidence for budding of human immunodeficiency virus type 1 selectively from glycolipid-enriched membrane lipid rafts', *J Virol,* 74 (7), 3264-72.

Nguyen, T. H., et al. (1998), 'Amphotropic retroviral vectors displaying hepatocyte growth factor-envelope fusion proteins improve transduction efficiency of primary hepatocytes', *Hum Gene Ther,* 9 (17), 2469-79.

Nosjean, O., Briolay, A., and Roux, B. (1997), 'Mammalian GPI proteins: sorting, membrane residence and functions', *Biochim Biophys Acta,* 1331 (2), 153-86.

Ory, D. S., Neugeboren, B. A., and Mulligan, R. C. (1996), 'A stable human-derived packaging cell line for production of high titer retrovirus/vesicular stomatitis virus G pseudotypes', *Proc Natl Acad Sci U S A,* 93 (21), 11400-6.

Paar, M., et al. (2007), 'Effects of viral strain, transgene position, and target cell type on replication kinetics, genomic stability, and transgene expression of replication-competent murine leukemia virus-based vectors', *J Virol,* 81 (13), 6973-83.

Pariente, N., et al. (2007), 'A novel dual-targeted lentiviral vector leads to specific transduction of prostate cancer bone metastases in vivo after systemic administration', *Mol Ther,* 15 (11), 1973-81.

Park, F. (2003), 'Correction of bleeding diathesis without liver toxicity using arenaviral-pseudotyped HIV-1-based vectors in hemophilia A mice', *Hum Gene Ther,* 14 (15), 1489-94.

Passineau, M. J., et al. (2011), 'Ultrasound-assisted non-viral gene transfer to the salivary glands', *Gene Ther,* 18 (4), 424.

Patlolla, A., Patlolla, B., and Tchounwou, P. (2010), 'Evaluation of cell viability, DNA damage, and cell death in normal human dermal fibroblast cells induced by functionalized multiwalled carbon nanotube', *Mol Cell Biochem,* 338 (1-2), 225-32.

Pickl, W. F., Pimentel-Muinos, F. X., and Seed, B. (2001), 'Lipid rafts and pseudotyping', *J Virol,* 75 (15), 7175-83.

Pinaud, F., et al. (2009), 'Dynamic partitioning of a glycosyl-phosphatidylinositol-anchored protein in glycosphingolipid-rich microdomains imaged by single-quantum dot tracking', *Traffic,* 10 (6), 691-712.

Pornillos, O., et al. (2003), 'HIV Gag mimics the Tsg101-recruiting activity of the human Hrs protein', *J Cell Biol,* 162 (3), 425-34.

Raty, J. K., et al. (2007), 'Non-invasive Imaging in Gene Therapy', *Mol Ther,* 15 (9), 1579-86.

Rifkin, M. R. and Landsberger, F. R. (1990), 'Trypanosome variant surface glycoprotein transfer to target membranes: a model for the pathogenesis of trypanosomiasis', *Proc Natl Acad Sci U S A,* 87 (2), 801-5.

Rodrigues, T., et al. (2007), 'Purification of retroviral vectors for clinical application: biological implications and technological challenges', *J Biotechnol,* 127 (3), 520-41.

Rooney, I. A., Heuser, J. E., and Atkinson, J. P. (1996), 'GPI-anchored complement regulatory proteins in seminal plasma. An analysis of their physical condition and the mechanisms of their binding to exogenous cells', *J Clin Invest,* 97 (7), 1675-86.

Rooney, I. A., et al. (1993), 'Physiologic relevance of the membrane attack complex inhibitory protein CD59 in human seminal plasma: CD59 is present on extracellular organelles (prostasomes), binds cell membranes, and inhibits complement-mediated lysis', *J Exp Med,* 177 (5), 1409-20.

Roux, P., Jeanteur, P., and Piechaczyk, M. (1989), 'A versatile and potentially general approach to the targeting of specific cell types by retroviruses: application to the infection of human cells by means of major histocompatibility complex class I and class II antigens by mouse ecotropic murine leukemia virus-derived viruses', *Proc Natl Acad Sci U S A,* 86 (23), 9079-83.

Ryu, B. Y., et al. (2008), 'The block to membrane fusion differs with the site of ligand insertion in modified retroviral envelope proteins', *J Gen Virol,* 89 (Pt 4), 1049-58.

Saifuddin, M., et al. (1994), 'Host cell components affect the sensitivity of HIV type 1 to complement-mediated virolysis', *AIDS Res Hum Retroviruses,* 10 (7), 829-37.

--- (1997), 'Human immunodeficiency virus type 1 incorporates both glycosyl phosphatidylinositol-anchored CD55 and CD59 and integral membrane CD46 at levels that protect from complement-mediated destruction', *J Gen Virol,* 78 (Pt 8), 1907-11.

--- (1995), 'Role of virion-associated glycosylphosphatidylinositol-linked proteins CD55 and CD59 in complement resistance of cell line-derived and primary isolates of HIV-1', *J Exp Med,* 182 (2), 501-9.

Sakoda, T., et al. (2007), 'Lentiviral vector-mediated gene transfer to endotherial cells compared with adenoviral and retroviral vectors', *Prep Biochem Biotechnol,* 37 (1), 1-11.

Sandrin, V., et al. (2002), 'Lentiviral vectors pseudotyped with a modified RD114 envelope glycoprotein show increased stability in sera and augmented transduction of primary lymphocytes and CD34+ cells derived from human and nonhuman primates', *Blood,* 100 (3), 823-32.

Santoni de Sio, F. R., et al. (2006), 'Proteasome activity restricts lentiviral gene transfer into hematopoietic stem cells and is down-regulated by cytokines that enhance transduction', *Blood,* 107 (11), 4257-65.

Schellingerhout, D. and Bogdanov, A. A., Jr. (2002), 'Viral imaging in gene therapy noninvasive demonstration of gene delivery and expression', *Neuroimaging Clin N Am,* 12 (4), 571-81, vi-vii.

Segura, M. M., Kamen, A., and Garnier, A. (2008a), 'Purification of retrovirus particles using heparin affinity chromatography', *Methods Mol Biol,* 434, 1-11.

Segura, M. M., et al. (2010), 'New protocol for lentiviral vector mass production', *Methods Mol Biol,* 614, 39-52.

--- (2008b), 'Identification of host proteins associated with retroviral vector particles by proteomic analysis of highly purified vector preparations', *J Virol,* 82 (3), 1107-17.

Shah, K., et al. (2004), 'Molecular imaging of gene therapy for cancer', *Gene Ther,* 11 (15), 1175-87.

Shaw, A. S. (2006), 'Lipid rafts: now you see them, now you don't', *Nat Immunol,* 7 (11), 1139-42.

Sheridan, C. (2011), 'Gene therapy finds its niche', *Nat Biotechnol,* 29 (2), 121-8.

Skountzou, I., et al. (2007), 'Incorporation of glycosylphosphatidylinositol-anchored granulocyte- macrophage colony-stimulating factor or CD40 ligand enhances immunogenicity of chimeric simian immunodeficiency virus-like particles', *J Virol,* 81 (3), 1083-94.

Snitkovsky, S. and Young, J. A. (2002), 'Targeting retroviral vector infection to cells that express heregulin receptors using a TVA-heregulin bridge protein', *Virology,* 292 (1), 150-5.

Snitkovsky, S., et al. (2001), 'Targeting avian leukosis virus subgroup A vectors by using a TVA-VEGF bridge protein', *J Virol,* 75 (3), 1571-5.

--- (2000), 'A TVA-single-chain antibody fusion protein mediates specific targeting of a subgroup A avian leukosis virus vector to cells expressing a tumor-specific form of epidermal growth factor receptor', *J Virol,* 74 (20), 9540-5.

Somia, N. V., Zoppe, M., and Verma, I. M. (1995), 'Generation of targeted retroviral vectors by using single-chain variable fragment: an approach to in vivo gene delivery', *Proc Natl Acad Sci U S A,* 92 (16), 7570-4.

Spitzer, D., et al. (2003), 'Green fluorescent protein-tagged retroviral envelope protein for analysis of virus-cell interactions', *J Virol,* 77 (10), 6070-5.

Strang, B. L., et al. (2004), 'Characterization of HIV-1 vectors with gammaretrovirus envelope glycoproteins produced from stable packaging cells', *Gene Ther,* 11 (7), 591-8.

Subbiah, R., Veerapandian, M., and Yun, K. S. (2010), 'Nanoparticles: functionalization and multifunctional applications in biomedical sciences', *Curr Med Chem,* 17 (36), 4559-77.

Tai, C. K., et al. (2003), 'Antibody-mediated targeting of replication-competent retroviral vectors', *Hum Gene Ther,* 14 (8), 789-802.

Tunster, S. J., Van De Pette, M., and John, R. M. (2011), 'BACs as tools for the study of genomic imprinting', *J Biomed Biotechnol,* 283013.

Vakeva, A., et al. (1994), 'High-density lipoproteins can act as carriers of glycophosphoinositol lipid-anchored CD59 in human plasma', *Immunology,* 82 (1), 28-33.
van der Zande, M., et al. (2011), 'Carbon nanotubes in animal models: a systematic review on toxic potential', *Tissue Eng Part B Rev,* 17 (1), 57-69.
Verhoeyen, E. and Cosset, F. L. (2004), 'Surface-engineering of lentiviral vectors', *J Gene Med,* 6 Suppl 1, S83-94.
Waehler, R., Russell, S. J., and Curiel, D. T. (2007), 'Engineering targeted viral vectors for gene therapy', *Nat Rev Genet,* 8 (8), 573-87.
Warden, C., Tang, Q., and Zhu, H. (2011), 'Herpesvirus BACs: past, present, and future', *J Biomed Biotechnol,* 2011, 124595.
Watson, D. J., et al. (2002), 'Targeted transduction patterns in the mouse brain by lentivirus vectors pseudotyped with VSV, Ebola, Mokola, LCMV, or MuLV envelope proteins', *Mol Ther,* 5 (5 Pt 1), 528-37.
Williams, S. L., Eccleston, M. E., and Slater, N. K. (2005a), 'Affinity capture of a biotinylated retrovirus on macroporous monolithic adsorbents: towards a rapid single-step purification process', *Biotechnol Bioeng,* 89 (7), 783-7.
Williams, S. L., et al. (2005b), 'Affinity recovery of Moloney Murine Leukaemia Virus', *J Chromatogr B Analyt Technol Biomed Life Sci,* 820 (1), 111-9.
Wong, L. F., et al. (2004), 'Transduction patterns of pseudotyped lentiviral vectors in the nervous system', *Mol Ther,* 9 (1), 101-11.
Wong, S. and Kwon, Y. J. (2011), 'Synthetically functionalized retroviruses produced from the bioorthogonally engineered cell surface', *Bioconjug Chem,* 22 (2), 151-5.
Yang, G., et al. (2006a), 'Retrovirus molecular conjugates: a versatile and efficient gene transfer vector system for primitive human hematopoietic progenitor cells', *Cancer Gene Ther,* 13 (5), 460-8.
Yang, H., et al. (2008a), 'Gamma-retroviral vectors enveloped with an antibody and an engineered fusogenic protein achieved antigen-specific targeting', *Biotechnol Bioeng,* 101 (2), 357-68.
Yang, L., et al. (2006b), 'Targeting lentiviral vectors to specific cell types in vivo', *Proc Natl Acad Sci U S A,* 103 (31), 11479-84.
--- (2008b), 'Engineered lentivector targeting of dendritic cells for in vivo immunization', *Nat Biotechnol,* 26 (3), 326-34.
Ye, K., et al. (2004), 'Tagging retrovirus vectors with a metal binding peptide and one-step purification by immobilized metal affinity chromatography', *J Virol,* 78 (18), 9820-7.
Zavada, J. (1982), 'The pseudotypic paradox', *J Gen Virol,* 63 (Pt 1), 15-24.
Zavorotinskaya, T. and Albritton, L. M. (2001), 'Two point mutations increase targeted transduction and stabilize vector association of a modified retroviral envelope protein', *Mol Ther,* 3 (3), 323-8.
Zeng, Y., et al. (2009), 'High-efficiency labeling of sialylated glycoproteins on living cells', *Nat Methods,* 6 (3), 207-9.
Zhang, X. Y., La Russa, V. F., and Reiser, J. (2004), 'Transduction of bone-marrow-derived mesenchymal stem cells by using lentivirus vectors pseudotyped with modified RD114 envelope glycoproteins', *J Virol,* 78 (3), 1219-29.
Zhao, Y., et al. (1999), 'Identification of the block in targeted retroviral-mediated gene transfer', *Proc Natl Acad Sci U S A,* 96 (7), 4005-10.

Ziegler, L., et al. (2008), 'Targeting lentiviral vectors to antigen-specific immunoglobulins', *Hum Gene Ther,* 19 (9), 861-72.

Zielske, S. P. and Gerson, S. L. (2003), 'Cytokines, including stem cell factor alone, enhance lentiviral transduction in nondividing human LTCIC and NOD/SCID repopulating cells', *Mol Ther,* 7 (3), 325-33.

4

The Glucocorticoid Receptor in Retroviral Infection

Victor Solodushko and Brian Fouty
University of South Alabama,
U.S.A.

1. Introduction

The hope that delivering genes to ailing tissues and organs can treat disease more effectively than drugs or surgery, has fueled the intense interest in gene therapy. Potential uses of gene therapy include replacing mutated genes with healthy ones, inactivating improperly functioning mutated genes, or introducing new genes into the body to help fight a specific disease. While the concept of gene therapy is easy to understand, technical difficulties have limited its practical use. Delivered genes that function admirably in cell culture may not function correctly in vivo, may have unexpected consequences on intracellular signaling pathways, or may transform cells raising the risk of iatrogenic malignancy.

Retroviruses play a central role in gene delivery applications because they have a high infection efficiency and are able to induce stable mutagenesis in eukaryotic cells (Yi et al., 2005; Somia & Verma, 2000; Thomas et al., 2003). Stable incorporation of retroviral DNA into the host genome is advantageous, since long-term expression of the transgene, usually a requirement for prolonged therapeutic efficacy, is possible. While they are currently being used for *in vitro* and (animal) *in vivo* studies, the clinical use of retroviral vectors to deliver genes is still in its infancy. Among the reasons for the slow progress in adapting retroviruses to deliver genes are the concerns over potential adverse events when introduced into humans and a limited understanding of the mechanisms that affect retroviral function and expression in infected (target) cells.

Both wild type and genetically modified retroviruses rely on the host cell to assist during its life cycle. Retroviral infection of cells, followed by integration of its genome into the host genome, is not always a certain process, however, and cellular and extracellular processes can influence these events. Therefore, while retroviral gene delivery is generally successful, the impact of viral infections on target cells remains less predictable and can be considered, basically uncontrollable. Despite the care with which viral vectors are generated, researchers ultimately rely on random events that can yield both positive and negative outcomes.

In most eukaryotic cells, steroid hormones regulate a wide variety of physiological functions ranging from inflammation to pregnancy. There are five major classes of steroid hormones: glucocorticoids, mineralocorticoids, estrogens, androgens, and progestins. Steroid hormones from each class can complex with their specific receptors, and often with other transcription factors, to recognize DNA sequences called response elements. This mechanism of gene regulation by steroids is so potent and universal throughout the biosphere that it is not surprising that retroviruses have exploited the host nuclear steroid receptor regulatory system to expand their own genomes and improve their overall functionality.

While most steroid hormone receptor systems could be utilized by retroviruses during target cell infection, the strongest evidence exists for an important role of the glucocorticoid receptor (GR) in this process. This review focuses on the role of the nuclear glucocorticoid receptor in controlling retroviral infection and function and highlights its potential importance in retroviral-based gene therapy applications.

2. Retroviral vectors for gene therapy

Retroviruses belong to the family *Retroviridae* which consists of a large and diverse group of viruses classified into seven genera. Within each genera retroviruses are structurally and functionally similar and further classified based on a computer analysis of their genome. Only two of them, gamma-retroviruses and lentiviruses, are commonly used as vectors for gene therapy, however. The murine leukemia virus (MLV) is the prototypical gamma-retroviral backbone that has been modified to generate different gene delivery vectors, whereas the human immunodeficiency virus type 1 (HIV-1) provides the standard backbone for most lentiviral vectors. Both types of retroviruses (gamma-retroviruses and lentiviruses) have been used to generate stable genetic modification in host cells through the chromosomal integration of the transferred vector genomes. This ability to stably modify target cell genomes is useful not only for research purposes, but also for clinical gene therapy strategies intended to correct genetic defects. An important difference between gamma-retroviruses and lentiviruses is that gamma-retroviruses can only infect dividing cells whereas lentiviruses can infect both dividing and quiescent cells. To date, gamma-retroviral and lentiviral vectors have been used in more than 300 clinical trials targeting various diseases (Telesnitsky, 2010).

All retroviral genomes are non-segmented and typically consist of at least 4 genes: *gag, pro, pol* and *env*. The *gag* gene encodes the major structural polyprotein Gag which is both necessary and sufficient for the assembly of non-infectious and immature viral-like particles. The *pro* gene encodes the viral protease that is responsible for facilitating the maturation of viral particles. Products of the *pol* gene include reverse transcriptase, RNase H and integrase, all critical for the successful integration of the viral genome into the host genome. *Env* encodes the viral surface glycoprotein and transmembrane proteins that mediate cellular receptor binding and membrane fusion. There are additional genes (called accessory genes) that are present in some, but not all, gamma-retroviruses and lentiviruses. These accessory genes are involved in regulating the synthesis and processing of viral RNA and other replicative functions. For the HIV-1 based viruses, these additional genes include: Vif, *Vpr, Vpu, Tat, Rev,* and *Nef* (Malim & Emerman, 2008).

The retroviral genome is flanked by two long terminal repeat (LTR) sequences at both the 5′- and 3′- ends. In the integrated virus (provirus) each LTR consists of three regions: 1) the R sequence, 2) the U3 region, and 3) the U5 region. The R region is a short (18-250nt) sequence which forms a direct repeat at both ends of the genome, and is flanked upstream by the U3 region and downstream by the U5 region in the integrated virus. The U3 is a unique non-coding segment of 200-1,200nt that forms the 5′ end of the virus after reverse transcription. It contains the enhancer elements responsible for transcription of the integrated virus. The U5 is a unique, non-coding region of 75-250nt which is the first part of the genome to be reverse transcribed, forming the 3′ end of the provirus genome. Both U3 and U5 sequences are required for viral integration. The Primer Binding Site (PBS) is an 18nt sequence complementary to the 3' end of the specific tRNA primer used by the virus to begin reverse transcription. Downstream from the PBS is the packaging signal (*psi*) sequence that allows completed RNA transcripts to be packaged into budding viral cores. Polypurine Tract (PPT) is a short (~10nt) run of A/G residues responsible for initiating (+)strand synthesis during reverse transcription. The 5′ LTR is the control center for gene expression and contains both promoter and regulatory elements that can be responsive to both viral and cellular trans-activating factors. The 3′ LTR functions as a transcription terminator and a polyadenylation signal that leads to the development of a mature viral transcript.

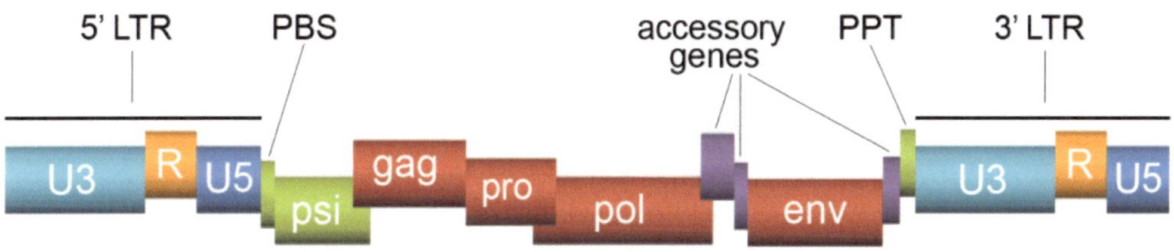

Fig. 1. Schematic representation of the retroviral genome.

For gene delivery applications both gamma-retroviral and lentiviral genomes are initially modified to meet certain criteria (Lech & Somia, 2008). This includes removal of *gag, pol* and *env* to prevent the provirus from generating infectious particles in target cells. This makes them safer and therefore more suitable to deliver genes than wild type viruses. Other parts of the viral genome, such as PBS and PPT, cannot be removed if the vector is to remain functional, however. In addition, while both the LTRs and the *psi* sequence can be partially truncated or modified, they must be present for the virus to function.

A critical difference therefore, between wild type retroviruses and modified retroviruses used in research applications, is the ability of the wild type to generate infectious particles, a trait the retroviral vectors lack. The modifications required to make retroviruses safer, however, can impact enhancer and promoter elements within the LTR and thus make direct comparisons between the behavior of wild type and modified retroviral vectors difficult. Specific to this review, modifications within the LTR promoter of both gamma-retroviruses and lentiviruses can alter the activity of the nuclear GR-regulatory pathway, yielding potentially conflicting experimental results depending on the vector and cell type.

3. Glucocorticoid receptor regulatory system

The glucocorticoid receptor (GR) is also known as NR3C1 (nuclear receptor subfamily 3, group C, member 1) and is encoded by the *NR3C1* gene located on chromosome 5 (5q31) in humans (Hollenberg et al., 1985; Francke & Foellmer, 1989; Lu et al., 2006; Rhen & Cidlowski, 2005). The GR is expressed in almost every cell in the body and upon binding to glucocorticoids, regulates genes controlling development, metabolism, and immune response.

In the absence of the glucocorticoid hormone, the GR resides, inactive, in the cytosol, complexed with a variety of proteins (Pratt et al., 2006). When glucocorticoids bind to the GR it can lead to either gene transactivation or gene transrepression (Buckingham, 2006; Hayashi et al., 2004). Transactivation usually involves homodimerization of the receptor followed by its translocation into the nucleus via active transport. The activated GR binds to specific DNA sequences called glucocorticoid response elements (GRE), which are short sequences of DNA within the promoter of a gene that are able to bind GR complexes and regulate transcription. The GRE's sequence is most commonly a pair of inverted repeats separated by a short linker, indicating that the receptor binds as a homodimer. Half-sites GRE are also present and usually bind monomeric GR. These half-sites are only weakly activated by GR complexes, but can also have inhibitory effects, leading to transrepression.

Nuclear factor-kappaB (NFκB) and the activator protein-1 (AP-1) are two important transcription factors that are negatively regulated by the nuclear GR signaling pathway. In the absence of activated GR, NFκB and AP-1 are able to translocate into the nucleus and transactivate target genes by binding to specific DNA sequences that correspond to each transcription factor. Activated GR can complex with either of these transcription factors, however, and prevent them from binding their target genes, repressing genes that are normally upregulated by NFκB or AP-1. GR-mediated transrepression of NFkB can also occur through GR's binding to NFκB's response elements, thus preventing transactivation (Hermoso & Cidlowski, 2003; Nissen & Yamamoto, 2000; Tuckermann et al., 1999).

NFkB regulates the expression of well over 100 genes, the majority of which participate in the host immune response (Ghosh et al., 1998). These proteins include cytokines and chemokines, receptors required for immune recognition, proteins involved in antigen presentation, and adhesion receptors involved in transmigration across blood vessel walls. Because of its extensive role in immune action, NFkB has been termed the central mediator of the immune response (Hiscott et al., 2001). The ability of activated GR to block NFkB's transactivation of these genes is likely important in mediating the immunosuppressive effect of glucocorticoids (Ito et al., 2001).

GRE are present in the genomes of most gamma-retroviruses (Bruland et al., 2003a, Rodriguez & Goff, 2010, Pages et al., 1995) and HIV-1 based lentiviruses (Ghosh, 1992; Mitra et al., 1995; Hapgood & Tomasicchio, 2010). NFkB response elements are generally absent in gamma-retroviruses, but present in HIV-1, making GR-mediated regulation of lentiviral vectors derived from the HIV-1 backbone more complex. The presence of GRE and NFkB response elements in the retroviral genome suggests that glucocorticoids can exert influence on the viral-host cell interaction. Defining the role of GR on the retroviral lifecycle may not only provide clues on how to combat retroviral infections, but also provide alternate strategies for adapting retroviral vectors for gene delivery.

4. Effects of activated glucocorticoid receptors on gamma-retroviral and lentiviral promoters

The prominence of GRE in the gamma- and lentiviral genomes suggests that their life cycles are dependent on the host's GR regulatory system (Rusmevichientong & Chow, 2010). Glucocorticoids stimulate gamma-retroviral promoter activity in multiple cell types. Synthetic corticosteroid hormones stimulated MLV transgene expression in primary bone marrow stromal cells (Jaalouk et al., 2000). The synthetic glucocorticoid, dexamethasone, increased gamma-retroviral LTR promoter activity in pulmonary artery endothelial and smooth muscle cells and also in 293 cells as evidenced by an increased expression of the reporter protein, GFP, in infected cells (Solodushko et al., 2009) Most published evidence suggests that the usual effect of glucocorticoids on gamma-retroviral promoter activity is positive (Mitra et al., 1995).

The effect of GR on the lentiviral promoter is more complicated than its effect on gamma-retroviruses, however. Activation of the GR can enhance lentivirus functionality. H9V3 cells transfected with the reporter HIV-1 LTR did show increased transgene expression in the presence of glucocorticoids (Kolesnitchenko & Snart, 1992). HIV-1 infected lymphoid and monocytoid cell lines treated with cortisol or dexamethasone also increased HIV-1 gene expression and virus production in vitro, a process that required the presence of the GRE (Soudeyns et al., 1993). In addition, glucocorticoid administration has also been associated with increased HIV-1 promoter activity leading to increased virus replication and AIDS progression in infected individuals (Kino et al., 2000; Soudeyns et al., 1993).

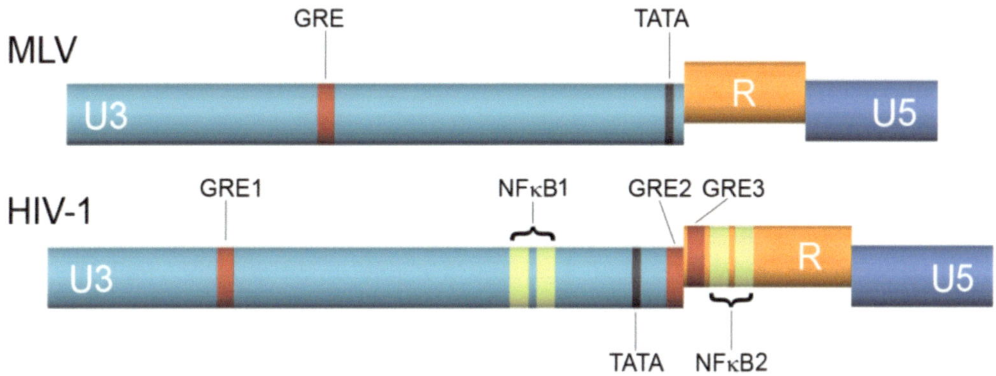

Fig. 2. Schematic representation of binding sites for activated GR in the LTR of MLV (gamma-retrovirus) and HIV-1 (lentivirus). In MLV GR can bind GRE resulting in transactivation. In HIV-l GR can bind GRE1 generally resulting in transactivation and GRE2 and GRE3 (both half sites) leading to transrepression. Activated GR can also directly interact with HIV-1 NFkB binding sites resulting in transrepression of the viral promoter.

Lentiviruses contain both stimulatory and inhibitory GRE sites though and therefore activated GR can cause different effects depending on the cell type. The first GRE (GRE1) is located between −264 and −259 relative to the transcriptional start site and can generally be considered a stimulatory GRE. The other GREs (GRE2 and 3) are half sites and are positioned between −6 and −1 and between +15 and +20, respectively, relative to the transcriptional start site (Mitra et al., 1995; Berkhout et al., 1989). Both GRE half-sites (2 and 3) are shown to be negative regulators of the viral promoter (Meijsing et al., 2009).

In addition to its ability to signal through the GRE, the GR signaling pathway can also regulate lentiviral (although not gamma-retroviral) behavior through its interaction with the NFkB and AP-1 pathway. Activated GR can interfere with NFkB signaling either by directly interacting with NFkB response sites or by binding with NFkB proteins (thus blocking its ability to enhance the lentiviral LTR). As shown in figure 2 two NFkB response sequences (NFkB1) in the HIV-1 U3 region are located between GRE1 and the TATA box. Wild type HIV-1 that lacks both of the NFkB binding sites is replication-incompetent; returning one or both NFkB elements restores the virus's ability to replicate (Ross et al., 1991).

The active binding sites for NFkB, however, are not limited to the enhancing region but can be found downstream of the transcription initiation site. In addition to this double NFkB site in the U3 region, another double NFkB binding site is present in the R region of the lentiviral LTR (NFκB2). This site is also active and contributes to the GR and NFκB response and is involved in activating the LTR in response to mitogenic stimuli (Mitra et al., 1995; Berkhout et al., 1989; Logan et al., 2004; Kilareski et al., 2009). The p50-p65-NFκB complex can bind both of these sites and enhance expression of HIV-1 genes. Further downstream, three AP-1 binding sites in U5 may also potentiate NFkB-dependent responses in integrated proviruses (Logan et al., 2004; Kilareski et al., 2009). Figure 2 shows the only direct binding sites for GR in retroviral LTR.

Thus the GR is a regulatory factor that can influence HIV-1 activity through multiple mechanisms, not only by its direct binding to the GRE, but also through its effects on NFkB and AP-1 signaling pathways. These influences can be both positive and negative. (Hapgood & Tomasicchio, 2010; Kino et al., 1999; Ayyavoo et al., 1997a; Mirani et al., 2002) The overall effect of glucocorticoids on lentiviral promoter activity, therefore, can be difficult to predict. This may explain the confusing, and often contradictory, results on the effect of glucocorticoids on HIV-1 progression obtained by different research groups (Kino et al., 2000).

5. Viral protein R potentiates the effect of glucocorticoid receptor

In contrast to the relatively simple ways that gamma-retroviruses induce host cell infection, lentiviruses have evolved multiple strategies to induce a persistent infection in host cells. HIV-1 in particular, employs several strategies that rely on an array of virally encoded accessory proteins, including Vif, Vpr, Vpu, and Nef. Collectively, these proteins appear to manipulate host cell biology to ensure a favorable cellular environment for viral replication, transmission, dissemination, and immune evasion (Malim & Emerman, 2008). One of them in particular, the 14-kDa HIV-1 viral protein R (Vpr), down-regulates the expression of genes involved in cell cycle/proliferation, DNA repair, tumor antigen presentation by the host cell, and immune activation factors, and upregulates many ribosomal and structural proteins required for viral propagation (Janket et al., 2004; Levy et al., 1994; Wu et al., 1995, Sherman et al., 2000). These changes can occur in the absence of other viral gene products, suggesting that Vpr can mediate its proviral effects partially, or perhaps solely, through modulation of the target cell environment (Ayyavoo et al., 1997a).

Vpr protein is present in high titers in the serum of AIDS patients and can be efficiently taken up from the extracellular medium by cells *in vitro* in a process that occurs independent of other HIV-1 proteins and also independent of cellular receptors. Following cellular uptake, Vpr can have multiple actions on the host cell GR signaling pathway, an interaction that can affect both the host cell and the virus. Two highly conserved leucine-rich domains within Vpr resemble the GR coactivator signature motif which allows Vpr to activate the GR in the absence in glucocorticoids (Sherman et al., 2000). As a result, the activated Vpr-GR complex translocates into the nucleus and induces the expression of glucocorticoid-responsive genes in a similar direction to that seen with dexamethasone in either the host cell or the viral promoters (Muthumani et al., 2006). Vpr can also activate the HIV-1 promoter without GR, directly binding to the viral SP-1 site in complexes with other activators (Kino et al., 2002, Kino et al., 2000, Amini et al., 2004). Thus, Vpr can stimulate the retroviral promoter leading to increased virus production and virion maturation. Experimentally it has been shown to induce virus expression in the peripheral blood mononuclear cells of HIV-infected individuals (Levy et al., 1994) and can directly induce T-cell receptor-triggered apoptosis. This effect, central to the ability of HIV-1 to deplete T cells, can be prevented by the inhibitory steroid hormone mifepristone (Ayyavoo et al., 1997b; Fakruddin & Laurence, 2005). In addition to its effect on the lentiviral and the host cell promoters, Vpr also enhances expression of the beta-retroviral mouse mammary tumor virus (MMTV) promoter suggesting that Vpr could be used as an enhancer in retroviruses other than lentiviruses (Kino et al., 2002).

Vpr interaction with the host cell's GR and subsequent ability to transactivate the HIV-1 LTR directly (i.e. in the absence of glucocorticoids), can be blocked by mifepristone. Mifepristone, also known as RU-486 is an abortifacient that has both anti-progestin and anti-glucocorticoid activity. It can bind and activate the GR-alpha primarily, but recent work suggests that it can also bind and translocate the GR-beta into the nucleus of Cos1 and U2OS cells, leading to upregulation of a number of genes (Lewis-Tuffin et al., 2007). In vitro, mifepristone was able to inhibit Vpr-mediated translocation of the HIV nucleoprotein preintegration complex into the host cell nucleus and block Vpr-induced apoptosis, cytokine production and T-cell proliferation (Schafer et al., 2006). This and other experimental observations led to the hypothesis that mifepristone could reduce viral synthesis in infected cells and therefore could reduce the pace of infection in vivo. A clinical trial examining the anti-HIV activity and safety of mifepristone on viral load, disease progression, and survival in HIV-1 infected individuals was begun in 2006 (Clinical trial number: NCT00352911). Final results of that trial have not yet been released, but interim results suggest no benefit of mifepristone in the primary endpoint of reducing HIV viral load at 28 days (Para et al., 2010).

6. Role of glucocorticoid receptor in immune resonance, retroviral release and integration capability

Glucocorticoids are among the most commonly prescribed drugs worldwide due to their profound anti-inflammatory and immunosuppressive activity (Herold et al., 2006; Kim et al., 2001; Janket et al., 2004). They control homeostasis of T cell monocytes/macrophages, osteoclasts, and dendritic cells by inducing their apoptosis or inhibiting maturation. Most, if not all, of these effects are mediated through their interactions with the GR (Herold et al., 2006). Activated GR can interfere with the signaling pathways of AP-1 and NFκB, two key host transcription factors that regulate expression of pro-inflammatory genes and other genes involved in immune responses (Hapgood & Tomasicchio, 2010; De Bosscher et al., 2003; Smoak & Cidlowski, 2004)

Vpr enhances the immunosuppressive effect of endogenous and therapeutic glucocorticoids (Mirani et al., 2002; Kino et al., 1999). Vpr administered extracellularly potentiated the glucocorticoid-induced suppression of mRNA expression and secretion of IL-12 by dendritic cells (Kim et al., 2001). Vpr also potentiated the glucocorticoid-induced inhibition of other immunologically important cytokines such as IL-2, IL-10, TNF alpha and IL-4, all of which are NFκB -dependent (Fakruddin & Laurence, 2005). Both the GR and Vpr are involved in the apoptosis in T cells and dendritic cells (Hapgood & Tomasicchio, 2010; Bruland et al., 2003b). In addition, patients with AIDS and normal cortisol secretion have manifestations compatible with glucocorticoid hypersensitivity of the immune system, such as suppression of innate and cellular immunity.

Since the GR plays an important role in regulating viral promoter activity it is not surprising that it also affects viral particle production. Dexamethasone can stimulate the gamma-retroviral promoter in viral producing cells (i.e. HEK 293 packaging cells) significantly increasing viral release into the cultured medium, a strategy that can be used to increase the viral titer for gene delivery applications (Solodushko et al., 2009). A similar effect can be seen with lentiviruses, but this is dependent on the formulation of glucocorticoid used and cell type infected. Hydrocortisone increased the efficacy of HIV-1 infection in fresh normal human peripheral blood mononuclear leukocytes whereas other corticosteroids (dexamethasone) and sex hormones, had no effect (Markham et al., 1986).

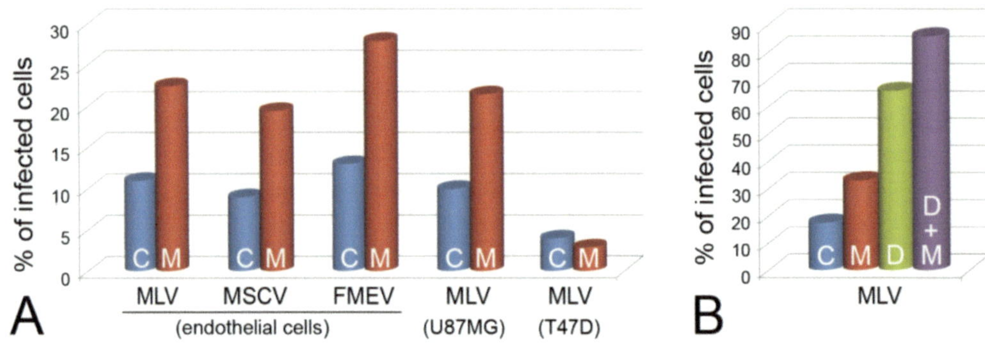

Fig. 3. A: The anti-glucocorticoid and anti-progestin agent, mifepristone, increased the integration efficiency of three gamma-retroviruses: moloney murine leukemia virus (MLV), murine stem cell virus (MSCV) and friend murine embryonic stem cell virus (FMEV). Target cells included: lung microvascular endothelial cells (expressing both functioning glucocorticoid (GR) and progesterone (PR) receptors), U87MG cells (lacking functioning GR) and T47D cells (lacking functioning PR). This effect was independent of viral titer. B: Infection efficiency of endothelial cells with MLV under four conditions: (C) control, no steroid treatment at time of virus propagation and infection; (D) virus was propagated and target cells were infected in the presence of glucocorticoid dexamethasone; (M) virus was propagated with no steroids and target cells were infected in the presence of mifepristone; (D+M) virus was propagated in the presence of dexamethasone followed by infection of target cells in the presence of dexamethasone and mifepristone.

We and others have demonstrated that dexamethasone can stimulate the gamma-retroviral LTR promoter and increase viral particle production in packaging cell lines. This effect could be blocked by the progestin and glucocorticoid antagonist, mifepristone. In a novel observation, we demonstrated that mifepristone could increase the infection efficiency of gamma-retroviruses in a number of different target cells including (human, rat, and mouse) vascular endothelial and smooth muscle cells, and epithelial cells. This effect was independent of viral titer. Later studies demonstrated that mifepristone had no effect on viral entry, viral survival or viral DNA synthesis, but increased gamma-retroviral infection efficiency by facilitating viral integration into the host genome (figure 3A). This effect appeared to be due to mifepristone's anti-glucocorticoid, but not its anti-progestin, activity since T47D cells lacking functioning GR did not demonstrate increased infection efficiency in the presence of mifepristone, whereas U87MG cells lacking functional progesterone receptors, did. Mifepristone had no effect on lentiviral integration into host cells, however. These results suggest that inhibition of the GR enhances retroviral integration into the host genome and indicates that cells may have a natural protection again retroviral infection that may be reduced by glucocorticoid receptor antagonists (Solodushko & Fouty, 2010).

Based on these observations, we demonstrated that gamma-retroviral infection of target cells can be maximized by first incubating packaging cells with dexamethasone to increase the viral titre in the supernatant and then incubating target cells with mifepristone to improve integration of virus into the host genome (figure 3B) (Solodushko & Fouty, 2010).

The predominantly cytoplasmic localization of the GR appears to be a specific obstacle for HIV replication by preventing its migration into the nucleus where it can complete the infectious process. The presence of both endogenous and exogenous glucocorticoids tends to increase the lentiviral infection efficiency of target cells. Resting peripheral mononuclear blood cells are not easily infected with HIV-1 due to a block, prior to integration, of the provirus into the host genome. Proviral integration increases after addition of a GR ligand (such as hydrocortisone or dexamethasone). This effect is confined to an early time period after incubation of the cells with the virus and requires the presence of the GR and the GR binding viral protein Vpr (Wiegers et al., 2008).

7. Lessons for retroviral gene therapy

Due to safety concerns, retroviral vectors are made replication incompetent by the removal of the *gag, pol* and *env* genes. As a result, while retroviral vectors are still capable of transducing cells and expressing the foreign (delivered) gene, they cannot produce infectious viral particles due to the lack of structural and enzymatic genes. To generate the retroviral vectors needed to deliver genes of interest to target cells, the *gag, pol* and *env* genes are stably introduced into retroviral-packaging (producing) cells. The presence of functioning LTRs, PBS, psi and PPT are required and sufficient for the proper function of most gamma-retroviral vectors whereas additional trans and cis elements are required for the proper function of lentiviruses. The genetic modifications required to transform wild type gamma-retroviruses and lentiviruses into vectors suitable for use in research and clinical trials can significantly alter their response to environmental signals. Since the retroviral life cycle is dependent somewhat on the function of the GR in host cells, retroviral gene delivery vectors derived from wild type retroviruses are also regulated by GR activity.

While many regions of the wild type retroviral backbones genome can be altered to meet the demands of gene delivery, essential parts of the viral genome must be retained to allow transgene expression and vector (virus) production. An intact R and U5 regions of the LTR promoter are required for the virus to work. Parts of the U3 (enhancer) region of the promoter can be modified, deleted or replaced by other sequences, without significantly decreasing virus functionality, however. The U3 region of most retroviruses contains GRE and, in the case of lentiviruses, NFkB response elements as well. Removing these response elements will still allow the virus to function, but will alter its responsiveness to GR signaling pathways. Therefore vectors with full length LTR or truncated LTR that retain these GR responsive sequences, will behave like wild type viruses in response to GR activation whereas vectors in which they have been removed will appear non-responsive to GR activation.

The promoters of gamma-retroviral vectors with completely functional GRE are strongly stimulated when exposed to GR. This enhancing effect of activated GR on the LTR promoter in gamma-retroviruses can be exploited to increase viral production by packaging cells and also to increase expression of reporter or therapeutic genes in target cells once the viral genome is integrated. The net effect of activated GR (due to either glucocorticoids or Vpr) on LTR activity in lentiviruses is less predictable, however, due to the opposing effects of GR on the GRE and NFkB regulatory segments. Published data indicate that glucocorticoids can have either positive or negative effects on the LTR promoter in lentiviruses depending on the cell type, glucocorticoid formulation, and vector being studied (Soudeyns et al., 1993; Kolesnitchenko & Snart, 1992; Kino et al., 2000; Mitra et al., 1995).

For the HIV-1 based vector, most of the accessory genes (*Vif, Vpr, Vpu, Nef*) as well as *Tat* and *Rev* have been deleted for safety reasons or separated from the packaging construct. Despite these deletions, this modified virus can still function as a gene delivery vector.

While the absence of Vpr does not interfere with infection efficiency in most cell types, this protein can potentiate transduction of macrophages (Amado & Chen, 1999; Heinzinger et al., 1994), muscle, and liver cells (Kafri et al., 1997; Blomer et al., 1997). In addition, Vpr is a known activator of lentiviral and cellular promoters and can also enhance activity of the MMLV LTR promoter by directly binding to p300/CBP coactivators (Kino et al., 2002). Since Vpr is deleted in most lentiviral vectors, its ability to enhance activation of the viral LTR and the host promoters is also eliminated. Vpr can enter cells independent of the virus, however, and can activate retroviral vectors even if it is not included in the vector. Vpr can block NFkB and AP-1 signaling, thus inducing immune suppression which increases the likelihood of successful retroviral stable infection of host cells *in vivo*. When using third generation lentiviral vectors which lack Vpr, some investigators have delivered Vpr separately to increase the chances of a successful infection.

Self-inactivating (SIN) retroviral vectors are ones in which a region of the 3'LTR that contains an enhancing region of the viral promoter is deleted. The complementary region in the 5'LTR is replaced by a promoter to allow transcription of the full-length viral genome. After integration into the host genome, the retroviral LTR becomes inactive allowing increased transgene expression from another internal promoter. This allows the placement of a stronger promoter such as cytomegalovirus (CMV) to increase transgene expression, or alternatively, to allow site-specific activation of the transgene such as when the internal promoter is the endothelial promoter, Tie2, which will only allow transgene expression in endothelial cells. Originally SIN vectors were thought to be safer for gene therapy because they lacked the retroviral enhancer element and therefore do not continue to replicate within the host genome. There is some debate about whether this is true or not, however (Bosticardo et al., 2009; Yu et al., 1986).

In SIN vectors, the role of the GR on viral promoter activity is further reduced because the GREs within the U3 region are also removed. To combat this limitation, the excised GRE can be restored within the second internal promoter. Even without restoring GREs in SIN vectors, however, activated GR continue to have an effect on lentiviral behavior due to the presence of GRE and NFkB responsive sequences in regions other than U3 (Soudeyns et al., 1993; Hapgood & Tomasicchio, 2010; Mitra et al., 1995; Berkhout et al., 1989; Logan et al., 2004; Kilareski et al., 2009). GR, in cooperation with other regulatory proteins, can bind these sites and enhance AP-1 signaling since several AP-1 binding sites are present not only in U3, but in the U5 region of HIV-1 also. Since the R and U5 regions are not significantly altered in retroviral vectors due to their importance in viral function, these NFkB and AP-1 sites remain relatively intact even in SIN lentiviral vectors and therefore may contribute to residual LTR transcriptional activity (Logan et al., 2004; Kilareski et al., 2009; Logan et al., 2004)

Depending on the type of internal promoter used in SIN vectors, their enhancers may also have GRE or NFkB response elements. The most robust and popular internal promoters used in lentiviral vectors (such as CMV or SV-40) may also contain NFkB binding sites that increase promoter activity when NFkB is bound (Ross et al., 1991). Lentiviral Vpr can also increase the activity of CMV, SV-40 and many other internal promoters (Hiscott et al., 2001; Roux et al., 2000; Kim et al., 2007). Glucocorticoids can have different effects on these internal retroviral promoters if they are used with an intact LTR promoter, however, and this appears to be a function of cell type. For example, in bone marrow cells infected with a retroviral construction that contains a full length LTR and a second internal SV-40 promoter (which does not contain the GRE), dexamethasone suppresses SV-40 promoter activity, whereas in retrovirus-infected fibroblasts infected with the same retroviral vector, dexamethasone increased SV-40 activity (Akahane et al., 2002). Therefore, retroviral vectors with internal promoters should be designed individually depending on the cell type that needs to be infected and the effect of glucocorticoids on these vectors needs to be tested in each cell type. Understanding the distinct effects of modified vectors in different cell types is important for successful gene therapy (Derecka et al., 2006).

8. Conclusions

Gamma-retroviruses and lentiviruses are the most commonly used vectors for in vitro and in vivo gene delivery and both are responsive to activated GR. The GR signaling pathway is an important regulator of retroviral functionality through both its effects on the retrovirus and its effects on the target cell. In addition to its effects on the host cell and the retrovirus, glucocorticoids and activated GR can also dampen cellular immunity. This is particularly important when retroviruses are used as gene delivery vehicles *in vivo*. Once these wild type viruses are modified for gene delivery applications, however, the direction and magnitude of this GR response can be altered. Depending on what areas of the retroviral genome are changed, the effects of GR activation can vary greatly. In addition, the cell type infected contributes to the GR response making predictions about the effects of GR activators (i.e. glucocorticoids and Vpr) in specific cell types, difficult. Retroviral vectors therefore, need to be designed for a specific purpose and cell type and they must also be tested within the cell of interest under the conditions of interest to confirm the desired effect.

9. Acknowledgements

This work was supported, in part, by an American Heart Association Grant-in-Aid from the Greater Southeast Affiliate (09GRNT2260914).

10. References

Akahane, M., Kuriyama, S., Ohgushi, H., Akahane, T., Kawamura, K., Watanabe, S., Funakoshi, F., Yoshiji, H., Ikenaka, K. & Takakura, Y. (2002). Enhancing and suppressing effects of dexamethasone on transgene expression in vitro. *Int J Mol Med,* Vol. 10, No. 1, pp. 107-12.

Amado, R.G. & Chen, I.S. (1999). Lentiviral vectors--the promise of gene therapy within reach? *Science,* Vol. 285, No. 5428, pp. 674-6.

Amini, S., Saunders, M., Kelley, K., Khalili, K. & Sawaya, B.E. (2004). Interplay between HIV-1 Vpr and Sp1 modulates p21(WAF1) gene expression in human astrocytes. *J Biol Chem,* Vol. 279, No. 44, pp. 46046-56.

Ayyavoo, V., Mahalingam, S., Rafaeli, Y., Kudchodkar, S., Chang, D., Nagashunmugam, T., Williams, W.V. & Weiner, D.B. (1997a). HIV-1 viral protein R (Vpr) regulates viral replication and cellular proliferation in T cells and monocytoid cells in vitro. *J Leukoc Biol,* Vol. 62, No. 1, pp. 93-9.

Ayyavoo, V., Mahboubi, A., Mahalingam, S., Ramalingam, R., Kudchodkar, S., Williams, W.V., Green, D.R. & Weiner, D.B. (1997b). HIV-1 Vpr suppresses immune activation and apoptosis through regulation of nuclear factor kappa B. *Nat Med,* Vol. 3, No. 10, pp. 1117-23.

Berkhout, B., Silverman, R.H. & Jeang, K.T. (1989). Tat trans-activates the human immunodeficiency virus through a nascent RNA target. *Cell,* Vol. 59, No. 2, pp. 273-82.

Blomer, U., Naldini, L., Kafri, T., Trono, D., Verma, I.M. & Gage, F.H. (1997). Highly efficient and sustained gene transfer in adult neurons with a lentivirus vector. *J Virol,* Vol. 71, No. 9, pp. 6641-9.

Bosticardo, M., Ghosh, A., Du, Y., Jenkins, N.A., Copeland, N.G. & Candotti, F. (2009). Self-inactivating retroviral vector-mediated gene transfer induces oncogene activation and immortalization of primary murine bone marrow cells. *Mol Ther,* Vol. 17, No. 11, pp. 1910-8.

Bruland, T., Lavik, L.A., Dai, H.Y. & Dalen, A. (2003a). A glucocorticoid response element in the LTR U3 region of Friend murine leukaemia virus variant FIS-2 enhances virus production in vitro and is a major determinant for sex differences in susceptibility to FIS-2 infection in vivo. *J Gen Virol,* Vol. 84, No. Pt 4, pp. 907-16.

Bruland, T., Lavik, L.A., Dai, H.Y. & Dalen, A. (2003b). Identification of Friend murine retrovirus-infected immune cells and studies of the effects of sex and steroid hormones in the early phase of infection. *APMIS,* Vol. 111, No. 9, pp. 878-90.

Buckingham, J.C. (2006). Glucocorticoids: exemplars of multi-tasking. *Br J Pharmacol,* Vol. 147 Suppl 1, pp. S258-68.

De Bosscher, K., Vanden Berghe, W. & Haegeman, G. (2003). The interplay between the glucocorticoid receptor and nuclear factor-kappaB or activator protein-1: molecular mechanisms for gene repression. *Endocr Rev,* Vol. 24, No. 4, pp. 488-522.

Derecka, K., Wang, C.K. & Flint, A.P. (2006). Interactions between the cytomegalovirus promoter and the estrogen response element: implications for design of estrogen-responsive reporter plasmids. *J Biomol Tech,* Vol. 17, No. 3, pp. 218-27.

Fakruddin, J.M. & Laurence, J. (2005). HIV-1 Vpr enhances production of receptor of activated NF-kappaB ligand (RANKL) via potentiation of glucocorticoid receptor activity. *Arch Virol,* Vol. 150, No. 1, pp. 67-78.

Francke, U. & Foellmer, B.E. (1989). The glucocorticoid receptor gene is in 5q31-q32 [corrected]. *Genomics,* Vol. 4, No. 4, pp. 610-2.

Ghosh, D. (1992). Glucocorticoid receptor-binding site in the human immunodeficiency virus long terminal repeat. *J Virol,* Vol. 66, No. 1, pp. 586-90.

Ghosh, S., May, M.J. & Kopp, E.B. (1998). NF-kappa B and Rel proteins: evolutionarily conserved mediators of immune responses. *Annu Rev Immunol,* Vol. 16, pp. 225-60.

Hapgood, J.P. & Tomasicchio, M. (2010). Modulation of HIV-1 virulence via the host glucocorticoid receptor: towards further understanding the molecular mechanisms of HIV-1 pathogenesis. *Arch Virol,* Vol. 155, No. 7, pp. 1009-19.

Hayashi, R., Wada, H., Ito, K. & Adcock, I.M. (2004). Effects of glucocorticoids on gene transcription. *Eur J Pharmacol,* Vol. 500, No. 1-3, pp. 51-62.

Heinzinger, N.K., Bukinsky, M.I., Haggerty, S.A., Ragland, A.M., Kewalramani, V., Lee, M.A., Gendelman, H.E., Ratner, L., Stevenson, M. & Emerman, M. (1994). The Vpr protein of human immunodeficiency virus type 1 influences nuclear localization of viral nucleic acids in nondividing host cells. *Proc Natl Acad Sci U S A,* Vol. 91, No. 15, pp. 7311-5.

Hermoso, M.A. & Cidlowski, J.A. (2003). Putting the brake on inflammatory responses: the role of glucocorticoids. *IUBMB Life,* Vol. 55, No. 9, pp. 497-504.

Herold, M.J., McPherson, K.G. & Reichardt, H.M. (2006). Glucocorticoids in T cell apoptosis and function. *Cell Mol Life Sci,* Vol. 63, No. 1, pp. 60-72.

Hiscott, J., Kwon, H. & Genin, P. (2001). Hostile takeovers: viral appropriation of the NF-kappaB pathway. *J Clin Invest,* Vol. 107, No. 2, pp. 143-51.

Hollenberg, S.M., Weinberger, C., Ong, E.S., Cerelli, G., Oro, A., Lebo, R., Thompson, E.B., Rosenfeld, M.G. & Evans, R.M. (1985). Primary structure and expression of a functional human glucocorticoid receptor cDNA. *Nature,* Vol. 318, No. 6047, pp. 635-41.

Ito, K., Jazrawi, E., Cosio, B., Barnes, P.J. & Adcock, I.M. (2001). p65-activated histone acetyltransferase activity is repressed by glucocorticoids: mifepristone fails to recruit HDAC2 to the p65-HAT complex. *J Biol Chem,* Vol. 276, No. 32, pp. 30208-15.

Jaalouk, D.E., Eliopoulos, N., Couture, C., Mader, S. & Galipeau, J. (2000). Glucocorticoid-inducible retrovector for regulated transgene expression in genetically engineered bone marrow stromal cells. *Hum Gene Ther,* Vol. 11, No. 13, pp. 1837-49.

Janket, M.L., Manickam, P., Majumder, B., Thotala, D., Wagner, M., Schafer, E.A., Collman, R.G., Srinivasan, A. & Ayyavoo, V. (2004). Differential regulation of host cellular genes by HIV-1 viral protein R (Vpr): cDNA microarray analysis using isogenic virus. *Biochem Biophys Res Commun,* Vol. 314, No. 4, pp. 1126-32.

Kafri, T., Blomer, U., Peterson, D.A., Gage, F.H. & Verma, I.M. (1997). Sustained expression of genes delivered directly into liver and muscle by lentiviral vectors. *Nat Genet,* Vol. 17, No. 3, pp. 314-7.

Kilareski, E.M., Shah, S., Nonnemacher, M.R. & Wigdahl, B. (2009). Regulation of HIV-1 transcription in cells of the monocyte-macrophage lineage. *Retrovirology,* Vol. 6, pp. 118.

Kim, K.D., Choe, Y.K., Choe, I.S. & Lim, J.S. (2001). Inhibition of glucocorticoid-mediated, caspase-independent dendritic cell death by CD40 activation. *J Leukoc Biol,* Vol. 69, No. 3, pp. 426-34.

Kim, K.I., Kang, J.H., Chung, J.K., Lee, Y.J., Jeong, J.M., Lee, D.S. & Lee, M.C. (2007). Doxorubicin enhances the expression of transgene under control of the CMV promoter in anaplastic thyroid carcinoma cells. *J Nucl Med,* Vol. 48, No. 9, pp. 1553-61.

Kino, T., Gragerov, A., Kopp, J.B., Stauber, R.H., Pavlakis, G.N. & Chrousos, G.P. (1999). The HIV-1 virion-associated protein vpr is a coactivator of the human glucocorticoid receptor. *J Exp Med,* Vol. 189, No. 1, pp. 51-62.

Kino, T., Gragerov, A., Slobodskaya, O., Tsopanomichalou, M., Chrousos, G.P. & Pavlakis, G.N. (2002). Human immunodeficiency virus type 1 (HIV-1) accessory protein Vpr induces transcription of the HIV-1 and glucocorticoid-responsive promoters by binding directly to p300/CBP coactivators. *J Virol,* Vol. 76, No. 19, pp. 9724-34.

Kino, T., Kopp, J.B. & Chrousos, G.P. (2000). Glucocorticoids suppress human immunodeficiency virus type-1 long terminal repeat activity in a cell type-specific, glucocorticoid receptor-mediated fashion: direct protective effects at variance with clinical phenomenology. *J Steroid Biochem Mol Biol,* Vol. 75, No. 4-5, pp. 283-90.

Kolesnitchenko, V. & Snart, R.S. (1992). Regulatory elements in the human immunodeficiency virus type 1 long terminal repeat LTR (HIV-1) responsive to steroid hormone stimulation. *AIDS Res Hum Retroviruses,* Vol. 8, No. 12, pp. 1977-80.

Lech, P. & Somia, N.V. (2008). Retrovirus vectors. *Contrib Nephrol,* Vol. 159, pp. 30-46.

Levy, D.N., Refaeli, Y., MacGregor, R.R. & Weiner, D.B. (1994). Serum Vpr regulates productive infection and latency of human immunodeficiency virus type 1. *Proc Natl Acad Sci U S A,* Vol. 91, No. 23, pp. 10873-7.

Lewis-Tuffin, L.J., Jewell, C.M., Bienstock, R.J., Collins, J.B. & Cidlowski, J.A. (2007). Human glucocorticoid receptor beta binds RU-486 and is transcriptionally active. *Mol Cell Biol,* Vol. 27, No. 6, pp. 2266-82.

Logan, A.C., Haas, D.L., Kafri, T. & Kohn, D.B. (2004). Integrated self-inactivating lentiviral vectors produce full-length genomic transcripts competent for encapsidation and integration. *J Virol,* Vol. 78, No. 16, pp. 8421-36.

Lu, N.Z., Wardell, S.E., Burnstein, K.L., Defranco, D., Fuller, P.J., Giguere, V., Hochberg, R.B., McKay, L., Renoir, J.M., Weigel, N.L., Wilson, E.M., McDonnell, D.P. & Cidlowski, J.A. (2006). International Union of Pharmacology. LXV. The pharmacology and classification of the nuclear receptor superfamily: glucocorticoid, mineralocorticoid, progesterone, and androgen receptors. *Pharmacol Rev,* Vol. 58, No. 4, pp. 782-97.

Malim, M.H. & Emerman, M. (2008). HIV-1 accessory proteins--ensuring viral survival in a hostile environment. *Cell Host Microbe,* Vol. 3, No. 6, pp. 388-98.

Markham, P.D., Salahuddin, S.Z., Veren, K., Orndorff, S. & Gallo, R.C. (1986). Hydrocortisone and some other hormones enhance the expression of HTLV-III. *Int J Cancer,* Vol. 37, No. 1, pp. 67-72.

Meijsing, S.H., Pufall, M.A., So, A.Y., Bates, D.L., Chen, L. & Yamamoto, K.R. (2009). DNA binding site sequence directs glucocorticoid receptor structure and activity. *Science,* Vol. 324, No. 5925, pp. 407-10.

Mirani, M., Elenkov, I., Volpi, S., Hiroi, N., Chrousos, G.P. & Kino, T. (2002). HIV-1 protein Vpr suppresses IL-12 production from human monocytes by enhancing glucocorticoid action: potential implications of Vpr coactivator activity for the innate and cellular immunity deficits observed in HIV-1 infection. *J Immunol,* Vol. 169, No. 11, pp. 6361-8.

Mitra, D., Sikder, S.K. & Laurence, J. (1995). Role of glucocorticoid receptor binding sites in the human immunodeficiency virus type 1 long terminal repeat in steroid-mediated suppression of HIV gene expression. *Virology,* Vol. 214, No. 2, pp. 512-21.

Muthumani, K., Choo, A.Y., Zong, W.X., Madesh, M., Hwang, D.S., Premkumar, A., Thieu, K.P., Emmanuel, J., Kumar, S., Thompson, C.B. & Weiner, D.B. (2006). The HIV-1 Vpr and glucocorticoid receptor complex is a gain-of-function interaction that prevents the nuclear localization of PARP-1. *Nat Cell Biol,* Vol. 8, No. 2, pp. 170-9.

Nissen, R.M. & Yamamoto, K.R. (2000). The glucocorticoid receptor inhibits NFkappaB by interfering with serine-2 phosphorylation of the RNA polymerase II carboxy-terminal domain. *Genes Dev,* Vol. 14, No. 18, pp. 2314-29.

Pages, J.C., Loux, N., Farge, D., Briand, P. & Weber, A. (1995). Activation of Moloney murine leukemia virus LTR enhances the titer of recombinant retrovirus in psi CRIP packaging cells. *Gene Ther,* Vol. 2, No. 8, pp. 547-51.

Para, M.F., Schouten, J., Rosenkranz, S.L., Yu, S., Weiner, D., Tebas, P., White, C.J., Reeds, D., Lertora, J., Patterson, K.B., Daar, E.S., Cavert, W. & Brizz, B. (2010). Phase I/II trial of the anti-HIV activity of mifepristone in HIV-infected subjects ACTG 5200. *J Acquir Immune Defic Syndr,* Vol. 53, No. 4, pp. 491-5.

Pratt, W.B., Morishima, Y., Murphy, M. & Harrell, M. (2006). Chaperoning of glucocorticoid receptors. *Handb Exp Pharmacol*, No. 172, pp. 111-38.

Rhen, T. & Cidlowski, J.A. (2005). Antiinflammatory action of glucocorticoids--new mechanisms for old drugs. *N Engl J Med*, Vol. 353, No. 16, pp. 1711-23.

Rodriguez, J.J. & Goff, S.P. (2010). Xenotropic murine leukemia virus-related virus establishes an efficient spreading infection and exhibits enhanced transcriptional activity in prostate carcinoma cells. *J Virol*, Vol. 84, No. 5, pp. 2556-62.

Ross, E.K., Buckler-White, A.J., Rabson, A.B., Englund, G. & Martin, M.A. (1991). Contribution of NF-kappa B and Sp1 binding motifs to the replicative capacity of human immunodeficiency virus type 1: distinct patterns of viral growth are determined by T-cell types. *J Virol*, Vol. 65, No. 8, pp. 4350-8.

Roux, P., Alfieri, C., Hrimech, M., Cohen, E.A. & Tanner, J.E. (2000). Activation of transcription factors NF-kappaB and NF-IL-6 by human immunodeficiency virus type 1 protein R (Vpr) induces interleukin-8 expression. *J Virol*, Vol. 74, No. 10, pp. 4658-65.

Rusmevichientong, A. & Chow, S.A. (2010). Biology and pathophysiology of the new human retrovirus XMRV and its association with human disease. *Immunol Res*, Vol. 48, No. 1-3, pp. 27-39.

Schafer, E.A., Venkatachari, N.J. & Ayyavoo, V. (2006). Antiviral effects of mifepristone on human immunodeficiency virus type-1 (HIV-1): targeting Vpr and its cellular partner, the glucocorticoid receptor (GR). *Antiviral Res*, Vol. 72, No. 3, pp. 224-32.

Sherman, M.P., de Noronha, C.M., Pearce, D. & Greene, W.C. (2000). Human immunodeficiency virus type 1 Vpr contains two leucine-rich helices that mediate glucocorticoid receptor coactivation independently of its effects on G(2) cell cycle arrest. *J Virol*, Vol. 74, No. 17, pp. 8159-65.

Smoak, K.A. & Cidlowski, J.A. (2004). Mechanisms of glucocorticoid receptor signaling during inflammation. *Mech Ageing Dev*, Vol. 125, No. 10-11, pp. 697-706.

Solodushko, V., Bitko, V. & Fouty, B. (2009). Dexamethasone and mifepristone increase retroviral infectivity through different mechanisms. *Am J Physiol Lung Cell Mol Physiol*, Vol. 297, No. 3, pp. L538-45.

Solodushko, V. & Fouty, B. (2010). Mifepristone increases gamma-retroviral infection efficiency by enhancing the integration of virus into the genome of infected cells. *Gene Ther*, Vol. 17, No. 10, pp. 1253-61.

Somia, N. & Verma, I.M. (2000). Gene therapy: trials and tribulations. *Nat Rev Genet*, Vol. 1, No. 2, pp. 91-9.

Soudeyns, H., Geleziunas, R., Shyamala, G., Hiscott, J. & Wainberg, M.A. (1993). Identification of a novel glucocorticoid response element within the genome of the human immunodeficiency virus type 1. *Virology*, Vol. 194, No. 2, pp. 758-68.

Telesnitsky, A. (2010). Retroviruses: Molecular Biology, Genomics and Pathogenesis. *Future Virol*, Vol. 5, No. 5, pp. 539-543.

Thomas, C.E., Ehrhardt, A. & Kay, M.A. (2003). Progress and problems with the use of viral vectors for gene therapy. *Nat Rev Genet*, Vol. 4, No. 5, pp. 346-58.

Tuckermann, J.P., Reichardt, H.M., Arribas, R., Richter, K.H., Schutz, G. & Angel, P. (1999). The DNA binding-independent function of the glucocorticoid receptor mediates repression of AP-1-dependent genes in skin. *J Cell Biol*, Vol. 147, No. 7, pp. 1365-70.

Wiegers, K., Schwarck, D., Reimer, R. & Bohn, W. (2008). Activation of the glucocorticoid receptor releases unstimulated PBMCs from an early block in HIV-1 replication. *Virology,* Vol. 375, No. 1, pp. 73-84.

Wu, B.Y., Woffendin, C., Duckett, C.S., Ohno, T. & Nabel, G.J. (1995). Regulation of human retroviral latency by the NF-kappa B/I kappa B family: inhibition of human immunodeficiency virus replication by I kappa B through a Rev-dependent mechanism. *Proc Natl Acad Sci U S A,* Vol. 92, No. 5, pp. 1480-4.

Yi, Y., Hahm, S.H. & Lee, K.H. (2005). Retroviral gene therapy: safety issues and possible solutions. *Curr Gene Ther,* Vol. 5, No. 1, pp. 25-35.

Yu, S.F., von Ruden, T., Kantoff, P.W., Garber, C., Seiberg, M., Ruther, U., Anderson, W.F., Wagner, E.F. & Gilboa, E. (1986). Self-inactivating retroviral vectors designed for transfer of whole genes into mammalian cells. *Proc Natl Acad Sci U S A,* Vol. 83, No. 10, pp. 3194-8.

Part 2

Adenoviral Vector

5

Adenoviral Vectors: Potential and Challenges as a Gene Delivery System

Suresh K. Mittal, AnneMarie Swaim and Yadvinder S. Ahi
Department of Comparative Pathobiology, Purdue University Center for Cancer Research, and Bindley Bioscience Center, Purdue University, West Lafayette, IN, USA

1. Introduction

Adenoviruses (AdV) have been well delineated and made into suitable vectors for gene transfer by their somewhat benign nature, broad tissue tropism, and the relative ease of manipulation of their genome. These viruses readily transduce both quiescent and dividing cells, are adaptable for large scale production and have certified cell lines that have been developed for purification. Nevertheless, these vectors are not recommended for all purposes. Currently, adenoviral vectors are more widely evaluated in applications where a short-term transgene expression is sought after (i.e., cancer and vaccines) (Jolly et al., 2008; Sharma et al., 2009b).

Rowe and colleagues in 1953 were the first to isolate AdV from adenoidal tissue and to describe the spontaneous degeneration of primary cell lines from whence they were derived (Rowe WP et al., 1953). A similar virus was isolated from an epidemic of respiratory illness in U.S. military recruits in 1954 (Hilleman MR & Werner JH, 1954). In 1956, the viruses were named adenoviruses after the tissue from which they were isolated (Enders et al., 1956). Their anti-tumor potential was explored in the clinical treatment of cervical carcinoma following AdV inoculation not long after 1956 (Huebner et al., 1956). Despite this initial use, it took several years following the advent of recombinant technology before the therapeutic potential of AdV was truly realized. Since then, adenoviral vectors have received much attention as gene transfer agents and currently are being tested in a wide variety of gene therapy applications.

There are more than 120 AdV that infect a wide host range including mammalian, avian, and reptile species. AdV are divided into four genera: Atadenovirus, Aviadenovirus, Mastadenovirus, and Siadenovirus. Mastadenovirus serotypes which infect humans are placed in groups (A-F) or subgenera. Initial parameters for grouping were based on patterns of hemagglutination from various animal species; now the grouping is based on DNA homology. Some of these genera are being engineered for use as AdV vectors.

The *Adenoviridae* family is characterized by a linear, double-stranded DNA genome that is encapsulated in an icosohedral shell of protein that measures 70 to 90 nm in diameter. Virions of AdV are comprised of 13% DNA and 87% protein (Rux & Burnett, 2004; San & Burnett, 2003). Their genome is approximately 35-38 kilobases in size. The majority of the viral capsid encompasses three proteins: fiber, penton base and hexon. Fiber and penton base proteins are necessary for receptor binding and cell internalization, whereas hexon proteins form most of the viral capsid. These three proteins are also crucial targets of virus neutralizing antibodies.

AdV infections are common in humans and have relatively benign sequelae. Primarily, they are the etiologic agents that cause upper and lower respiratory infections. However, they do infect other tissues such as the eyes, gastrointestinal and urinary tracts, brain, heart, kidney, and liver where they pose minor health risks. Individuals with a normal immune system have self-limiting infections without notable clinical sequelae. Yet immunocompromised individuals may develop conditions more frequently associated with uncommon variants (i.e., group B, serotype 35). During infection, adenoviral DNA is not usually integrated into host cell chromosomes thereby minimizing concerns regarding insertional mutagenesis or potential germ line risks. The clinical mildness of a natural AdV infection is probably attributed to their immunogenicity which has made these viruses popular as gene transfer vectors. In spite of this positive side of their immunogenicity, these viruses without considerable modifications may not be useful for applications that necessitate long-term expression since they do not incorporate into the host genome.

1.1 Advantages of AdV vectors

There are several factors that contribute to the advantages of AdV-based vectors. The molecular mechanisms underlying the AdV genome and its life cycle have been extensively studied which has facilitated molecular manipulations of the viral genome in plasmid form. Only the packaging signal and the inverted terminal repeat (ITR) (approximately 300bp) are essential to package nearly 105% of the total AdV genome. This facilitates a decrease in the occurrence of replication-competent recombinants while also permitting introduction of a large transgene cassette (up to approx. 35kb) into the AdV virion. Additional benefits include relatively simple and reliable manufacturing methods, high levels of expression in various replicating and non-replicating tissues even at low temperatures, delineation of its toxicity profile, minimized risk of genomic insertional mutagenesis due to its episomal persistence in the nucleus, and extensive knowledge of the effects pertaining to vector genome uptake following a particular route of administration. Also, AdV vectors have demonstrated the ability to prime and boost T- and B-cell responses (Pinto et al., 2003; Vemula & Mittal, 2010). Most importantly, safety has been demonstrated in the therapeutic application of AdV vectors in a number of clinical trials (Sharma et al., 2009b).

AdV vectors can be generated to express multiple proteins from various expression cassettes located within the genome of the AdV. Vaccine formulations that exploit the advantages of these AdV vectors increase the potency and reduce the prospective costs. Also the use of multi-gene expression technology permits flexibility in vaccine design regarding rapid antigen swapping after AdV vector development. A prerequisite for such an AdV vector is that it must adequately express multiple antigens (Jolly et al., 2008). Finally, while some may view the transient nature of AdV vectors to be a disadvantage, it does have beneficial medical applications. AdV vectors have demonstrated therapeutic potential in treating various forms of cancer, infectious disease, and tissue remodeling.

1.2 Disadvantages of AdV vectors

Transient expression of the transgene by AdV vectors can be a disadvantage for gene therapy applications where continous expression of the trangene is necessary for a desired therapeutic effect. Due to the promiscuous nature of AdV biodistribution following systemic administration, targeting of the AdV vector to only a specific cell type is a considerable challenge.

AdV vectors at a very high dose could lead to significant toxicity. Expression of viral proteins by the AdV vector and activation of innate immunity are partially responsible for this *in vivo* toxicity. The deadly potential of AdV *in vivo* toxicity was highlighted after the intravascular delivery of an AdV to a patient enrolled in a clinical trial in 1999. A large dose of vector was administered into the hepatic artery of the patient recruited in a partial ornithine transcarbamylase (OTC) deficiency clinical trial. This large dose resulted in liver dysfunction and death due to multiple organ failure (Raper et al., 2003). The investigators concluded that the toxicity was due to the 'extremely high dose' (3.8×10^{13} virus particles) of AdV causing a saturation of the available AdV receptors on hepatocytes and the subsequent spread of the vector to other organs. The patient's death was thought to be due to strong activation of an innate immune response. This unfortunate event has led to new guidelines for the validation of new technologies.

AdV are a common human pathogen, especially human adenovirus 5 (HAdV5); therefore, *in vivo* delivery of AdV may be hampered due to pre-existing vector immunity in the majority of human population. Although low levels of vector immunity can be quelled by increasing the dose of administered AdV vector without increasing toxic side effects (Pratt et al., 2010), the issue of pre-existing vector immunity is a cause for concern. Challenges also exist in correlating the protective outcomes of the quality of T cell responses over the quantity of T cells that are stimulated by different immunization protocols and vector strategies. Priming with some AdV vectors stimulates transgene-specific immune responses that have a low correlation with type I interferon (IFN) production; the reduced levels are associated with reduced transgene expression. Reduced IFN also hampers quality T cell responses and B cell differentiation into effector plasma cells. However, too much type I IFN results in clearance by innate effector systems and poor transgene expression. Thus, type I IFN responses must be rigidly controlled to attain therapeutic efficacy (Draper & Heeney, 2010).

2. AdV induced innate immune response

The AdV vector-mediated acute toxicity subsequent to intravascular inoculation is known to be a direct result of potent activation of the innate immune system - a desirable outcome for the purpose of vaccine development or cancer immunotherapy (Muruve, 2004). The activated immune system in these scenarios also results in the induction of a stronger immune response against the desired antigen or cancer cells. However, this strong immune reaction remains an obstacle for AdV-mediated gene therapy since the danger of severe toxicity prevents administration of the dose necessary to achieve the desirable therapeutic effect. The immune system activation follows a dose-dependent pattern and is independent of viral gene expression. Immune system activation is manifested as severe liver inflammation, thrombocytopenia, and systemic flu-like symptoms such as fever and myalgias (Raper et al., 2002). The severe inflammatory response is also associated with poor target cell tranduction and loss of viral genome and transgene expression within two to three weeks post administration (Yang et al., 1994).

The initial host response to AdV vectors occurs within minutes after systemic administration and may last from several hours to days. It is characterized by elevated serum levels of proinflammatory cytokines such as tumor necrosis factor- α (TNF- α), IL-

6, IL-1β, IFN-γ, and chemokines such as macrophage inhibitory protein (MIP)-2, IFN-γ inducible protein 10 (IP-10), RANTES, MIP-1α, MIP-1β and monocyte chemoattaractant protein 1 ((MCP-1) (Muruve et al., 2004). Induction of inflammatory response to viral pathogens proceeds through opsonization, uptake of opsonized viral particles, antigen processing and presentation, and, finally, the release of inflammatory cytokines. Likewise, high doses of systemically administered AdV vectors result in activation of splenic dendritic cells (DCs) and macrophages inducing the production of inflammatory cytokines such as IL-6, IL-12 and TNF-α. Depletion of tissue macrophages and DCs prevents the production of the aforementioned cytokines, indicating a central role of these innate effectors in the acute inflammatory response (Kuzmin et al., 1997; Lieber et al., 1997; Zhang et al., 2001). Recently, an *in vitro* study using co-culture of epithelial cells and macrophages demonstrated the dependence of AdV-induced inflammatory response on the activation of macrophages through interactions with epithelial cells where the activation was mediated by NF-κB. AdV infection of the co-culture resulted in cytotoxicity, expression of inflammatory cytokines and chemokines, NOS and ROS generation and activation of inflammatory transcription factors (Lee et al., 2010). However, the nature of macrophage and epithelial cell interaction and their implications during AdV infection *in vivo* remain to be elucidated.

Neutrophils also seem to play an important role in AdV-induced acute inflammation. The chemokines, MCP-1, RANTES and MIP-1β, upregulate the neutrophil chemoattaractant chemokine MIP-2 which then recruits neutrophils to the liver. Recruitment of neutrophils and rapid induction of C-C and C-X-C chemokines correlates with acute liver injury and histopathological changes (Muruve et al., 1999). Moreover, AdV vectors are shown to activate endothelium in post-sinusoidal venules and promote P and E selectin-mediated rolling. This is followed by adhesion mediated through interactions between α4-integrin on the neutrophil surface and vascular cell adhesion molecule-1 (VCAM-1) on endothelial cells (Li et al., 2002). Blocking of either leukocyte rolling and adhesion or neutrophil depletion results in lower expression of the proinflammatory gene expression implying a central role of neutrophils in AdV-induced liver inflammation (Liu et al., 2003b). The neutrophils are recruited to the liver where they take up AdV particles in a complement receptor 1 (CR1)- and Fc receptor-dependent manner sequestering the AdV particles away from target cells (Cotter et al., 2005). How the neutrophil sequestration of AdV particles affects the vector-induced innate immune response calls for further exploration. Although other types of leukocytes such as monocytes and macrophages are also recruited to the liver, neutrophils constitute more than 70% of the total leukocytes in the liver following systemic AdV administration.

Natural killer (NK) cells are another cell type activated and populated to the liver following AdV infection and are directly associated with liver injury. Type 1 IFNs, produced in response to viral infection, promote activation of NK cells which mediate clearance of AdV genome and lowers transgene expression. Pre-treatment with anti-NK cells antibodies enhances AdV genome persistence, prolongs transgene expression and dampens the innate immune-mediated liver injury (Liu et al., 2003a; Zhu et al., 2007). A very interesting strategy to mitigate the impact of AdV-induced innate immune response would be to transiently remove the effector cells of the innate immune system, such as neutrophil and NK cells. Alternatively, in the light of evidence of IFN-γ-mediated NK cell activation, transient suppression of type 1 IFN response prior to AdV administration might also be beneficial (Zhu et al., 2007).

Several studies in the recent past have focused on delineating the molecular mechanisms governing AdV-mediated activation of the innate immune system. This system, being the first line of defense against invading pathogens, has evolved a highly conserved repertoire of 'pattern recognition receptors (PRRs)' which specifically identify 'pathogen-associated molecular patterns (PAMPs)' (Kumar et al., 2009). A variety of PRRs, including Toll-like receptors (TLRs), RIG-1-like receptors (RLRs) and Nod-like receptors (NLRs), are employed for the recognition of all types of pathogens ranging from bacteria, fungi, viruses and protozoa.

2.1 Role of TLR signaling in AdV-induced innate immune response

Depending on the cell type, the sensing of AdV by innate immune response is mediated by both TLR-dependent and independent pathways and appears to be very complex (Appledorn et al., 2008b; Cerullo et al., 2007; Nociari et al., 2007; Zhu et al., 2007). Among the members of the TLR family, four are known to recognize viral nucleic acids: TLR3 (dsRNA), TLR7, TLR8 (ssRNA) and TLR9 (dsDNA). The myeloid differentiation primary response gene 88 (MyD88), a TLR Adaptor protein for downstream activation of signaling cascades such as MAPK and NF-κB pathways, is necessary to initiate an AdV-induced proinflammatory cytokine and chemokine response (Hartman et al., 2007a; Hartman et al., 2007b). TLR9 is spatially and temporally co-localized with AdV as it is expressed in endosomes and is specifically upregulated during AdV infection. As a result, it effectively recognizes unmethylated CpG motifs in dsDNA released after proteolytic degradation of AdV particles within endosomes and initiates a signaling cascade through MyD88 in plasmacytoid DCs (pDCs). This culminates with their maturation and the production of high levels of type 1 IFNs as witnessed during AdV infection. The type 1 IFN production in pDCs is TLR9/MyD88-dependent, as opposed to non-pDCs which recognize AdV DNA through a cytosolic sensor different from TLR9. Significant amounts of type 1 IFNs are produced with an AdV infection. In addition to the activation of NK cells, the type 1 IFNs play a crucial role in the AdV-mediated activation of innate immune response by enhancing production of proinflammatory cytokines IL-6 and IL-12 (Zhu et al., 2007). TLR2 also plays a crucial role regulating AdV-induced innate immune response by mediating the rapid activation of MAPK and NF-kB pathways which are linked to induction of inflammatory cytokine and chemokine gene expression. Specifically, TLR2 is required for sustained late phase induction of these pathways; initial activation is TLR2 independent (Appledorn et al., 2008b; Tibbles et al., 2002).

The induction of chemokines MCP-1 and RANTES depends solely on TLR-9 within one hour post-infection (hpi), but relies on both TLR2 and TLR9 at eight hpi. Collectively, TLR2 and TLR9 play crucial roles through the differential induction of cytokines and chemokines. However, the induction of chemokines independent of both TLR2 and TLR9, was discovered to be MyD88-dependent at beth early and late time points suggesting the involvement of different MyD88- dependent sensors in the full spectrum induction of innate immune response (Appledorn et al., 2008b).

As noted above, AdV infection of non-pDCs such as conventional DCs (cDCs), macrophages and fibroblasts stimulates production of significant amounts of type 1 IFNs, proinflammatory cytokines and chemokines through phosphorylation of interferon regulatory factor (IRF)-3. The activation of IRF-3 occurs as a result of the recognition of AdV DNA by a yet unidentified cytosolic DNA sensor which promotes phosphorylation of IRF-3. The phosphorylation initiates IRF-3 dimerization and translocation to the nucleus where it causes transcriptional activation of several IRF-3 responsive inflammatory cytokine and chemokine genes (Hiscott, 2007; Nociari et al., 2007). However, AdV vectors can also induce IRF-3 phosphorylation directly through the capsid-cell membrane interactions prior to the endosomal escape of viral DNA, thereby providing an additional IRF-3 activation signal for stronger IFN and inflammatory response (Nociari et al., 2009). Evidently, AdV infection induces type 1 IFN response through multiple pathways and, therefore, causes a very strong activation of IFN responsive genes which might explain the powerful induction of innate immune response following AdV infection.

The NALP3 protein, a type of Nod-like receptor, plays an important role in cytosolic sensing of AdV DNA and the subsequent induction of proinflammatory IL-1β response. However, NALP3 is a general sensor for any kind of dsDNA including viral, bacterial, or even host (mammalian DNA) (Martinon et al., 2009). AdV DNA was shown *in vitro* to activate NALP3 signaling events through apoptosis-associated speck-like protein containing caspase recruitment domain (ASC), the adaptor protein for NALP3, resulting in the recruitment of the inflammatory caspase-1 into the molecular complex called the inflammasome which activates caspase-1. The activated caspase-1 initiates the proteolytic cleavage of pro-IL-1β into an active and secreted form of IL-1β. A similar response was detected upon infection with first generation AdV vectors, helper-dependent (HD) AdV vectors, and by transfecting cells with AdV DNA implying that the nature of DNA did not affect inflammasome activation. However, empty capsids failed to elicit a similar response suggesting that mere internalization of the capsid proteins was not enough for the inflammatory response. Furthermore, NALP-, ASC- and caspase-1-deficient mice systemically injected with AdV vectors developed only a blunted inflammatory response in the liver and showed a remarkable reduction in the expression of NF-kB regulated pro-inflammatory genes confirming the role of NALP3 and inflammasome in AdV-induced innate immune response (Muruve et al., 2008). Furthermore, recognition of AdV DNA through endosomally expressed TLR9 upregulated expression of NALP3, ASC and pro-IL-1β thereby tuning the cellular environment for a stronger IL-1β response.(Barlan et al., 2011)

2.2 AdV interactions with blood factors

In addition to immune responses, successful gene therapy will depend on organ specific delivery and an adequate expression level of the gene of interest. Following intravascular delivery, AdV vectors first come in contact with blood and its components. Considering the diverse cell types and myriad of proteins with roles in processes as complex as immune response, coagulation, cell signaling and others, it is not surprising that interactions between AdV vectors and blood components are pivotal in shaping the biodistribution profile of intravascularly delivered AdV and, also, the complexity of the ensuing host immune response (Parker et al., 2008). Therefore, a thorough understanding of AdV and blood factor interactions is advantageous in devising novel strategies to preclude deleterious interactions and to efficiently target vector delivery to the organ.

Based on *in vitro* experiments, the classical pathway for AdV internalization involves a primary interaction of fiber knob domain with Coxsackievirus and adenovirus receptor (CAR) resulting in viral attachment to cell surface, followed by a secondary interaction of the RGD motif on a penton base with integrins promoting internalization of the attached virus via receptor-mediated endocytosis. However, the *in vivo* biodistribution pattern cannot be attributed to knob-CAR interaction alone since CAR follows a ubiquitous expression profile, whereas the majority of intravascularly delivered AdV is sequestered primarily in the liver. Further, HAdV5 vectors modified by inserting retargeting peptides and ablated for CAR binding fail to efficiently retarget to intended sites (Nicklin et al., 2005). These observations suggest involvement of CAR-independent pathways of cellular transduction *in vivo* by AdV. Heparan sulfate proteoglycans (HSPG) and LDL receptor-related proteins (LRP) were identified as alternative receptors for AdV transduction of liver cells. Initially, the blood coagulation factor IX and complement factor C4BP were shown to bind to HAdV5 and HAdV35 fiber knobs and bridge them to HSPG and LRP, thereby providing a 'CAR-independent' pathway of AdV infection *in vivo*.

Transduction of Kupffer cells which sequester the majority of the AdV transducing the liver is CAR-independent; hepatocytes rely on CAR-dependent, as well as CAR-independent, pathways for AdV uptake (Shayakhmetov et al., 2005). Consequently, abrogation of the factor IX- and factor C4BP-mediated AdV transduction can be an effective strategy for precluding AdV sequestration in Kupffer cells which contributes significantly to a proinflammatory cytokine and chemokine response to systemic administration of AdV vectors (Lieber et al., 1997; Manickan et al., 2006). Preventing Kupffer cell transduction can simultaneously provide dual benefits for effective liver gene therapy by mitigating the innate immune response and enhancing hepatocyte transduction through greater bioavailability of the vector.

The Vitamin K-dependent blood coagulation factors FVIII, FIX, FX and protein C also appear to play crucial roles in hepatocyte transduction through interactions with the HAdV5 viral capsid. Of note, these coagulation factors contain a conserved domain with an identical, defined structure comprising of a γ-carboxyglutamate (Gla)-EGF-1-EGF-2-serine protease domain which supposedly arose due to gene duplication. All of these factors significantly enhance hepatocyte transduction *in vitro* with factors FX and protein C being more efficient than factors FVIII and FIX through mediating interactions between the capsid, and the alternate AdV receptors, HSPGs and LRP. Interestingly, the factors did not exert an additive effect on transduction as they all seem to bind at a common site on the capsid and, therefore, might have an overlapping role in mediating AdV entry. Depletion of vitamin K-dependent blood coagulation factors in mice through warfarin treatment prior to intravascular AdV administration resulted in a remarkable reduction in hepatocyte transduction. This effect could be reversed by restoring physiological levels of factor FX just prior to AdV inoculation (Parker et al., 2006). The relevance of factor FX - hexon interaction to AdV vector biology is justified by swapping the hypervariable regions (HVRs) of HAdV5 with those from HAdV48, a non-factor FX-binding serotype, which absolutely abrogates the interaction and also decreases the hepatocyte transduction by more than 150-fold. The interaction between factor FX and the capsid hexon is calcium-dependent and mediated by the (Gla)-EGF1 domain of factor FX and the HVRs of hexons. No other capsid proteins play any role in the factor FX-capsid interaction. Furthermore, the hexon from all human AdV serotypes does not bind factor FX equally; serotypes 5, 2, 50 and 16 show strong binding, while serotypes 35 and 3 show weak binding, and serotypes 26 and 48 show no binding (Waddington et al., 2008). Construction of hexon swapped AdV vectors should be performed accordingly, keeping in mind the factor FX binding ability of the serotype and the intended clinical use of the vector. While constructing AdV vectors targeted to specific sites, tissue-specific fiber modifications must be accompanied by appropriate hexon HVR modifications large enough to ablate factor FX binding yet small enough to allow the chimeric virus rescue.

A recent study suggested that AdV sequestration in the liver is a collective result of a defined set of molecular mechanisms occurring in a redundant, sequential and synergistic pathway (Di Paolo et al., 2009). In addition to the trapping of intravascular AdV by Kupffer cells and hepatocytes through interactions with blood factors, the AdV penton base-β3-integrin interaction becomes predominant in the absence of other virus clearance mechanisms. Combined treatment with chlodronate liposomes and warfarin removes Kupffer cells and inactivates vitamin K-dependent blood factor, prevents AdV entry into Kupffer cells and hepatocytes, and, therefore, might force AdV to accumulate in the liver sinusoidal space. Here the interaction between penton base RGD motif and β3-integrin may promote AdV uptake by sinusoidal endothelial cells (Di Paolo et al., 2009). These observations led to the proposal of a three step, dose-dependent model of AdV sequestration in the liver. At low doses, Kupffer cells are the primary niche for AdV retained in the liver. When the dose is higher and exceeds Kupffer cell capacity, the excess AdV enter hepatocytes in a blood factor-dependent manner. At an even higher dose, both Kupffer cells and hepatocytes become fully loaded, and AdV start entering sinusoidal epithelial cells. Following these principles, complete elimination of liver retention of systemically delivered AdV through simultaneous blocking of all three mechanisms might enhance the bioavailability of AdV vectors for gene therapy applications of extrahepatic organs and preclude induction of innate immune-mediated hepatotoxicity from reaching dangerous levels.

3. Adaptive immune responses to AdV vectors

AdV vector-mediated transduction *in vivo* results in efficient but transient transgene expression in various organs with the exception of those in newborn, immunocompromised or immunodeficient animals. The loss of transgene expression is attributed to a low basal level expression of AdV proteins despite the absence of E1A and E1B (Yang et al., 1994). Apart from induction of a strong innate immune response, AdV vectors also elicit adaptive immune responses directed towards the capsid components. The induction of adaptive immunity is profoundly influenced by the activated innate immune response (Descamps & Benihoud, 2009). The AdV-specific cellular immune response is induced through the uptake of AdV particles by antigen-presenting cells such as macrophages and DCs and the presentation of peptides derived from capsid proteins through MHC class I and class II pathways. Subsequently, the CTLs recognize and destroy the host cells displaying AdV-specific peptides, thereby leading to diminished transgene expression in immunocompetent hosts (Schagen et al., 2004). Macrophages also play a role in transporting AdV to draining lymph nodes, where AdV-specific B lymphocytes are activated resulting in an AdV-specific humoral immune response comprising of anti-AdV antibodies directed against capsid proteins (Junt et al., 2007).

The HD-AdV vectors, due to a lack of all viral genes, effectively remain unseen by the immune system and consequently cause a severely attenuated adaptive immune response. However, a transgene-specific immune response can be induced causing elimination of the host cells expressing the target protein in addition to antibody-mediated clearance of secreted target protein from circulation. The problem of anti-transgene immunity is unique and no less confounding than vector-associated primary complications since immunity may vary with the nature of transgene, animal model or even individual (Brown et al., 2004). On the positive side, HD-AdV vector-based gene therapy studies in various mouse and rat models of diseases such as diabetes, hemophilia, familial hypercholesterolemia, ornithine transcarbamylase deficiency, and Crigler Najjar syndrome produced favorable results through long-term phenotypic correction implying transgene-specific immunity may not be a significant hindrance (Seiler et al., 2007).

3.1 Significance of pre-existing vector immunity

More than 80% of the human population has been exposed to one or more serotypes among over fifty different serotypes of human AdV (Harvey et al., 1999; Xiang et al., 2006). The adjuvant effect of AdV results in development of strong anti-viral humoral and cellular immune responses in the pre-exposed individuals. These neutralizing antibodies are serotype-specific and are directed toward the viral capsid proteins. Similarly, the AdV-specific CD8+ T cells against both viral structural and non-structural proteins as well as the transgene will eliminate AdV-transduced cells (Tang et al., 2006). In the absence of pre-existing immunity, re-administration of homologous vector mimics vector administration in the presence of pre-existing immunity. Therefore, first and second generation AdV vectors are not suitable for correction of disorders requiring multiple vector inoculations and are limited to only those applications requiring short-term transgene expression or circumvention of vector immunity, either natural or induced. The presence of anti-AdV antibodies also enhances AdV uptake by DCs and macrophages via interaction with the Fc-receptor (FcR), but without a consequent increase in transgene expression. Pre-immunization with homologous vectors has been shown to exacerbate vector-induced hepatotoxicity and increase mortality rates (Vlachaki et al., 2002) which might be the indirect consequences of stronger innate immune activation.

4. Evolution of AdV vector systems

Despite early observations, it took several years following the advent of recombinant technology before the therapeutic potential of AdV was truly realized. The first generation AdV vectors (FGAdV) have a deleted early region (E) 1 (E1). The E1 region has two subunits E1A and E1B (Dormond et al., 2009). E1A deletions impair vector replication, down regulate transactivation of other early units, and deregulate cell cycle controls. However, this deletion does permit transgene expression capacity up to 5kb. E1B primarily inhibits apoptotic cell signaling. Most of these vectors also have a deletion in E3, which does not hinder *in vitro* growth but adds 3kb worth of transgene capacity. The different types of AdV vectors are described below and illustrated in Figure 1.

The Frank Graham Laboratory in 1977 developed a human embryonic kidney-derived 293 cell line that expresses the E1 gene products *in trans* thereby enabling the production of the first recombinant AdV (rAdV) in a helper-free environment (Graham et al., 1977). The 293 cell line used in vector manufacturing has nucleotides 1-4344 of the left end of the AdV genome which provides considerable overlap in the sequences with conventional vectors. These overlapping sequences within the cell promote homologous recombination between the vector and the AdV sequences which can generate replication-competent AdV (RCAdV) recombinants during the process of amplification.

Currently, the FDA has ruled that there must be less than one RCA per 3 x 10^{10} vector particles (Jolly et al., 2008). New cell lines, such as PER.C6 (Fallaux et al., 1998) and SL0036 (Howe et al., 2006), have been developed which abrogate sequence overlap and reduce RCAdV occurrence. Another method to diminish sequence overlap and reduce RCAdV risk has been to transfer a protein encoding gene into the cell genome which encodes for pIX, a minor AdV capsid protein (Hehir et al., 1996). The introduction of stuffer DNA into the E3 region is an additional method which increases the FGAdV DNA size but renders the system unpackageable in E1-recombined viral DNA progeny.

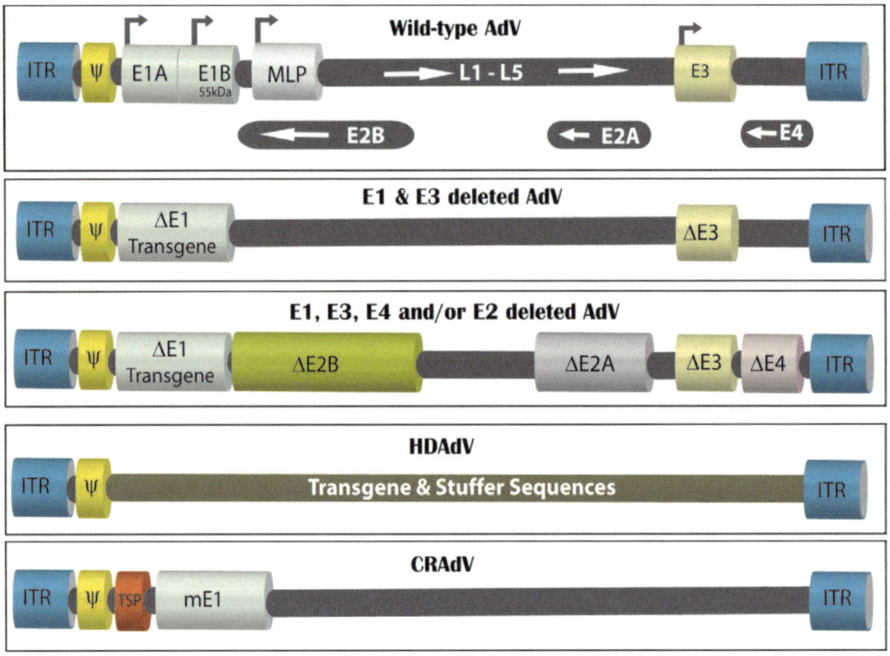

Fig. 1. Representative Diagram of the wild type AdV genome and different deletions in the various AdV vector constructs. E1 - E4: early transcription regions; L1 - L5: late transcription regions; ITRs: inverted terminal repeats; ψ: packaging signal; mE1: mutated E1; TSP: tumor-specific promoter.

In order to reduce the *in vivo* toxicity associated with the FGAdV, the second generation AdV vectors (SGAdV) were developed with additional deletions in their vector constructs. The initial E1 or E1/E3 deletions are supplemented with full or partial deletions in E2 and/or E4. Complementing cell lines are designed to constitutively express the matching E2/E4 region, but isolating these cell lines is a time-consuming process. The propagation of these vector constructs is less likely to generate RCAdV but will also have a lower yield. Although production possesses its own problems, it ultimately limits effects on immunogenicity resulting in the loss of interest for these multiple regions-deleted vectors (Lusky et al., 1998; Morral et al., 2002; O'Neal et al., 1998). Ultimately, long term expression and added safety were not attained with SGAdV (Dormond et al., 2009).

The further deletions of viral encoding genes that were gradually introduced to address safety concerns gave rise to the third generation AdV vectors (TGAdV). TGAdV lack all non-essential viral sequences. The TGAdV or helper-dependent AdV (HD-AdV) rely on helper-dependent systems in order to be generated. Along with the packaging signals, the inverted terminal repeats (ITRs) of AdV are required *in cis* to initiate replication (Grable & Hearing, 1992). Non-coding stuffer DNA is introduced into the 36kb of space that is available for transgene insertion. Helper functions are furnished by FGAdV which are also referred to as helper AdV. Initially, this class of AdV yielded a low number of TGAdV and a high level of contamination from helper AdV (Kochanek, 1999; Mitani et al., 1995). The purification of TGAdV from FGAdV by density gradient is a difficult task (Kumar-Singh & Chamberlain, 1996; Mitani et al., 1995; Parks & Graham, 1997). To facilitate better separation, the size of TGAdV should not exceed 32 kb which permits a better separation from the 36 kb FGAdV.

A recombinase system has been introduced into the TGAdV platform in order to reduce the amount of contamination (Hardy et al., 1997; Lieber et al., 1996; Parks et al., 1996). Adding a recombinase recognition site next to the packaging signal of the helper AdV yields an unpackageable FGAdV while co-infecting into HEK293 cells that constitutively express the respective recombinase. Currently, three recombinase systems have been employed: (1) Cre/LoxP, (2) FLP/frt and (3) C31/attB-attP (Alba et al., 2007; Ng et al., 2001; Umana et al., 2001). The two latter systems possess similar potential for the removal of FGAdV (Ng et al., 2001; Umana et al., 2001). Certain sequences on the TGAdV genome influence the yield. The stuffer DNA that is selected is of non-coding human DNA origin with minimized repeating sequences (Parks et al., 1999; Sandig et al., 2000; Schiedner et al., 2002). A promoter in the E4 region has provided amplification enhancement to TGAdV (Sandig et al., 2000). Additional amplification has been accomplished by the strategic development of FGAdV (Zhou et al., 2002). Sequence homology between packaging signals of the FGAdV and TGAdV should be avoided in order to limit the recombination events (Hardy et al., 1997; Sandig et al., 2000).

Complementary cell lines used in the production of TGAdV were derived from those that produce FGAdV and SGAdV. Furthermore, these cell lines express the respective recombinase enzyme such as Cre, FLP, or C31 (Alba et al., 2007; Ng et al., 2001; Umana et al., 2001). Generating competent cell lines that amplify TGAdV, while limiting FGAdV contamination has been difficult. Investigators have demonstrated that FGAdV contamination is due to the AdV-mediated shutoff of the host cell (Hartigan-O'Connor et al., 2002). The appearance of RCAs in TGAdV preparations has been attributed to a low level of FGAdV serving as helper AdV. Yet, production methods that necessitate that two viral constructs be present during serial passages increases the incidence of RCA. The use of PERC.6, a cell line which minimizes homology (Sakhuja et al., 2003), and the addition of stuffer DNA into the E3 region of FGAdV DNA (Parks et al., 1996) which limits encapsidation are useful solutions to minimizing RCAs.

Some AdV constructs have been changed to focus on the targeting potential instead of deleting multiple regions. Various methods are based on the rationale of expanding the otherwise limited tropism of the AdV while also reducing the potential toxicity seen in non-target tissue during over expression thereby improving the odds for systemic delivery. There are two approaches used in targeting: the modification of the virion to specifically transduce targeted cells or the use of gene regulation to restrict transgene expression to desired tissues. Tissue restriction modifications can be accomplished by genetically modifying the fiber-knob structure or through the covalent binding of a "bridging" molecule to the virion (Fattori et al., 2006; Folgori et al., 2006; Gherardi et al., 2003; Heeney et al., 2000; Lemckert et al., 2005; Liu et al., 2009; Shiver et al., 2002; Yu et al., 2008). Modification possibilities are limitless and range from the addition of de novo peptides or fiber-knob hybrids that combine other human and nonhuman AdV to exploitation of common receptor-ligand interactions to variations in RGD or similar motifs (Jolly et al., 2008). The bridging molecule method is advantageous since multiple antibodies and ligands can be implemented to form bispecific (target and AdV) bridges between the vector and the target cell type. Despite the advantages, each bispecific molecule and virion combination will possess unique effects, distribution, and toxicity profiles which will have to be defined both individually and as a constituent of a biological complex used in clinical data for drug trials. Retargeted or unique serotype vectors may prove efficacious in bypassing anti-vector immunity which could otherwise disturb transgene delivery used in

vaccine applications. Promising preclinical data with canine and nonhuman primate AdV exists (Alejo et al., 2006; Beveridge et al., 2007; McElrath et al., 2008).
Transcriptional targeting is achieved by placing a gene of interest under the control of a tissue- or tumor-specific promoter. This construct possesses potential for desired long term gene expression especially when small levels of expression in nontargeted cells can significantly impact potency or toxicity. One of the first constructs implemented in a human lung cancer cell line used the carcinoembryonic antigen promoter (CEA) to drive expression of the thymidine kinase gene derived from the herpes simplex virus (Liu et al., 2008a). Other promoters have been used which possess similar efficacy while simultaneously reducing the vector toxicity (Geiben-Lynn et al., 2008; Jego et al., 2003).
Conditionally replicating AdV vectors (CRAdV) have been implemented in cancer therapeutics because lysis of solid tumor masses requires a replicating vector in order to penetrate and spread through the tumor cells (Everts & van der Poel, 2005). The first class of deletion mutant CRAdV was designed so that a portion of E1 remains intact. Either E1A or E1B are mutated in order to confer replicative capacity only in human tumor cells which possess an impaired retinoblastoma tumor suppressor (Rb) or p53 gene. The second class of CRAdV possesses a tissue specific promoter upstream of E1A which restricts replication only in the target cells. Class 1 and 2 CRAdV have been adequately produced in E1-containing cell lines. RCAdV-preventing cell lines such as HeLA or A549 have also been implemented in CRAdV production (Longley et al., 2005; Yuk et al., 2004).

5. AdV vectors as a gene therapy tool

One of the important applications of gene therapy is the treatment of patients with monogenic recessive disorders by delivery of the mutated or non-functional gene. Hemophilia, cystic fibrosis and muscular dystrophies are some of the several thousand inherited disorders that can, in principle, be corrected by gene therapy. The various techniques used for delivery of therapeutic genes include viral vectors, physical methods, chemical methods and naked nucleic acids. A successful gene therapy program requires an efficient gene delivery system and targeting of a specific cell type without dissemination of the therapeutic gene to other cells thereby allowing longer persistence and adequate expression of the replaced gene. In the case of viral vectors, the host immune response may become a significant barrier to gene delivery and impede the overall success of the gene therapy effort.
AdV-based vectors were initially thought to be very promising candidates for gene therapy applications for genetic disorders. However, the progress of AdV vectors have been hampered by vector immunity and the toxicity induced by AdV vectors following systemic administration. The pre-existing anti-AdV neutralizing antibodies in the majority of the human population induced following natural exposure to AdV clears the AdV vectors soon after systemic administration. In the absence of pre-existing anti-AdV antibodies, the AdV vectors persist longer following initial inoculation. Repeated administration results in development of a neutralizing antibody response similar to natural infection preventing subsequent inoculations with the same vector from being effective.
The death of the patient in the ornithine transcarbamylase (OTC) clinical trial (Raper et al., 2003) and the results of several subsequent pre-clinical trials shifted the focus of AdV research towards the molecular mechanisms underlying AdV-induced innate immune pathways leading to development of AdV vectors, such as HD-AdV vectors, particularly suited for gene therapy applications. These HD-AdV vectors, due to the deletion of most of

the viral genome, can accommodate inserts as large as 36 Kb, making them the vector of choice for delivering very large genes, multiple genes or ta tissue-specific regulatory promoter which may be very long (Shi et al., 2002; Shi et al., 2006). The host cells transduced by HD-AdV vectors do not express the viral proteins and, therefore, cells carrying HD-AdV are not recognized by the host immune system resulting in longer persistence and transgene expression.

5.1 HD-AdV for liver gene therapy

The liver is the most affected organ in several genetic diseases including Crigler-Najjar syndrome and OTC deficiency. HD-AdV vectors have shown tremendous promise for liver directed gene therapy in several pre-clinical studies in small and large animal models. Their abilities to support long-term transgene expression, low chronic toxicity, natural liver tropism of AdV vectors and the fenestrated structure of liver endothelium allowing efficient hepatocyte transduction are the main factors (Brunetti-Pierri et al., 2008; Dimmock et al., 2011; Toietta et al., 2005). HD-AdV vectors were shown to be very effective for liver gene therapy in Gunn rats, the animal model for Crigler-Najjar syndrome. A single injection of a HD-AdV vector expressing uridine diphospho-glucuronosyl transferase 1A1 (UGT1A) was sufficient to induce life-long normalization of hyperbilirubinemia (Toietta et al., 2005). Similarly, an HD-AdV vector expressing canine glycogen-6-phosphatase was able to correct the hypoglycemia and prolong survival up to seven months in a mouse model of glycogen storage disease type 1 (Koeberl et al., 2007). Results of several other studies have supported the clinical utility of HD-AdV vectors in the gene therapy of liver diseases (Brunetti-Pierri et al., 2008; Gau et al., 2009; Hu et al., 2011; McCormack, Jr. et al., 2006; Oka et al., 2007).

However, the prospects of liver directed gene therapy using HD-AdV vectors are hampered by the high vector doses necessary to result in efficient hepatocyte transduction. Such high doses may not be clinically relevant for human use. A non-linear relation is observed between the vector dose and hepatocyte transduction; at low doses, there is very little to undetectable transgene expression, yet there are disproportionately high levels of transgene expression when vector dose is increased (Morral et al., 2002; Sullivan et al., 1997) with the Kupffer cells sequestering more than 85% of the intravascularly administered AdV vectors. AdV vectors also associate with platelets, red blood cells and other binding components in circulation resulting in eventual elimination of the vector. Sequestration by Kupffer cells and binding to the blood components determines the 'threshold dose' which must be administered for efficient hepatocyte transduction. Unfortunately, such high doses precipitate acute toxicity due to activation of the innate immune system and might result in the death of patient as observed during the human clinical trial for gene therapy of OTC deficiency (Raper et al., 2003). This conundrum warrants a thorough understanding of mechanisms underlying AdV-mediated innate immune system induction and calls for development of novel strategies to achieve high level hepatocyte transduction at clinically relevant doses.

5.2 HD-AdV for brain gene therapy

Due to the complexity of tissue organization in the nervous system, treatment of neurological disorders imposes a huge challenge to both healthcare providers and clinical researchers alike. HD-AdV gene therapy is currently being employed in preclinical trials as well as in animal models in the cases of brain cancer, sensory neuronopathies, neurodegenerative diseases, and multiple sclerosis, to name a few. Despite pre-exposure to

AdV, the sustained transgene expression in the brain for at least one year (Barcia et al., 2007) and the ability to infect the cells of the central nervous system renders HD-AdV vectors particularly appealing for brain gene therapy.

5.2.1 Gliomas

The tumor originating from glial cells is called a glioma which is highly lethal and associated with a median survival of mere 9-12 months (Furnari et al., 2007). Among gliomas, Glioblastoma multiforme (GBM) is the most common and so far incurable; aggressive primary brain cancer in adults has a median survival time of 15-21 months (Grossman et al., 2010). GBM is highly invasive with a limited potential for complete resection and a high recurrence rate owing to its resistance towards conventional chemotherapy and radiotherapy. A combination of HD-AdV-TK (cytotoxic herpes simplex type 1 thymidine kinase/HSV1-TK) and HD-AdV vector encoding Flt3L (human soluble fms-like tyrosine kinase ligand 3) under the control of a tightly regulatable mCMV-TetOn expression system (HC-AdV-TetOn-Flt3L29–31) was tried in rats bearing GBM (Muhammad et al., 2010). As a result of intratumoral administration of HD-AdV vectors, tumor cells were rapidly removed from the brain, and ~70% of the animals showed a reduction in the tumor mass within thirty days of the treatment leading to a long-term survival rate. The treatment also ensured the safety of the protocol with a one-year follow-up indicating the lack of behavioral deficits, chronic inflammation in the brain or alteration in the brain architecture. Furthermore, in order to lower the vector dose and improve production yield, a bi-cistronic HD-AdV vector has been developed "that encodes both constitutively expressed HSV1-TK and inducible Flt3L from a single HD-AdV vector genome" - the first one of its kind (Puntel et al., 2010).

5.2.2 Sensory neuronopathies

Dorsal root ganglion (DRG) neuron dysfunction is commonly associated with a number of sensory neuronopathies, and therefore, DRG comprises the target of choice for their treatment. Undesirable side effects of conventional treatments can be minimized by targeted gene delivery towards DRG neurons (Waehler et al., 2007). Fiber modified HD-AdV vectors have been engineered to specifically target DRG neurons in mice (Terashima et al., 2009) and were also tested in *Hexb–/–* mice, an animal model exhibiting neurological impairment leading to death before the age of twenty weeks (Sango et al., 2002). DRG-targeted HD-AdV vectors were injected through an intra-thecal route and were shown to have a significantly higher transduction of DRG neurons compared to unmodified HD-AdV vectors. Testing in Hexb–/– mice also showed production of β-hexosaminidase in the original Hexb-deficient mice as well as a reversal of gangliosidosis and improvement in peripheral sensory dysfunction (Terashima et al., 2009).

5.2.3 Neurodegenerative diseases

A helper-dependent canine AdV (CAdV-2) vector was designed and tested by Soudais et al (2003) and was proposed to be useful in the treatment of neurodegenerative diseases (Soudais et al., 2004). The advantages associated with this particular vector include preferential transduction of the neurons and retrograde transportation through the axons. Due to the chronic nature of neurodegenerative diseases, it is of particular interest whether the treatment can be offered over a long period of time. HD-AdV vectors have been administered into the cerebrospinal fluid (CSF) of non-human primates through lumbar puncture, and it was shown that the intervention allowed a long-lasting (three months) infection of the neuroepithelial cells without any systemic or local toxicity (Butti et al., 2008).

5.2.4 Multiple sclerosis

The ability of HD-AdV vectors to express anti-inflammatory molecules can be useful in inflammatory disorders of the central nervous system. Experimental autoimmune encephalomyelitis (EAE) is an animal model of multiple sclerosis that has been adopted for pre-clinical studies. HD-AdV vectors expressing IL-4 were administered into the CSF of immunocompetent mice that allowed transduction of neuroepithelial cells and prolonged (five months) transgene expression without any adverse effects (Butti et al., 2008).

6. AdV vectors for cancer therapy

Not long after the discovery of existence of AdV, AdV were noted for their oncolytic nature in the clinical treatment of cervical carcinoma. Since that time, AdV have shown promise in the cancer vaccine field and currently offer a variety of methodologies which are being implemented to combat various forms of cancer (Table 1). The field of cancer vaccinology is fraught with complications since an effectively persistent immune response must be stimulated. One complication lies in the fact that immune tolerance must be overcome against self-antigens. These self-antigens, which are weak stimulators of the immune system or completely lack the ability to be immunogenic in an immunocompromised environment, pose quite a hurdle in the cancer vaccine development.

AdV	Condition	Intervention	Route of Inoculation	Phase	Sponsor
		Cancer			
Replication defective AdV5 [E1-, E2b-]-CEA(6D) [ETBX-011]	Advanced or metastatic malignancies expressing CEA (colon cancer, lung cancer, breast cancer)	Biological: Ad5 CEA Vaccine	s.q.	I	Etubics Corp.
Replication defective, Adv/CMV.rhENDO (AdVE10A)	Head and Neck Squamous Carcinoma Nasopharyngeal Carcinoma	Drug: E10A Drug: Cisplatin Drug: Paclitaxel	i.t.	II	Sun Yat-sen University
Replication defective E1-,E3-deleted HAdV5/CD40L gene driven by RSV promoter	Bladder cancer	Genetic: AdCD40L	Intravesical	I / II	Uppsala University
E1a and E1b-deleted CRrAdV5-p53 (SCH-58500)	recurrent, or progressive glioblastoma multiforme, anaplastic astrocytoma, or anaplastic mixed glioma	Biological: recombinant adenovirus-p53 SCH-58500	i.t.	I	National Cancer Institute (NCI)

AdV	Condition	Intervention	Route of Inoculation	Phase	Sponsor
Infectivity enhanced CRAdV5/tk (GliAtak) (PancAtak) (ProstAtak)	malignant glioma, glioblastoma multiforme, anaplastic astrocytoma, pancreatic cancer, prostate cancer	Biological: AdV-tk Drug: Valacyclovir + Standard Chemo-/Radio- therapy	i.t.	II	Advantagene Inc.
Replication defective E1a/E1b/E3 HAdV5.IL2 into autologous neuroblastoma cells	Neuroblastoma	Biological: autologous neuroblastoma vaccine	s.q.	I / II	Baylor College of Medicine
AdV.IFNgamma (TG1042)	Relapsing primary cutaneous B-Cell Lymphoma	Genetic: Adenovirus Interferon gamma	intralesional	II	Transgene
Replication-defective E1/E3-deleted AdVHer2/neu under the control of MMTV promoter transduced into DC	breast neoplasm	Biological: CD34+ derived DCs	intradermal	I	Hamilton Health Sciences Corporation
E1/E2a/E3-deleted HDAdV expressing rat Her2/neus	metastatic breast cancer, recurrent breast cancer	Biological: adenoviral vector encoding rat Her-2/neu	intradermal	I	Ontario Clinical Oncology Group (OCOG)
Replication deficient, E1/E3 deleted rAdV/RSV-hIL12 gene	primary metastatic breast cancer spread to liver	Biological: adenovirus-mediated human interleukin-12	i.t.	I	Mount Sinai School of Medicine
Replication-incompetent Ad-sig-hMUC-1/ecdCD40L vaccine	MUC-1 positive cancer cells in metastatic breast cancer	Biological: Ad-sig-hMUC-1/ecdCD40L vaccine	s.q.	I	University of California, Los Angeles
Replication defective, recombinant Ad.hIFNbeta gene	Colorectal carcinoma metastases	Drug: Ad.hIFNbeta (BG0001, IDEC-201)	i.v.	I / II	Biogen Idec
Replication-deficient (E1, E3 and E4 deleted) AdV containing TNF-alpha gene under control of radiation inducible promoter	Esophageal cancer	Genetic: TNFerade	i.t.	II	GenVec
Replication-deficient E1/E3 deleted rAdcuCD40L	Esophageal neoplasms	Genetic: AdcuCD40L	i.t.	I / II	Weill Medical College of Cornell University
(INGN 201) (Advexin®)HAd5CMV/p53	Head and Neck Cancer: premalignant carcinoma of the oral cavity or pharynx	Biological: Ad5CMV-p53 gene	oral rinse	I / II	M.D. Anderson Cancer Center
HAd5F35.LMP1/LMP2-DC	Head and Neck Cancer: metastatic nasopharyngeal cancer	Biological: Ad5F35-LMP1/LMP2-transduced autologous DC Drug: celecoxib	intradermal	II	NCC Head and Neck Clinic

AdV	Condition	Intervention	Route of Inoculation	Phase	Sponsor
Replication defective AdV w/TK, TK99UN suicide gene therapy	Carcinoma, hepatocellular	Genetic: TK99UN	i.t.	I	Instituto Cientifico y Tecnologico de Navarra, Universidad de Navarra
AdVhAFP	Locoregionally pre-treated hepatocellular carcinoma	Drug: AFP + GM-CSF Plasmid Prime and AdV/hAFP Boost	i.m.	I / II	University of Pittsburgh
AdV.p53-DC	Extensive Stage Small Cell Lung Cancer	Biological: Autologous DC transduced w/ AdVp53 + chemo Drug: w/ or w/o all trans retinoic acid (ATRA)	intradermal	II	H. Lee Moffitt Cancer Center and Research Institute
E1b 55kD-, E3- HAdV5/RSV-TK	Cutaneous Metastatic Malignant Melanoma	Biological: adenovirus RSV-TK Drug: ganciclovir	Intra-lesional	I	National Human Genome Research Institute (NHGRI)
Replication-defective AdV.IFNalpha gene	Malignant Pleural Mesothelioma	Drug: SCH 921015 + chemotherapy	intrapleural infusion	0	Abramson Cancer Center of the University of Pennsylvania
Replication-defective AdV.TNFalpha controlled by chemoraditation inducible promoter	unresectable locally advanced pancreatic cancer.	Genetic: TNFerade 5-FU	i.t.	III	GenVec
CRhAdV5/SSTR/TK.RGD (imaging gene/infectivity enhanced suicide gene)	ovarian cancer	Genetic: Ad5.SSTR/TK.RGD Drug: Ganciclovir (GCV)	Intra-peritoneal	I	University of Alabama at Birmingham
Replication defective AdVhIL12	prostatic neoplasms prostate cancer	Genetic: Il-12 gene	prostatic injection	I	Baylor College of Medicine
Ad-REIC/Dkk-3	Prostate cancer	Biological: Ad-REIC/Dkk-3	prostatic injection	I	Momotaro-Gene Inc.
Replication competent AdV5-yCD/mut TKSR39 rep-ADP	Prostate cancer	Biological: Ad5-yCD/mutTKSR39rep-ADP Radiation: IMRT	prostatic injection	II / III	Henry Ford Health Systems
		Gene Therapies			
Replication deficient AdGVVEGF121cDNA	Coronary Artery Disease	Genetic: AdGVVEGF121cDNA	Intra-myocardial	FU on Phase I	Weill Medical College of Cornell University

AdV	Condition	Intervention	Route of Inoculation	Phase	Sponsor
Replication deficient E1, E4 deleted HAdV5OTCcDNA	Ornithine Transcarbamylase Deficiency Disease	Genetic: AdV Vector-Mediated Gene Transfer	Femoral arterial placement of a hepatic intraarterial catheter	I	FDA Office of Orphan Products Development
Replication deficient E1 deleted rHAd5-CB-CFTR	Cystic Fibrosis	Genetic: Ad5-CB-CFTR	nasal cavity	I	National Center for Research Resources (NCRR)
E1 deleted, E3 substituted (d1309) AdV5/OTC	Amino Acid Metabolism, Inborn Errors	Behavioral: Protein and calorie controlled diet	i.v.	I	National Center for Research Resources (NCRR)
Replication deficient, E1, E3 and E4 deleted, AdV/PEDF (pigment epithelium-derived factor) protein	Macular Degeneration	Drug: AdGVPEDF.11D	intravitreal injection into one eye	I	GenVec
Replication deficient deleted for all of E1a, most of E1b, and E3 sequences AdV/VEGF-D gene and a biodegradable local delivery device (collar) made of collagen	End Stage Renal Disease	(RAVE trial) Procedure: Graft placement surgery plus Trinam therapy	Near anasto-mosis	III	Ark Therapeutics Ltd
Replication deficient, E1-,E3-deleted AdV5/PDGF-B	Varicose Ulcer	Drug: Ad5/PDGF-B	intra-ulcer injection	I	National Institute of Arthritis and Musculoskeletal and Skin Diseases (NIAMS)
Replication-deficient AdV/VEGF-D	Angina Pectoris Myocardial Infarction	Biological: VEGF-D gene transfer	endocardial injection system	I	Kuopio University Hospital
Replication-defective E1 deleted HAdV5/hAQP1	Parotid Salivary Dysfunction	Gene Transfer Drug: AdhAQP1	catheter into parotid	I	National Institute of Dental and Craniofacial Research (NIDCR)
Infectious Diseases					
Mix of 2 Replication-deficient, recombinants (Ebola-rAd5) encoding GP from Zaire and SudanGulu strains	Ebola Hemorrhagic Fever	Drug: VRC-EBOADV018-00-VP	i.m.	I	National Institute of Allergy and Infectious Diseases (NIAID)
ADhVN1203/04.H5	Pandemic Influenza	Pandemic Influenza Vaccine	Oral ingestion of enteric capsule	I	Vaxin Inc.

AdV	Condition	Intervention	Route of Inoculation	Phase	Sponsor
Replication-Competent, recombinant AdV4/H5N1 (Ad4-H5-Vtn)	Avian Influenza	Biological: Ad4-H5-Vtn	Oral ingestion of enteric capsule	I	PaxVax, Inc.
Live, Replication-deficient rAdV35 (E1-, partially deleted E3encoding fusion protein of the Mycobacterium tuberculosis antigens	Tuberculosis	Biological: AERAS-402	i.m.	I / II	Aeras Global TB Vaccine Foundation
Replication incompetent, multiclade rAdV5 VRC-HIVADV014-00-VP	HIV	Biologicals: VRC-HIVDNA016-00-VP; VRC-HIVADV014-00-VP; VRC-DILUENT013-DIL-VP; VRC-HIVADV014-00-VP placebo	i.m. via Bioinjector	I / II	National Institute of Allergy and Infectious Diseases (NIAID)
AdV.ZFN/CCR5 (SB-728-T)	HIV	Biological: ZFN modified T cells	Infusion of apheresed T cells	I	University of Pennsylvania
Replication defective MRK Ad5 HIV-1 gag	HIV	Biological: MRK Ad5 HIV-1 gag vaccine	i.m.	II	National Institute of Allergy and Infectious Diseases (NIAID)
rAd26.ENVA.01	HIV	Biologicals: Ad26.ENVA.01 (rAd26); Placebo Vaccine	i.m.	I	National Institute of Allergy and Infectious Diseases (NIAID)
rAd35, rAd5	HIV	DNA Vaccine; DNA Vaccine placebo; rAd35; rAd35 placebo; rAd5; rAd5 placebo	i.m.	I	National Institute of Allergy and Infectious Diseases (NIAID)
rAd5	HIV	Biological: NYVAC-B (poxvirus) Biological: Placebo Biological: rAd5	i.m.	I	HIV Vaccine Trials Network
Replication defective simian Ad	HIV	Biological: MVA.HIVconsv low dose Other: Placebo low dose Biological: MVA.HIVconsv high dose Other: Placebo high dose	i.m.	I	University of Oxford

AdV	Condition	Intervention	Route of Inoculation	Phase	Sponsor
Ad26.ENVA.01, Ad35-ENV	HIV	Biological: Ad35-ENV vaccine Biological: Ad26.ENVA.01 vaccine Biological: Placebo Control	i.m.	I	International AIDS Vaccine Initiative

DC=dendritic cell; h=human; LMP= latent membrane protein; PEDF = pigment epithelium-derived factor protein; OTC: ornithine transcarbamylase; r=recombinant; VEGF=Vascular Endothelial Growth Factor D; SSTR=somatostatin receptor type 2

Table 1. Clinical Trials of AdV vectors

6.1 Tumor suppressor therapies

Several genes (p53, Rb,BRCA1, PTEN, etc) regulate the cell cycle and apoptotic pathways. The cellular machinery can inhibit tumor formation by suppressing aberrant cellular proliferation. Several malignancies have a loss-of-function mutation in one or more of the cell cycle control genes. Gene delivery can rescue a cell from a tumor phenotype by restoring the dysfunctional gene or a tumor-suppressor gene. One of the most extensively studied tumor suppressor genes, p53, is mutated in more than 50% of all human malignancies. The administration of wild-type p53 through gene transfer with a replication-defective AdV has demonstrated significant tumor suppression (Roth, 2006). The repair of p53 activity also has impaired angiongenic activity, inhibited the growth of nontransduced cells and directed a local immune response against tumor cells. In addition, replacement of p53 increased the vulnerability of tumor cells to chemotherapy and radiotherapy by reestablishing pro-apoptotic pathways. Furthermore, the potency of an anti-tumor response is enhanced when p53 gene replacement therapy is supplemented with available cytotoxic chemotherapeutics (El-Deiry, 2003). The first AdV gene therapy construct for the treatment of cancer has been approved by the State Food and Drug Administration (SFDA) of China. This AdV construct contains a p53 expression cassette in the deleted E1 region and has demonstrated remarkable synergistic effects when combined with radio-/chemotherapy, surgery, or hyperthermia for the management of cancer (Peng, 2005).

Another way to inhibit tumor growth is to manipulate ligand-receptor interactions. AdV have been engineered to deliver ligands to oncogenic receptors in the form of antibodies against the receptor or by mimicking natural interactions. Peptides with either natural or recombined ligand moieties have been particularly efficacious in receptor-ligand mimicry (Pasquale, 2010). Receptor-ligand interactions typically lead to down-regulation of that receptor either directly or through signal transduction complexes. One example is the EphA2 receptor, a tyrosine kinase protein, which is elevated in breast (Zelinski et al., 2001), prostate (Walker-Daniels et al., 1999), pancreatic, (Van Geer et al., 2010) and many other cancers. Thus, EphA2 is a good therapeutic candidate for treating cancer. Under normal conditions, the EphA2 receptor is localized at intracellular junctions where it binds to its membrane-anchored ligand, EphrinA1, resulting in phosphorylation of the receptor. E-cadherin, a cell adhesion molecule, is also able to phosphorylate EphA2 and aid in proper localization of the receptor. In many cancer cells, EphA2 is over expressed, unphosphorylated and unable to bind to its ligands due to its altered localization (Kinch & Carles-Kinch, 2003; Zantek et al., 1999). Monoclonal antibodies directed against EphA2 have been used in order to mimic ligand-induced downregulation. These antibodies caused elevated levels of EphA2 phosphorylation which encouraged its degradation (Carles-Kinch et al., 2002). AdV-mediated delivery of the secretory form of EphrinA1 produced autophosphorylation, degradation, and subsequent inhibition of tumor growth and metastasis (Noblitt et al., 2004; Noblitt et al., 2005). Likewise, AdV-mediated antibodies directed against ErbB2 (HER2/neu) demonstrated that ErbB2 down-regulation increased apoptosis and cytotoxicity both *in vitro* and *in vivo* (Arafat et al., 2002; Jiang et al., 2006).

6.2 CRAdV therapy

An effective approach to cancer therapy is the use of RCAdV that selectively replicate inside a tumor and ultimately kill tumor cells while leaving normal cells intact. As previously mentioned, therapeutic CRAdV are either engineered by deletion mutagenesis or engineered for the tumor- or tissue-specific replication by use of transcriptional regulatory elements (TREs).

6.2.1 Deletion mutation of CRAdV

CRAdV have expanded our knowledge regarding AdV proteins and how they interact with cellular proteins. E1 proteins of AdV adjust cell cycle controls in order to promote virus replication. The product of the E1A gene binds to the wild type Rb protein which causes the release and activation of E2F, a transcription factor (Whyte et al., 1988). Once E2F is activated, the transcription of S phase entry genes facilitates the hijacking of cellular machinery involved in AdV replication (Flint & Shenk, 1997). Additionally, E2F transactivates the p14ARF gene which increases p53 levels within the cell by inhibiting its degradation by murine double minute 2 (MDM2) (Bates et al., 1998). Although increased p53 levels can cause cellular apoptosis or arrest of the cell cycle, it also inhibits viral replication. To circumvent this replication inhibition, AdV E1B 55 kDa proteins work with E4 open reading from (ORF) 6 to bind to p53 and inactivate it preventing apoptosis and permitting virus replication and spread (Dobner et al., 1996; Yew & Berk, 1992). A *bcl-2*-related protein, E1B 19 kDa, also prevents apoptosis stimulated by E1A (Boyd et al., 1994; Rao et al., 1992). This knowledge combined with known tumor suppressor genes (i.e., p53 and Rb), tumor-associated antigens (CEA) or specialized promoters has facilitated the development of efficacious CRAdV.

The first CRAdV to enter clinical trials was ONYX-15 (also known as dl1520), a E1B 55kDa/E3B deleted vector. This mutant CRAdV selectively replicates in cancer cells that possess a defective p53 while leaving cells with intact p53 alone. It has undergone numerous clinical trials (Phase I to III) to test its therapeutic potential in head and neck squamous cell carcinoma, glioblastoma, hepatocellular carcinoma, colorectal carcinoma, sarcomas, ovarian, pancreatic, and hepatobiliary cancer (Aghi & Martuza, 2005; Kirn, 2001). Data indicate that ONYX-15 is safe and selective for cancer (Kirn & Thorne, 2009), but the strategy has failed to demonstrate extensive therapeutic effects or significant systemic spread (Liu et al., 2008b). Other oncolytic vectors that possess the same E1B/E3B mutations have exhibited the same capabilities, but only H101 was finally approved by the Chinese SFDA for use in combination with chemotherapy to treat late-stage refractory nasopharyngeal cancer (Kirn et al., 2008; Liu et al., 2008b).

There is a weak correlation between p53 status and cellular susceptibility to E1B/E3B mutant CRAdV (Geoerger et al., 2002; Hay et al., 1999; Rothmann et al., 1998). Some researchers have observed that when E1B 55kDa binds to p53, AdV-mediated death is followed by a productive infection (Dix et al., 2000; Hall et al., 1998). Others argue that the preferential killing by ONYX-15 types may be due to infectivity variances of the vector, permissiveness, upregulation of AdV early proteins (Steegenga et al., 1999), p14ARF failure (Ries et al., 2000), mutation features of p53 (Hann & Balmain, 2003), or late export of viral RNA (O'Shea et al., 2004) rather than solely the status of p53 (Sharma et al., 2009b). Replication of ONYX-15 is attenuated when compared with wild-type virus (Dix et al., 2001) which may be attributable to other E1B functions such as translation, nuclear exports of late viral mRNA, and compromised inhibition of host cell protein synthesis (Babiss & Ginsberg, 1984). Other mutations have been identified in the E1B 55 kDa protein that enhanced selectivity for tumors without hindering viral replication (Shen et al., 2001).

An alternative method involves the use of CRAdV mutants that possess a deletion in E1A and Rb-binding domain (CR-2) which ultimately targets cancers that have aberrant Rb pathways (Fueyo et al., 2000; Heise et al., 2000). When anti-tumor potential is compared between E1B mutations and CR-2 deletion vectors which do not inhibit vector replication in cancerous cells, the CR-2 vectors demonstrate better efficacy *in vivo* and *in vitro* (Alemany & Curiel, 2001). There are safety concerns, however, that exist with CR-2 deletion vectors since their replication is not restricted to cancer cells alone (Heise et al., 2000). Incorporation of tumor-specific promoters which restrict viral gene expression (i.e., ONYX-411) or the incorporation of Arg-Gly-Asp(RGD) motifs are beneficial to enhancing tumor cell selectivity and safety (Johnson et al., 2002; Page et al., 2007).

CRAdV targeting CEA-expressing malignancies in the colon, lung, and breast tissues have been successful and are in Phase I clinical trials with HAd5[E1-,E2b-]-CEA(6D) or ETBX-011. The HAdV5 has been engineered to express the CEA protein which is found in some cancerous cells. The goal is to direct the immune system to target cancer cells producing CEA. [http://clinicaltrials.gov/ct2/show/NCT01147965]

6.2.2 Transcriptional regulation of CRAdV

Another class of CRAdV replaces viral promoters that control vital transcriptional units with transcription regulating elements (TREs). Transcriptional targeting drives selection according to the vector gene expression and replication parameters set in motion by the TREs. The most obvious gene to be selected for TRE regulation is E1A since it is responsible for viral replication and adaptations which favor virus replication in the host cell environment. CN706 was the first TRE-regulated AdV to demonstrate potent anti-tumor effects (Rodriguez et al., 1997). In this construct, E1A expression was under the control of the prostate-specific antigen (PSA)-derived minimal enhancer/promoter which permitted selective replication in PSA-expressing prostate cells. Several promising TREs under investigation today include those that regulate expression of human telomerase reverse transcriptase (hTERT), transcription factor E2F, alpha-fetoprotein (AFP), and many more which tailor vector replication to be selective for a specific tumor phenotype.

Leaky replication has been observed in normal cells even though a single essential viral gene is under exogenous control. To improve tumor specificity and safety of CRADV, other essential viral genes (e.g., E1B, E2, E4) can be manipulated (Brunori et al., 2001; Doronin et al., 2001; Kawashima et al., 2004; Kuppuswamy et al., 2005; Li et al., 2005). A more complete list is available in a previous review (Sharma et al., 2009b). Other deletion mutations have been made in an effort to exploit specific oncolytic potentials while also retaining the replicative capacity of the virus. However, more work is warranted in all areas of CRAdV development before they can be used commercially. Additional safety features should include external regulation of oncolytic CRAdV through activation of inducible promoter systems such as TET or MMTV promoters (Avvakumov & Mymryk, 2002; Chong et al., 2002; Fechner et al., 2003). Furthermore, tissue-specific promoters can regulate where the vector replicates (Hernandez-Alcoceba et al., 2000; Hsieh et al., 2002). Radiation, chemical or heat-inducible promoters have also been employed to restrict transgene expression (Lee et al., 2001; Rasmussen et al., 2002).

Various regulatory elements have been fused in order to artificially design promoters which restrict TRE size while also preserving or amplifying rigid control of vector replication (Nettelbeck et al., 2000; Nettelbeck, 2008). In one artificial design, bidirectional promoters that simultaneously exert control over two key viral genes (i.e., E1A/E1B or E1A/E4) have been applied. Another promoter concept includes a dual-specific hybrid with regulatory elements that react to a hypoxic environment and estrogen thereby conferring greater discriminatory capabilities to oncolytic CRAdV (Hernandez-Alcoceba et al., 2002). Engineering of these transcriptionally-regulated CRAdV is an onerous task and poses several limitations due to the variety of viral and non-viral factors which can influence the response of the heterologous promoter. Safety concerns arise when *cis*-acting enhancer elements or cryptic transcription initiation sites lie in the left ITR or packaging signal. These regions that are upstream of E1A can influence transcriptional read-through of the E1A or transgene region even in the presence of a TRE (Yamamoto et al., 2003). Other elegant designs which address the limitations include the insertion of additional transcriptional terminators or insulators which are upstream of heterologous promoters, orientation changes of the E1A expression cassette, or the translocation of the packaging signal from the left ITR to the right ITR.

Post-transcriptional methods which control mRNA stability or translation are also under investigation for CRAdV development. Within the tumor microenvironment, proliferative signals are the driving force for expression of specific tumor-associated proteins. Expression of these proteins is boosted partially by the stabilization of mRNA by a 3'UTR which is regulated by an activated mitogen-activated protein kinase (P-MAPK) pathway. The 3'UTR regulates mRNA stability in several genes; hence, ligation of the 3'UTR with crucial AdV genes confers the vector with the ability to better target tumors (Sharma et al., 2009b).

No CRAdV have currently been developed that completely lack the ability to replicate or cause some toxicity in normal cells. They do however confer a great deal of selectivity and safety. Future conceptions should involve the enhancement of tumor-specific replication.

6.3 Suicide gene therapy

Suicide gene therapy selectively orchestrates a gene-directed enzyme for prodrug therapy (GDEPT) to deliver chemotherapeutic moieties to specific tumors. Nontoxic drugs (i.e., chemotherapeutic agents) are converted by AdV loaded with a GDEPT into cytotoxic agents within the tumor. Classic chemotherapy is often harmful to normal cells and, thus, promotes deleterious effects with the high doses needed for maintaining therapeutic indices. Since nontoxic prodrugs can be administered without harmful side effects to normal cells, this is a preferred methodology for chemotherapeutic delivery.

Two suicide genes which have been well characterized include the herpes simplex virus, type I thymidine kinase (HSV-TK) and the Escherichia coli, cytosine deaminase (CD) genes. HSV-TK phosphorylates ganciclovir (GCV) which cooperates with DNA polymerase to interfere with DNA synthesis ultimately leads to cell death in rapidly dividing cells. CD transforms 5-fluorocytosine (5-FC) into a very toxic metabolite 5-fluorouracil (5-FU), which is a frequently used chemotherapeutic (Aghi et al., 1998). Although direct toxicity is imparted by GDEPT-mediated cell death, there is also significant growth inhibition/killing of uninfected neighboring tumor cells due to the transfer of the toxic drug. The causes of this event are hypothesized to involve transfer via gap junctions or diffusion and stimulation of an anti-tumor response against lysed tumor cells (Lumniczky & Safrany, 2006).

Replication-defective AdV were initially used in GDEPT but demonstrated poor anti-tumor efficacy. RCAdV have had a better outcome, and the combination of suicide genes with standard therapies has further enhanced anti-tumor efficacy. However, GDEPT loaded AdV must be administered intratumorally in order to protect normal cells from cytotoxic events.

Other methods have evolved which can be used alone or in combination with the methods described above. The transductional targeting of tumors, the selective expression of suicide genes, or the addition of tumor specific promoters to AdV essential genes have improved anti-tumor potential of AdV vectors. These suicide gene/prodrug combinations are under investigation in both preclinical and clinical trials. Better dosage regimens and vaccination protocols must be formulated in order to improve the therapeutic potential of this system.

Another approach to consider for improvement involves thorough documentation of the kinetics of the prodrug and vector transgene expression. Timing prodrug administration in order to maximize benefits is of crucial importance. One novel method that has been proposed involves sequential administration of prodrug 5-FC followed by GCV. This double suicide gene therapy produced significant synergistic cytotoxicity. Avoidance of premature cell death is of critical importance since AdV will not be able to replicate. If virus proliferation is inhibited, yield will decrease markedly affecting the benefit of AdV-mediated suicide gene therapy (Sharma et al., 2009b).

6.4 Cancer immunotherapy

An intact immune system is capable of recognizing and eliminating tumor cells in the body; however, cancer cells possess the ability to evade immune detection. Tumor cells have several methods to avoid immune detection which include but are not limited to the release of immunosuppressive or anti-inflammatory proteins, flawed antigen presentation and processing caused by mutations within the mechanisms of antigen presentation or decreased expression of MHC molecules. The ineffectual anti-tumor immune response (humoral or cell-mediated) along with the progression of immunosuppression during oncogenesis demonstrates how the immune system needs to be magnified and specificity-modified to target tumor cells and the process of oncogenesis. The objective of cancer immunotherapy is to stimulate an endogenous immune response against already established or rapidly developing tumors. AdV have been employed to promote an immune response against cancerous cells by transporting immunostimulatory molecules or by arming dendritic cells (DC) with the appropriate tumor-associated antigen (TAA) (Sharma et al., 2009b).

6.4.1 Delivery of cytokines/co-stimulatory molecules via AdV

The administration of cytokines augments the cytokine environment within the tumor cell while also rallying immune cells to elicit an anti-tumor response. Many cytokines and membrane bound receptors (IL-12, IL-2, IFN-gamma, CD40L, etc) are very potent immunomodulators but elicit systemic toxicity during exogenous delivery. They also have a short half-life *in vivo* and are maintained at subtherapeutic levels at the tumor site. AdV loaded with cytokine expressing genes which are delivered intratumorally have demonstrated increased patient survival and decreased tumor growth. IL-2 suppresses tumor growth by stimulating cell-mediated killing activities in cytotoxic T lymphocytes (CTLs), lymphokine-activated killer (LAK) cells, or tumor infiltrating lymphocytes (TILs) (Eberlein & Schoof, 1991). A few clinical trials have exploited the potential of IL-2 in order to build an immune response to eventually kill tumor cells. IL-12 is another cytokine under investigation which elicits a potent anti-tumor response when administered locally by stimulating proliferation and cytotoxicity of CTLs and natural killer (NK) cells. A replication defective AdV (AdV.TNF) which does not target any particular tumor-associated antigen but rather expresses TNF-α under a chemoradiation-inducible promoter is in Phase III of clinical trials. The AdV.TNF is administered intratumorally along with radiation and 5-FU to induce an anti-tumor response. Co-stimulatory molecules, such as CD40L, have also demonstrated an ability to suppress tumor growth and are in Phase I/II of clinical trials (Habib-Agahi et al., 2007; Kikuchi & Crystal, 1999; Loskog et al., 2004; Martinet et al., 2000; Xu et al., 2005; Yoshida et al., 2003).

6.4.2 AdV Infection of DCs facilitate cancer immunotherapy

DCs are efficient and specialized APCs which present MHC-tagged epitopes to T cells in order to generate a specific immune response. These cells have been modified by AdV *ex vivo* so that the DCs either present TAA to effector cells of the immune system and/or introduce various immunomodulatory genes (i.e., cytokines or co-stimulatory receptors). Several of the anti-cancer therapies utilizing AdV have coupled the vector with the DC's abilities in order to generate an effective anti-tumor therapy. This method offers several advantages: (1) the AdV demonstrates adjuvant activity and has the ability to activate DCs and promote maturation which facilitates the induction of strong anti-tumor response (Geutskens et al., 2000; Kanagawa et al., 2008) , (2) AdV expression of TAA within DCs permits processing and loading onto both MHCI and MHCII molecules which stimulates the appropriate and relatively persistent activation of CD8+/CD4+ responses (Xia et al., 2006), and (3) *ex vivo* treatment of DCs with AdV evades any potential problems with pre-existing vector immunity (Wan et al., 1999).

7. AdV vaccines for infectious diseases

Significant advancements have been made in recombinant viral-vaccine strategies for infectious disease. AdV vaccines have demonstrated remarkable levels of T cell immunogenicity. AdV possess the ability to prime the immune response to target a transgene. This immune response can be boosted to high levels with a second vector that is recombined with the target antigen or with a serotype from a heterologous AdV (Jolly et al., 2008).

7.1 HIV vaccines

HIV is a constantly evolving virus that is an imposing challenge in the realm of engineering vaccines. The goal of HIV-1 vaccines is to reduce viral load, prolong survival, and minimize transmission. Vaccines that induce the HIV-1-specific cellular immune response have a delicate balance to maintain with regard to population preservation and selective stimulation. The vaccine construct should preserve the CD4+ T cell population and also increase the degree to which the CD8+ and CD4+ T cells recognize and bind HIV-1 antigens such as Gag and Pol. In addition, an elevated titer of neutralizing antibodies which possess high-avidity for the native trimeric Env protein of the virus needs to be attained.

A HAdV5-based HIV-1 vaccine was tested in humans in a Phase II trial to evaluate the risk for acquiring HIV infection. Unfortunately this trial was halted because the monitoring board determined that the vaccine was not able to demonstrate protection (Buchbinder et al., 2008; McElrath et al., 2008; Priddy et al., 2008). Future goals are focused on additional optimization of vaccine immunogens and technologies (Bradac & Dieffenbach, 2009). Since other researchers report the ability to induce a high level of cell-mediated immune response in non-HIV formulations, this is the time to apply this proof of principle to the area of HIV vaccine research.

In other areas of research, an AdV vector with chimeric fiber is used to infect autologous T cells to facilitate HIV therapy. This chimeric fiber contains both the HAdV5 fiber tail and the HAdV35 fiber shaft and knob domains (Perez et al., 2008). Due to its specificity to CCR5, CD4+ T-cells treated with this vector are relatively resistant to HIV infection. The data, while preliminary, are encouraging. Also, the modified CD4+ T cells treated with this vector are well-tolerated and engraft, replicate, and persist within the body after a single infusion. They behave like unmodified T-cells in so much as they migrate to the gut mucosa where they undergo selective expansion (Barouch, 2010). When used in combination with conventional anti-HIV therapies, this strategy might prove beneficial.

Different immunization strategies include a prime-boost approach with AdV-modified vaccinia virus Ankara (MVA) or heterologous HAdV5 and HAdV35 regimens or triple combinations which further elicit both T and B cell responses. The use of HAdV26 and HAdV35 in a prime-boost approach has shown promise in avoiding pre-existing vector immunity (Barouch, 2010). Immunization with HAdV26-Gag and HAdV35-Gag resulted in increased levels of CD127, CD62L, and Bcl-2 on T cells compared to HAdV5-Gag inoculation. These markers are indicative of improved functioning in T lymphocytes. There is also increased proliferation potential as well as increased antigen specificity.

7.2 Malaria vaccines

Malaria is characterized by several molecular interactions between the parasite and host during the parasite's incubation. An effective malaria vaccine will vigorously induce protective antibody and T cell responses to various malaria antigens that are expressed during the parasite's differentiation at the various life stages. Currently a mixture of two HAdV-5 vectors which express the pre-erthrocytic-stage malaria antigen circumsporozoite protein (CSP) or blood-stage malaria antigen apical membrane antigen 1 (AMA1) have demonstrated some success and are in Phase I/II of clinical trials. After immunization, human volunteers had a remarkable response to each antigen. Depletion studies determined that the response was due to a mixed population of CD8+ and CD4+ T cells. The CD8+ T cell lineage was five times greater than the CD4+phenotype when IFN-γ secreting cells were assayed within the response population (Draper & Heeney, 2010).

Another malaria vaccine platform involves the use of rAdV of rarer human serotypes or of non-human origin. These designs are engineered in such a way as to avoid pre-existing vector immunity against HAdV5. Some preclinical trials investigate priming with one AdV (i.e., HAdV5) and boosting with a heterologous AdV (i.e., HAdV35). Another strategy uses chimpanzee AdV serotype 63 (AdVCh63). AdVCh63 expresses the pre-erthrocytic-stage antigen thrombospondin-related adhesion protein combined with a multi-epitope string (ME-TRAP). A preclinical study utilizing a HAdV5 vector for priming followed with a boost by a MVA vector to promote the antibody and T cell responses. This particular HAdV5-MVA protocol used vectors that had been recombined with blood-stage malaria antigen merozoite surface protein 1 (MSP1) which induces a T cell response which was partially effective against the liver-stage infection (Draper et al., 2009) and a protective antibody response effective against the blood-stage infection (Draper et al., 2008). Future studies will have to address the immunogenicity problems of the AdV system that may exist when it is used in a target population of African children between the ages of one and six. This age group lives in a highly endemic region for malaria. It has already been shown that vector immunogenicity, provided by sequential immunization with two attenuated poxvirus vectors, was less effective in affording protection when immunized children were compared with naturally immune adults in Africa and malaria-naïve volunteers from developed countries (Bejon et al., 2006).

7.3 Tuberculosis (TB) vaccines

AdV vaccine programs are being investigated for human TB, but these programs are slightly hindered due to the absence of a good experimental model for humans during challenge. Currently, *M. bovis* BCG is being developed as a representative challenge for human *M. tuberculosis* (Draper & Heeney, 2010). The AdV in clinical trials for *M. tuberculosis* aims to circumvent vector immunity by utilizing HAdV35 in place of HAdV5. AERAS-402 utilizes a live, replication-deficient rHAdV35 that expresses a fusion protein of three Mycobacterium tuberculosis antigens, 85A, 85B, and 10.4 (Radosevic et al., 2007). This platform has demonstrated safety and efficacy in adults that were primed by BCG or recombinant BCG. The system intends to increase T cell-mediated immunity and, thus, protection from tuberculosis. Preclinical studies are exploring the potential of aerosolized delivery for AERAS-402 in an attempt to intensify mucosal immunity to provide greater protection against *M. tuberculosis* infection. However, in order to address these issues, more preclinical data needs to be collected from non-human primates.

7.4 Influenza vaccines

The establishment of an influenza vaccine that protects against multiple strains is a major undertaking and a long sought after goal. Given the current circumstances of the seasonal emergence of new permutations of influenza, the past pandemic involving the 2009 H1N1 influenza type A strain, and the possibility of highly pathogenic avian influenza to attain pandemic potential, accomplishing this goal is imperative. Inducing variant-specific antibody responses against the surface antigens, hemagglutinin and neuraminidase, is not the best way to combat influenza viruses which are constantly changing their surface proteins due to antigenic drift. Initiating a strong T cell response in addition to neutralizing antibody response to conserved T and B cell epitopes is important for protection against influenza variants.

AdV-based influenza vaccines provide particular advantages over egg-based influenza vaccines due to their low production costs and the quick and easy manufacturing of a substantial amount in validated cell lines. Replication-competent as well as replication-defective AdV vectors have been developed to express distinct influenza antigens. Each construct has been evaluated for its immunogenicity and efficacy in a variety of animal models, and a few formulations have been evaluated for the safety and efficacy in clinical trials in humans.

Immunization of mice with an AdV expressing the HA gene from swine influenza virus - A/Swine/Iowa/1999 (H3N2) resulted in high levels of influenza-specific neutralizing antibodies. Also, the immunization led to partial protection against a lethal challenge with a heterologous virus [A/HK/1/1968 (H3N2)] (Tang et al., 2002). Intranasal or epicutaneous immunization of humans with a replication-defective AdV encoding the HA gene of A/PR/8/1934 (H1N1) influenza virus resulted in a fourfold increase in hemagglutination inhibition (HI) titers in 83% of the participants (Van Kampen et al., 2005). The presence of pre-existing vector immunity did not seem to have a significant impact on the resultant hemagglutinin (HA)-specific immune response.

A replication defective HAdV5 influenza A (HAd-H5HA) vaccine containing the HA gene from HK/156/97 (H5N1) was evaluated for immunogenicity and protection in a mouse model (Hoelscher et al., 2006). The immunization resulted in the development of epitope-specific CD8 T cells and virus neutralizing antibodies. HAd-H5HA expresses HA from H5N1 influenza strain A/Hong Kong/156/1997 (HK/156/97) and is administered intramuscularly or intranasally. This vaccine construct provided complete protection to mice when challenged with homologous (HK/156/97) or heterologous (VN/1203/04) H5N1 influenza virus challenge indicating that HAd-H5HA afforded cross-protection to antigenically distinct strains of highly pathogenic H5N1. Immunized mice with HAd-H5HA were fully protected following challenge with a homologous H5N1 virus even after one year following immunization (Hoelscher et al., 2007). Inclusion of the HA genes from clade 1 and clade 2 H5N1 influenza viruses and the NP gene from one of the clades in the AdV-based vaccine resulted in expanded protection (Hoelscher et al., 2008). A replication-defective AdV vector expressing the HA gene from a H5N1 influenza virus has been tested in a Phase 1 clinical trial. The replication competent HAdV4 vector-based vaccine containing the HA gene of a H5N1 virus induced both humoral and mucosal antibodies as well as a cellular immune response when administered in a enteric capsule (Palkonyay, 2009).

An AdV vector provokes both humoral and cellular immune responses. If an AdV is engineered to carry multiple genes from different influenza strains, this will enhance the cross-protective efficacy against multiple strains. An AdV that is loaded with cross-reactive potential will provide a stockpiling option to address the vaccine need for a potential H5N1-based pandemic influenza (Vemula & Mittal, 2010).

7.5 Filovirus vaccine

In the effort to battle Ebola and Marburg viruses, a Phase I study has been completed using a mixture of two replication-deficient, rAdV5 (Ebola-rAdV5) encoding glycoproteins (GP) from Zaire and Sudan-Gulu strains, as well as the nucleoprotein (NP) of filovirus. It demonstrated excellent pre-clinical results with 100% protection in monkeys, but, apparently, it did not do well in human clinical trials (Martin et al., 2006). Virus neutralizing antibodies that were specific for the virus strains used in the trial were undetectable in the persons vaccinated. It was also determined that NP was not necessary for inclusion in the vaccine construct and may actually dampen the protective immune response (Sullivan et al., 2006).

8. Improving adenovirus based gene transfer- strategies for immune evasion

Staggering innate and adaptive immune responses have undoubtedly limited the therapeutic potential of AdV based gene transfer. However, the extensive promise that Ad vectors offer for improving human and animal health has fueled tremendous interest in acquiring a deeper understanding of molecular mechanisms underlying the immune activation. Several promising innovative strategies to eliminate or minimize the acute inflammatory responses induced by AdV vectors, as well as to circumvent the vector immunity in order to prolong the vector persistence in host are being developed.

8.1 Immunosuppression and immunomodulation

Elimination of a significant fraction of intravascularly administered AdV vectors within initial twenty-four hours is attributed to elements of non-specific innate immune response, particularly the liver Kupffer cells, acting as a buffer against invading pathogen. Hepatocyte transduction occurs only after the saturation of kupffer cells at higher doses (Di Paolo et al., 2009). Removal of Kupffer cells is expected to result in higher hepatocyte transduction efficiency. In fact, transient depletion of macrophages prior to vector inoculation using pre-treatment with gadolinium chloride ($GdCl_3$) or dicholoromethylene bisphosphate (Cl_2MBP) not only reduces the initial vector clearance, but also seem to prolong the long-term transgene expression, possibly through attenuating the vector-specific adaptive immune responses (Kuzmin et al., 1997; Lieber et al., 1997). Although an effective macrophage depletion strategy may not be able to prevent vector elimination entirely since other mechanisms are also involved, this strategy might be used effectively in combination with other immune suppression methods.

The anti-vector humoral and cytotoxic immune responses are primarily responsible for preventing long-term transgene expression and act by eliminating the vector-transduced cells. Several studies have shown that treatment with non-specific immunosuppressive agents such as cyclosporine A, cyclophosphamide, deoxyspergualin, dexamethasone and FK506 at the time of vector administration in presence of pre-existing immunity can suppress progression of humoral and/or cellular immune response and prolong the persistence of transgene in the host (Kaplan & Smith, 1997; Kuriyama et al., 2000; Seregin et al., 2009; Smith et al., 1996; Thomas et al., 2008). Similar effects can be obtained through transient immunosuppression by using specific antibodies targeted against molecules such as T lymphocyte antigens, CD4, CD40, or CD86 to block the receptor-ligand interaction (Chirmule et al., 2000; Haegel-Kronenberger et al., 2004; Ye et al., 2000). Many AdV vector applications require administration of high vector doses and, therefore, necessitate prevention or mitigation of an AdV-induced acute inflammatory response. Simultaneous administration of suppressor of cytokine signaling 1 (SOCS-1) results in generalized lower serum levels of cytokines, including IL-6, MCP-1, RANTES and TNF-α (Sakurai et al., 2008). Other studies have targeted suppression of specific cytokines, for example, TNF-α (Wilderman et al., 2006) and IFN-α/β (Zhu et al., 2007) resulted in significant reduction of the inflammatory response. Interestingly, a regimen for the inhibition of multiple cytokines at same time may have an additive or synergistic effect on inhibition of the inflammatory response. However, caution must be exercised for interpreting the results of such studies as species-specific variations may exist, and the observation made in animal models may not be replicated in humans. Each immunosuppressive or immunomodulatory approach needs to be thoroughly evaluated for potential side effects before their transition to clinical trials. Additionally, although transient, a generalized immunosuppression might render the patients more vulnerable to other diseases.

8.2 Vector modifications

Strategies involving vector modifications impose lesser risk to the host than those that involve attenuating or modifying host immune responses. Vector modifications can be achieved through several different strategies, each with its own advantages and disadvantages, and will vary pertinent to the specific application. Vector modifications can consist of many alternatives such as (1) those intended to ablate interactions between AdV and its primary and/or secondary receptor, (2) fiber knob modifications to retarget vector to specific cell types, (3) replacement of fibers using serotype chimerism, (3) covalent modifications, (4) vector pseudotyping, and (5) vector microencapsulation.

8.2.1 Fiber knob modification

Binding of the HAdV5 fiber knob domain to CAR on the cell surface is the foremost step in virus entry. Multiple strategies are available for altering the natural biodistribution pattern of AdV vectors and retargeting them to specific cell types. Complexing the vector with a bi-specific antibody for recognizing the fiber knob or a specific cell surface molecule will serve the dual purpose of ablating knob-CAR interaction and targeting the modified vector to an alternative receptor (Curiel, 1999; Mizuguchi & Hayakawa, 2004). Alternatively, the vector can be treated with a CAR ectodomain-single chain antibody targeted against a tissue-specific antigen. The CAR ectodomain will bind to the fiber knob preventing interaction between CAR on cell surface. The single chain antibody will retarget the vector to the specific cell type (Li et al., 2009). *In vivo*, the fiber knob domain also interacts with coagulation factor IX and factor C4BP, targeting AdV vectors to HSPGs and LRP on hepatocytes and Kupffer cells. Consequently, fiber knob modifications might also ablate these interactions, thereby reducing liver transduction and subsequent hepatotoxicity (Shayakhmetov et al., 2005).

8.2.2 Serotype chimerism

Chimeric AdV vectors are most commonly constructed by replacing the knob domain or whole fiber with one from an alternative AdV serotype. Remarkable similarities among fibers of different Ad serotypes allows for the 'fiber chimerism'. Since the subgroup B viruses use cell surface molecules other then CAR as their primary attachment receptor, it is credible to replace HAdV5 fiber knob with one of a subgroup B virus, or vice versa, and expect a shift in vector biodistribution. Expectedly, fibers from subgroup B AdV have been successfully used for constructing HAdV5-based fiber chimeric vectors with an altered biodistribution pattern compared to HAdV5 alone. For example, HAdV5 carrying a fiber knob from HAdV16p, a subgroup B virus, showed greater transduction of cardiovascular and synovial tissues (Havenga et al., 2001). Similarly, HAdV5 with fiber from HAdV35, another subgroup B virus, showed enhanced transduction of hematopoeitic cells and human pancreatic cancer cells *in vitro* (Shayakhmetov et al., 2000; Toyoda et al., 2008).

Alternatively, the replacement of only the knob domain instead of the whole fiber has also been evaluated. A HAdV5 vector with fiber knob domain from HAdV3 proved to be remarkably efficient for gene transfer in animal models of breast cancer, ovarian cancer, gastric cancer and renal cancer and also showed good oncolytic ability (Ranki & Hemminki, 2010). A recent study explained the possibility of exploiting non-human AdV vectors for constructing fiber chimerism. Replacing the HAdV5 shaft and knob domains of HAdV5 with those from a bovine AdV ablated the vector interaction with blood factors IX and X and the subsequent HSPG-mediated hepatocyte transduction. As a result, serum levels of many of the pro-inflammatory cytokines and chemokines at early time points after the intravascular inoculation were significantly reduced (Rogee et al., 2010).

The major capsid protein hexon of HAdV5 interacts with factor X and mediates hepatocyte transduction. Being the most abundant capsid protein, it is expected to contribute significantly to non-CAR-dependent tropism. However, not all AdV serotypes bind factor X, and therefore, have variable hepatocyte transduction profiles *in vivo*. Chimeric HAdV5 27 vectors whose HVRs were replaced with HVRs of HAdV26 or HAdV27, which do not bind factor X, ablated factor X binding and showed a reduced hepatocyte transduction at a comparatively high dose (10^{11} vp/mouse). However, a greater degree of macrophage transduction was observed, giving a possible reason for the concomitant higher degree of proinflammatory cytokine and chemokine response following intravascular administration of the hexon chimeric HAdV5 vector. Interestingly, inserting HAdV35 fiber in place of native fiber of this chimeric HAdV5 vector dramatically increased lung transduction by more than 16000 times compared to the vector with HAdV5 fiber (Alba et al., 2010). Such a vector may prove very useful for lung gene therapy applications. Furthermore, this study also highlighted an interesting possibility of combining hexon and fiber chimerism to construct novel vectors with decreased immunogenicity and suitability for a particular application. Recently, another study reported a chimeric HAdV5 vector with the hexon from HAdV3. This chimeric vector showed ablation for factor X binding, which translated into reduced liver transduction and enhanced anti-tumor activity, owing to greater bioavailability of the vector for tumor transduction (Short et al., 2010).

8.3 Covalent modification of Ad capsid

Covalent modification of AdV capsids is an attractive alternative to genetic modification for preventing induction of immune responses and the acute toxicity following systemic administration. Addition of chemical groups to AdV capsids masks the natural immunodominant epitopes and the molecular patterns required for interaction with Ad-neutralizing antibodies along with the pattern recognition receptors, thereby preventing antibody-mediated vector clearance and induction of innate immune responses. Several standardized methods for covalent modifications are available for the generation of high titer stocks of modified vectors. Furthermore, simultaneous modification of a large number of capsid amino acids is feasible with covalent modification which may not be possible through genetic modification. Multiple studies have reported the so-called 'stealth AdV vectors' modified with synthetic polymers, for example, polyethylene glycol (PEG) (Kreppel & Kochanek, 2008). In accordance with the above principles, covalently modified AdV vectors have been shown to prevent or attenuate the induction of innate and adaptive immune responses, as well as, to evade pre-existing AdV-neutralizing antibodies (Croyle et al., 2002; Croyle et al., 2005). In addition, the use of bifunctional PEG allows for tissue-specific targeting of AdV vectors by coupling one functional group to capsid proteins and another functional group to a ligand of a specific tissue receptor (Park et al., 2008).

8.4 Alternative Ad vectors

Since AdV-neutralizing antibodies are serotype-specific and the prevalence of some of the HAdV serotypes in the human population is rare, HAdV vectors derived from the rare HAdV serotypes can potentially circumvent the pre-existing vector immunity, and, therefore, be more effective than vectors derived from common HAdV serotypes such as HAdV5. Vector systems based on HAdV serotypes in all subgroups have been reported (Appledorn et al., 2008a).

8.5 Non-human Ad vectors

Vectors based on nonhuman AdV serotypes are very promising candidates to serve as gene delivery vehicles and are frequently derived from AdV infecting bovine, porcine, ovine and chimpanzee. The nonhuman AdV do not cause disease in humans and are not neutralized by the HAdV-specific neutralizing antibodies (Moffatt et al., 2000; Sharma et al., 2010; Singh et al., 2008). In addition, nonhuman AdV vectors have been shown to transduce human cells in culture and express transgene (Bangari et al., 2005; Bangari & Mittal, 2004; Farina et al., 2001; Klonjkowski et al., 1997; Mittal et al., 1995; Rasmussen et al., 1999). Advances in the past decade signify the potential of nonhuman AdV vectors as effective gene delivery vehicles without any significant toxicity and interference from pre-existing immunity. A bovine AdV serotype 3 (BAdV3) vector has been shown to possess low liver tropism, prolonged vector genome persistence and, thereby, higher transgene expression than a HAdV5 vector in the heart, lungs, and kidneys of mice following intravenous inoculation (Sharma et al., 2009a). The humoral as well as cellular immune responses generated against various non-human AdV are expected to be non cross-neutralizing (Sharma et al., 2010). Sequential use of alternative non-human AdV-derived vectors might prolong the transgene expression and, therefore, the desired therapeutic effect.

9. Conclusion

The future of AdV vectors is very promising. Much research has been conducted on the various constructs of the vectors with the hope of finding therapies that will enable specific targeting of diseased cells or tumors thereby causing minimum harm to surrounding cells or organs. With continued research on the mechanisms of AdV gene expression and tissue tropism, the medical and scientific communities have great reason to anticipate breakthroughs in cancer and vaccine therapies.

10. Acknowledgement

This work was supported by Public Health Service grants AI059374 and CA110176 from the National Institute of Allergy and Infectious Diseases, and the National Cancer Institute, respectively. We are thankful to Jane Kovach for her secretarial assistance.

11. References

Aghi et al (1998) *J.Natl.Cancer Inst.* 90,5, pp.370-380
Aghi & Martuza (2005) *Oncogene* 24,52, pp.7802-7816
Alba et al (2010) *Blood* 116,15, pp.2656-2664
Alba et al (2007) *Virology* 367,1, pp.51-58
Alejo et al (2006) *Proc.Natl.Acad.Sci.U.S.A* 103,15, pp.5995-6000
Alemany & Curiel (2001) *Gene Ther.* 8,17, pp.1347-1353
Appledorn et al (2008a) *Gene Ther.* 15,12, pp.885-901
Appledorn et al (2008b) *J.Immunol.* 181,3, pp.2134-2144
Arafat et al (2002) *Gene Ther.* 9,4, pp.256-262
Avvakumov & Mymryk (2002) *J.Virol.Methods* 103,1, pp.41-49
Babiss & Ginsberg (1984) *J.Virol.* 50,1, pp.202-212
Bangari & Mittal (2004) *Virus Res.* 105,2, pp.127-136

Bangari et al (2005) *Biochem.Biophys.Res.Commun.* 327,3, pp.960-966
Barcia et al (2007) *Mol.Ther.* 15,12, pp.2154-2163
Barlan et al (2011) *J.Virol.* 85,1, pp.146-155
Barouch, DH . Alternative Serotype Adenovirus Vectors. (4-14-2011). Available from: http://www.hivvaccineenterprise.org/conference_archive/2010/pdf-presentations/Wednesday/Symposium-02/BarouchD.pdf
Bates et al (1998) *Nature* 395,6698, pp.124-125
Bejon et al (2006) *PLoS.Clin.Trials* 1,6, pp.e29
Beveridge et al (2007) *Eur.J.Immunol.* 37,11, pp.3089-3100
Boyd et al (1994) *Cell* 79,2, pp.341-351
Bradac & Dieffenbach (2009) *IDrugs.* 12,7, pp.435-439
Brown et al (2004) *J.Thromb.Haemost.* 2,1, pp.111-118
Brunetti-Pierri et al (2008) *J.Gene Med.* 10,8, pp.890-896
Brunori et al (2001) *J.Virol.* 75,6, pp.2857-2865
Buchbinder et al (2008) *Lancet* 372,9653, pp.1881-1893
Butti et al (2008) *Gene Ther.* 15,3, pp.233-238
Carles-Kinch et al (2002) *Cancer Res.* 62,10, pp.2840-2847
Cerullo et al (2007) *Mol.Ther.* 15,2, pp.378-385
Chirmule et al (2000) *J.Virol.* 74,7, pp.3345-3352
Chong et al (2002) *Mol.Ther.* 5,2, pp.195-203
Cotter et al (2005) *J.Virol.* 79,23, pp.14622-14631
Croyle et al (2002) *Hum.Gene Ther.* 13,15, pp.1887-1900
Croyle et al (2005) *Gene Ther.* 12,7, pp.579-587
Curiel (1999) *Ann.N.Y.Acad.Sci.* 886:158-71.,158-171
Descamps & Benihoud (2009) *Curr.Gene Ther.* 9,2, pp.115-127
Di Paolo et al (2009) *Mol.Ther.* 17,4, pp.675-684
Dimmock et al (2011) *Hum.Gene Ther.* 22,4, pp.483-488
Dix et al (2001) *J.Virol.* 75,12, pp.5443-5447
Dix et al (2000) *Cancer Res.* 60,10, pp.2666-2672
Dobner et al (1996) *Science* 272,5267, pp.1470-1473
Dormond et al (2009) *Biotechnol.Adv.* 27,2, pp.133-144
Doronin et al (2001) *J.Virol.* 75,7, pp.3314-3324
Draper et al (2009) *Cell Host.Microbe* 5,1, pp.95-105
Draper & Heeney (2010) *Nat.Rev.Microbiol.* 8,1, pp.62-73
Draper et al (2008) *Nat.Med.* 14,8, pp.819-821
Eberlein & Schoof (1991) *Compr.Ther.* 17,1, pp.49-56
El-Deiry (2003) *Oncogene* 22,47, pp.7486-7495
ENDERS et al (1956) *Science* 124,3212, pp.119-120
Everts & van der Poel (2005) *Cancer Gene Ther.* 12,2, pp.141-161
Fallaux et al (1998) *Hum.Gene Ther.* 9,13, pp.1909-1917
Farina et al (2001) *J.Virol.* 75,23, pp.11603-11613
Fattori et al (2006) *Gene Ther.* 13,14, pp.1088-1096
Fechner et al (2003) *Gene Ther.* 10,19, pp.1680-1690
Flint & Shenk (1997) *Annu.Rev.Genet.* 31,177-212

Folgori et al (2006) *Nat.Med.* 12,2, pp.190-197
Fueyo et al (2000) *Oncogene* 19,1, pp.2-12
Furnari et al (2007) *Genes Dev.* 21,21, pp.2683-2710
Gau et al (2009) *Mol.Ther.* 17,7, pp.1155-1163
Geiben-Lynn et al (2008) *Clin.Vaccine Immunol.* 15,4, pp.691-696
Geoerger et al (2002) *Cancer Res.* 62,3, pp.764-772
Geutskens et al (2000) *Gene Ther.* 7,16, pp.1410-1416
Gherardi et al (2003) *J.Virol.* 77,12, pp.7048-7057
Grable & Hearing (1992) *J.Virol.* 66,2, pp.723-731
Graham et al (1977) *J.Gen.Virol.* 36,1, pp.59-74
Grossman et al (2010) *Clin.Cancer Res.* 16,8, pp.2443-2449
Habib-Agahi et al (2007) *Int.Immunol.* 19,12, pp.1383-1394
Haegel-Kronenberger et al (2004) *Gene Ther.* 11,3, pp.241-252
Hall et al (1998) *Nat.Med.* 4,9, pp.1068-1072
Hann & Balmain (2003) *J.Virol.* 77,21, pp.11588-11595
Hardy et al (1997) *J.Virol.* 71,3, pp.1842-1849
Hartigan-O'Connor et al (2002) *Hum.Gene Ther.* 13,4, pp.519-531
Hartman et al (2007a) *Virology* 358,2, pp.357-372
Hartman et al (2007b) *J.Virol.* 81,4, pp.1796-1812
Harvey et al (1999) *Hum.Gene Ther.* 10,17, pp.2823-2837
Havenga et al (2001) *J.Virol.* 75,7, pp.3335-3342
Hay et al (1999) *Hum.Gene Ther.* 10,4, pp.579-590
Heeney et al (2000) *J.Med.Primatol.* 29,3-4, pp.268-273
Hehir et al (1996) *J.Virol.* 70,12, pp.8459-8467
Heise et al (2000) *Nat.Med.* 6,10, pp.1134-1139
Hernandez-Alcoceba et al (2002) *Hum.Gene Ther.* 13,14, pp.1737-1750
Hernandez-Alcoceba et al (2000) *Hum.Gene Ther.* 11,14, pp.2009-2024
Hilleman MR & Werner JH (1954) *Proc Soc Exp Biol Med* 85,183-188
Hiscott (2007) *J.Biol.Chem.* 282,21, pp.15325-15329
Hoelscher et al (2006) *Lancet* 367,9509, pp.475-481
Hoelscher et al (2007) *Clin.Pharmacol.Ther.* 82,665-671
Hoelscher et al (2008) *J.Inf.Dis.* 197,8, pp.1185-1188
Howe et al (2006) *Virology* 345,1, pp.220-230
Hsieh et al (2002) *Cancer Res.* 62,11, pp.3084-3092
Hu et al (2011) *Proc.Natl.Acad.Sci.U.S.A* 108,5, pp.2082-2087
Huebner et al (1956) *Cancer* 9,6, pp.1211-1218
Jego et al (2003) *Immunity.* 19,2, pp.225-234
Jiang et al (2006) *Clin.Cancer Res.* 12,20 Pt 1, pp.6179-6185
Johnson et al (2002) *Cancer Cell* 1,4, pp.325-337
Jolly et al (2008)39-59 9780470184585
Junt et al (2007) *Nature* 450,7166, pp.110-114
Kanagawa et al (2008) *Virology* 374,2, pp.411-420
Kaplan & Smith (1997) *Hum.Gene Ther.* 8,9, pp.1095-1104
Kawashima et al (2004) *Clin.Cancer Res.* 10,1 Pt 1, pp.285-292

Kikuchi & Crystal (1999) *Hum.Gene Ther.* 10,8, pp.1375-1387
Kinch & Carles-Kinch (2003) *Clinical & Experimental Metastasis* 20,1, pp.59-68
Kirn (2001) *Gene Ther.* 8,2, pp.89-98
Kirn & Thorne (2009) *Nat.Rev.Cancer* 9,1, pp.64-71
Kirn et al (2008) *Cancer Res.* 68,7, pp.2071-2075
Klonjkowski et al (1997) *Hum.Gene Ther.* 8,17, pp.2103-2115
Kochanek (1999) *Hum.Gene Ther.* 10,15, pp.2451-2459
Koeberl et al (2007) *Mol.Ther.* 15,7, pp.1253-1258
Kreppel & Kochanek (2008) *Mol.Ther.* 16,1, pp.16-29
Kumar et al (2009) *Biochem.J.* 420,1, pp.1-16
Kumar-Singh & Chamberlain (1996) *Hum.Mol.Genet.* 5,7, pp.913-921
Kuppuswamy et al (2005) *Gene Ther.* 12,22, pp.1608-1617
Kuriyama et al (2000) *Int.J.Cancer* 85,6, pp.839-844
Kuzmin et al (1997) *Gene Therapy* 4,4, pp.309-316 0969-7128
Lee et al (2010) *Immunol.Lett.* 134,1, pp.93-102
Lee et al (2001) *Cancer Gene Ther.* 8,6, pp.397-404
Lemckert et al (2005) *J.Virol.* 79,15, pp.9694-9701
Li et al (2009) *Cancer Res.* 69,2, pp.554-564
Li et al (2005) *Cancer Res.* 65,5, pp.1941-1951
Li et al (2002) *Eur.J.Immunol.* 32,12, pp.3443-3452
Lieber et al (1996) *J.Virol.* 70,12, pp.8944-8960
Lieber et al (1997) *J.Virol.* 71,11, pp.8798-8807
Liu et al (2008a) *J.Virol.* 82,10, pp.4844-4852
Liu et al (2009) *Nature* 457,7225, pp.87-91
Liu et al (2003a) *Hum.Gene Ther.* 14,7, pp.627-643
Liu et al (2003b) *Human Gene Therapy* 14,7, pp.627-643 1043-0342
Liu et al (2008b) *Methods Mol.Biol.* 433,243-258
Longley et al (2005) *Cytotechnology* 49,2, pp.161-171 0920-9069
Loskog et al (2004) *J.Immunol.* 172,11, pp.7200-7205
Lumniczky & Safrany (2006) *Pathol.Oncol.Res.* 12,2, pp.118-124
Lusky et al (1998) *J.Virol.* 72,3, pp.2022-2032
Manickan et al (2006) *Mol.Ther.* 13,1, pp.108-117
Martin et al (2006) *Clin.Vaccine Immunol.* 13,11, pp.1267-1277
Martinet et al (2000) *J.Natl.Cancer Inst.* 92,11, pp.931-936
Martinon et al (2009) *Annu.Rev.Immunol.* 27,229-265
McCormack, Jr. et al (2006) *J.Thromb.Haemost.* 4,6, pp.1218-1225
McElrath et al (2008) *Lancet* 372,9653, pp.1894-1905
Mitani et al (1995) *Proc.Natl.Acad.Sci.U.S.A* 92,9, pp.3854-3858
Mittal et al (1995) *J.Gen.Virol.* 76,Pt 1, pp.93-102
Mizuguchi & Hayakawa (2004) *Hum.Gene Ther.* 15,11, pp.1034-1044
Moffatt et al (2000) *Virology* 272,1, pp.159-167
Morral et al (2002) *Hum.Gene Ther.* 13,1, pp.143-154
Muhammad et al (2010) *Clin.Pharmacol.Ther.* 88,2, pp.204-213
Muruve (2004) *Hum.Gene Ther.* 15,12, pp.1157-1166

Muruve et al (1999) *Hum.Gene Ther.* 10,6, pp.965-976
Muruve et al (2004) *J.Virol.* 78,11, pp.5966-5972
Muruve et al (2008) *Nature* 452,7183, pp.103-107
Nettelbeck (2008) *J.Mol.Med.* 86,4, pp.363-377
Nettelbeck et al (2000) *Trends Genet.* 16,4, pp.174-181
Ng et al (2001) *Mol.Ther.* 3,5 Pt 1, pp.809-815
Nicklin et al (2005) *Mol.Ther.* 12,3, pp.384-393
Noblitt et al (2004) *Cancer Gene Ther.* 11,11, pp.757-766
Noblitt et al (2005) *Cancer Gene Ther.* 12,1, pp.46-53
Nociari et al (2009) *J.Virol.* 83,9, pp.4081-4091
Nociari et al (2007) *J.Virol.* 81,8, pp.4145-4157
O'Neal et al (1998) *Hum.Gene Ther.* 9,11, pp.1587-1598
O'Shea et al (2004) *Cancer Cell* 6,6, pp.611-623
Oka et al (2007) *Gene Ther.* 14,3, pp.191-202
Page et al (2007) *Am.J.Obstet.Gynecol.* 196,4, pp.389-389
Palkonyay (2009)
Park et al (2008) *Biochem.Biophys.Res.Commun.* 366,3, pp.769-774
Parker et al (2008) *Curr.Opin.Mol.Ther.* 10,5, pp.439-448
Parker et al (2006) *Blood* 108,8, pp.2554-2561
Parks et al (1999) *J.Virol.* 73,10, pp.8027-8034
Parks et al (1996) *Proc.Natl.Acad.Sci.U.S.A* 93,24, pp.13565-13570
Parks & Graham (1997) *J.Virol.* 71,4, pp.3293-3298
Pasquale (2010) *Nat.Rev.Cancer* 10,3, pp.165-180
Peng (2005) *Hum.Gene Ther.* 16,9, pp.1016-1027
Perez et al (2008) *Nat.Biotechnol.* 26,7, pp.808-816
Pinto et al (2003) *J.Immunol.* 171,12, pp.6774-6779
Pratt et al (2010) *Clin.Vaccine Immunol.* 17,4, pp.572-581
Priddy et al (2008) *Clin.Infect.Dis.* 46,11, pp.1769-1781
Puntel et al (2010) *J.Virol.* 84,12, pp.6007-6017
Radosevic et al (2007) *Infect.Immun.* 75,8, pp.4105-4115
Ranki & Hemminki (2010) *Viruses-Basel* 2,10, pp.2196-2212 1999-4915
Rao et al (1992) *Proc.Natl.Acad.Sci.U.S.A* 89,16, pp.7742-7746
Raper et al (2003) *Mol.Genet.Metab* 80,1-2, pp.148-158
Raper et al (2002) *Hum.Gene Ther.* 13,1, pp.163-175
Rasmussen et al (2002) *Cancer Gene Ther.* 9,11, pp.951-957
Rasmussen et al (1999) *Hum.Gene Ther.* 10,16, pp.2587-2599
Ries et al (2000) *Nat.Med.* 6,10, pp.1128-1133
Rodriguez et al (1997) *Cancer Res.* 57,13, pp.2559-2563
Rogee et al (2010) *Gene Ther.* 17,7, pp.880-891
Roth (2006) *Expert.Opin.Biol.Ther.* 6,1, pp.55-61
Rothmann et al (1998) *J.Virol.* 72,12, pp.9470-9478
Rowe WP et al (1953) *Proc Soc Exp Biol Med* 84,570-573
Rux & Burnett (2004) *Hum.Gene Ther.* 15,12, pp.1167-1176
Sakhuja et al (2003) *Hum.Gene Ther.* 14,3, pp.243-254

Sakurai et al (2008) *J.Immunol.* 180,7, pp.4931-4938
San & Burnett (2003) *Curr.Top.Microbiol.Immunol.* 272,57-94
Sandig et al (2000) *Proc.Natl.Acad.Sci.U.S.A* 97,3, pp.1002-1007
Sango et al (2002) *Neuropathol.Appl.Neurobiol.* 28,1, pp.23-34
Schagen et al (2004) *Crit Rev.Oncol.Hematol.* 50,1, pp.51-70
Schiedner et al (2002) *J.Virol.* 76,4, pp.1600-1609
Seiler et al (2007) *Curr.Gene Ther.* 7,5, pp.297-305
Seregin et al (2009) *Mol.Ther.* 17,4, pp.685-696
Sharma et al (2009a) *Virus Res.* 143,2, pp.184-194
Sharma et al (2010) *Gene Ther.* 17,5, pp.634-642
Sharma et al (2009b) *Curr.Drug ther.* 4,2, pp.117-138
Shayakhmetov et al (2005) *J.Virol.* 79,12, pp.7478-7491
Shayakhmetov et al (2000) *J.Virol.* 74,6, pp.2567-2583
Shen et al (2001) *J.Virol.* 75,9, pp.4297-4307
Shi et al (2006) *J.Gene Med.* 8,4, pp.442-451
Shi et al (2002) *Hum.Gene Ther.* 13,2, pp.211-224
Shiver et al (2002) *Nature* 415,6869, pp.331-335
Short et al (2010) *Mol.Cancer Ther.* 9,9, pp.2536-2544
Singh et al (2008) *Mol.Ther.* 16,5, pp.965-971
Smith et al (1996) *Gene Ther.* 3,6, pp.496-502
Soudais et al (2004) *FASEB J.* 18,2, pp.391-393
Steegenga et al (1999) *Oncogene* 18,36, pp.5032-5043
Sullivan et al (1997) *Hum.Gene Ther.* 8,10, pp.1195-1206
Sullivan et al (2006) *PLoS.Med.* 3,6, pp.e177
Tang et al (2006) *Virology* 350,2, pp.312-322
Tang et al (2002) *Arch.Virol.* 147,11, pp.2125-2141
Terashima et al (2009) *J.Clin.Invest* 119,7, pp.2100-2112
Thomas et al (2008) *Mol.Ther.* 16,10, pp.1665-1673
Tibbles et al (2002) *J.Virol.* 76,4, pp.1559-1568
Toietta et al (2005) *Proc.Natl.Acad.Sci.U.S.A* 102,11, pp.3930-3935
Toyoda et al (2008) *Int.J.Oncol.* 33,6, pp.1141-1147
Umana et al (2001) *Nat.Biotechnol.* 19,6, pp.582-585
Van Geer et al (2010) *Int.J.Oncol.* 36,1, pp.233-244
Van Kampen et al (2005) *Vaccine* 23,8, pp.1029-1036
Vemula & Mittal (2010) *Expert.Opin.Biol.Ther.* 10,10, pp.1469-1487
Vlachaki et al (2002) *Mol.Ther.* 6,3, pp.342-348
Waddington et al (2008) *Cell* 132,3, pp.397-409
Waehler et al (2007) *Nat.Rev.Genet.* 8,8, pp.573-587
Walker-Daniels et al (1999) *Prostate* 41,4, pp.275-280
Wan et al (1999) *Int.J.Oncol.* 14,4, pp.771-776
Whyte et al (1988) *Nature* 334,6178, pp.124-129
Wilderman et al (2006) *Mol.Ther.* 13,5, pp.910-917
Xia et al (2006) *Cell Res.* 16,3, pp.241-259
Xiang et al (2006) *Emerg.Infect.Dis.* 12,10, pp.1596-1599

Xu et al (2005) *Gene Ther.* 12,20, pp.1526-1533
Yamamoto et al (2003) *J.Virol.* 77,2, pp.1633-1637
Yang et al (1994) *Proc.Natl.Acad.Sci.USA* 91,10, pp.4407-4411
Ye et al (2000) *Gene Ther.* 7,20, pp.1761-1767
Yew & Berk (1992) *Nature* 357,6373, pp.82-85
Yoshida et al (2003) *Cancer Immunol.Immunother.* 52,2, pp.97-106
Yu et al (2008) *Vaccine* 26,48, pp.6124-6131
Yuk et al (2004) *Biotechnol.Bioeng.* 86,6, pp.637-642
Zantek et al (1999) *Cell Growth Differ.* 10,9, pp.629-638
Zelinski et al (2001) *Cancer Res.* 61,5, pp.2301-2306
Zhang et al (2001) *Mol.Ther.* 3,5 Pt 1, pp.697-707
Zhou et al (2002) *J.Gene Med.* 4,5, pp.498-509
Zhu et al (2007) *J.Virol.* 81,7, pp.3170-3180

6

Adenovirus-Based Gene Therapy for Cancer

Changqing Su
Department of Molecular Oncology
Eastern Hepatobiliary Surgical Hospital
The Second Military Medical University, Shanghai
P. R. China

1. Introduction

The concept of gene therapy is defined as a biomedical technology to treat diseases with functional genes or therapeutic genes by transferring these genes into cells. According to the most comprehensive source of information on worldwide gene therapy clinical trials available on the internet from "The Journal of Gene Medicine" clinical trial site (http://www.wiley.com/genmed/clinical), there are 1060 clinical trials (64.5%) for cancer treatment among the total 1644 trials updated June 2010, and most of them (23.8%) use adenovirus as vector. However, gene therapy goes through one of gains and losses since the very day of its naissance. Until late 2009, gene therapy received a series of great achievements after years of silence. The journal, Science, appraised 10 breakthroughs of the Year 2009, in which the seventh was gene therapy. It brings us a rekindled hope for overcoming the genetic diseases including cancer.

Adenoviral vectors have been used extensively in cancer gene therapy (Su et al., 2008; Yang et al., 2007). Most of them are replication-deficient (Yang, 1995). The first generated replication-deficient adenovirus lacks the E1 and E3 regions. The second and third ones also contain E2 and/or E4 deletions (Andrews et al., 2001; Thomas et al., 2003). Because the replication-deficient adenoviruses can not replicate, they express the foreign therapeutic genes only in the cells that are initially infected. Synchronously, they also lack a specificity target to cancer cells (Kurihara et al., 2000). These problems may decrease the therapeutic effect on cancer cells and result in toxicity to normal cells. Therefore, development of a novel tumor-targeting adenoviral vector is needed to enhance the efficiency and specificity of transgene expression. Oncolytic adenoviruses are promising as therapeutic agents in cancer treatment. These viruses are genetically modified to target, infect and replicate in cancer cells causing them to lyse with an improved, superior efficacy compared to non-replicating adenoviral vector which lacks the E1 genes. Here, combined with the studies of our group (Fang et al., 2009, 2010; He et al., 2009, 2010; Hu et al., 2010; Ma et al., 2009; Su et al., 2004, 2006a, 2006b, 2008a, 2008b), we review the development of oncolytic adenovirus-based gene therapy for cancer, and figured the potential prospects of gene therapy in cancer treatment.

2. Adenovirus gene therapy

The strategy of virotherapy, a method for the treatment of cancer with viruses, has been revitalized since the appearance of a series of novel conditionally replicating adenoviruses

(CRAds), also known as oncolytic adenoviruses (Alemany et al., 2000). These tumor-selective replicating viruses were designed to replicate preferentially in cancer cells, but not in normal cells. The infection, replication and oncolytic abilities of CRAds were targeted specifically to cancer cells and had little or no influence on the normal cells (Kirn et al., 2001). After infecting one cancer cell and replicating in it, the viruses replicate and lyse the infected cell, and the progeny virions are released and infect the rest neighboring cancer cells. These cycles of infections and replications carry on repeatedly, making a chain reaction to facilitate viral spread within the cancer tissues till all cancer cells are destroyed (Ramachandra et al., 2001).

As antitumor therapeutic agents, CRAds are accordingly armed with incontestable advantages and is superior to replication-deficient adenovirus. There are a number of ongoing preclinical or clinical trials with oncolytic adenoviruses in treatment of a variety of cancers, such as OBP-301 (Telomelysin) in lung and prostate cancers, Ad-dl922-947, Ad-Onyx-015, Ad-Onyx-017, Ad-vKH1 and AdEHE2F in breast, colon, head and neck cancers (Bazan-Peregrino et al., 2008; Ouchi et al., 2009). A product of Onyx Pharmaceuticals (Richmond, CA), ONYX-015, is a replicative virus studied in clinical trials for several years. It is a chimeric human group C adenovirus (Ad2 and Ad5) modified by deletion between nucleotides 2496 and 3323 in the E1B region encoding the 55-kDa protein which binds the tumor suppressor protein p53. ONYX-015 has an ability to selectively replicate in and kill many human malignant tumor cells with mutations of p53 gene (Bischoff et al., 1996; Khuri et al., 2000).

Although the replicative viruses have many advantages to exert antitumor efficacy, they also have limitations in cancer therapy. Durable responses in clinical trials with replicative viruses, including ONYX-015, as single oncolytic agents have not been very encouraging (Ganly et al., 2000). It is not unexpected that a virus utilizing one of many mechanisms, such as p53 pathway, to promote its replication does not have enough power to destroy all cancer cells. This intrinsic limitation of targeted therapies mandates devotion to developing a series of selectively replicating viruses targeted to different tumorigenesis pathways, and to refining on replicative viruses with higher specificity, lower toxicity and stronger oncolytic efficacy for different tumors and different patients.

In order that viruses will specifically infect cancer cells, and the viral replication can be carefully controlled for the purpose of killing cancer cells safely and effectively, a cancer-specific expression and transportation system is required. One attempt to achieve CRAd is to modify adenovirus by partial deletion of viral genes (Biederer et al., 2002; Ring, 2002). The representative of this type of CRAd is ONYX-015. Moreover, many cancers have their own special markers whose expression is controlled by the particular cis-acting elements and trans-acting factors. Another attempt to achieve CRAd is to place viral replicative genes under the control of cancer-specific promoters. Although these tissue- or cancer-specific promoters can provide the restricted viral replication in cancer cells by controlling the expression of viral replicative genes, their shortcomings are obvious and cannot be ignored. Firstly, they are limited to a narrow range of cancers expressing the targeted tumor markers, and cannot be used for treatment of cancers of different origins. Secondly, most of them are much weaker than commonly used viral promoters such as cytomegalovirus (CMV) or SV40 early promoter (Gu et al., 2002). The expression of the genes driven by these specific promoters is generally in lower levels, thus attenuating their effects in cancer therapy (Su et al., 2004).

Many attempts have been made to improve both the antitumor potency and biosafety of approaches combining viral oncolytic therapy and transgene therapy. Genetic re-engineering of CRAds by incorporating therapeutic payloads may yield mutually supportive antitumor effects. CRAd replication selectively amplifies therapeutic transgene expression in cancer cells (Haviv et al., 2001; Nanda et al., 2001), and transgene expression synchronously increases the spread of viral progeny within a tumor cell mass (Hermiston & Kuhn, 2002; Van Beusechem et al., 2002). It has been shown that the approach combining gene therapy with oncolytic virotherapy is more effective than their use individually. Many therapeutic transgenes have exhibited antitumor efficacy in experimental models, including cytotoxic genes, suicide genes, tumor suppressor genes, apoptosis-inducing genes, angiogenesis-inhibiting genes and immunostimulatory genes (Haviv & Curiel, 2003; Lam & Breakefield, 2001). Some strategies have employed CRAds armed with immunostimulatory genes to enhance their overall antitumor activity. Heat shock proteins (HSPs) play important roles in eliciting innate and adaptive immunity by chaperoning peptides for antigen presentation to antigen-presenting cells and providing endogenous danger signalling. The recombinant oncolytic adenoviruses overexpressing the HSP70 protein can accordingly eradicate primary tumors, as well as inhibit the growth of established metastatic tumors in mice as a result of their capacity to induce individual tumor-specific immune responses (Huang et al., 2003). Although a few achievements have recently been made in the field of cancer gene therapy, great effort is still needed to select effective transgenes with more efficacy against cancers, and modify adenoviral vectors with more biosafety and specificity (Su et al., 2006a).

2.1 Modification of adenovirus E1a gene for CRAds

CRAds are genetically modified to express the wild type of E1a (wE1a) and showed good cytolytic effect in various human cancers (Hong et al., 2008; Liao et al., 2007; Su et al., 2006b, 2008a, 2008b), which binds to cellular regulators and mediates a series of genetic events, for instance, suppression of transformation, tumorigenicity and cancer metastatic ability (Kim et al., 2007). In addition, the E1a antitumor effect may be involved in many genetic factors in cancer cells, including E1a-induced apoptosis (Radke et al., 2008), Ela-enhanced sensitivity to chemotherapeutics and radiation (Sánchez-Prieto et al., 1996), E1a-triggered accumulation of p53 product and the E1a-mediated down-regulation of the oncogene Neu (ErbB-2/HER2) expression (Bartholomeusz et al., 2005; Madhusudan et al., 2004). Neu protein is a member of epidermal growth factor receptor (EGFR) and is commonly overexpressed in many human solid cancers, eg. in breast and primary liver cancer. E1a-mediated down-regulation of Neu expression in cancer cells could inhibit cancer cell proliferation and progression. Indeed, E1a-targeted gene therapy has been tested in clinical trials in cancer patients (Yoo et al., 2001). Moreover, during adenovirus infection, E1a protein interacts with a number of cellular proteins, thereby has an important role in facilitating viral replication.

The wE1a protein consists of three conserved regions (CR1, CR2, and CR3). These regions have different functions for viral antitumor effect and its replication. CR1 and CR2 are known to act through several cellular transcription factors, such as E2F, AP1, ATF, ETF, Sp1, CBP/p300, P/CAF, and USF, that interact with E1a-inducible promoters (Hale & Braithwaite, 1999). The N-terminus of CR1 is also required for the transcriptional activation, expression and stability of p53, and induces p53-dependent apoptosis (Itamochi et al., 2007). The CR2 domain binds to retinoblastoma tumor suppressor (Rb) protein, resulting in an inhibition of E2F transcription factors, and activating genes for cell cycle progression (Berk,

2005). The CR3 is a transcriptional activation domain that associates with CtIP, Sur2, CtBP (Bruton et al., 2007, 2008). However, any modification of the E1a gene which would optimise its antitumor efficacy without any significant negative effect on viral replication still needs to be investigated.

For increasing the wE1a antitumor efficacy without decreasing its effect on viral replication, the 870-bp wE1a gene was modified by deleting parts of the E1a CR2 (amino acid residues 125 to 128) and CR3 (amino acid residues 140 to 185) to yield a novel 720-bp truncated minimal-E1a gene (mE1a). The mE1a gene was introduced into an oncolytic adenoviral vector lacking the E1b genes, placing it under the control of human telomerase reverse transcriptase (hTERT) promoter, creating AdDC315-mE1a. The experiments showed that the vector was shown to give a high expression of mE1a protein in all cancer cell lines tested, including HepGII, A549, SGC-7901, Hela, MCF-7, HT-29, and also in HepGII xenograft models in nude mice where the expression was stable throughout the experiment (35 days). In AdDC315-mE1a treated cell lines and the xenografted tumors, the mE1a protein expression was selective in various cancer cell lines, but expression was negative or only weakly positive in the normal cells (Fang et al., 2009).

The truncated mE1a gene was also proved to have capacities to down-regulate Neu expression, and also support adenoviral replication for the oncolytic vector as well as the wE1a gene. But there is a difference between the mE1a gene and wE1a gene, the mE1a gene can release Rb protein efficiently and preserve the Rb function. The Rb pathway is frequently defective by phosphorylation of Rb protein (pRb). When the cancer cells are infected with adenoviruses, the Rb protein also can be inactivated by combination with the E1a-CR2 domains (Nemajerova et al., 2008). Both the phosphorylation and combination of Rb protein resulted in the release of E2F factor, thus the E2F activity is high in cancer cells. The oncolytic adenovirus with a deletion of 24 bp in Rb-binding region of the E1a protein (amino acids 122–129) is sufficient to prevent binding to and inactivation of the Rb protein, but it has little effect on the functions of the E1a protein that are necessary for effective viral replication in cancer cells (Fueyo et al., 2000). The results demonstrated that the mE1a gene with a small deletion of 125-128 amino acid residules in Rb-binding region has a diminished binding affinity to Rb and can preserve Rb function.

The adenovirus E1a can render the adenovirus-infected cells susceptible to DNA damage from chemotherapy and radiation. Interestingly, normal cells appear to be unaffected by E1a protein (Sánchez-Prieto et al., 1996). Most oncolytic adenoviruses have been engineered by holding E1a gene expression. Thereby, in addition to their oncolytic effects, E1a protein endows oncolytic adenovirus with higher antitumor potency. Since the 1990s, oncolytic adenoviruses with E1a expression were utilized to treat cancer patients from Phase I to Phase III. In 2004, China approved one kind of oncolytic adenovirus, H101, to market. Clinical data showed that H101 is well tolerable and has good efficacy when combined with chemotherapy in some cancer treatment modalities (Yu & Fang, 2007). For the purpose of optimizing the therapeutic efficacy of wE1a, the small truncated E1a variant, mE1A, is proved to be capable of down-regulating Neu expression and supporting adenovirus replication in the mE1a-expressed cancer cells. It has a particular strongpoint to boost Rb function differed from the wE1a gene. Thereby, the mE1a-supported oncolytic adenovirus is endowed with more effective effects on tumor growth suppression, cell cycle arrest and cancer cell apoptosis as demonstrated in hepatocarcinoma xenografts in nude mice (Fang et al., 2009).

2.2 Modification of tumor-selective promoters for CRAds

Several tissue- and cell-specific promoters that are more active in the particular cancer cells, but inactive or only weakly active in the cancer-originating somatic cells, have been identified and exploited to construct CRAds or target gene transportation and expression in cancers, such as the carcinoembryonic antigen (CEA) promoter in colorectal and lung cancer (Osaki et al., 1994), the DF3/MUC1 antigen promoter in breast cancer (Kurihara et al., 2000), the E2F transcriptional factor promoter in cancers with a defective pRb/E2F/p16 pathway (Johnson et al., 2002; Ramachandra et al., 2001; Tsukuda et al., 2002), the α-fetoprotein promoter in hepatocellular cancer (Ohashi et al., 2001), the prostate-specific antigen (PSA) promoter in prostate cancer (Rodriguez et al., 1997) and the L-plastin promoter in ovarian and bladder cancers (Peng et al., 2001). These cancer-specific promoters can provide CRAds the selective replication in corresponding cancer cells and demonstrate antitumor activity in preclinical models and clinical trials. However, most of them limit to target a narrow range of cancers expressing the corresponding tumor antigen, thus attenuating their efficacy in cancer therapy. More efforts should be put in seek the tumor-selective promoters targeting a wide range of human cancers.

2.2.1 The hTERT promoter-regulated CRAds

A number of gene therapeutic approaches have been proposed to kill cancer cells or inhibit growth of caners by targeting telomerase (Hodes, 2001). Telomerase, a unique enzyme that synthesizes telomeric repeats, is highly activated in immortalized cell lines and most of the malignant tumors, but is inactive in normal somatic cells (Cong et al., 1999; Kim et al., 1994; Shay & Bacchetti, 1997). Telomerase activation has been regarded as a crucial step in cellular carcinogenesis, and it is the broadest spectrum molecular marker of malignancies found. More detailed analyses of telomerase activity in normal and malignant cells suggested that telomerase is active in most cancers, more than 85% of human primary cancers exhibit telomerase activity (Nowak et al., 2003; Saretzki et al., 2002), but not in normal tissues except hematopoietic stem cells and germ cells in the ovary and testis (Kim et al., 1994; Yui et al., 1998). With these properties, telomerase is an ideal target for cancer gene therapy and has attracted an intense interest in recent years. The studies have established a possibility that the manipulation of telomerase function may have an important role in cancer therapeutic intervention. Based on the knowledge on the structure and function of telomere and telomerase, a number of approaches have been proposed to inhibit the growth and division of caner cells by targeting the telomerase (Hodes, 2001).

Telomerase is a ribonucleoprotein complex composed of the telomerase RNA (hTR), the telomerase associated protein and the telomerase reverse transcriptase (hTERT). By cloning of the hTR and hTERT components to clarify the mechanism of telomerase activation, it has been demonstrated that hTR is expressed in both telomerase-positive and -negative cells, but hTERT is expressed only in telomerase-positive cells but not in telomerase-negative cells. Transferring hTERT gene into telomerase-negative cells can induce telomerase activation in these cells (Nakayama et al., 1998; Weinrich et al., 1997). A strong correlation is established between hTERT expression and telomerase activity. These findings strongly suggest that the hTERT component is the key determinant of human telomerase activity, and utilizing hTERT promoter to drive antitumoral genes in cancer gene therapy can target to and selectively kill the cancer cells with positive telomerase activity, without affecting the normal cells with negative telomerase activity (Koga et al., 2000; Poole et al., 2001).

The hTERT promoter has been cloned and identified (Cong et al., 1999; Horikawa et al., 1999). It is highly G/C-rich and lacks TATA and CAAT boxes, and has several binding sites for transcriptional factors, including the transcriptional activating factors Myc (Eickbush, 1997), SP1 (Kyo et al., 2000), and the transcriptional repressing factors Mad1 (Gunes et al., 2000), p53 (Xu et al., 2000), MZF2 (Fujimoto et al., 2000). By measuring the transcriptional activity of a series of constructs containing unidirectionally deleted fragments of the hTERT promoter, some investigators discovered that a 181 bp fragment upstream of the transcriptional start site is the smallest core promoter essential for transcriptional activation of hTERT gene (Abdul-Ghani et al., 2000; Takakura et al., 1999). The expression of c-Myc oncoprotein markedly induces the transcriptional activity of the hTERT promoter in the endogenous hTERT-negative cells, and induces 3- to 7-fold increase of the hTERT promoter activity in the hTERT-positive cell lines (Horikawa et al., 1999). The mechanism of c-Myc protein up-regulating the hTERT promoter activity is probably through the E-box motifs (CACGTG) within the hTERT core promoter. It has been shown that although SP1 factor is over-expressed in the telomerase-negative normal somatic cells and its binding to the specific sites promotes the start of hTERT gene transcription, by comparison, the major determinant regulating the hTERT gene expression is the transcriptional factors that combined with E-box motifs. In addition to the E-box (-187 bp to -182 bp) upstream of the transcriptional start site (Horikawa et al., 1999), there is another E-box (+22 bp to +27 bp) downstream of the transcriptional start site (Horikawa et al., 2002). This downstream E-box mediates the activation or repression of hTERT gene transcription by binding c-Myc or Mad1 transcriptional factors, respectively (Greenberg et al., 1999; Gunes et al., 2000). The current research demonstrated that the downstream E-box is a target for down-regulating the hTERT activity in the telomerase-negative cells. But this downstream E-box changes to the binding site for up-regulating the hTERT gene transcription in the telomerase-positive cells when it combines with the transcriptional activating factors such as the upstream stimulatory factor (USF), a member of Myc family (Horikawa et al., 2002). Therefore, the expression of the hTERT gene determining the telomerase activity is firmly controlled by many factors including the transcriptional activating and repressing factors, and the regulatory sites mainly locate in the promoter region of the hTERT gene.

Some current studies showed that the hTERT promoter which was used to construct CRAds by controlling the E1a gene demonstrated a sufficient activity for viral effective replication in cancer cells (Huang et al., 2003; Irving et al., 2004; Kawashima et al., 2004; Zou et al., 2004). To further improve the specificity of hTERT promoter, the activity of hTERT core promoter could be enhanced significantly in the majority of the cancer cell lines by inserting the adenovirus E1a TATA box downstream of the hTERT promoter (Wirth et al., 2003). A CRAd, CNHK300, in which the hTERT promoter is used to replace the original regulatory elements of E1a gene and to control the E1a gene expression, can target to the telomerase-positive cancer cells and replicate in them, resulting in oncolysis, when the progeny virions are released and infect the adjacent cancer cells, they will not affect the normal cells negative for telomerase activity. Another interesting approach developed an oncolytic adenovirus AdEHT2 in which a minimal dual-specificity promoter that responds to estrogens and hypoxia was used to control the viral E1a gene, and the hTERT core promoter was introduced into the E4 region of AdEHT2 (Hernandez-Alcoceba et al., 2002). Their experiments of viral replication and cytotoxicity showed that AdEHT2 was not attenuated in telomerase-negative cells when these cells were infected under hypoxia conditions. It was postulated that the good expression of the adenoviral E1a gene activated by hypoxia was sufficient to promote the viral replication. They also held that the E1a protein can potentially stimulate the hTERT promoter in the E4 region directly or as a consequence of the cell cycle activation. Although the E4-deleted adenovirus was attenuated, a low level of the E4 open reading frame expression could support its replication under the condition that the rest transcriptional units of the virus were activated. Based on the published data and the current study, it is reasonable to conclude that the tight regulation of the adenoviral E1a gene is crucial for the replication of the virus.

One of the major concerns was the potential toxicity of hTERT promoter-regulated CRAds to stem cells or other normal cells, although there were evidences suggesting that the toxic effects caused by the use of the hTERT promoter on normal cells may be transient (Chiu et al., 1996), and could be prevented by using the adenoviral vectors which infect stem cells poorly (Gu et al., 2000). The toxicity assay was performed in BALB/c mice by sequential intravenous injections of the hTERT promoter-regulated CRAds and the control virus (wild adenovirus type 5, wAd5). The main objective is to investigate whether the replicative adenovirus has toxicity to liver cells after systemic delivery. The results suggested that the hTERT promoter-regulated CRAds are less toxic than wAd5 after intravenous administration. They are well tolerated at a low dosage that was equal to the therapeutic dosage for the treatment of the transplantation tumors of nude mice. Even at a high dosage of hTERT promoter-regulated CRAds, mice showed no signs of toxicity in terms of mortality, liver enzyme levels and hepatocyte morphology, no replication of viruses was found in liver tissues by E1a immunohistochemistry, and only slight granular or hydropic degeneration of hepatocytes could be observed. Meanwhile, wAd5 displayed both a certain mortality and liver toxicity. All mice died at a high dosage of wAd5, and the therapeutic dosage induced an obvious increase of liver enzymes and evidence of cytopathic effects on liver tissues. Therefore, the toxic effect of hTERT promoter-regulated CRAds is much weakened compared with wAd5 by the use of the hTERT promoter (Su et al., 2004, 2006b, 2008a; Wang et al., 2008).

2.2.2 The E2F promoter-regulated CRAds

The loose control of cell cycle is a key feature of cancer cell proliferation. Much evidence suggests that the Cyclin/Cyclin-dependent kinase (CDK)/P16/retinoblastoma protein (Rb)/E2F pathway is the major link for cell cycle control. Cyclin D1 activates CDK4 and promotes the phosphorylation of Rb protein, which makes the E2F transcriptional factor released from Rb-E2F complex. Then the E2F transcriptional factor activates the transcription of many important cell cycle regulatory genes, and promotes tumorigenesis. P16 is known as a negative regulator of cell cycle, which can block cell cycle progression from G1 to S phase by binding to CDK4 and inhibiting the action of Cyclin D1 (Coqueret, 2002; Ortega et al., 2002). It was found that the inactivation of Cyclin D/ CDK/ P16/ Rb/ E2F pathway is a common characteristic of most solid cancers (Gemin et al., 2005; Johnson et al., 2002; Tsukuda et al., 2002). This pathway is an ideal target for cancer gene therapy and has attracted an intense interest in recent years.

As described above, cancer cells with the deficiency of Cyclin /CDK/P16/Rb/E2F pathway have high activity of E2F transcriptional factor, thus this important factor is defined as a crucial target in cancer treatment. A CRAd, AdEHE2F, in which the expression of E4 gene is controlled by the E2F promoter, had been generated for breast cancer treatment (Post et al., 2003). The tight regulation of E4 expression correlated with the viral ability to selectively replicate and kill cancer cells. Current study constructed an E2F promoter-regulated CRAd which was armed with the p16 gene, AdE2F-p16. By controlling the E1a gene expression with the E2F promoter, AdE2F-p16 achieved a desired specificity to target cancer cells, while the normal cells were spared. The luciferase assay suggested that the E2F promoter had a high activity in cancer cells but not in normal cells. The data from in vitro experiments showed that AdE2F-p16 specifically replicated and induced E1a expression in cancer cells. Due to the viral replication, AdE2F-p16 more efficiently expressed P16 than the replication-deficient adenovirus AdCMV-p16 in cancer cells. Thereby, AdE2F-p16 overcomes the disadvantages of low transfer rate and poor gene expression compared with the replication-deficient adenovirus vectors. In summary, the E2F promoter-regulated, p16-armed CRAd can mediate the effective expression of transgene in cancer cells, and displays a satisfactory therapeutic effect for cancer (Ma et al., 2009).

To further investigate the molecular mechanisms of P16-induced apoptosis, the consequential study found that the adenovirus-mediated P16 reactivation lead to an inhibition of Akt signaling pathway and a downregulation of survivin expression in hepatocellular carcinoma cells (Hu et al., 2010). P16 and survivin are a pair of incompatible factors in the cell cycle and cell apoptosis regulation. Cyclin D1 and P16 eventually regulate cell cycle by interacting with CDK4 (Ai et al., 2005). CDK4 and survivin are co-localized mainly in nuclei of the P16-deficient hepatocellular carcinoma cells. But when cancer cells re-express P16, the P16 protein competes with survivin for CDK4 binding and transports CDK4 from nuclei to cytoplasm. The translocation of CDK4 from nuclei to cytoplasm illuminates that its function to accelerate cell proliferation is weakened. Interestingly, it is found an important molecular event that the nuclear survivin is reduced obviously in cancer cells after P16 re-expressed. The localization of survivin in cancer cells exerts different functions. The nuclear survivin is involved in promoting cell proliferation, whereas the cytoplasmic survivin may participate in controlling cell survival (Connell et al., 2008; Li et al., 2005; Liu & Matsuura, 2005). Accordingly, survivin promotes cell proliferation and inhibits cell apoptosis by competitively interacting with CDK4, and the P16-induced decrease of the amount of survivin and CDK4 in nuclei contributes to the inhibition of cell cycle progression and induction of detachment-induced apoptosis (anoikis) in cancer cells. This new insight into P16 function would help in designing better strategies for cancer gene therapy.

2.3 Utilization of antitumor transgenes

CRAds can be designed to function as therapeutic gene delivery vehicles by incorporating antitumor transgenes, and their antitumor efficacy is thus increased by the combination of antitumor gene therapy and oncolytic viral therapy (Chen et al., 2005; Nagayama et al., 2003; Post et al., 2003; Su et al., 2006a). Previous studies confirmed the antitumor activity of various vectors carrying cytokine genes, such as interferons (Belardelli & Gresser, 1996), tumor necrosis factors (Zhang et al., 1996), drug-sensitive gene HSV-tk (Steele, 2000), antiangiogenesis genes (Fang et al., 2010). When these therapeutic genes were inserted into the genome of CRAds, they were selectively and highly expressed in cancer cells as a result of the cancer-selective replication of CARds, which further enhanced therapeutic effect targeting cancer cells without toxicity to normal tissues or cells.

2.3.1 CRAd with interferon-gamma (IFN-γ) gene

Interferons (IFNs) are the first cytokines to be applied clinically in treatment of human cancers, and have anti-proliferative effects and immune modulatory activity. They have also been shown to inhibit angiogenesis and suppress tumor vascularization (Dvorak & Gresser, 1989; Fathallah-Shaykh et al., 2000; Singh et al., 1995). Among IFNs, IFN-γ is vital to the promotion of tumor surveillance in immunocompetent hosts and activates macrophages to nonspecifically lyse cancer cells through various mechanisms (Baratin et al., 2001; Guadagni et al., 1994). IFN-γ can enhance antitumor immune response by upregulating major histocompatibility complex class I expression and accentuating the migration of specific and non-specific immune cells to necrotic areas which develop spontaneously in large tumors (Khorana et al., 2003; Merritt et al., 2004; Peyregne et al., 2004). Gene transfer of IFN-γ inhibits neovascularization of tumors by inducing apoptosis of endothelial cells (Kowalczyk et al., 2003), suggesting that IFN-γ represses tumor growth by the dual mechanisms of inhibition of angiogenesis and elicitation of an immunotherapeutic response.

In clinical trials, only high concentration of IFN-γ product in tumor tissues yields antiangiogenic effects and immune response. Unfortunately, high concentration of IFN-γ product is associated with significant toxic effects, including fever, endocrine dysfunction, thrombocytopenia, and hepatic toxicity (Jonasch & Haluska, 2001). Therefore, its toxicity limits the administration of high concentration of this agent. Based on dual antitumor features of the IFN-γ gene and tumor-selective replication of viruses, CRAds armed with the IFN-γ gene could amplify transgene copies in tumor cells and produce high local concentration of IFN-γ product in tumor tissues. This strategy could thus yield multiple antitumor effects including oncolysis, antiangiogenesis, and induction of immune response. Even in immunodeficient animals, delivery of IFN-γ can partially restore significant immune activity (Wu et al., 2001).

In tumor models of nude mice, the IFN-γ gene-armed CRAd exhibited efficient antitumor activity against tumor xenografts. Many extensive foci of necrosis appeared in virus-treated tumor specimens. Around the necrotic foci, there were cancer cells positive for adenoviral capsid protein in tumor tissues, suggesting the selective replication and oncolytic effect of the IFN-γ gene-armed CRAd in cancer cells. The number of microvessels was clearly decreased in tumor tissues, which may be one of the mechanisms of IFN-γ-mediated antitumor responses in mice. Since suppressing tumor angiogenesis could lead to tumor starvation and regression (Folkman, 1998), decreasing the number of microvessels in tumor tissues might strongly suppress tumor growth. The present study found that more effective antitumor immune responses were exhibited when the IFN-γ gene-armed CRAd was used in immunocompetent hosts than in immunodeficient animals, because the host immune system was intact to support the full function of IFN-γ. After treated with the IFN-γ gene-armed CRAd, the increase in numbers of LCA+, CD4+, and CD8+ lymphocytes and the ratio of CD4+/CD8+ in tumor tissues accounted for the enhancement of immune responses to cancer cells (Su et al., 2006a). It is hypothesized that the combination of oncolytic virotherapy and immune gene therapy would enhance antitumor efficacy in both immunodeficient and immunocompetent hosts, and obtained results strongly supporting this hypothesis.

2.3.2 CRAd with antiangiogenesis gene

Increasing evidence suggests that the solid tumors and their metastasis are angiogenesis dependent. Angiogenesis is a complex process that includes the activation, proliferation, and migration of endothelial cells. This process involves in the formation of vascular tubes and networks. Antiangiogenic therapy attempts to stop new microvessels from forming around tumors and to break up the existing network of abnormal capillaries that feed the cancerous mass, finally mediates the inhibition of cancer growth.

Endostatin, a 20-kDa C-terminal fragment of collagen XVIII, is the most potent angiogenesis inhibitor and specifically inhibits endothelial cell proliferation and migration, induces apoptosis of vascular endothelial cells (Lai et al., 2007; Li et al., 2008; Ning et al., 2008), and has been demonstrated to be with antitumor effect in many solid tumors, and without toxicity, immunogenesis or resistance. The adenovirus vector carrying a secretable form of mouse endostatin, Av3mEndo, mediated the secreted expression of endostatin from Av3mEndo-transduced mammalian cells and showed a potential inhibition of endothelial cell migration in vitro. A single intravenous administration of Av3mEndo in mice could result in prolonged and elevated levels of circulating endostatin, partial inhibition of vascular endothelial growth factor (VEGF)-induced angiogenesis, and in 25% of mice the complete prevention of tumor growth (Chen et al., 2000). The CRAd, AdSu-hE, in which a chimeric promoter of HER2 enhancer and hTERT promoter was used to drive the E1a gene, a cytomegalovirus promoter to control the human endostatin gene. In vivo intratumoral delivery of the CRAd to pre-established hepatocellular carcinoma tumors in nude mice induced a significant tumor reduction and, in some cases resulted in a complete tumor regression (Fang et al., 2010).

Canstatin, a novel matrix-derived inhibitor of angiogenesis, was described as being at least 10-fold more active than endostatin (Kamphaus et al., 2000; Narazaki & Tosato, 2006). Experiments demonstrated that recombinant canstatin can potently inhibit endothelial cell proliferation, migration, and induce apoptosis in vitro. Moreover, it can successfully suppress the growth of implanted human xenografts of renal cell carcinoma and prostate tumors through antiangiogenesis effect (Kamphaus et al., 2000). The canstatin gene was inserted into an E1B-55kDa-deleted adenovirus vector and constructed an adenovirus, CRAd-Cans. It showed markedly improved inhibitory effects on the growth of the pancreatic cancer in mice with a prolonged survival rate through the mechanisms of oncolytic and anti-angiogenesis effects (He et al., 2009).

2.3.3 CRAd with tumor suppression gene

P16 is known as a negative regulator of cell cycle, which can block cell cycle progression from G1 to S phase by binding to CDK4 and inhibiting the action of Cyclin D1 (Canepa et al., 2007; Coqueret, 2002). It was found that the P16 inactivation is a frequent molecular event in most cancers. The mechanisms of P16 inactivation include the homozygous deletion, point mutation and 5′-CpG island methylation (Ortega et al., 2002). Due to the P16 inactivation, cancer cells show growth superiority and high malignancy. Reactivation of P16 by transferring the p16 gene into cancer cells induced cell G1 arrest and apoptosis (Chen et al., 2005), suggesting that the p16 gene may have a good future application in cancer gene therapy. The E2F promoter-regulated CRAd armed with the p16 gene, AdE2F-p16, was constructed (Ma et al., 2009). With the selective replication of AdE2F-p16 under the control of the E2F promoter, AdE2F-p16 expressed P16 with high levels in cancer cells. The improved antitumor efficacy of AdE2F-p16 was shown in human gastric cancer model in nude mice. The viral selective replication resulted in enhanced oncolysis, and p16 expression induced cancer cell apoptosis, suggesting that the combined effects led to the tumor growth inhibition in mouse models.

The p53 gene is one of the most important tumor suppressor gene. It plays an important role in cancer gene therapy, which has received preclinical validation by developing anticancer agents that specifically reactivate P53 function (Martins et al., 2006). To explore the efficacy of wild type p53 reactivation as a tumor therapy, some investigators demonstrated that restoring endogenous P53 expression in mice led to regression of autochthonous lymphomas through cellular apoptosis pathway and sarcomas through cellular senescence in mice, but without affecting normal tissues (Ventura et al., 2007). By RNA interference (RNAi) to conditionally regulate endogenous P53 expression in a mosaic mouse model of liver carcinoma, it was found that even brief reactivation of endogenous P53 in p53-deficient tumors could produce complete tumor regressions through the induction of a cellular senescence that was associated with differentiation and upregulation of inflammatory cytokines (Xue et al., 2007). These studies indicated that the p53-triggered tumor regression is not only due to the cellular apoptosis but the cellular senescence program, which is dependent on the tumor types. The transfer of wide type p53 gene is an important method to cure the p53-deficient cancers (Swisher & Roth, 2002; Weill et al., 2000). A previous study demonstrated the enhanced antitumor effect of CRAd with the wild type p53 gene in the treatment of glioma (Van Beusechem et al., 2002). The tumor-specific CRAds carrying the wide type p53 gene, SG600-p53, can selectively replicate in tumor cells, whereas hardly replicated in normal cell lines, suggesting that SG600-p53 has a high selectivity to cancer cells and a low toxicity to normal cells. SG600-p53 expressed P53 with high efficiency in cancer cells. Both the high selectivity of viral replication and high efficiency of P53 expression ensured the efficient oncolytic effect and inhibition effect on cancer cells. In NCI-H1299 tumor xenografts in nude mice, SG600-p53 achieved the significant antitumor efficacy. By pathological examination, administration of SG600-p53 resulted in cancer cell apoptosis. It is concluded that the CRAd carrying p53 gene, as a more potent and safer antitumor agent, could provide a new strategy for cancer biotherapy.

3. Problems and prospects

The achievements of success in adenovirus-based gene therapy bring forth new hope to treat cancer. Many countries worldwide invested heavily in cancer gene therapy, however, there are few products used in clinic because of their low efficacy. The differences between the in vitro and in vivo experiments, basic technology and clinical application should be further investigated. More worrying about the long-term toxicity of transgene vector also limits the wide utilization of gene therapy. These problems existed and exist, but they can not counteract the developments and prospects of gene therapy. The traditional strategies for cancer treatment, including surgery, chemotherapy and radiation, are difficult to eradicate the root of various cancers, the gene therapy absolutely searches for the roots cause of carcinogenesis, and corrects the genetic defects in transformed cells. Further investigations on the carcinogenesis mechanism, signal transduction and genetic characteristic of cancer cells will promote the development and breakthrough of cancer gene therapy in the future.

4. References

Abdul-Ghani, R., Ohana, P., Matouk, I., Ayesh, S., Ayesh, B., Laster, M., Bibi, O., Giladi, H., Molnar-Kimber, K., Sughayer, M. A., De Groot, N. & Hochberg, A. (2000). Use of transcriptional regulatory sequences of telomerase (hTER and hTERT) for selective killing of cancer cells, *Mol. Ther.* 2(6): 539-544.

Ai, M. D., Li, L. L., Zhao, X. R., Wu, Y., Gong, J. P. & Cao, Y. (2005). Regulation of survivin and CDK4 by Epstein-Barr virus encoded latent membrane protein 1 in nasopharyngeal carcinoma cell lines, *Cell Res.* 15(10):777-784.

Alemany, R., Balagué, C. & Curiel, D. T. (2000). Replicative adenoviruses for cancer therapy, *Nat. Biotechnol.* 18(7): 723-727.

Andrews, J. L., Kadan, M. J., Gorziglia, M. I., Kaleko, M. & Connelly, S. (2001). Generation and characterization of E1/E2a/E3/E4-deficient adenoviral vectors encoding human factor VIII, *Mol. Ther.* 3(3):329-336.

Baratin, M., et al. (2001). Regression of primary hepatocarcinoma in cancer-prone transgenic mice by local interferon-gamma delivery is associated with macrophages recruitment and nitric oxide production, *Cancer Gene Ther.* 8(3):193-202.

Bartholomeusz, C., Itamochi, H., Yuan, L. X., Esteva, F. J., Wood, C. G., Terakawa, N., Hung, M. C. & Ueno, N. T. (2005). Bcl-2 antisense oligonucleotide overcomes resistance to E1A gene therapy in a low HER2-expressing ovarian cancer xenograft model, *Cancer Res.* 65(18):8406-8413.

Bazan-Peregrino, M., Carlisle, R. C., Hernandez-Alcoceba, R., Iggo, R., Homicsko, K., Fisher, K. D., Halldén, G., Mautner, V., Shen, Y. & Seymour, L. W. (2008). Comparison of molecular strategies for breast cancer virotherapy using oncolytic adenovirus, *Hum. Gene Ther.* 19(9): 873-886.

Belardelli, F. & Gresser, I. (1996). The neglected role of type I interferon in the T-cell response: implications for its clinical use, *Immunol. Today* 17(8):369-372.

Berk, A. J. (2005). Recent lessons in gene expression, cell cycle control, and cell biology from adenovirus, *Oncogene* 24(52):7673-7685.

Biederer, C., Ries, S., Brandts, C. H. & McCormick, F. (2002). Replication-selective viruses for cancer therapy, *J. Mol. Med.* 80(3):163-175.

Bischoff, J. R., Kirn, D. H., Williams, A., Heise, C., Horn, S., Muna, M., Ng, L., Nye, J. A., Sampson-Johannes, A., Fattaey, A. & McCormick, F. (1996). An adenovirus mutant that replicates selectively in p53-deficient human tumor cells, *Science* 274(5286):373-376.

Bruton, R. K., Pelka, P., Mapp, K. L., Fonseca, G. J., Torchia, J., Turnell, A. S., Mymryk, J. S. & Grand, R. J. (2008). Identification of a second CtBP binding site in adenovirus 5 E1A conserved region 3, *J. Virol.* 82(17):8476-8486.

Bruton, R. K., Rasti, M., Mapp, K. L., Young, N., Carter, R. Z., Abramowicz, I. A., Sedgwick, G. G., Onion, D. F., Shuen, M., Mymryk, J. S., Turnell, A. S. & Grand, R. J. (2007). C-terminal-binding protein interacting protein binds directly to adenovirus early region 1A through its N-terminal region and conserved region 3, *Oncogene* 26(53):7467-7479.

Canepa, E. T., Scassa, M. E., Ceruti, J. M., Marazita, M. C., Carcagno, A. L., Sirkin, P. F. & Ogara, M. F. (2007). INK4 proteins, a family of mammalian CDK inhibitors with novel biological functions, *IUBMB Life* 59(7):419-426.

Chen, C. T., Lin, J., Li, Q., Phipps, S. S., Jakubczak, J. L., Stewart, D. A., Skripchenko, Y., Forry-Schaudies, S., Wood, J., Schnell, C. & Hallenbeck, P. L. (2000). Antiangiogenic gene therapy for cancer via systemic administration of adenoviral vectors expressing secretable endostatin, *Hum. Gene Ther.* 11(14):1983-1996.

Chen, F., Li, Y., Lu, Z., Gao, J. & Chen, J. (2005). Adenovirus-mediated Ink4a/ARF gene transfer significantly suppressed the growth of pancreatic carcinoma cells, *Cancer Biol. Ther.* 4(12):1348-1354.

Chiu, C. P., Dragowska, W., Kim, N. W., Vaziri, H., Yui, J., Thomas, T. E., Harley, C. B. & Lansdorp, P. M. (1996). Differential expression of tolemerase activity in hematopoietic progenitors from adult human bone marrow, *Stem Cells* 14(2):239-248.

Cong, Y. S., Wen, J. & Bacchetti, S. (1999). The human telomerase catalytic subunit hTERT: organization of the gene and characterization of the promoter, *Hum. Mol. Genet.* 8(1):137-142.

Connell, C. M., Wheatley, S. P. & McNeish, I. A. (2008). Nuclear survivin abrogates multiple cell cycle checkpoints and enhances viral oncolysis, *Cancer Res.* 68(19):7923-7931.

Coqueret, O. (2002). Linking cyclins to transcriptional control, *Gene* 299(1-2):35-55.

Dvorak, H. F. & Gresser, I. (1989). Microvascular injury in pathogenesis of interferon-induced necrosis of subcutaneous tumors in mice, *J. Nat. Cancer Inst.* 81(7):497-502.

Eickbush, T. H. (1997). Telomerase and retrotransposons: which came first? *Science* 277(5328): 911-912.

Fang, L., Huang, Y., Hu, X., Sun, L., He, X., Hu, H., Pu, Y., Cao, X., Luo, H., Pan, S., Gu, J. & Su, C. (2009). A truncated minimal-E1a gene with potency to support adenoviral replication mediates antitumor activity by down-regulating Neu expression and preserving Rb function, *Chem. Biol. Interact.* 181(1):1-7.

Fang, L., Pu, Y. Y., Hu, X. C., Sun, L. J., Luo, H. M., Pan, S. K., Gu, J. Z., Cao, X. R. & Su, C. Q. (2010). Antiangiogenesis gene armed tumor-targeting adenovirus yields multiple antitumor activities in human HCC xenografts in nude mice, *Hepatol. Res.* 40(2):216-228.

Fathallah-Shaykh, H. M., Zhao, L. J., Kafrouni, A. I., Smith, G. M. & Forman, J. (2000). Gene transfer of IFN-gamma into established brain tumors represses growth by antiangiogenesis, *J. Immunol.* 164(1):217-222.

Folkman, J. (1998). Antiangiogenic gene therapy, *Proc. Natl. Acad. Sci. U S A* 95(16):9064-9066.

Fueyo, J., Gomez-Manzano, C., Alemany, R., Lee, P. S., McDonnell, T. J., Mitlianga, P., Shi, Y. X., Levin, V. A., Yung, W. K. & Kyritsis, A. P. (2000). A mutant oncolytic adenovirus targeting the Rb pathway produces antiglioma effect in vivo, *Oncogene* 19(1):2–12.

Fujimoto, K., Kyo, S., Takakura, M., Kanaya, T., Kitagawa, Y., Itoh, H., Takahashi, M. & Inoue, M. (2000). Identification and characterization of negative regulatory elements of the human telomerase catalytic subunit (hTERT) gene promoter: possible role of MZF-2 in transcriptional repression of hTERT, *Nucleic Acids Res.* 28(13):2557-2562.

Ganly, I., Kirn, D., Eckhardt, G., Rodriguez, G. I., Soutar, D. S., Otto, R., Robertson, A. G., Park, O., Gulley, M. L., Heise, C., Von Hoff, D. D., Kaye, S. B. & Eckhardt, S. G. (2000). A phase I study of Onyx-015, an E1B attenuated adenovirus, administered intratumorally to patients with recurrent head and neck cancer, *Clin. Cancer Res.* 6(3):798-806.

Gemin, A., Sweet, S., Preston, T. J. & Singh, G. (2005). Regulation of the cell cycle in response to inhibition of mitochondrial generated energy, *Biochem. Biophys. Res. Commun.* 332(4):1122-1132.

Greenberg, R. A., O'Hagan, R. C., Deng, H., Xiao, Q., Hann, S. R., Adams, R. R., Lichtsteiner, S., Chin, L., Morin, G. B. & Depinho, R. A. (1999). Telomerase reverse transcriptase gene is a direct target of c-Myc but is not functionally equivalent in cellular transformation, *Oncogene* 18(5):1219-1926.

Gu, J., Andreeff, M., Roth, J. A. & Fang, B. (2002). hTERT promoter induces tumor-specific Bax gene expression and cell killing in syngenic mouse tumor model and prevents systemic toxicity, *Gene Ther.* 9(1):30-37.

Gu, J., Kagawa, S., Takakura, M., Kyo, S., Inoue, M., Roth, J. A. & Fang, B. (2000). Tumor-specific transgene expression from the human telomerase reverse transcriptase promoter enables targeting of the therapeutic effects of the bax gene to cancers, *Cancer Res.* 60(19):5359-5364.

Guadagni, F., Roselli, M., Schlom, J. & Greiner, J. W. (1994). In vitro and in vivo regulation of human tumor antigen expression by human recombinant interferons: a review, *Int. J. Biol. Markers* 9(1):53-60.

Gunes, C., Lichtsteiner, S., Vasserot, A.P. & Englert, C. (2000). Expression of the hTERT gene is regulated at the level of transcriptional initiation and repressed by Mad1, *Cancer Res.* 60(8):2116-2121.

Hale, T. K. & Braithwaite, A. W. (1999). The adenovirus oncoprotein E1a stimulates binding of transcription factor ETF to transcriptionally activate the p53 gene, *J. Biol. Chem.* 274(34):23777-23786.

Haviv, Y. S., Blackwell, J. L., Li, H., Wang, M., Lei, X. & Curiel, D. T. (2001). Heat shock and heat shock protein 70i enhance the oncolytic effect of replicative adenovirus, *Cancer Res.* 61(23):8361-8365.

Haviv, Y. S. & Curiel, D. T. (2003). Engineering regulatory elements for conditionally-replicative adeno-viruses, *Curr. Gene Ther.* 3(4):357-385.

He, X., Liu, J., Yang, C., Su, C., Zhou, C., Zhang, Q., Li, L., Wu, H., Liu, X., Wu, M. & Qian, Q. (2010). 5/35 fiber-modified conditionally replicative adenovirus armed with p53 shows increased tumor-suppressing capacity to breast cancer cells. *Hum. Gene Ther.* doi:10.1089/hum.2010.058.

He, X., Su, C., Wang, X., Pan, X., Tu, Z., Gong, Y., Gao, J., Liao, Z., Jin, J., Wu, H., Man, X. & Li, Z. (2009). E1B-55kD-deleted oncolytic adenovirus armed with canstatin gene yields an enhanced anti-tumor efficacy on pancreatic cancer, *Cancer Lett.* 285(1):89-98.

Hermiston, T. W. & Kuhn, I. (2002). Armed therapeutic viruses: strategies and challenges to arming oncolytic viruses with therapeutic genes, *Cancer Gene Ther.* 9(12):1022-1035.

Hernandez-Alcoceba, R., Pihalja, M., Qian, D. & Clarke, M. F. (2002). New oncolytic adenoviruses with hypoxia- and estrogen receptor-regulated replication, *Human Gene Ther.* 13(14):1737-1750.

Hodes, R. (2001). Molecular targeting of cancer: telomeres as targets, *Proc. Natl. Acad. Sci. U S A* 98(14):7649-7651.

Hong, S., Paulson, Q. X. & Johnson, D. G. (2008). E2F1 and E2F3 activate ATM through distinct mechanisms to promote E1A-induced apoptosis, *Cell Cycle* 7(3):391-400.

Horikawa, I., Cable, P. L., Afshari, C. & Barrett, J. C. (1999). Cloning and characterization of the promoter region of human telomerase reverse transcriptase gene, *Cancer Res.* 59(4):826-830.

Horikawa, I., Cable, P. L., Mazur, S. J., Appella, E., Afshari, C. A. & Barrett, J. C. (2002). Downstream E-box-mediated regulation of the human telomerase reverse transcriptase (hTERT) gene transcription: evidence for an endogenous mechanism of transcriptional repression, *Mol. Biol. Cell* 13(8):2585-2597.

Hu, H., Li, Z., Chen, J., Wang, D., Ma, J., Wang, W., Li, J., Wu, H., Li, L., Wu, M., Qian, Q., Chen, J. & Su, C. (2010). P16 reactivation induces anoikis and exhibits antitumor potency by downregulating Akt/Survivin signaling in hepatocellular carcinoma cells, *Gut* doi:10.1136/gut.2010.220020.

Huang, T. G., Savontaus, M. J., Shinozaki, K., Sauter, B. V. & Woo, S. L. C. (2003). Telomerase-dependent oncolytic adenovirus for cancer treatment, *Gene Ther.* 10(15):1241-1247.

Huang, X. F., Ren, W., Rollins, L., Pittman, P., Shah, M., Shen, L., Gu, Q., Strube, R., Hu, F. & Chen, S. Y. (2003). A broadly applicable, personalized heat shock protein-mediated oncolytic tumor vaccine, *Cancer Res.* 63(21):7321-7329.

Irving, J., Wang, Z., Powell, S., O'Sullivan, C., Mok, M., Murphy, B., Cardoza, L., Lebkowski, J. S. & Majumdar, A. S. (2004). Conditionally replicative adenovirus driven by the human telomerase promoter provides broad-spectrum antitumor activity without liver toxicity, *Cancer Gene Ther.* 11(3):174-185.

Itamochi, H., Kigawa, J., Kanamori, Y., Oishi, T., Bartholomeusz, C., Nahta, R., Esteva, F. J., Sneige, N., Terakawa, N. & Ueno, N. T. (2007). Adenovirus type 5 E1A gene therapy for ovarian clear cell carcinoma: a potential treatment strategy, *Mol. Cancer Ther.* 6(1):227-235.

Jonasch, E. & Haluska, F. G. (2001). Interferon in oncological practice: review of interferon biology, clinical applications, and toxicities, *Oncologist* 6(1):34-55.

Johnson, L., Shen, A., Boyle, L., Kunich, J., Pandey, K., Lemmon, M., Hermiston, T., Giedlin, M., McCormick, F. & Fattaey, A. (2002). Selectively replicating adenoviruses targeting deregulated E2F activity are potent, systemic antitumor agents, *Cancer Cell* 1(4):325-337.

Kamphaus, G. D., Colorado, P. C., Panka, D. J., Hopfer, H., Ramchandran, R., Torre, A., Maeshima, Y., Mier, J. W., Sukhatme, V. P. & Kalluri, R. (2000). Canstatin, a novel matrix-derived inhibitor of angiogenesis and tumor growth, *J. Biol. Chem.* 275(2):1209-1215.

Kawashima, T., Kagawa, S., Kobayashi, N., Shirakiya, Y., Umeoka, T., Teraishi, F., Taki, M., Kyo, S., Tanaka, N. & Fujiwara, T. (2004). Telomerase-specific replication-selective virotherapy for human cancer, *Clin Cancer Res.* 10(1 Pt 1):285-292.

Khorana, A. A., Rosenblatt, J. D., Sahasrabudhe, D. M., Evans, T., Ladrigan, M., Marquis, D., Rosell, K., Whiteside, T., Phillippe, S., Acres, B., Slos, P., Squiban, P., Ross, M. & Kendra, K. (2003). A phase I trial of immunotherapy with intratumoral adenovirus-interferon-gamma (TG1041) in patients with malignant melanoma, *Cancer Gene Ther.* 10(4):251-259.

Khuri, F. R., Nemunaitis, J., Ganly, I., Arseneau, J., Tannock, I. F., Romel, L., Gore, M., Ironside, J., Macdougall, R. H., Heise, C., Randlev, B., Gillenwater, A. M., Bruso, P., Kaye, S. B., Hong, W. K. & Kirn, D. H. (2000). A controlled trial of intratumoral ONYX-015, a selectively-replicating adenovirus, in combination with cisplatin and 5-fluorouracil in patients with recurrent head and neck cancer, *Nat. Med.* 6(8):879-885.

Kim, J., Kim, J. H., Choi, K. J., Kim, P. H. & Yun, C. O. (2007). E1A- and E1B-Double mutant replicating adenovirus elicits enhanced oncolytic and antitumor effects, *Hum. Gene Ther.* 18(9):773-786.

Kim, N. W., Piatyszek, M. A., Prowse, K. R., Harley, C. B., West, M. D., Ho, P. L., Coviello, G. M., Wright, W. E., Weinrich, S. L. & Shay, J. W. (1994). Specific association of human telomerase activity with immortal cells and cancer, *Science* 266(5193):2011-2015.

Kirn, D., Martuza, R. L. & Zwiebel, J. (2001). Replication-selective virotherapy for cancer: Biological principles, risk management and future directions, *Nat. Med.* 7(7):781-787.

Koga, S., Hirohata, S., Kondo, Y., Komata, T., Takakura, M., Inoue, M., Kyo, S. & Kondo, S. (2000). A novel telomerase-specific gene therapy: gene transfer of caspase-8 utilizing the human telomerase catalytic subunit gene promoter, *Hum. Gene Ther.* 11(10):1397-1406.

Kowalczyk, D. W., Wlazlo, A. P., Giles-Davis, W., Kammer, A. R., Mukhopadhyay, S. & Ertl, H. C. (2003). Vaccine-induced CD8+ T cells eliminate tumors by a two-staged attack, *Cancer Gene Ther.* 10(12): 870-878.

Kurihara, T., Brough, D. E., Kovesdi, I. & Kufe, D. W. (2000). Selectivity of a replication-competent adenovirus for human breast carcinoma cells expressing the MUC1 antigen, *J. Clin. Invest.* 106(6): 763-771.

Kyo, S., Takakura, M., Taira, T., Kanaya, T., Itoh, H., Yutsudo, M., Ariga, H. & Inoue, M. (2000). Sp1 cooperates with c-Myc to activate transcription of the human telomerase reverse transcriptase gene (hTERT), *Nucleic Acids Res.* 28(3):669-677.

Lai, L. J., Xiao, X. & Wu, J. H. (2007). Inhibition of corneal neovascularization with endostatin delivered by adeno-associated viral (AAV) vector in a mouse corneal injury model, *J. Biomed. Sci.* 14(3):313-22.

Lam, P. Y. & Breakefield, X. O. (2001). Potential of gene therapy for brain tumors, *Hum. Mol. Genet.* 10(7):777-787.

Li, F., Yang, J., Ramnath, N., Javle, M. M. & Tan, D. (2005). Nuclear or cytoplasmic expression of survivin: what is the significance? *Int. J. Cancer* 114(4):509-512.

Li, X., Liu, Y., Lee, S., Gardner, T., Jeng, M & Kao, C. (2008). Prostate-restricted replicative adenovirus expressing human endostatin-angiostatin fusion gene exhibiting dramatic antitumor efficacy, *Clin. Cancer Res.* 14(1): 291-299.

Liao, Y., Yu, D. & Hung, M. C. (2007). Novel approaches for chemosensitization of breast cancer cells: the E1A story, *Adv. Exp. Med. Biol.* 608:144-169.

Liu, F. & Matsuura, I. (2005). Inhibition of Smad antiproliferative function by CDK phosphorylation. *Cell Cycle* 4(1):63-66.

Ma, J., He, X., Wang, W., Huang, Y., Chen, L., Cong, W., Gu, J., Hu, H., Shi, J., Li, L. & Su, C. (2009). E2F promoter-regulated oncolytic adenovirus with p16 gene induces cell apoptosis and exerts antitumor effect on gastric cancer, *Digest. Dis. Sci.* 54(7):1425-1431.

Madhusudan, S., Tamir, A., Bates, N., Flanagan, E., Gore, M. E., Barton, D. P., Harper, P., Seckl, M., Thomas, H., Lemoine, N. R., Charnock, M., Habib, N. A., Lechler, R., Nicholls, J., Pignatelli, M. & Ganesan, T. S. (2004). A multicenter Phase I gene therapy clinical trial involving intraperitoneal administration of E1A-lipid complex in patients with recurrent epithelial ovarian cancer overexpressing HER-2/neu oncogene, *Clin. Cancer Res.* 10(9): 2986-2996.

Martins, C. P., Brown-Swigart, L. & Evan, G. I. (2006). Modeling the therapeutic efficacy of p53 restoration in tumors, *Cell* 127(7):1323-34.

Merritt, R. E., Yamada, R. E., Crystal, R. G. & Korst, R. J. (2004). Augmenting major histocompatibility complex class I expression by murine tumors in vivo enhances antitumor immunity induced by an active immunotherapy strategy, *J. Thorac. Cardiovasc. Surg.* 127(2):355-364.

Nagayama, Y., Nakao, K., Mizuguchi, H., Hayakawa, T. & Niwa, M. (2003). Enhanced antitumor effect of combined replicative adenovirus and nonreplicative adenovirus expressing interleukin-12 in an immunocompetent mouse model, *Gene Ther.* 10(16):1400-1403.

Nakayama, J., Tahara, H., Tahara, E., Saito, M., Ito, K., Nakamura, H., Nakanishi, T., Tahara, E., Ide, T. & Ishikawa, F. (1998). Telomerase activation by hTRT in human normal fibroblasts and hepatocellular carcinomas, *Nat. Genet.* 18(1):65-68.

Nanda, D., Vogels, R., Havenga, M., Avezaat, C. J., Bout, A. & Smitt, P. S. (2001). Treatment of malignant gliomas with a replicating adenoviral vector expressing herpes simplex virus-thymidine kinase, *Cancer Res.* 61(24):8743-8750.

Narazaki, M. & Tosato, G. (2006). Canstatin: an inhibitor of angiogenesis and tumor growth revisited, *Cancer J.* 12(2):110-112.

Nemajerova, A., Talos, F., Moll, U. M. & Petrenko, O. (2008). Rb function is required for E1A-induced S-phase checkpoint activation, *Cell Death Differ.* 15(9):1440-1449.

Ning, T., Yan, X., Lu, Z. J., Wang, G. P., Zhang, N. G., Yang, J. L., Jiang, S. S., Wu, Y., Yang, L., Guan, Y. S. & Luo, F. (2009). Gene therapy in orthotopic lung cancer murine model with angiogenesis inhibitor, endostatin, *Hum. Gene Ther.* 20(2):103-111.

Nowak, J., Januszkiewicz, D., Lewandowski, K., Nowicka-Kujawska, K., Pernak, M., Rembowska, J., Nowak, T. & Wysocki, J. (2003). Activity and expression of human telomerase in normal and malignant cells in gastric and colon cancer patients, *Eur. J. Gastroenterol. Hepatol.*15(1):75-80.

Ohashi, M., Kanai, F., Tateishi, K., Taniguchi, H., Marignani, P. A., Yoshida, Y., Shiratori, Y,, Hamada, H. & Omata, M. (2001). Target gene therapy for alpha-fetoprotein-producing hepatocellular carcinoma by E1B55k-attenuated adenovirus, *Biochem. Biophys. Res. Commun.* 282(2):529-535.

Ortega, S., Malumbres, M. & Barbacid, M. (2002). Cyclin D-dependent kinases, INK4 inhibitors and cancer, *Biochim. Biophys. Acta* 1602(1):73-87.

Osaki, T., Tanio, Y., Tachibana, I., Hosoe, S., Kumagai, T., Kawase, I., Oikawa, S. & Kishimoto, T. (1994). Gene therapy for carcinoembryonic antigen-producing human lung cancer cells by cell type-specific expression of herpes simplex virus thymidine kinase gene, *Cancer Res.* 54(20):5258-5261.

Ouchi, M., Kawamura, H., Urata, Y. & Fujiwara, T. (2009). Antiviral activity of cidofovir against telomerase-specific replication-selective oncolytic adenovirus, OBP-301 (Telomelysin), *Invest. New Drugs* 27(3):241-245.

Peng, X. Y., Won, J. H., Rutherford, T., Fujii, T., Zelterman, D., Pizzorno, G., Sapi, E., Leavitt, J., Kacinski, B., Crystal, R., Schwartz, P. & Deisseroth, A. (2001). The use of the L-plastin promoter for adenoviral-mediated, tumor-specific gene expression in ovarian and bladder cancer cell lines, *Cancer Res.* 61(11): 4405-4413.

Peyregne, V., Quash, G., Isaac, S., Chantepie, J., Akiba, H., Scoazec, J. Y. & Gilly, F. N. (2004). Survival after gamma interferon intratumoral injections in a model of hepatocarcinoma, *Hepatogastroenterology* 51(58):1115-1120.

Poole, J. C., Andrews, L. G. & Tollefsbol, T. O. (2001). Activity, function, and gene regulation of the catalytic subunit of telomerase (hTERT), *Gene* 269(1-2):1-12.

Post, D. E., Khuri, F. R., Simons, J. W. & van Meir, E. G. (2003). Replicative oncolytic adenoviruses in multimodal cancer regimens, *Hum. Gene Ther.* 14(10):933-946.

Radke, J. R., Siddiqui, Z. K., Miura, T. A., Routes, J. M. & Cook, J. L. (2008). E1A oncogene enhancement of caspase-2-mediated mitochondrial injury sensitizes cells to macrophage nitric oxide-induced apoptosis, *J. Immunol.* 180(12):8272-8279.

Ramachandra, M., Rahman, A., Zou, A., Vaillancourt, M., Howe, J. A., Antelman, D., Sugarman, B., Demers, G. W., Engler, H., Johnson, D. & Shabram, P. (2001). Re-engineering adenovirus regulatory pathways to enhance oncolytic specificity and efficacy, *Nat. Biotechnol.* 19(11):1035-1041.

Ring, C. J. (2002). Cytolytic viruses as potential anti-cancer agents, *J. Gen. Virol.* 83(Pt 3):491-502.

Rodriguez, R., Schuur, E. R., Lim, H. Y., Henderson, G. A., Simons, J. W. & Henderson, D. R. (1997). Prostate attenuated replication competent adenovirus (ARCA) CN706: a selective cytotoxic for prostate-specific antigen-positive prostate cancer cells, *Cancer Res.* 57(13):2559-2563.

Sánchez-Prieto, R., Quintanilla, M., Cano, A., Leonart, M. L., Martin, P., Anaya, A. & Ramón y Cajal, S. (1996). Carcinoma cell lines become sensitive to DNA-damaging agents by the expression of the adenovirus E1A gene, *Oncogene* 13(5):1083-1092.

Saretzki, G., Petersen, S., Petersen, I., Kolble, K. & Von Zglinicki, T. (2002). hTERT gene dosage correlates with telomerase activity in human lung cancer cell lines, *Cancer Lett.* 176(1):81-91.

Shay, J. W. & Bacchetti, S. (1997). A survey of telomerase activity in human cancer, *Eur. J. Cancer* 33(5):787-791.

Singh, R. K., Gutman, M., Bucana, C. D., Sanchez, R., Llansa, N. & Fidler, I. J. (1995). Interferons alpha and beta down-regulate the expression of basic fibroblast growth factor in human carcinomas, *Proc. Natl. Acad. Sci. U S A* 92(10):4562–4566.

Steele, T. A. (2000). Recent developments in the virus therapy of cancer, *Proc. Soc. Exp. Biol. Med.* 223(2):118-127.

Su, C., Cao, H., Tan, S., Huang, Y., Jia, X., Jiang, L., Wang, K., Chen, Y., Long, J., Liu, X., Wu, M., Wu, X. & Qian, Q. (2008a). Toxicology profiles of a novel p53-armed replication-competent oncolytic adenovirus in rodents, felids and nonhuman primates, *Toxicol. Sci.* 106(1):242-250.

Su, C., Na, M., Chen, J., Wang, X., Liu, Y., Wang, W., Zhang, Q., Li, L., Long, J., Liu, X., Wu, M., Fan, X. & Qian, Q. (2008b). Gene-viral cancer therapy using dual-regulated oncolytic adenovirus with antiangiogenesis gene for increased efficacy, *Mol. Cancer Res.* 6(4):568-575.

Su, C., Peng, L., Sham, J., Wang, X., Zhang, Q., Chua, D., Liu, C., Cui, Z., Xue, H., Wu, H., Yang, Q., Zhang, B., Liu, X., Wu, M. & Qian, Q. (2006a). Immune gene-viral therapy with triplex efficacy mediated by oncolytic adenovirus carrying interferon-gamma gene yields efficient antitumor activity in immunodeficient and immunocompetent mice, *Mol. Ther.* 13(5):918-927.

Su, C., Sham, J., Xue, H., Wang, X., Chua, D., Cui, Z., Peng, L., Li, L., Jiang, L., Wu, M. & Qian, Q. (2004). Potent antitumoral efficacy of a novel replicative adenovirus cnhk300 targeted to the telomerase-positive cancer cells, *J. Cancer Res. Clin. Oncol.* 130(10):591-603.

Su, C., Wang, X., Chen, J., Liu, Y., Wang, W., Li, L., Wu, M. & Qian, Q. (2006b). Antitumor activity of an hTERT promoter-regulated tumor-selective oncolytic adenovirus in human hepatocellular carcinoma, *World J. Gastroenterol.* 12(47):7613-7620.

Swisher, S. G. & Roth, J. A. (2002). p53 Gene therapy for lung cancer, *Curr. Oncol. Rep.* 4(4):334-40.

Takakura, M., Kyo, S., Kanaya, T., Hirano, H., Takeda, J., Yutsudo, M. & Inoue, M. (1999). Cloning of human telomerase catalytic subunit (hTERT) gene promoter and identification of proximal core promoter sequences essential for transcriptional activation in immortalized and cancer cells, *Cancer Res.* 59(3):551-557.

Thomas, C. E., Ehrhardt, A. & Kay, M. A. (2003). Progress and problems with the use of viral vectors for gene therapy, *Nat. Rev. Genet.* 4(5):346-358.

Tsukuda, K., Wiewrodt, R., Molnar-Kimber, K., Jovanovic, V. P. & Amin, K. M. (2002). An E2F-responsive replication-selective adenovirus targeted to the defective cell cycle in cancer cells: potent antitumoral efficacy but no toxicity to normal cell, *Cancer Res.* 62(12):3438-3447.

Van Beusechem, V. W., van den Doel, P. B., Grill, J., Pinedo, H. M. & Gerritsen, W. R. (2002). Conditionally replicative adenovirus expressing p53 exhibits enhanced oncolytic potency, *Cancer Res.* 62(21):6165-6171.

Ventura, A., Kirsch, D. G., McLaughlin, M. E., Tuveson, D. A., Grimm, J., Lintault, L., Newman, J., Reczek, E. E., Weissleder, R. & Jacks, T. (2007). Restoration of p53 function leads to tumour regression in vivo, *Nature* 445(7128):606-607.

Wang, X., Su, C., Cao, H., Li, K., Chen, J., Jiang, L., Zhang, Q., Wu, X., Jia, X., Liu, Y., Wang, W., Liu, X., Wu, M. & Qian, Q. (2008). A novel triple-regulated oncolytic adenovirus carrying p53 gene exerts potent antitumor efficacy on common human solid cancers, *Mol. Cancer Ther.* 7(6):1598-1603.

Weill, D., Mack, M., Roth, J., Swisher, S., Proksch, S., Merritt, J. & Nemunaitis, J. (2000). Adenoviral-mediated p53 gene transfer to non-small cell lung cancer through endobronchial injection, *Chest* 118(4):966-970.

Weinrich, S. L., Pruzan, R., Ma, L., Ouellette, M., Tesmer, V. M., Holt, S. E., Bodnar, A. G., Lichtsteiner, S., Kim, N. W., Trager, J. B., Taylor, R. D., Carlos, R., Andrews, W. H., Wright, W. E., Shay, J. W., Harley, C. B. & Morin, G. B. (1997). Reconstitution of human telomerase with the template RNA component hTR and the catalytic protein subunit hTRT, *Nat. Genet.* 17(4):498-502.

Wirth, T., Zender, L., Schulte, B., Mundt, B., Plentz, R., Rudolph, K. L., Manns, M., Kubicka, S., Kühnel, F. (2003). A telomerease-dependent conditionally replicating adenovirus for selective treatment of cancer, *Cancer Res.* 63(12):3181-3188.

Wu, M., Hussain, S., He, Y. H., Pasula, R., Smith, P. A. & Martin, W. J. 2nd. (2001). Genetically engineered macrophages expressing IFN-gamma restore alveolar immune function in scid mice, *Proc. Natl. Acad. Sci. U S A* 98(25):14589–14594.

Xu, D., Wang, Q., Gruber, A., Bjorkholm, M., Chen, Z., Zaid, A., Selivanova, G., Peterson, C., Wiman, K. G. & Pisa, P. (2000). Downregulation of telomerase reverse transcriptase mRNA expression by wild type p53 in human tumor cells, *Oncogene* 19(45):5123-5133.

Xue, W., Zender, L., Miething, C., Dickins, R. A., Hernando, E., Krizhanovsky, V., Cordon-Cardo, C. & Lowe, S. W. (2007). Senescence and tumour clearance is triggered by p53 restoration in murine liver carcinomas, *Nature* 445(7128): 656-660.

Yang, C., Cirielli, C., Capogrossi, M. C. & Passaniti, A. (1995). Adenovirus-mediated wild-type p53 expression induces apoptosis and suppresses tumorigenesis of prostatic tumor cells. *Cancer Res.* 55(19):4210-4213.

Yang, Z. R., Wang, H. F., Zhao, J., Peng, Y. Y., Wang, J., Guinn, B. A. & Huang, L. Q. (2007). Recent developments in the use of adenoviruses and immunotoxins in cancer gene therapy, *Cancer Gene Ther.* 14(7):599-615.

Yoo, G. H., Hung, M. C., Lopez-Berestein, G., LaFollette, S., Ensley, J. F., Carey, M., Batson, E., Reynolds, T. C. & Murray, J. L. (2001). Phase I trial of intratumoral liposome E1A gene therapy in patients with recurrent breast and head and neck cancer, *Clin. Cancer Res.* 7(5):1237-1245.

Yu, W. & Fang, H. (2007). Clinical trials with oncolytic adenovirus in China, *Curr. Cancer Drug Targets* 7(2):141-148.

Yui, J., Chiu, C. P. & Lansdorp, P. M. (1998). Telomerase activity in candidate stem cells from fetal liver and adult bone marrow, *Blood* 91(9):3255-3262.

Zhang, J. F., Hu, C., Geng, Y., Selm, J., Klein, S. B., Orazi, A. & Taylor, M. W. (1996). Treatment of a human breast cancer xenograft with an adenovirus vector containing an interferon gene results in rapid regression due to viral oncolysis and gene therapy, *Proc. Natl. Acad. Sci. U S A* 93(9):4513-4518.

Zou, W., Luo, C., Zhang, Z., Liu, J., Gu, J., Pei, Z., Qian, C. & Liu, X. (2004). A novel oncolytic adenovirus targeting to telomerase activity in tumor cells with potent, *Oncogene* 23(2):457-464.

Recombinant Adenovirus Infection of Human Dendritic Cells

William C. Adams and Karin Loré
Center for Infectious Medicine, Department of Medicine, Karolinska Institutet, Stockholm, Sweden

1. Introduction

Recombinant Adenoviruses (rAd) are widely used as gene delivery vectors in gene therapy and vaccination (Hall et al., 2010, Liu, 2010). These replication incompetent vectors have established safety in humans and possess a number of advantages, such as that high viral titres can be produced efficiently. Several different human rAd types are being intensively investigated in clinical trials for their usefulness. In addition, there is an ever-expanding body of literature covering basic virology of Ad and interactions with host immune and other cells. It is important to understand how rAd vectors interact with specific cells of the immune system in order to improve their clinical efficacy. In particular, studies on the interaction of rAd and professional antigen presenting cells (pAPC), which specialize in recognizing pathogens and initiating a cascade of events that lead to specific immunity, are highly relevant. The most potent type of pAPC are dendritic cells (DC) that possess a unique ability to prime adaptive immune responses (Palucka & Banchereau, 1999, Palucka et al., 2010). rAd vectors likely contact DC early following inoculation and thus these cells may play a major role in regulating immunity towards the vector itself and encoded transgenes.

This chapter will include a review of the current literature on the interactions between DC and rAd vectors reported by ourselves and others, in addition to a presentation of novel data. We will first summarize the phenotype and function of specific human DC subsets and methods to isolate or differentiate DC, which are crucial tools to study the interplay of DC and rAd vectors in physiologically relevant systems. Further, we will discuss basic virological aspects of rAd including vector generation and cellular receptor usage among different rAd species. While a multitude of receptors have been described for rAd, we will focus on those relevant for DC. In addition to how rAd vectors bind and infect DC, the extent by which different rAd types infect different DC subsets will be examined. Finally we will give an overview of the functional response of DC to rAd vectors, including maturation, cytokine production, and antigen presentation. Understanding how human DC sense and respond to rAd vectors will assist in guiding the use of these gene delivery vehicles in their many different clinical applications.

2. Human dendritic cells

2.1 Function in innate and adaptive immunity

DC participate centrally in the initiation of immune responses towards foreign antigen and in this way link the innate and adaptive arms of the immune system (Palucka & Banchereau,

1999). During the steady state, DC have an immature phenotype, possess high endocytic capacity, and express a diverse array of pathogen recognition receptors (PRR) to sense extracellular and intracellular foreign antigen. Recognition of specific viral nucleic acid signatures by cytosolic and endosomal PRR enables DC to initiate downstream signalling cascades that lead to phenotypic maturation and production of cytokines such as type-1 interferons (IFN) (Pichlmair & Reis e Sousa, 2007). DC activation is also characterized by upregulation of chemokine receptors that facilitate their migration from the periphery to the spleen or lymph nodes, the primary sites for presentation of antigens, to activate antigen-naïve T lymphocytes. The morphological and phenotypic changes that occur upon maturation endow DC with a notable capacity to activate lymphocytes in an antigen specific manner (Steinman & Witmer, 1978). Specifically, DC have a unique capacity to present foreign peptides on MHC (major histocompatibility complex) I and II to activate both cytotoxic CD8+ T cells and helper CD4+ T cells, respectively. In addition to efficient induction of antigen-specific T cell responses, DC are also becoming increasingly appreciated for their role in shaping the function of innate immune cells such as NK cells (Medzhitov, 2007). Since DC have a multifaceted role in both innate and adaptive immunity, they likely respond to and influence the efficacy of rAd vector administration. While DC may facilitate the induction of systemic immunity towards vector transgenes, local immune responses may in contrast blunt the desired effect of the delivered gene. Part of the diversity in DC function is attributable to the presence of distinct DC subsets present in blood and other tissues.

2.2 Overview of DC subsets, phenotype, and function

Human DC are classified into subsets based on characteristics such as surface phenotype, anatomical location, cytokine and maturation profiles, and the capacity to present antigen to activate antigen specific lymphocytes. In this section, we will describe the phenotypes and functions of subsets of DC derived from human blood and skin.

2.2.1 Blood DC subsets

Human DC from blood can be broadly separated into three distinct subsets: plasmacytoid DC (pDC) and two types of myeloid DC (mDC) (Ueno et al., 2011, Ziegler-Heitbrock et al., 2010) (Table I). These subsets are distinguished by their unique expression of different blood DC antigens (BDCA) (Dzionek et al., 2000, Palucka et al., 2010). mDC are CD1c+ (BDCA-1+), while pDC co-express CD303 (BDCA-2) and CD304 (BDCA-4) (Table I). Another recently identified mDC subset expressing CD141+ (BDCA-3) is notably adept at presenting exogenous foreign peptides on MHC I molecules, in a process termed cross-presentation (Bachem et al., 2010, Crozat et al., 2010, Jongbloed et al., 2010, Poulin et al., 2010). Because there is very limited data on the interaction of rAd vectors and the CD141+ mDC subsets this chapter will focus on pDC and CD1c+ mDC. While mDC and pDC are similar in that they share several classical DC functions, such as mechanisms for efficient uptake of antigen, expression of PRR, ability to phenotypically mature, migrate and activate naïve T cells, they also differ in a number of critical aspects. For example, their expression repertoire of PRR differs. mDC express toll like receptors (TLR) 1 through 8, and 10 whereas pDC express TLR 7 and 9. mDC are generally considered more potent antigen presenting cells, while pDC specialize in the production of rapid and copious type-1 IFN (IFNα/β) and may thus have a particularly important role in viral immunity (Liu, 2005). Both pDC and mDC are also defined as being mostly CD14- (Fig. 1). A surrogate for DC of myeloid lineage may also be differentiated *in vitro* from CD14+ monocytes (termed monocytes derived DC or MDDC). These cells lose CD14 expression, but concurrently gain expression of CD1a and DC-specific intercellular adhesion molecule-3-grabbing non-integrin (DC-SIGN) (Table I and Fig. 2). It is currently unclear whether MDDC represent any single primary DC subset, but recent a report indicates that they in part mimic skin resident interstitial dermal DC in that they produce similar cytokines and express DC-SIGN (Klechevsky et al., 2008). In **section 2.3** we will briefly discuss the methods for differentiating MDDC *in vitro* and isolating mDC and pDC from blood.

	DC Subset	Phenotype	Cytokines Produced	Selection method	Culture media
Blood Subsets	**CD1c+ Myeloid DC (mDC)**	**CD1c+ (BDCA-1)** CD11c+ CD14+/- HLA-DR+	IL-12p70 TNF IL-6	anti-CD1c magnetic microbeads with positive selection on Automacs (Miltenyi)	RPMI media 10 % fetal calf sera GM-CSF
Blood Subsets	**Plasmacytoid DC (pDC)**	**CD303+ (BDCA-2)** **CD304+ (BDCA-4)** CD123+ (IL-3Rα) CD14- HLA-DR+	IFNα/β IL-6	anti-CD304 magnetic microbeads with positive selection on Automacs (Miltenyi)	RPMI media 10 % fetal calf sera IL-3
in vitro derived	**Monocyte derived DC (MDDC)**	**CD1a+** **CD209+ (DC-SIGN)** HLA-DR+ CD14-	IL-12p70 TNF IL-6	Monocyte isolation followed by 6 day culture with IL-4 and GM-CSF	RPMI media 10 % fetal calf sera GM-CSF + IL-4
Cutaneous Subsets	**Dermal Interstitial DC (dDC)**	**CD209+/- (DC-SIGN)** **CD14+/-** HLA-DR+ CD1a +/-	TNF IL-1 IL-6 IL-12p40	Collagenase digestion of skin or GM-CSF induced migration from dermal skin layer	RPMI media 10 % fetal calf sera
Cutaneous Subsets	**Epidermal Langerhans Cells (LC)**	**CD207+ (Langerin)** CD1a+ HLA-DR+	TNF IL-1 IL-15 IL-8	Collagenase digestion of skin or GM-CSF induced migration from dermal skin layer	RPMI media 10 % fetal calf sera

Table 1. Overview of DC, phenotype, cytokines, methods for selection, and culturing.

2.2.2 Cutaneous DC subsets

Cutaneous DC are commonly divided into two main subsets based on the tissue in which they reside in steady state conditions: dermal interstitial DC (dDC) resident in the dermal layer, and Langerhans cells (LC) resident in the epidermal layer. Both subsets express HLA-DR and are of myeloid origin. LC are distinguished by expression of Langerin and CD1a, while dDC consist of a more diverse population based on differential expression of DC-SIGN, CD1a and CD14 (Bond et al., 2009, Klechevsky et al., 2008). A more complete phenotypic characterization of these cells is provided in Table I. The unique roles that each of these skin DC play in detecting viral infection and initiating immune responses likely depends on both the route of inoculation and the nature of the particular virus (Palucka et al., 2010). It has been shown that dDC, in particular the CD14+ subset, stimulate humoral immunity (i.e. antibody producing B cells) while LC specialize at inducing cellular immunity (i.e. cytotoxic CD8+ T cells) (Klechevsky et al., 2008). The methods for isolating cutaneous DC subsets from healthy skin tissue will be briefly discussed in **section 2.3.3**.

2.3 Differentiation and isolation of DC from blood and skin

2.3.1 Isolation of primary blood DC subsets

We have developed methods that yield significant numbers of highly pure and immature CD303+ pDC and CD1c+ mDC (Adams et al., 2009, Douagi et al., 2009, Lore, 2004, Lore et al., 2003). These cells allow for studies of more physiologically relevant primary human DC than *in vitro* surrogate DC (i.e. MDDC). As discussed earlier, isolation of pDC and mDC is facilitated by differential BDCA expression. A series of sequential separations is necessary to yield sorted cells of high purity. We have developed two means of first enriching DC and monocytes from the total peripheral blood mononuclear cell (PBMC) population: (i) aphaeresis of donor leukocytes followed by counterflow centrifugation elutriation to separate monocytes and lymphocytes based on cell size and sedimentation density (Lore et al., 2003, Lore et al., 2005), or (ii) treatment of PBMC with RosetteSep CD14+ enrichment kit (Lambert et al., 2009). Both these methods result in a fraction of cells highly enriched of monocytes and DC, and depleted of lymphocytes. Subsequently, the pDC are positively selected by staining with anti-CD304 monoclonal antibodies (mAb) directly conjugated to magnetic microbeads (Miltenyi). Since a subset of B cells expresses CD1c, these cells are depleted by staining with anti-CD19 mAb directly conjugated to magnetic microbeads (Miltenyi). mDC may thereafter be positively selected with mAb against CD1c. Cell separation based on magnetic microbead conjugated mAb can be performed using either an AutoMacs instrument or manually with appropriate selection columns (Miltenyi). This sequential magnetic sorting procedure results in the isolation of highly pure CD123 expressing CD304+ pDC and CD11c expressing CD1c+ mDC (Fig. 1). pDC and mDC are then cultured in complete media supplemented with IL-3 and GM-CSF, respectively. These rare subsets of DC isolated from blood display an immature phenotype that is consistent with the established literature (Ziegler-Heitbrock et al., 2010). Important to note is that although pDC may be isolated with anti-CD303 mAb, ligation of this receptor with the currently available clones (Miltenyi) attenuates type-1 IFN production (Dzionek et al., 2001), TLR9 induced phenotypic maturation, and optimal antigen presentation (Jahn et al., 2010).

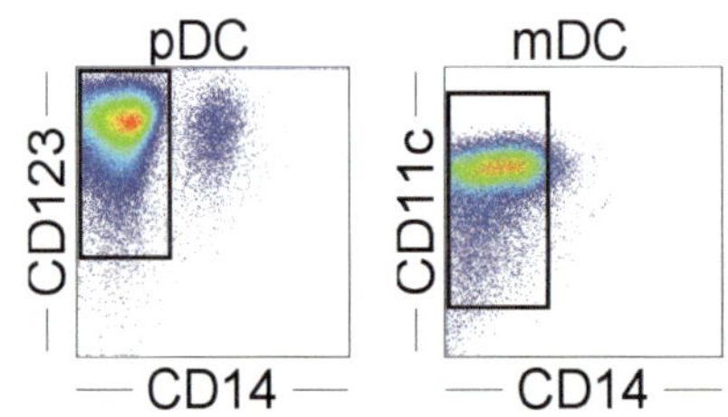

Fig. 1. Phenotype and purity of human pDC and mDC sorted from blood.

pDC and mDC were positively selected on an AutoMacs after staining with anti-CD304 and anti-CD1c mAb conjugated directly to magnetic microbeads, respectively (Miltenyi). Freshly isolated pDC or mDC were stained with anti-CD123 or anti-CD11c, respectively, and anti-CD14 mAbs (BD Biosciences). Surface expression was evaluated using flow cytometry (BD FACS Calibur) and data was analyzed with FlowJo software (Treestar).

2.3.2 Differentiation of monocyte derived DC

Due to the rarity of DC subsets in blood and skin an alternative method was developed to more readily study DC (Sallusto & Lanzavecchia, 1994). This method to *in vitro* generate

MDDC from monocytes significantly accelerated investigations of human DC function. Here, primary monocytes are isolated from PBMC fractions. Highly pure CD14+ monocytes are obtained either by collection of plastic-adherent cells or treatment of PBMC with RosetteSep CD14+ enrichment kit (Stem Cell Technologies) (Adams et al., 2009, Lambert et al., 2009). Subsequent culture of monocytes with recombinant human interleukin (IL)-4 and granulocyte macrophage-colony stimulating factor (GM-CSF) at optimal concentrations over 6 days induces monocytes to differentiate into MDDC that display CD1a, DC-SIGN, HLA-DR, but lack CD14 (Fig. 2).

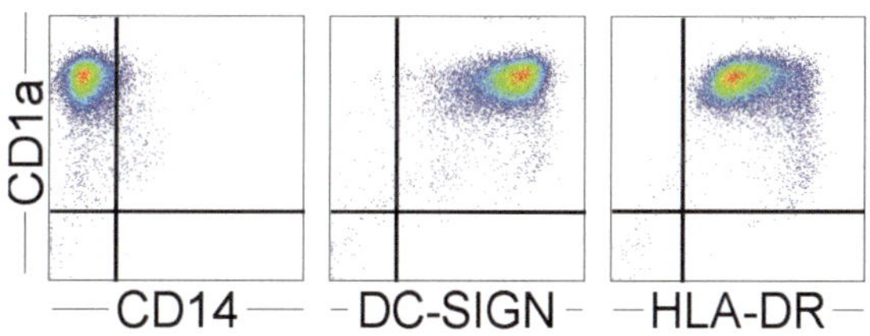

Fig. 2. Phenotype of human DC differentiated from primary monocytes with GM-CSF and IL-4 over six days.

Human PBMC were treated with RosetteSep CD14+ enrichment kit to isolate monocytes, which were then cultured for 6 days in the presence of IL-4 (4 ng/ml) and GM-CSF (4 ng/ml). On day 6, the cells were washed, stained with anti-CD14, anti-DC-SIGN, anti-HLA-DR, and anti-CD1a mAbs (BD Biosciences). Surface expression was evaluated using flow cytometry and data was analyzed with FlowJo software.

2.3.3 Isolation of skin DC subsets

We have recently described methods to isolate DC subsets from healthy skin tissue obtained after reconstructive plastic surgery (Bond et al., 2009). These methods employ a skin graft mesher (Zimmer) that mechanically expands skin in a net-like fashion and increases the accessibility of dispase, an enzyme that separates the dermal and epidermal layers, to penetrate the tissue. After dispase treatment, these layers can then be physically teased apart with forceps. This step is followed by incubation with collagenase, which enzymatically disrupts the collagen fibers and thereby the tissue integrity. After sequential filtering steps, this method results in single cell suspensions enriched for dDC and LC from the dermis and epidermis, respectively. In an alternative method to isolate skin DC, the separated layers are incubated with collagenase and GM-CSF, which induces the cells to migrate from the tissue and into the media. Suspensions of the cells typically consist of a higher percentage of DC, but which may display a more mature phenotype compared to DC isolated with collagenase alone. Regardless of maturation state, the harvested LC are identified by uniform and high expression of HLA-DR, CD1a and Langerin. dDC express HLA-DR, but exhibit differential expression of CD1a and CD14 (Bond et al., 2009). These techniques allow for efficient isolation of significant numbers of skin DC useful for investigations of rAd infection.

3. Recombinant adenovirus vectors

3.1 Background

The family of human Adenoviruses (*Adenoviridae*) consists of at least 50 different subtypes divided into seven species and causes a diverse array of acute human diseases (Arnberg,

2009). The virion has an icosohedral non-enveloped capsid containing fibers spikes protruding from each vertice that encapsulates a double stranded linear DNA genome. The complete high resolution structure of the 150 megadalton Ad viron has recently been solved (Liu et al., 2010, Reddy et al., 2010) and provides critical insights into the virology of Ad. The genome organization and capsid structure are relatively conserved amongst Ad species, but receptor usage, cellular and tissue tropism, and activation of immune cells differs. Recombinant Adenoviruses (rAd), rendered replication incompetent by removal of viral early genes (e.g. E1, E3, and E4), have steadily gained prominence as vectors in various gene therapy and vaccine applications (Liu, 2010, Patterson et al., 2009). The use of rAd as gene delivery vehicles is driven largely by the extensive characterization of Ad virology and the ability to produce high titers of replication incompetent virus that encode for relatively large foreign gene inserts. Transduction of many cell types by rAd leads to transcription of the inserted transgene and high production of its encoded protein, especially when the transgene is under control of an optimized promoter element. Moreover, replication incompetent rAd vectors have proven safe in both pre-clinical toxicology and clinical trials (Catanzaro et al., 2006, Sheets et al., 2008). rAd type 5 (rAd5) of species C has been used most widely, but due to various limitations such as common pre-existing antibody mediated immunity, alternative Ad species (e.g. B) are now being investigated and employed (Abbink et al., 2007). Thus, investigation of these alternative Ad species, which are often less well characterized compared to rAd5 in terms of their specific receptor usage and ability to transduce different cells, is highly warranted and will hopefully expand their usefulness in gene therapy and vaccination.

3.2 Generation of recombinant adenovirus vectors

Replication incompetent rAd vectors can be efficiently generated in mammalian packing cells lines and are the type in common use (He et al., 1998). These vectors are rendered replication incompetent by genetic deletion of early genes, which are transcribed early in the virus life cycle and are required for viral replication. Numerous packaging cell lines, such as PER.C6 or 293-ORF6, have been developed that provide deleted early genes *in trans*. rAd5 and rAd35 vectors have capacity for foreign transgenes of up to 7.5 kb under control of a CMV promoter (McVey et al., 2010). This type of promoter has been found to be the most active in human DC (Papagatsias et al., 2008). However, these authors noted that promoter type strongly affected transgene expression, and promoter activity was dependent on cell type. Thus, cell lines may neither accurately represent promoter activity nor predict gene expression in primary immune cells. Viral expression cassettes typically also include SV40 polyadenylation signals to further enhance expression of the transgene. Transgenes encoding fluorescent proteins can be used to follow viral infection. These current methods result in the generation of high viral titre stocks with severely limited viral replication.

3.3 Receptor usage

3.3.1 Primary cellular attachment receptors

Ad use a variety of cellular attachment receptors that are determined both by cell type and the virus species (reviewed by (Arnberg, 2009)). Furthermore, receptor usage may be substantially different depending on the host species; such as between human and mice. Therefore, for the purposes of this chapter, we will focus on the receptors expressed by human DC that have been or may be implicated in rAd infection. Table II provides an overview of described and potential receptors on human DC for selected Ad types. It is well established that species B Ad35 requires the complement regulatory protein CD46 to attach to and infect a variety of human cells (Gaggar et al., 2003). The trimeric fiber knob protein mediates high affinity and avidity binding of rAd35 to a region within the extracellular short consensus repeats (SCR)1 and 2 of CD46 (Nemerow et al., 2009, Wang et al., 2007, Wang et al., 2008). In fact, all species B rAd probably use CD46 except types 3 and 7 (Marttila et al., 2005). We have previously confirmed these findings by showing that rAd35 requires CD46 to infect pDC and mDC (Lore et al., 2007). Using anti-CD46 mAb directed against the known binding regions of the rAd35 knobs we demonstrated that CD46 attachment was required for rAd35 infection. CD46 is ubiquitously expressed on all nucleated cells and it is therefore likely that rAd35 infects or at least binds to a range of cells. In addition to its role as a complement regulatory protein, CD46 regulates immune cell function through putative signalling domains within its cytoplasmic tails (Kemper & Atkinson, 2007, Wang et al., 2000). Thus, CD46 using rAd vectors, such as rAd35, may modulate immune cells through receptor interactions. For example, CD46 engagement drives the differentiation of CD4+ T cells to a regulatory phenotype (Kemper et al., 2003).

Contrary to rAd35, the receptors used by the species C Ad5 to infect human DC are less clear. While the coxsackie-adenovirus receptor (CAR) is the described receptor for rAd5 on epithelial cells (Bergelson et al., 1997), blood DC were found to not express this receptor at levels detectable by flow cytometry (Lore et al., 2007). However, we have found that CAR plays a minor role in mediating rAd5 infection of skin DC, which express CAR (Adams et al., 2009). Thus, rAd5 may infect DC, especially blood DC, in a CAR-independent manner. To this end, several CAR-independent pathways for rAd5 infection have been suggested. Lactoferrin (Lf), an iron-binding protein present in abundance at mucosal sites and in many bodily fluids, was shown to facilitate epithelial cell infection by species C Ad (Johansson et al., 2007). We expanded on this report and found that Lf strongly enhanced rAd5 infection of all tested blood and skin DC subsets (Adams et al., 2009). Of particular interest in the application of rAd5 as a gene therapy or vaccine vector was the mechanism by which Lf facilitated infection. Lf species with high mannose type *N*-linked glycans mediated rAd5 infection via binding to DC-SIGN. As mentioned earlier, this receptor is expressed by both MDDC and a subset of skin resident dDC. Thus, Lf represents a mechanism to mediate rAd5 infection of CAR- human DC and may provide a means to enhance the infection of DC both *in vitro* and *in vivo*. Coagulation factors also play a critical role in mediating *in vivo* tropism of rAd5 vectors, especially after intravenous administration (Kalyuzhniy et al., 2008, Waddington et al., 2008). High affinity Ad5 hexon protein interactions with coagulation factor X (FX) mediate liver tropism through high efficiency transduction of hepatocytes in mice. These studies illustrate that cellular tropism may be determined by binding events that occur independent of the classical Ad knob-receptor interactions. It is currently unknown to what extent these soluble factors mediate infection of human DC *in vivo*, but this will be important to determine in future studies. In murine DC, a region within the rAd5 fiber-shaft facilitates infection in a heparin dependent manner (Cheng et al., 2007). It will be critical to determine whether this receptor usage also exists in DC. These authors also found that rAd5 mutants with ablated CAR binding retained their ability to infect murine DC, which supports our earlier findings that Ad5 infects human DC, albeit to a lesser extent than rAd35, in the absence of CAR.

Adenovirus Type	Species	Receptors or mediators	Receptor expressed on DC	Reference
Ad5	C	CAR	Blood: no	Bergelson et al.,1997; Lore et al., 2007
			skin: yes	Adams et al., 2009
		Lactoferrin	yes	Johansson et al., 2007; Adams et al., 2009
		FX	n.d.	Kalyuzhniy et al., 2008; Waddington et al., 2008
		Heparin	n.d.	Cheng et al., 2007
Ad35	B(2)	CD46	yes	Gaggar et al., 2003; Marttila et al., 2005; Lore et al., 2007
Ad37	D	GD1a glycan	n.d.	Nilsson et al., 2011
Ad3	B(1)	Desmoglein	n.d	Wang et al., 2011
		CD80/CD86	n.d.	Short et al., 2004; Short et al., 2006

n.d.: not determined

Table 2. Definitive and potential receptors on human DC for select Ad types.

Finally, increased vector transduction of DC has been tested by genetically modifying rAd vectors to target DC expressing CD40 (Korokhov et al., 2005b) and DC-SIGN (Korokhov et al., 2005a, Maguire et al., 2006). Targeting DC in this manner led to greater transduction efficiency of DC by retargeted rAd vectors compared to unmodified vectors. These reports are reminiscent of how Lf also enhanced infection through DC-SIGN (Adams et al., 2009). In conclusion, rAd vectors may be retargeted through genetic modification of the capsid structure or other soluble proteins to more efficiently infect DC, but it remains to be determined how effective such strategies are *in vivo*.

3.3.2 Secondary cellular receptors

A secondary interaction with cellular $\alpha v/\beta 3$ and $\alpha v/\beta 5$ integrins and RGD motifs of the Ad penton bases facilitates membrane penetration and internalization of Ad particles (Wickham et al., 1993). $\alpha v \beta 5$ integrins may even be sufficient to allow rAd infection when CAR is not present (Lyle & McCormick, 2010). However, mutant rAd with ablated integrin binding retained their ability to infect murine DC, which indicates that such interactions are not necessary on DC (Cheng et al., 2007). It will be important to further elucidate the role of integrins in mediating rAd infection of DC, particularly since the expression may differ between DC subsets and host species. β_3 integrins displayed by mouse macrophages are the major initiators of innate immune response towards Ad vectors *in vivo* (Di Paolo et al., 2009). In that study, binding of RGD motifs to integrins induce IL-1α independent of membrane penetration. This report highlights how Ad interactions with receptors may, in addition to mediating cellular attachment, influence immunity independent of infection (Shayakhmetov et al., 2010).

3.3.3 Other potential cellular attachment receptors on DC

The co-stimulatory receptors, CD80 and CD86, involved in the antigen presentation process have been implicated as receptors for Ad3 (Short et al., 2004, Short et al., 2006). These findings are relevant for DC since they display these markers whereas most other cells do not. As will be discussed in more detail in **section 5.1**, surface CD80 and CD86 levels increase on DC during phenotypic maturation. Whether CD80 and CD86 can act as candidate receptors for Ad3 on DC, needs to be confirmed. A recent report demonstrates that Ad3 binds the desmoglein receptor (Wang et al., 2011), although it is unknown if this receptor is expressed on DC and can facilitate infection. GD1a glycan was recently identified as the receptor for Ad37, although again the relevance of this receptor for DC infection has not yet been studied (Nilsson et al., 2011). Taken together, these data highlight the importance of understanding how rAd vectors used in gene therapy interact with immune cells. In particular, certain interactions with DC may have positive or negative consequences on immunity generated towards the rAd vector.

4. Susceptibility of DC to rAd infection

4.1 Methods for testing DC susceptibility *in vitro*

As previously discussed, there is significant complexity in the receptor usage of rAd vectors derived from different species or types, which likely results in vast differences in their ability to infect DC. What particular cells are infected with rAd after vector delivery is largely unknown. Whether expression of vector transgenes in all or specific cells of the heterogeneic DC population is desired or not may also depend on the specific gene therapy or vaccine application. It is thus important to determine the susceptibility of primary human DC subsets to rAd. We have developed methods to monitor rAd infection in DC (Adams et al., 2009, Lore et al., 2007). In these assays, freshly isolated DC are exposed to rAd vectors encoding green fluorescence protein (GFP) reporter transgene. Following receptor binding and penetration of the cellular membrane, the virus traffics to and enters the nucleus where replication occurs. Since the vectors are optimized for expression of the transgene, GFP may be expressed in susceptible cells. GFP expression can then be used as a surrogate marker of productive rAd infection. We have included examples here to demonstrate how the method is performed and how it can be used to compare the capacity of different rAd types to infect MDDC (Fig. 3), mDC and pDC (Fig. 4*A*), and LC and dDC (Fig. 4*B*). In these experiments, the DC were exposed to different inocula of rAd types 35 or rAd5, or rAd26. After 24 h, the cells were stained for surface markers to examine phenotype simultaneously with GFP by

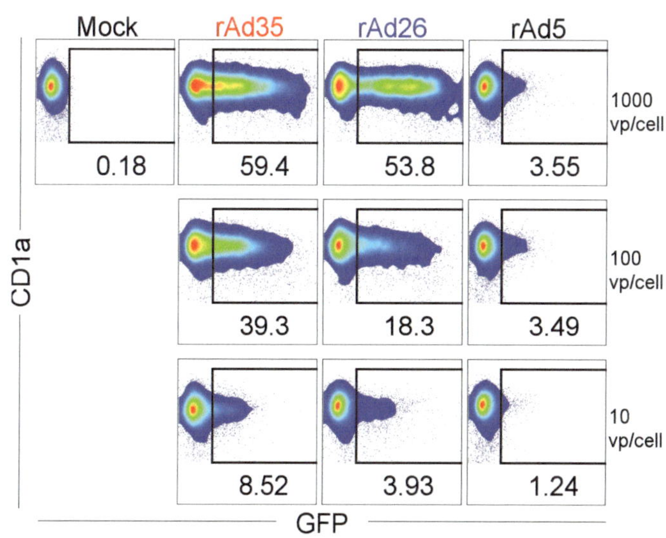

Fig. 3. Flow cytometry analysis of GFP transgene expression in human MDDC.

flow cytometry. GFP+ cells can be detected at earlier time points (≥ 8 hours), but the level of infection usually peaks around 24 hours. We have previously optimized these methods in pDC and mDC with similar results as presented here (Lore et al., 2007). Here, we confirmed these findings in all the mentioned DC (Fig. 3-4). In **section 4.2** of this chapter we will discuss the major differences observed between the susceptibility of DC subsets to different rAd species.

MDDC were exposed to rAd types 35, 26, and 5 encoding GFP at the indicated inocula (virus particles (vp) per cell). After 24 hours, the cells were washed and stained with directly conjugated anti-CD1a and anti-CD14 mAbs (BD Biosciences). Expression of surface markers and GFP was evaluated using flow cytometry and data was analyzed with FlowJo software.

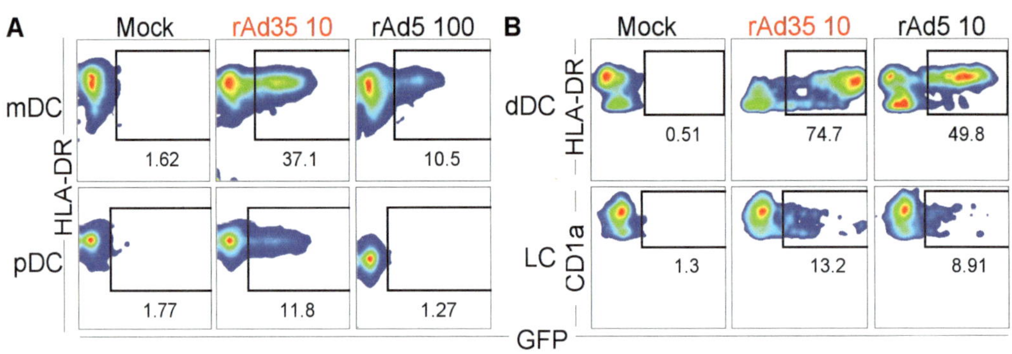

Fig. 4. Flow cytometry analysis of GFP transgene expression in human blood and skin DC subsets.

Freshly isolated (A) mDC and pDC or (B) dDC and LC were exposed to rAd35 or 5 encoding GFP at the indicated inocula (infectious virus particles (ip) per cell). After 24 hours, the cells were washed and stained with directly conjugated anti-CD1a or anti-HLA-DR mAbs (BD Biosciences). Expression of surface marker and GFP was evaluated using flow cytometry and data was analyzed with FlowJo software.

4.2 Notable differences in DC infection between rAd species

There may be important implications for gene delivery vehicles that differentially target DC. We have reported previously on the capacity of rAd vectors to infect primary human DC and MDDC (Adams et al., 2009, Lore et al., 2007). In these studies we have compared the species C rAd5 and species B rAd35, which are widely used as gene delivery vehicles. As discussed in **section 3.3**, a major difference between these viruses is their receptor usage. rAd35 uses CD46 as a primary attachment receptor, while rAd5 uses CAR to infect CAR+ cells. A flow cytometric analysis of surface marker expression revealed that pDC, mDC, and MDDC express high levels CD46, but have undetectable levels of CAR (Adams et al., 2009, Lore et al., 2007). Moreover, exposure of rAd35 encoding GFP led to a greater frequency of GFP+ pDC and mDC when compared to rAd5 (Fig. 4*A*). These differences have been observed by others as well (Ophorst et al., 2004, Rea et al., 2001) and are in agreement with data presented here that rAd35 infects MDDC (Fig. 3) and the cutaneous dDC and LC (Fig. 4*B*) more efficiently than rAd5. Others have also found that rAd35 infects skin emigrating DC more efficiently than rAd5 (de Gruijl et al., 2006). Here, we also show new data that species D rAd26 infected MDDC to about the same degree as rAd35 (Fig. 3). On this note, the specific receptor used by rAd26 for infection is still controversial and there are diverging reports implicating either CD46 (Abbink et al., 2007) or CAR (Chen et al., 2010). rAd5 infection of DC occurred in the absence of CAR expression and neutralizing anti-CAR mAb had no effect on infection (Lore et al., 2007). Unlike blood DC, subsets of cutaneous DC display CAR and blocking CAR has a noticeable but incomplete reduction of rAd5 infection (Adams et al., 2009). We also show here that dDC were substantially more susceptible to both rAd5 and 35 infection than donor matched LC (Fig. 4*B*). Another report found that LC were more susceptible to rAd infection compared to dDC when using skin DC differentiated from CD34+ haematopoietic stem cells *in vitro* (Rozis et al., 2005). These differing studies highlight the complexicity in comparing data generated using different sources of DC. It is criticial to perform detailed characterizations of the phenotypes and functions of the DC in each culture system to be able to relate it to how accurately they represent DC *in vivo*. The level of maturation should be carefully monitored since it may substantially affect DC susceptibility to rAd infection. Finally, even though rAd5 infects DC to a lesser extent than rAd35, it was recently shown that CD11c+ DC were indispensable for generating strong transgene specific CD8+ T cell responses in mice (Lindsay et al., 2010). This shows that DC recognition of rAd vectors plays a crucial role in mediating immunity and that it may be beneficial in gene therapy to retarget rAd to not infect DC in order to minimize insert specific immunity.

5. rAd induced activation of DC

5.1 Phenotypic maturation

As mentioned earlier in this chapter, phenotypic maturation is an important differentiation step in which DC convert from an immature resting state to an activated state with increased capacity to process and present foreign antigen. Maturation licenses DC to activate naïve T cells through expression of co-stimulatory molecules concurrently with presentation of foreign peptides on MHC molecules. Mature DC upregulate activating members of the B7 family (CD80 and CD86) that provide co-stimulation through CD28 engagement and optimally activate naïve T cells. DC also upregulate MHC class II (HLA-DR) and CD40 that activates both T and B cells through CD40L. There are also many more molecules that positively and negatively regulate DC mediated activation of T cells that are outside the scope of this chapter. Flow cytometry analysis of these surface markers is the most common and instructive method to assess maturation as it quantifies the change in expression on the surface of DC, which is indicative of the strength by which DC can activate T cells. We have found that different rAd types have vastly different capacities to induce phenotypic maturation of DC. For example, the species B rAd35 was found to induce maturation of primary human DC subsets, while rAd5 was not (Lore et al., 2007). In fact, while very high doses of rAd5 did not induce differentiation, a dose of only a few rAd35 particles per DC induced strong maturation. rAd35 induced upregulation of the maturation markers CD80, CD83, CD86, HLA-DR, and CD40 (Lore et al., 2007)(Adams and Loré, unpublished data). The maturation caused by rAd35 is comparable to that induced by strong maturation stimuli such as the TLR4 ligand lipopolysaccharide and the TLR7/8 using imidazoquinolines. While others have found rAd5 activates DC (Philpott et al., 2004), there may be important differences in the source of DC and viral dose between studies. Receptor usage may be linked to the capacity of different rAd types to induce maturation. Although the mechanisms of cellular entry may differ between Ad species and cell type (Hall et al., 2010), it is likely that viral nucleic acids could signal through endosomal or cytosolic expressed PRR and thereby initiate DC maturation. It is currently unclear why or how certain Ad species induce maturation while others do not. However, one potential explanation may be that species C and B Ads have different kinetics of endosomal retention and escape to the cytosol following receptor mediated endocytosis, which thereby affect PRR recognition in these compartments (Miyazawa et al., 2001). *In vivo*, maturation of mDC induced by rAd vectors was dependent on type-1 IFN signalling (Hensley et al., 2005), indicating that phenotypic maturation of DC may be induced directly through infection or facilitated indirectly through cytokine production. However, it is currently unknown what PRR are responsible for rAd mediated DC maturation.

5.2 Cytokine induction

In addition to phenotypic maturation, DC also produce numerous cytokines in response to foreign antigen exposure. In this regard, DC subsets differ in the specific cytokines they produce (Table I). Whereas mDC secrete IL-12p70, pDC possess a unique ability to rapidly secrete abundant type-1 interferons (IFNα/β) following viral infection (Swiecki et al., 2010). Like many other viruses Ads can potently induce systemic IFNα/β *in vivo*. We have previously used three methods to measure cytokines levels in DC: (i) enzyme-linked immunosorbent assay (ELISA), (ii) intracellular cytokine staining with flow cytometry, and (iii) quantitative RT-PCR (Douagi et al., 2009, Lore et al., 2007). DC cytokine production may also be measured *in situ* (Lore et al., 1998, Lore et al., 2001), but this method has not been combined with rAd infection. There are benefits and drawbacks to each of these techniques, which is why the appropriate method should be selected depending on the study aim. ELISA is highly sensitive and useful when the purity of the sorted cells is high, as is the case with sorted primary DC. This method quantifies secreted cytokines, but does not measure production on a per cell basis. Intracellular staining does allow for such assessment however. In this method the use of pharmacological inhibitors of protein secretion (e.g. Brefeldin A) enables detection of cytokines by causing their accumulation within the cells in which they are produced. Subsequent fixation and saponin-mediated cell membrane permeabilization enables staining of intracellular accumulated cytokines and detection by flow cytometry. This method is particularly useful for detecting cytokines in unsorted cell populations or when measuring GFP expression simultaneously (Fig. 5). Since several common pharmacological agents, such as monensin and chloroquine, may interfere with rAd infection or PRR signalling (Adams and Loré, unpublished data), they should be tested rigorously to avoid unwanted effects on DC function.

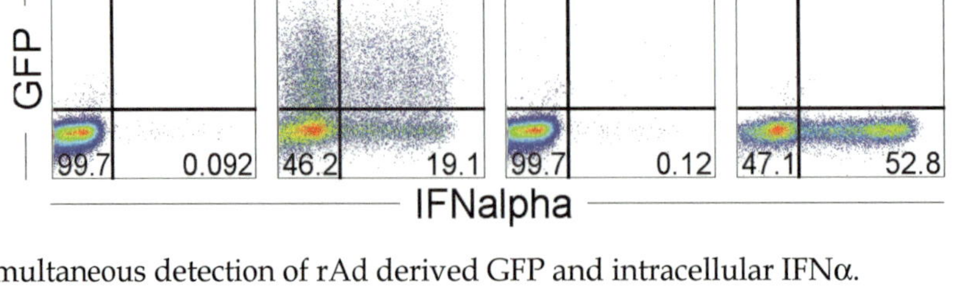

Fig. 5. Simultaneous detection of rAd derived GFP and intracellular IFNα.

pDC were exposed to rAd35-GFP, rAd5-GFP (100 ip/cell), or a TLR7/8-ligand (1 μg/ml) for 8 hours with Brefeldin A present for the last 7 hours. The cells were then washed, fixed and permeabilized with BD cytofix/cytoperm kit, and stained for anti-CD123 (BD) and anti-IFNα (Interferon Source). GFP expression was evaluated simultaneously with IFNα by flow cytometry (BD FACS LSR II) and data was analyzed with FlowJo software.

Intracellular IFNα, accumulated during the last 7 hours of stimulation by Brefeldin A, can be readily detected in pDC exposed to rAd35 (Lore et al., 2007). To add to our previous study we show here the simultaneous detection of the frequencies of infected (GFP+) and IFNα producing cells (Fig. 5). rAd35 again induced almost as much IFNα as the positive control, a TLR7/8-ligand, whereas rAd5 neither infected nor induced IFNα in pDC. We also observed four distinct groups of pDC following rAd35 exposure: GFP-, GFP+, GFP+/IFNα+, or IFNα+ (Fig. 5). Since DC may be infected with rAd even though no GFP is detected, this may explain why PDC make IFNα in the absence of GFP expression. Differential kinetics of GFP and IFNα production may also partly explain the observed expression pattern. Nevertheless, the strong induction of IFNα by pDC is an important parameter to study in the context of rAd infection. Type-1 IFN induction in PBMC was shown to be a feature unique to CD46 using Ads (Iacobelli-Martinez & Nemerow, 2007). In that study, IFNα/β production was dependent on endosomal TLR9 signalling. While rAd35 induces IFNα/β in pDC *in vitro*, there may be multiple sources of systemic IFNα/β, especially for non-CD46 using Ads. For example, murine splenic mDC are the major source of IFNα/β *in vivo* following inoculation of Ad3 or Ad5, independent of TLR and cytosolic nucleic acid receptor (RIG-I like) signalling (Fejer et al., 2008). Moreover, virus associated RNA synthesized by RNA polymerase III may also contribute to systemic type-1 IFN production after rAd immunization (Yamaguchi et al., 2010). Nevertheless, potent transgene-specific CD8+ T cell responses are mounted in the absence of intact type-1 IFN signalling (Hensley et al., 2005). IFNα likely has beneficial effects for vaccination in driving adaptive immunity, whereas in gene therapy antiviral properties of IFNα may blunt rAd mediated gene delivery.

RT-PCR is an alternative and sensitive method to quantify cytokine gene transcription (Douagi et al., 2009). However, this method requires highly pure populations of sorted cells and does not allow for cytokine measurement on a per cell basis. In addition, it is important to consider that detection of RNA may not correlate with protein translation and functional cytokine secretion.

5.3 Antigen presentation

When rAd are used in either gene therapy or vaccine vector applications, it is crucial to determine the immune responses to the transgene. Following vaccination the goal is to induce strong transgene immunity, while for gene therapy such immune responses may blunt the intended effect of the transgene. As such, we have previously studied *in vitro* the capacity of rAd vectors to activate transgene specific memory T cells (Lore et al., 2007). To be able to measure antigen-presentation of the transgene we developed rAd5 or rAd35 vectors encoding the immunodominant pp65 antigen of CMV. These rAd encoding pp65 were exposed to freshly isolated pDC or mDC for 24 hours to allow for sufficient time for transgene presentation and the DC were then added to autologous sorted CD4+ or CD8+ T cells from donors with known pre-existing T cell responses to CMV pp65. We found that rAd exposed DC were able to activate antigen (pp65)-specific memory T cells equivalently to antigen matched overlapping pp65 peptide pools. Importantly, rAd35 vectors more efficiently activated memory T cells compared to rAd5. While infected DC likely display rAd-derived peptide on class I to activate CD8 T cells, the mechanisms for class II presentation to activate CD4+ T cells are less clear. Nevertheless, these studies indicate that rAd5 and rAd35 exposed DC are able to present Ad encoded antigen and stimulate antigen specific T cells. Future studies should also evaluate how rAd vectors influence DC priming of naive T cells. These findings have important implications in clinical applications and depend on whether immune responses towards the transgene are desired or not (Zaiss et al., 2009).

6. Conclusions

In this chapter we have reviewed the basic concepts relating to the infection of primary human DC. Studying the interactions between clinically relevant rAd vectors and multiple subsets of pAPC is instructive for guiding the use of these delivery vectors *in vivo*. While studies in rodents, such as mice, may offer clues to how rAd vectors are recognized *in vivo*, there are notable biological differences between humans and mice (Mestas & Hughes, 2004). While receptors for viral nucleic acid may be similar in these species, the expression patterns within DC subsets are quite different. Additionally, the primary viral attachment receptors for human rAd species are likely different between their natural human hosts and mice; for example, mice do not express the species B receptor CD46. This likely has a significant impact on tissue and cellular tropism as well as innate viral recognition. For these reasons, it is crucial to study the interaction of rAd on immune cells from the host species (i.e. humans) with which the viruses co-evolved. To this end, isolating phenotypically immature primary human DC from both blood and skin tissue provides highly relevant cells with which to study the interactions between innate immune cells and different recombinant rAd species. Using GFP reporter transgenes, the susceptibility of different DC subsets can be monitored *in vitro*, as can the subsequent induction of DC activation (i.e. phenotypic maturation and cytokine production). Following infection and induction of maturation, DC become specialized to activate antigen-specific lymphocytes, which can also be tested *in vitro*. While it may be important to exploit the induction of innate immune responses to drive development of transgene specific adaptive immunity in a vaccine setting, the opposite is likely desired for locally targeted gene therapy. In both clinical applications it is evermore crucial to gain a more complete understanding of the human immune response raised against rAd vectors.

7. Acknowledgments

The rAd vectors described in this chapter were provided by Crucell, The Netherlands or GenVec Inc, USA. The authors wish to acknowledge Drs. Anna Smed-Sörensen and Kerrie Sandgren (Karolinska Institutet) and the Depts. of Transfusion Medicine and Surgery (Karolinska University Hospital) for technical assistance with donor apheresis and elutriations and skin specimens. This study was supported by the Swedish International Development Agency (Sida), the Swedish Governmental Agency for Innovation Systems (Vinnova), the Swedish Research Council (Vetenskapsrådet), the Jeansson's Foundation, and the Swedish Society for Medicine.

8. References

Abbink, P., Lemckert, A. A., Ewald, B. A., Lynch, D. M., Denholtz, M., Smits, S., Holterman, L., Damen, I., Vogels, R., Thorner, A. R., O'Brien, K. L., Carville, A., Mansfield, K. G., Goudsmit, J., Havenga, M. J. & Barouch, D. H. (2007). Comparative seroprevalence and immunogenicity of six rare serotype recombinant adenovirus vaccine vectors from subgroups B and D. *J Virol* 81, 4654-63.

Adams, W. C., Bond, E., Havenga, M. J., Holterman, L., Goudsmit, J., Karlsson Hedestam, G. B., Koup, R. A. & Lore, K. (2009). Adenovirus serotype 5 infects human dendritic cells via a coxsackievirus-adenovirus receptor-independent receptor pathway mediated by lactoferrin and DC-SIGN. *J Gen Virol* 90, 1600-10.

Arnberg, N. (2009). Adenovirus receptors: implications for tropism, treatment and targeting. *Rev Med Virol* 19, 165-78.

Bachem, A., Guttler, S., Hartung, E., Ebstein, F., Schaefer, M., Tannert, A., Salama, A., Movassaghi, K., Opitz, C., Mages, H. W., Henn, V., Kloetzel, P. M., Gurka, S. & Kroczek, R. A. (2010). Superior antigen cross-presentation and XCR1 expression define human CD11c+CD141+ cells as homologues of mouse CD8+ dendritic cells. *J Exp Med* 207, 1273-81.

Bergelson, J. M., Cunningham, J. A., Droguett, G., Kurt-Jones, E. A., Krithivas, A., Hong, J. S., Horwitz, M. S., Crowell, R. L. & Finberg, R. W. (1997). Isolation of a common receptor for Coxsackie B viruses and adenoviruses 2 and 5. *Science* 275, 1320-3.

Bond, E., Adams, W. C., Smed-Sorensen, A., Sandgren, K. J., Perbeck, L., Hofmann, A., Andersson, J. & Lore, K. (2009). Techniques for time-efficient isolation of human skin dendritic cell subsets and assessment of their antigen uptake capacity. *J Immunol Methods* 348, 42-56.

Catanzaro, A. T., Koup, R. A., Roederer, M., Bailer, R. T., Enama, M. E., Moodie, Z., Gu, L., Martin, J. E., Novik, L., Chakrabarti, B. K., Butman, B. T., Gall, J. G., King, C. R., Andrews, C. A., Sheets, R., Gomez, P. L., Mascola, J. R., Nabel, G. J. & Graham, B. S. (2006). Phase 1 safety and immunogenicity evaluation of a multiclade HIV-1 candidate vaccine delivered by a replication-defective recombinant adenovirus vector. *J Infect Dis* 194, 1638-49.

Chen, H., Xiang, Z. Q., Li, Y., Kurupati, R. K., Jia, B., Bian, A., Zhou, D. M., Hutnick, N., Yuan, S., Gray, C., Serwanga, J., Auma, B., Kaleebu, P., Zhou, X., Betts, M. R. & Ertl, H. C. (2010). Adenovirus-based vaccines: comparison of vectors from three species of adenoviridae. *J Virol* 84, 10522-32.

Cheng, C., Gall, J. G., Kong, W. P., Sheets, R. L., Gomez, P. L., King, C. R. & Nabel, G. J. (2007). Mechanism of ad5 vaccine immunity and toxicity: fiber shaft targeting of dendritic cells. *PLoS Pathog* 3, e25.

Crozat, K., Guiton, R., Contreras, V., Feuillet, V., Dutertre, C. A., Ventre, E., Vu Manh, T. P., Baranek, T., Storset, A. K., Marvel, J., Boudinot, P., Hosmalin, A., Schwartz-Cornil, I. & Dalod, M. (2010). The XC chemokine receptor 1 is a conserved selective marker of mammalian cells homologous to mouse CD8alpha+ dendritic cells. *J Exp Med* 207, 1283-92.

de Gruijl, T. D., Ophorst, O. J., Goudsmit, J., Verhaagh, S., Lougheed, S. M., Radosevic, K., Havenga, M. J. & Scheper, R. J. (2006). Intradermal delivery of adenoviral type-35 vectors leads to high efficiency transduction of mature, CD8+ T cell-stimulating skin-emigrated dendritic cells. *J Immunol* 177, 2208-15.

Di Paolo, N. C., Miao, E. A., Iwakura, Y., Murali-Krishna, K., Aderem, A., Flavell, R. A., Papayannopoulou, T. & Shayakhmetov, D. M. (2009). Virus binding to a plasma membrane receptor triggers interleukin-1 alpha-mediated proinflammatory macrophage response in vivo. *Immunity* 31, 110-21.

Douagi, I., Gujer, C., Sundling, C., Adams, W. C., Smed-Sorensen, A., Seder, R. A., Karlsson Hedestam, G. B. & Lore, K. (2009). Human B cell responses to TLR ligands are differentially modulated by myeloid and plasmacytoid dendritic cells. *J Immunol* 182, 1991-2001.

Dzionek, A., Fuchs, A., Schmidt, P., Cremer, S., Zysk, M., Miltenyi, S., Buck, D. W. & Schmitz, J. (2000). BDCA-2, BDCA-3, and BDCA-4: three markers for distinct subsets of dendritic cells in human peripheral blood. *J Immunol* 165, 6037-46.

Dzionek, A., Sohma, Y., Nagafune, J., Cella, M., Colonna, M., Facchetti, F., Gunther, G., Johnston, I., Lanzavecchia, A., Nagasaka, T., Okada, T., Vermi, W., Winkels, G., Yamamoto, T., Zysk, M., Yamaguchi, Y. & Schmitz, J. (2001). BDCA-2, a novel plasmacytoid dendritic cell-specific type II C-type lectin, mediates antigen capture and is a potent inhibitor of interferon alpha/beta induction. *J Exp Med* 194, 1823-34.

Fejer, G., Drechsel, L., Liese, J., Schleicher, U., Ruzsics, Z., Imelli, N., Greber, U. F., Keck, S., Hildenbrand, B., Krug, A., Bogdan, C. & Freudenberg, M. A. (2008). Key role of splenic myeloid DCs in the IFN-alphabeta response to adenoviruses in vivo. *PLoS Pathog* 4, e1000208.

Gaggar, A., Shayakhmetov, D. M. & Lieber, A. (2003). CD46 is a cellular receptor for group B adenoviruses. *Nat Med* 9, 1408-12.

Hall, K., Blair Zajdel, M. E. & Blair, G. E. (2010). Unity and diversity in the human adenoviruses: exploiting alternative entry pathways for gene therapy. *Biochem J* 431, 321-36.

He, T. C., Zhou, S., da Costa, L. T., Yu, J., Kinzler, K. W. & Vogelstein, B. (1998). A simplified system for generating recombinant adenoviruses. *Proc Natl Acad Sci U S A* 95, 2509-14.

Hensley, S. E., Giles-Davis, W., McCoy, K. C., Weninger, W. & Ertl, H. C. (2005). Dendritic cell maturation, but not CD8+ T cell induction, is dependent on type I IFN signaling during vaccination with adenovirus vectors. *J Immunol* 175, 6032-41.

Iacobelli-Martinez, M. & Nemerow, G. R. (2007). Preferential activation of Toll-like receptor nine by CD46-utilizing adenoviruses. *J Virol* 81, 1305-12.

Jahn, P. S., Zanker, K. S., Schmitz, J. & Dzionek, A. (2010). BDCA-2 signaling inhibits TLR-9-agonist-induced plasmacytoid dendritic cell activation and antigen presentation. *Cell Immunol* 265, 15-22.

Johansson, C., Jonsson, M., Marttila, M., Persson, D., Fan, X. L., Skog, J., Frangsmyr, L., Wadell, G. & Arnberg, N. (2007). Adenoviruses Use Lactoferrin as a Bridge for CAR-Independent Binding to and Infection of Epithelial Cells. *J Virol* 81, 954-63.

Jongbloed, S. L., Kassianos, A. J., McDonald, K. J., Clark, G. J., Ju, X., Angel, C. E., Chen, C. J., Dunbar, P. R., Wadley, R. B., Jeet, V., Vulink, A. J., Hart, D. N. & Radford, K. J. (2010). Human CD141+ (BDCA-3)+ dendritic cells (DCs) represent a unique myeloid DC subset that cross-presents necrotic cell antigens. *J Exp Med* 207, 1247-60.

Kalyuzhniy, O., Di Paolo, N. C., Silvestry, M., Hofherr, S. E., Barry, M. A., Stewart, P. L. & Shayakhmetov, D. M. (2008). Adenovirus serotype 5 hexon is critical for virus infection of hepatocytes in vivo. *Proc Natl Acad Sci U S A* 105, 5483-8.

Kemper, C. & Atkinson, J. P. (2007). T-cell regulation: with complements from innate immunity. *Nat Rev Immunol* 7, 9-18.

Kemper, C., Chan, A. C., Green, J. M., Brett, K. A., Murphy, K. M. & Atkinson, J. P. (2003). Activation of human CD4+ cells with CD3 and CD46 induces a T-regulatory cell 1 phenotype. *Nature* 421, 388-92.

Klechevsky, E., Morita, R., Liu, M., Cao, Y., Coquery, S., Thompson-Snipes, L., Briere, F., Chaussabel, D., Zurawski, G., Palucka, A. K., Reiter, Y., Banchereau, J. & Ueno, H. (2008). Functional specializations of human epidermal Langerhans cells and CD14+ dermal dendritic cells. *Immunity* 29, 497-510.

Korokhov, N., de Gruijl, T. D., Aldrich, W. A., Triozzi, P. L., Banerjee, P. T., Gillies, S. D., Curiel, T. J., Douglas, J. T., Scheper, R. J. & Curiel, D. T. (2005a). High efficiency transduction of dendritic cells by adenoviral vectors targeted to DC-SIGN. *Cancer Biol Ther* 4, 289-94.

Korokhov, N., Noureddini, S. C., Curiel, D. T., Santegoets, S. J., Scheper, R. J. & de Gruijl, T. D. (2005b). A single-component CD40-targeted adenovirus vector displays highly efficient transduction and activation of dendritic cells in a human skin substrate system. *Mol Pharm* 2, 218-23.

Lambert, H., Vutova, P. P., Adams, W. C., Lore, K. & Barragan, A. (2009). The Toxoplasma gondii-shuttling function of dendritic cells is linked to the parasite genotype. *Infect Immun* 77, 1679-88.

Lindsay, R. W., Darrah, P. A., Quinn, K. M., Wille-Reece, U., Mattei, L. M., Iwasaki, A., Kasturi, S. P., Pulendran, B., Gall, J. G., Spies, A. G. & Seder, R. A. (2010). CD8+ T cell responses following replication-defective adenovirus serotype 5 immunization are dependent on CD11c+ dendritic cells but show redundancy in their requirement of TLR and nucleotide-binding oligomerization domain-like receptor signaling. *J Immunol* 185, 1513-21.

Liu, H., Jin, L., Koh, S. B., Atanasov, I., Schein, S., Wu, L. & Zhou, Z. H. (2010). Atomic structure of human adenovirus by cryo-EM reveals interactions among protein networks. *Science* 329, 1038-43.

Liu, M. A. (2010). Immunologic basis of vaccine vectors. *Immunity* 33, 504-15.

Liu, Y. J. (2005). IPC: professional type 1 interferon-producing cells and plasmacytoid dendritic cell precursors. *Annu Rev Immunol* 23, 275-306.

Lore, K. (2004). Isolation and immunophenotyping of human and rhesus macaque dendritic cells. *Methods Cell Biol* 75, 623-42.

Lore, K., Adams, W. C., Havenga, M., Precopio, M. L., Holterman, L., Goudsmit, J. & Koup, R. A. (2007). Myeloid and plasmacytoid dendritic cells are susceptible to recombinant adenovirus vectors and stimulate polyfunctional memory T cell responses. *J Immunol* 179, 1721-9.

Lore, K., Betts, M. R., Brenchley, J. M., Kuruppu, J., Khojasteh, S., Perfetto, S., Roederer, M., Seder, R. A. & Koup, R. A. (2003). Toll-like receptor ligands modulate dendritic cells to augment cytomegalovirus- and HIV-1-specific T cell responses. *J Immunol* 171, 4320-8.

Lore, K., Smed-Sorensen, A., Vasudevan, J., Mascola, J. R. & Koup, R. A. (2005). Myeloid and plasmacytoid dendritic cells transfer HIV-1 preferentially to antigen-specific CD4+ T cells. *J Exp Med* 201, 2023-33.

Lore, K., Sonnerborg, A., Spetz, A. L., Andersson, U. & Andersson, J. (1998). Immunocytochemical detection of cytokines and chemokines in Langerhans cells and in vitro derived dendritic cells. *J Immunol Methods* 214, 97-111.

Lore, K., Spetz, A. L., Fehniger, T. E., Sonnerborg, A., Landay, A. L. & Andersson, J. (2001). Quantitative single cell methods that identify cytokine and chemokine expression in dendritic cells. *J Immunol Methods* 249, 207-22.

Lyle, C. & McCormick, F. (2010). Integrin alphavbeta5 is a primary receptor for adenovirus in CAR-negative cells. *Virol J* 7, 148.

Maguire, C. A., Sapinoro, R., Girgis, N., Rodriguez-Colon, S. M., Ramirez, S. H., Williams, J. & Dewhurst, S. (2006). Recombinant adenovirus type 5 vectors that target DC-SIGN, ChemR23 and alpha(v)beta3 integrin efficiently transduce human dendritic cells and enhance presentation of vectored antigens. *Vaccine* 24, 671-82.

Marttila, M., Persson, D., Gustafsson, D., Liszewski, M. K., Atkinson, J. P., Wadell, G. & Arnberg, N. (2005). CD46 is a cellular receptor for all species B adenoviruses except types 3 and 7. *J Virol* 79, 14429-36.

McVey, D., Zuber, M., Ettyreddy, D., Reiter, C. D., Brough, D. E., Nabel, G. J., King, C. R. & Gall, J. G. (2010). Characterization of human adenovirus 35 and derivation of complex vectors. *Virol J* 7, 276.

Medzhitov, R. (2007). Recognition of microorganisms and activation of the immune response. *Nature* 449, 819-26.

Mestas, J. & Hughes, C. C. (2004). Of mice and not men: differences between mouse and human immunology. *J Immunol* 172, 2731-8.

Miyazawa, N., Crystal, R. G. & Leopold, P. L. (2001). Adenovirus serotype 7 retention in a late endosomal compartment prior to cytosol escape is modulated by fiber protein. *J Virol* 75, 1387-400.

Nemerow, G. R., Pache, L., Reddy, V. & Stewart, P. L. (2009). Insights into adenovirus host cell interactions from structural studies. *Virology* 384, 380-8.

Nilsson, E. C., Storm, R. J., Bauer, J., Johansson, S. M., Lookene, A., Angstrom, J., Hedenstrom, M., Eriksson, T. L., Frangsmyr, L., Rinaldi, S., Willison, H. J., Pedrosa Domellof, F., Stehle, T. & Arnberg, N. (2011). The GD1a glycan is a cellular receptor for adenoviruses causing epidemic keratoconjunctivitis. *Nat Med* 17, 105-9.

Ophorst, O. J., Kostense, S., Goudsmit, J., De Swart, R. L., Verhaagh, S., Zakhartchouk, A., Van Meijer, M., Sprangers, M., Van Amerongen, G., Yuksel, S., Osterhaus, A. D. & Havenga, M. J. (2004). An adenoviral type 5 vector carrying a type 35 fiber as a vaccine vehicle: DC targeting, cross neutralization, and immunogenicity. *Vaccine* 22, 3035-44.

Palucka, K. & Banchereau, J. (1999). Linking innate and adaptive immunity. *Nat Med* 5, 868-70.

Palucka, K., Banchereau, J. & Mellman, I. (2010). Designing vaccines based on biology of human dendritic cell subsets. *Immunity* 33, 464-78.

Papagatsias, T., Rozis, G., Athanasopoulos, T., Gotch, F., Dickson, G. & Patterson, S. (2008). Activity of different vaccine-associated promoter elements in human dendritic cells. *Immunol Lett* 115, 117-25.

Patterson, S., Papagatsias, T. & Benlahrech, A. (2009). Use of adenovirus in vaccines for HIV. *Handb Exp Pharmacol*, 275-93.

Philpott, N. J., Nociari, M., Elkon, K. B. & Falck-Pedersen, E. (2004). Adenovirus-induced maturation of dendritic cells through a PI3 kinase-mediated TNF-alpha induction pathway. *Proc Natl Acad Sci U S A* 101, 6200-5.

Pichlmair, A. & Reis e Sousa, C. (2007). Innate recognition of viruses. *Immunity* 27, 370-83.

Poulin, L. F., Salio, M., Griessinger, E., Anjos-Afonso, F., Craciun, L., Chen, J. L., Keller, A. M., Joffre, O., Zelenay, S., Nye, E., Le Moine, A., Faure, F., Donckier, V., Sancho, D., Cerundolo, V., Bonnet, D. & Reis e Sousa, C. (2010). Characterization of human DNGR-1+ BDCA3+ leukocytes as putative equivalents of mouse CD8alpha+ dendritic cells. *J Exp Med* 207, 1261-71.

Rea, D., Havenga, M. J., van Den Assem, M., Sutmuller, R. P., Lemckert, A., Hoeben, R. C., Bout, A., Melief, C. J. & Offringa, R. (2001). Highly efficient transduction of human monocyte-derived dendritic cells with subgroup B fiber-modified adenovirus vectors enhances transgene-encoded antigen presentation to cytotoxic T cells. *J Immunol* 166, 5236-44.

Reddy, V. S., Natchiar, S. K., Stewart, P. L. & Nemerow, G. R. (2010). Crystal structure of human adenovirus at 3.5 A resolution. *Science* 329, 1071-5.

Rozis, G., de Silva, S., Benlahrech, A., Papagatsias, T., Harris, J., Gotch, F., Dickson, G. & Patterson, S. (2005). Langerhans cells are more efficiently transduced than dermal dendritic cells by adenovirus vectors expressing either group C or group B fibre protein: implications for mucosal vaccines. *Eur J Immunol* 35, 2617-26.

Sallusto, F. & Lanzavecchia, A. (1994). Efficient presentation of soluble antigen by cultured human dendritic cells is maintained by granulocyte/macrophage colony-stimulating factor plus interleukin 4 and downregulated by tumor necrosis factor alpha. *J Exp Med* 179, 1109-18.

Shayakhmetov, D. M., Di Paolo, N. C. & Mossman, K. L. (2010). Recognition of virus infection and innate host responses to viral gene therapy vectors. *Mol Ther* 18, 1422-9.

Sheets, R. L., Stein, J., Bailer, R. T., Koup, R. A., Andrews, C., Nason, M., He, B., Koo, E., Trotter, H., Duffy, C., Manetz, T. S. & Gomez, P. (2008). Biodistribution and toxicological safety of adenovirus type 5 and type 35 vectored vaccines against human immunodeficiency virus-1 (HIV-1), Ebola, or Marburg are similar despite differing adenovirus serotype vector, manufacturer's construct, or gene inserts. *J Immunotoxicol* 5, 315-35.

Short, J. J., Pereboev, A. V., Kawakami, Y., Vasu, C., Holterman, M. J. & Curiel, D. T. (2004). Adenovirus serotype 3 utilizes CD80 (B7.1) and CD86 (B7.2) as cellular attachment receptors. *Virology* 322, 349-59.

Short, J. J., Vasu, C., Holterman, M. J., Curiel, D. T. & Pereboev, A. (2006). Members of adenovirus species B utilize CD80 and CD86 as cellular attachment receptors. *Virus Res* 122, 144-53.

Steinman, R. M. & Witmer, M. D. (1978). Lymphoid dendritic cells are potent stimulators of the primary mixed leukocyte reaction in mice. *Proc Natl Acad Sci U S A* 75, 5132-6.

Swiecki, M., Gilfillan, S., Vermi, W., Wang, Y. & Colonna, M. (2010). Plasmacytoid dendritic cell ablation impacts early interferon responses and antiviral NK and CD8(+) T cell accrual. *Immunity* 33, 955-66.

Ueno, H., Klechevsky, E., Schmitt, N., Ni, L., Flamar, A. L., Zurawski, S., Zurawski, G., Palucka, K., Banchereau, J. & Oh, S. (2011). Targeting human dendritic cell subsets for improved vaccines. *Semin Immunol.*

Waddington, S. N., McVey, J. H., Bhella, D., Parker, A. L., Barker, K., Atoda, H., Pink, R., Buckley, S. M., Greig, J. A., Denby, L., Custers, J., Morita, T., Francischetti, I. M., Monteiro, R. Q., Barouch, D. H., van Rooijen, N., Napoli, C., Havenga, M. J., Nicklin, S. A. & Baker, A. H. (2008). Adenovirus serotype 5 hexon mediates liver gene transfer. *Cell* 132, 397-409.

Wang, G., Liszewski, M. K., Chan, A. C. & Atkinson, J. P. (2000). Membrane cofactor protein (MCP; CD46): isoform-specific tyrosine phosphorylation. *J Immunol* 164, 1839-46.

Wang, H., Li, Z. Y., Liu, Y., Persson, J., Beyer, I., Moller, T., Koyuncu, D., Drescher, M. R., Strauss, R., Zhang, X. B., Wahl, J. K., 3rd, Urban, N., Drescher, C., Hemminki, A., Fender, P. & Lieber, A. (2011). Desmoglein 2 is a receptor for adenovirus serotypes 3, 7, 11 and 14. *Nat Med* 17, 96-104.

Wang, H., Liaw, Y. C., Stone, D., Kalyuzhniy, O., Amiraslanov, I., Tuve, S., Verlinde, C. L., Shayakhmetov, D., Stehle, T., Roffler, S. & Lieber, A. (2007). Identification of CD46 binding sites within the adenovirus serotype 35 fiber knob. *J Virol* 81, 12785-92.

Wang, H., Liu, Y., Li, Z., Tuve, S., Stone, D., Kalyushniy, O., Shayakhmetov, D., Verlinde, C. L., Stehle, T., McVey, J., Baker, A., Peng, K. W., Roffler, S. & Lieber, A. (2008). In vitro and in vivo properties of adenovirus vectors with increased affinity to CD46. *J Virol* 82, 10567-79.

Wickham, T. J., Mathias, P., Cheresh, D. A. & Nemerow, G. R. (1993). Integrins alpha v beta 3 and alpha v beta 5 promote adenovirus internalization but not virus attachment. *Cell* 73, 309-19.

Yamaguchi, T., Kawabata, K., Kouyama, E., Ishii, K. J., Katayama, K., Suzuki, T., Kurachi, S., Sakurai, F., Akira, S. & Mizuguchi, H. (2010). Induction of type I interferon by adenovirus-encoded small RNAs. *Proc Natl Acad Sci U S A* 107, 17286-91.

Zaiss, A. K., Machado, H. B. & Herschman, H. R. (2009). The influence of innate and pre-existing immunity on adenovirus therapy. *J Cell Biochem* 108, 778-90.

Ziegler-Heitbrock, L., Ancuta, P., Crowe, S., Dalod, M., Grau, V., Hart, D. N., Leenen, P. J., Liu, Y. J., MacPherson, G., Randolph, G. J., Scherberich, J., Schmitz, J., Shortman, K., Sozzani, S., Strobl, H., Zembala, M., Austyn, J. M. & Lutz, M. B. (2010). Nomenclature of monocytes and dendritic cells in blood. *Blood* 116, e74-80.

8

Harnessing the Potential of Adenovirus Vectored Vaccines

Peter Johannes Holst,
Jan Pravsgaard Christensen and Allan Randrup Thomsen
Department of International Health, Immunology and Microbiology, University of Copenhagen, Copenhagen, Denmark

1. Introduction

A range of infectious diseases and cancers are in theory preventable or treatable by vaccination, but have remained outside the reach of traditional vaccination. This may be because of special problems regarding the selection of appropriate target antigens or certain requirements regarding the quality of the vaccine induced response. In this context, the use of recombinant virus vectored vaccines may be a promising future concept that combines important features of live attenuated vaccines with greater safety and the ability to target any imaginable antigen. Among the virus vectors investigated for vaccine purposes, adenovirus vectors have received considerable attention and today stand among the most potent tools available for induction of antibody and CD8+ T cell responses in mice, primates and humans (Barefoot et al., 2008; Bett et al., 2010; Shiver et al., 2002). Adenovirus vectored vaccines has, however, also been implicated in one of the most spectacular HIV vaccine failures (Buchbinder et al., 2008), and some papers describe either undesirable attributes of the adenovirus induced T cell response or properties of vector specific responses, which may increase mucosal HIV transmission (Benlahrech et al., 2009; Perreau et al., 2008). The current review will attempt to describe the key features of adenovirus vectored vaccine induced immune responses, the mechanisms underlying induction of different response qualities, how the adenovirus vectors compare with other vaccination tools in the immunological arsenal, and how adenovirus vectors can be combined in heterologous vaccination regimens. A final section will be dedicated to potential future clinical application of adenovirus vectored vaccines.

2. Immune responses against adenovirus vectored vaccines - the issue of magnitude and functionality

Although scientific progress had been made using replication incompetent adenovirus vectors for vaccination since the late 1980's (Alkhatib & Briedis, 1988) (see figure 1 for a description of the principal immunological differences between replication competent and replication incompetent adenovirus vectors), the interest in this vector system exploded with the demonstration of antiviral efficacy against simian human immunodeficiency virus (SHIV) of a vaccine encoding SIV gag delivered by a human serotype 5 adenovirus vector in non-human primates (NHPs)(Shiver et al., 2002). The failure of modified vaccinia Ankara (MVA) or DNA vectors to achieve similar results only served to underscore the potency of the adenoviral vector system. However, several reports both preceding and in particularly following the spectacular failure of the MERCK STEP trial have highlighted that adenoviral vectored vaccines may induces a substantial, yet functionally impaired T cell response (Tatsis et al., 2007a), that in many cases nevertheless provide highly significant protection (Yang et al., 2006). In that context it is pertinent to note, that adenoviral vaccination seems to induce T cells with a phenotype more resembling that associated with a chronic infection than with a resolved acute and self-limiting infection. Importantly, although the kinetics and magnitude of the reported adenovirus induced CD8+ T cell responses vary considerably depending on the encoded antigen as well as the route and dose of immunization, the responses are unusually stable over time. Thus, memory T cell frequencies frequently stabilizes above 30% of the peak response, which contrast with the 5-10% usually found to be associated with acutely resolved infections (Abbink et al., 2007; Holst et al., 2007; Holst et al., 2010b; Tatsis et al., 2007a) (See figure 2 for a cartoon of the different immune response patterns and their associated phenotypic properties).

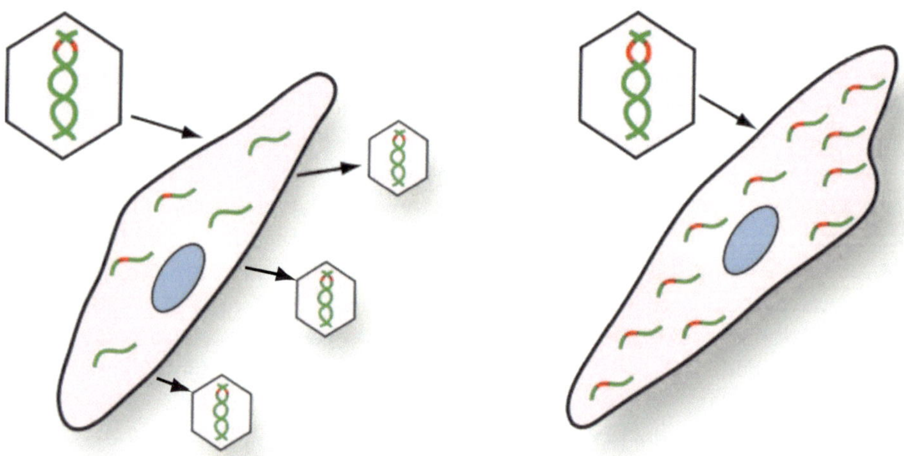

Fig. 1. **The principal differences between replication competent and replication incompetent viral vectors with regard to source of antigens.** Infection with a live replication competent vaccine vector (left side) or a replication incompetent vector (right side) differ markedly in the ability to present recombinant vaccine antigen. The replication competent vector has less cloning capacity (hence the small red fragment symbolizing recombinant antigen) and infection of a host cell results in many viral transcripts being produced, including those not containing the recombinant insert. On the positive side, the inoculum will be amplified (symbolized by the appearance of virus progeny), and present an ongoing infectious signature to the innate immune system. Replication incompetent vectors do not become amplified, but transcripts containing the recombinant insert dominate the transcription profile of the transduced cell. Other popular virus vectors such as vaccinia virus resemble replication competent adenovirus in the way in which they present antigen, whereas replication deficient variants, such as modified vaccinia Ankara (MVA), more resemble replication incompetent vectors (although with more non-recombinant gene expression)

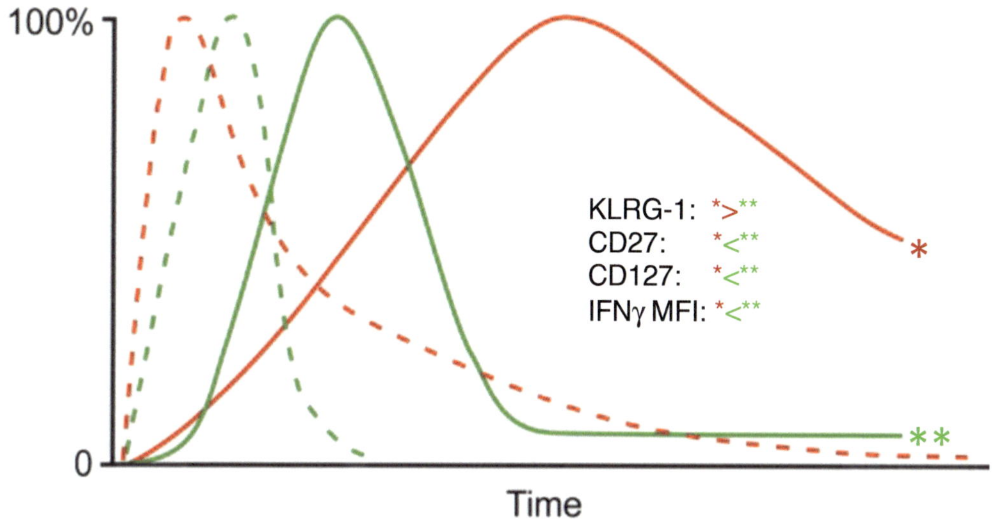

Fig. 2. **The principal time-course of antigen elimination and CD8+ T cell response after a self-limiting acute infection and an adenoviral vaccination.** Infection with an acute viral infection (green lines)) takes days to reach maximal antigen presentation (dashed green line) as viral replication is needed to amplify the inoculum. There is rapid and nearly complete elimination of the virus after the peak by the induced CD8+ T cell response (full green line) the time-course of which mimics the antigen curve with a few days delay. Vaccination with a replication incompetent adenoviral vector (red lines) is representing a bolus injection and the peak of antigen expression (dashed red line) is reached shortly after virus inoculation. Subsequently antigen presentation gradually declines over a protracted time-period. T cell expansion is delayed (full red line) and slowly reaches a peak as the majority of the antigen has been eliminated. The response then slowly declines, but is maintained at a high level relative to the peak response. The relative differences in the resulting memory T cell phenotype is inserted between the lines with color coding identifying the two populations.

2.1 Tissue transduction properties

The key to untangle these conflicting reports regarding the immunological properties of adenovirus vectors may lie in a better understanding of the mechanisms underlying the remarkable immunogenicity of adenoviral vectors and its relationship to route, dose and antigen presentation. To aid in this understanding we will first consider the unusual features of the adenoviral gene delivery system. Adenoviral vectors are not unique in their ability to target relevant populations of antigen presenting cells (Lindsay et al., 2010), but uniquely among all vaccine delivery technologies, adenoviral vectors have also received serious attention as vehicles of correctional or experimental gene therapy. Thus, adenoviral vectors can be used to transduce a large number of cell types, and intravenous or intramuscular application can lead to a situation where most liver cells or cells of the infected muscle are expressing vast amount of the transgene (Antinozzi et al., 1999; Jimenez-Chillaron et al., 1999; Okuyama et al., 1998). Thus, with the ability to transduce both professional APCs and vast numbers of tissue resident cells, adenoviruses are perfectly equipped to induce combined direct and cross-presentation of antigen to CD8+ T cells. In agreement with this notion, ubiquitous, keratinocyte specific and alveolar epithelial cell specific promoters have been used to induce CD8+ T cell responses towards the encoded antigen, and remarkably, no differences in the response level have been observed provided the administration route targeted cells with the relevant promoter activity (Prasad et al., 2001). Paradoxically, adenoviruses are extremely potent inducers of CD8+ T cells directed against the inserted transgene, yet induce levels of CD4+ T cell activation similar to that of naked DNA vaccines, which are much less efficient in tissue transduction (Wu et al., 2005). This is surprising because the ability to cross-prime CD8+ T cells implies that substantial amount of antigen are being released from dying cells, and this antigen would normally be expected to represent a good sources of peptides for MHC class II restricted presentation to CD4+ T cells. The reasons for this limited ability to induce CD4+ T cell responses are currently not understood. Unfortunately the study employing cell type specific promoters for antigen expression did not contain any data relating to the immunological potency, the kinetics of the response or the phenotype of the CD8+ T cells induced. This means, that while it is likely that both direct and cross-presentation contribute in the induction of the response, it has until recently been unclear what is the relative contribution of each type of antigen presentation pathway, how this contribution may differ between different antigens and how this may affect the phenotypes of the responding T cells. Recent work by our group (Holst et al., 2010b) and the group of Jonathan L. Bramson (Bassett et al., 2011; Finn et al., 2009; Yang et al., 2006) has now begun to address this issue in greater detail.

2.2 The issue of dose

Initially we discovered that increasing the dose of s.c. administered adenovirus from 10^9 to 10^{10} or 10^{11} particles, caused most of the increased inoculum to enter the systemic circulation and transduce the cells of the liver and spleen at levels comparable to those found after an i.v. administration (Holst et al., 2010b) (see figure 3). Intravenous administration was found to induce a slow response and require more vector for initiating a transgene specific response (10^{10} particles i.v., while 10^9 or less sufficed for s.c. administration). This is consistent with the notion that a key to a potent immune response is efficient priming in the local environment of the lymph nodes draining the injection site, and we were able to substantiate this suggestion by observing markedly impaired responses in L-selectin deficient mice after peripheral immunization using a moderate dose of adenovirus vectored vaccine (Holst PJ, Thomsen AR and Christensen JP, unpublished) (see figure 4A). However, after a considerable delay, i.v. administered adenovirus did induce a transgene specific CD8+ T cell response, which eventually surpassed the response following s.c. immunization in terms of cell numbers generated. For both routes of virus administration we found a positive correlation between the amount of vector reaching the systemic circulation and the magnitude of the response, whereas an inverse correlation was noted with regard to the quality of the response as measured by cytokine producing competence. These observations led us to suggest that dissemination of the vector was responsible for the apparent reduction in T cell quality in i.v. immunized mice. Bramson and co-workers had early on demonstrated that transgene expression after injection of moderate virus doses intramuscularly (i.m.) in the thigh were confined to the injection site and the draining lymph nodes (Yang et al., 2003). Recently, they took the mechanistic unraveling an important step further and demonstrated by surgical removal of the nodes that the full response depended on intact draining lymph nodes for more than 7 days post infection, but after 20 days they were no longer required. These results by themselves could have been an artifact reflecting the removal of antigen-specific CD8+ T cells sequestered in the draining lymph nodes rather than the abrogation of antigen presentation; yet they are consistent with the conclusions we drew from our experiments with L-selectin deficient mice. However, even in "denoded" mice, there was continuous T cell expansion for an additional 3 weeks, which could be abrogated by eliminating transcription of the transgene encoding gene using a doxycycline repressible system (Finn et al., 2009). This was interpreted by the authors to suggest that i.m. inoculation of adenovirus leads to extra nodal, but transgene expression dependent prolonged T cell expansion. To address this issue in detail they generated bone-marrow chimeric mice in which bone marrow cells from mice lacking the MHC element restricting the relevant transgene derived epitope was used for reconstitution of lethally irradiated WT mice. Using this system, they could confirm that epitopes restricted by MHC molecules only expressed by non-hematopoietic cells were driving late T cell expansion. This result was taken as evidence for non-hematopoietic antigen presentation by Bramson and co-workers and is referred to as such in the following; however, that this is the case has not been formally proven. Antigen could still be presented by professional antigen presenting cells which have acquired already peptide loaded MHC class I molecules from the surface of tissue resident, non-hematopoietic cells, a phenomenon coined by the phrase "cross-dressing" (see figure 4C) (Dolan et al., 2006). Nevertheless, the T cells maintained exclusively by so-called non-hematopoietic antigen presentation showed marked deficiencies in particular with respect to cytokine production, but also featured a more pronounced effector memory surface phenotype as compared with T cells generated in context of both hematopoietic and non-hematopoietic antigen-presentation. These phenotypic differences were roughly identical to those we had previously observed when comparing responses elicited by i.v. administration with those elicited by s.c. administration. Importantly, the dysfunctional T cells, be they induced by i.v immunization or non-hematopoietic priming were quite capable of performing cytotoxic activity. We also found i.v. primed T cells to be efficient in protection against vaccinia challenge (Holst et al., 2010b), whereas Bramson and co-workers found that non-hematopoietic primed T cells were partially effective against LCMV or melanoma (Bassett et al., 2011). Importantly, we also found the T cells induced by i.v. administration to be less capable of secondary expansion (Holst et al., 2010b), whereas Bramson and co-workers found non-hematopoietic and hematopoietic priming equally efficient in inducing memory T cells capable of undergoing secondary expansion (Bassett et al., 2011). However, the secondary expansion and protection data reported by Bramson and co-workers requires careful evaluation. The experiments were performed in vaccinated chimeras with and without hematopoietic antigen presentation of the relevant epitopes, and thus the adenovirus induced T cell priming as well as the antigen presentation taking place during the challenge phase would be affected. This might not be important during melanoma challenge, but certainly would impact the effector phase of the responses to infections with rapidly replicating viruses such as LCMV, vaccinia virus or influenza. Furthermore, as the capacity for protection was evaluated through the challenge of intact animals rather than by adoptive transfers of primed donor cells into naïve hosts, we do not know the phenotype of the cells actually responding. Importantly, during early primary expansion of OVA specific T cells hematopoietic and non-hematopoietic antigen presentation worked synergistically to increase CD8+ T cell numbers, but only hematopoietic antigen presentation supported sustained functionality as measured by cytokine competence (Bassett et al., 2011). Notably, beyond 20 days post vaccination only extra-nodal expansion contributed to the T cell response. This method of antigen presentation is highly important during the early memory phase of the response as cessation of antigen expression by a doxycycline regulated vector drastically reduced the magnitude of late memory responses (Finn et al., 2009). Our tools did not allow detailed control of antigen expression, but we also observed a continuous expansion of memory T cells from 20 to 60 days post vaccination following high-dose i.v. adenovirus vector administration (Holst et al., 2010b).

2.3 Model for adenovirus induced CD8+ T cell responses

Although there are differences between the studies of Bramson and coworkers using doxycycline repressible presentation of the ovalbumine derived SIINFEKL epitope and our own using adenovirus encoded β-galactosidase, in particular with regard to the kinetics of the induced response, the conclusions drawn in these reports are consistent. Taken together, these studies allows us to propose a mechanism by which adenoviral vector delivered antigen primes an immune response in part by directly transducing the available tissue resident dendritic cells and in part by transduction of the local tissue resident, non-hematopoietic cells. Regarding the antigen produced by cells at the injection site this may either be cross-presented via hematopoietic dendritic cells expressing the same MHC molecules as the tissue cells, be presented by the novel mechanism of "cross-dressing" described in Bassett et al.(Bassett et al., 2011), or be directly presented to the CD8+ T cells *in situ* (see figure 4 for a complete description of the different mechanisms potentially involved in the presentation of antigen). Increasing the inoculum leads to the systemic dissemination of viral vector and an altered balance between dendritic cell mediated lymph node presentation and presentation mediated by non-hematopoietic cells independent of the draining lymph nodes (see figure 3 for a description of the interrelation between virus dose and site of antigen presentation). This in turn leads to poorer cytokine producing competence. The relative importance of hematopoietic and non-hematopoietic antigen presentation at doses below ~10^9 particles is as yet undetermined, but some studies in mice and primates as well as humans have demonstrated the relative stability of the response within 10- fold variations of the inoculum (Bassett et al., 2011; Bett et al., 2010), and we have seen a plateau of the response between ~10^9 to ~10^8 particles administered s.c., with a gradual reduction of the magnitude of the response upon further dose reductions (Holst PJ, Thomsen AR and Christensen JP,unpublished and (Flatz et al., 2010)). A possible explanation for these plateaus could be that these doses are sufficient to target all the relevant professional antigen presenting cells present at the injection site, and that the major difference between the doses are in the degree of non-dendritic cell targeted transduction. As the non professional APC transduction leads to poorer cytokine producing competence and generation of more terminally differentiated cells, it is worth noticing that we have observed an increase in the ratio of CD127^{high} cells compared to KLRG1^{high} cells as the dose was further decreased (Holst PJ, Thomsen AR and Christensen JP, unpublished), and that termination of transgene expression after the acute response led to higher frequencies of central memory T cells, and higher CD27 expression, and a lower frequency of KLRG1 expression on the responding T cells (Finn et al., 2009).

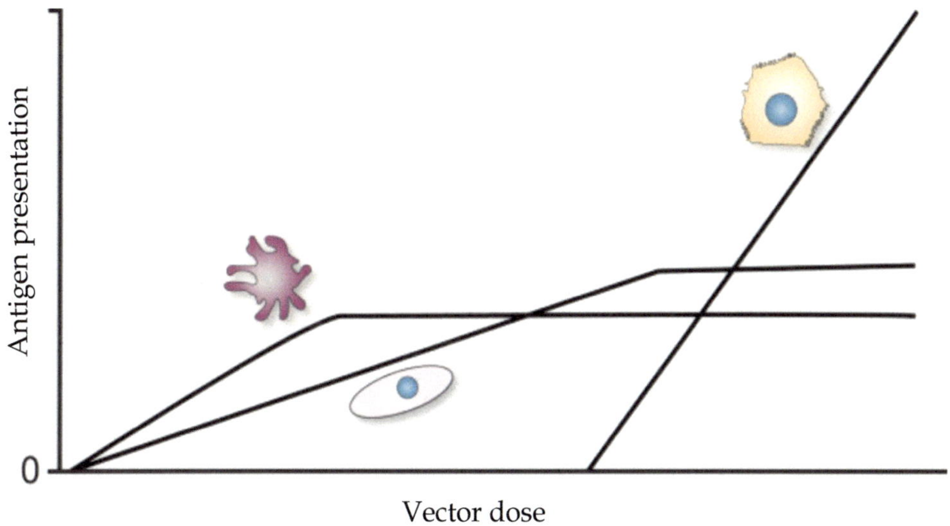

Fig. 3. **Relative contribution of antigen presentation from different cell types driving the CD8+ T cell expansion after peripheral administration of adenoviral vaccines.** Injection of increasing amounts of adenoviral vaccine initially results in a gradual and dose-dependent increase in the transduction of professional antigen presenting cells (APC, represented by a ruffled cell placed above the line to the left) and tissue resident parenchymal cells (represented by an oval cell placed below the line). The peak level of APC transduction is reached at a lower dose than is the parenchymal cell transduction and thus the ratio of APC to parenchymal cell transduction gradually declines. Increasing the dose further leads to spill-over into the systemic circulation causing transduction of central organs, particularly the liver (represented by a hepatocyte inserted next to the line at the top right corner).

The differences between the response patterns observed by us and by Bramson and co-workers deserve some consideration. Most remarkably, we find i.v. administration of 10^{10} particles (~$2x10^8$ IFU) of adenovirus to induce a response that becomes detectable in the spleen as late as between 30 and 60 days post vaccination whereas lower doses of virus given i.v. fail to induce any detectable response. Subcutaneous immunization induces an earlier response at lower doses. Bramson and co-workers on the other hand detect a response in the blood and spleen at 10 to 20 days post i.m. immunization with 10^7-10^8 pfu of adenovirus encoding SIINFEKL fused to luciferase (Bassett et al., 2011; Finn et al., 2009). This difference in the kinetics of the response after i.v. as compared to i.m. administration is not likely to be due to differences in antigen as Flatz et al.(Flatz et al., 2010) also noted a profound attenuation of the response after intravenously administration of $2.5x10^8$ pfu of adenovirus encoding the SIINFEKL containing ovalbumin sequence, whereas a potent response was observed at lower doses, all measured at 28 days post vaccination. Thus, whereas the difference between our report and the one of Flatz et al. (Flatz et al., 2010), who observed a strong response to low doses of ovalbumin encoding adenovirus, are likely due to the immunological potency of the encoded antigen (ovalbumin being a potent antigen, while β-galactosidase is a weak antigen), the differences between Flatz and Bramson must relate to the route of administration. In this regard it is interesting that we observed an early, transient cytokine competent CD8+ T cell response in the liver following i.v. administration;

this response seem to be associated with the transduction of liver cells, and it disappears before the systemic response can be measured in the spleen. The most likely explanation for this phenomenon is that the early transgene-specific T cell response is aborted within the liver parenchyma as previously reported for the adenovirus-specific response following i.v. immunization (Liu et al., 2001), and that systemic T-cell expansion can only occur after a reduction in transgene expression in the liver or when a lower inoculum has been used to induce the response as seen by Flatz et al.(Flatz et al., 2010). Based on our findings that peripheral virus administration leads to a marked increase in hepatic transduction when the dose is increased from 10^9 to 10^{10} particles, and that the entire increase in dose at 10^{11} particles enters the systemic circulation, we would think that working with peripheral administration of adenovirus at doses above 10^9 particles in murine systems entails a major risk for variability in response magnitude, kinetics and quality. The report from Tatsis et al.(Tatsis et al., 2007a) can be seen to support this conclusion as i.v. administration of 10^{10} adenoviral particles expressing LCMV glycoprotein gave a result midway between our results with i.v. administered β-gal at 10^{10} and s.c. administered β-gal at 10^{11} particles, whereas 10^{11} particles given i.m. induced a biphasic response. Hypothetically, the elimination of the first phase could be due to intrahepatic sequestration.

The delineation of adenovirus induced immune responses in hematopoietic and non-hematopoietic is recent, and the mechanisms of the non-hematopoietic antigen presentation is unknown. However, although non-hematopoietic antigen presentation is a novel finding for adenovirus induced immunizations, it is not the only system in which it is described. Thus, during allogenic bone marrow transplantation, non-hematopoietic antigen presentation contributes both to induction of T cells incapable of recall responses and functional exhaustion of T cells already generated (Flutter et al., 2010). What is special about the adenoviral immunization after a low dose injection is that it is taking place at a defined site and should in theory by highly amendable for studying. In any case, more attention should now be directed towards the events taking place at the site of adenovirus inoculation, because these appear to be crucial for both the immunological potency of adenoviral vectors and for excessive differentiation of adenovirus primed CD8+ effector T cells.

For non-hematopoietic antigen presentation to occur one must assume that either a local environment capable of causing naïve T cells activation is induced by the interaction of the immune system and persisting antigen, or that the antigen is transported to secondary lymphoid organs by macrophages or dendritic cells cross-dressed with loaded peptide/MHC complexes derived from dying (?) cells within the infected tissue (see figure 4 for an overview of potential mechanisms). Potentially, cross-dressing of APCs at the injection site could occur either through capture of exosomes by dendritic cells (Utsugi-Kobukai et al., 2003) or through a cell-contact dependent mechanism (Dolan et al., 2006), although it should be noted that recent studies have questioned the ability of exosomes to contribute to relevant responses against viral infections in vivo. However, in the latter case the antigens tested have been different and the sensitivity of the assays may have been rather low (Coppieters et al., 2009). That expression of foreign antigen following adenoviral vector injection contributes to an inflammatory infiltrate seems beyond question as no long term infiltrate can be seen following injection with vectors devoid of viral genes and a transgene which does not prime an immune response (Chen et al., 1997), yet the interest in such infiltrates have focused on their ability to clear gene therapy vectors rather than on their role in supporting immune responses. Thus, at present, we know the infiltrates contain CD4+ and CD8+ T cells, few macrophages but little else. In other systems, chronic or extended inflammation has been seen to induce lymphoid like structures within parenchymatous organs such as the CNS, kidneys (Moskophidis et al., 1987) and bronchi (Moyron-Quiroz et al., 2004), and such changes could possibly also take place following adenovirus immunizations. A more thorough understanding of the events occurring at the injection site could perhaps lead to strategies impeding excessive T cell differentiation without removing antigen stimulation and thus result in generation of even more potent vaccines.

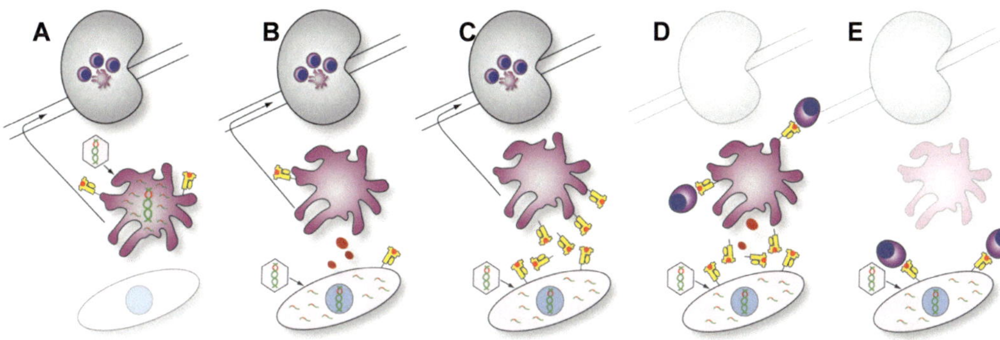

Fig. 4. **Overview of the potential antigen presentation mechanisms after adenoviral vaccination.** All the cartoons feature an oval tissue resident parenchymal cell in the bottom, a ruffled professional antigen presenting cell in the middle and a lymph node with afferent lymphatic vessels to the left. CD8+ T cells are drawn with a dark blue nuclei and dark purple cytoplasm. MHC class I molecules are yellow, whereas the presented recombinant antigen is red. Replication incompetent vectors are hexagonal containing double stranded DNA. **A) Direct presentation.** Professional APCs are directly transduced by the adenoviral vector, migrate to the draining lymph nodes and presents antigen synthesized within themselves to the CD8+ T cells. **B) Cross-presentation.** Tissue resident parenchymal cells are transduced and professional APCs take up the antigen, process it, migrate to the draining lymph node and on their own MHC molecules present the antigen to the CD8+ T cells. **C) Cross-dressing.** Tissue resident cell process and initially presents the antigen. However, somehow MHC/peptide complexes are released and taken up by APCs, which migrate to the draining lymph node and present the antigen to the CD8+ T cells on MHC molecules synthesized within the parenchymal cells. **D) Local presentation by APCs.** Tissue resident cells are transduced, but the antigen remains at the injection site. Resident and inflammatory APCs present antigen to CD8+ T cells locally, either from processing of tissue debris or from presentation of MHC molecules already loaded with antigen in the parenchymal cells. **E) Local presentation without APC's.** Tissue resident parenchymal cells are transduced, process the antigen and present it to CD8+ T cells locally on their own MHC class I molecules.

2.4 The issue of quality

The proposed model has profound implications for interpreting the existing literature and in appreciating the potential potency of adenoviral vectors for vaccination use. First of all, it partially explains why functionally exhausted T cells are a feature of increasing the dose beyond 10^9 particles (in mice). Secondly, as chronic non-hematopoietic antigen presentation cannot be avoided, it may also help explain why adenovirus induced CD8+ T cells tend to be more terminally differentiated than are T cells induced by live viral vaccines or MVA vectors. As murine studies reporting an exhausted phenotype of adenovirus induced CD8+ T cells have typically involved virus doses in the range of 10^{10}-10^{11} viral particles (Tatsis et al., 2007a; Yang et al., 2006), one might question the relevance of the results obtained when it comes to human or primate vaccination, where the virus dose is typically in the order of 10^{10}-10^{11} particles (Bett et al., 2010). In contrast to the studies using high doses of adenoviral vectors in mice, CD8+ T cells induced by adenoviral vaccination in primates and humans are cytokine competent and cytotoxic cells, but seemingly terminally differentiated effector-like cells are found in the circulation for extended periods of time. A key question in this respect is whether this should be of significant concern. In the opinion of these authors it should not. Under the premise that the adenoviral infection is not overdosed, the phenotype of adenovirus primed CD8+ T cells resemble that of T cells found in association with chronic, but well-controlled viral infections such as Epstein Barr virus infection in human (Ibegbu et al., 2005) and γ herpes virus-68 (MHV-68) infection in mice (Cush & Flano, 2011). A key cell surface marker in this context is KLRG1, the expression of which is often taken to indicate replicative senescence. However, in EBV infected humans it has been found that while KLRG1 is indeed expressed by terminally differentiated T cells, by no means all $KLRG1^{high}$ cells are end cells, but rather seem to represent a subset of memory cells associated with antigen persistence (Ibegbu et al., 2005). Along the same lines the meticulous study by Cush and Flãno (Cush & Flano, 2011) have clearly demonstrated that $KLRG1^{high}$ CD8+ T cells in MHV-68 infected mice are fully functional, can expand upon reactivation and provide even better protection against reinfection than do $KLRG\text{-}1^{low}$ cells with the same specificity. Furthermore, despite having predominantly an effector memory ($CD62L^{low}CD43^{low}$) phenotype, $KLRG1^{high}$ CD8+ T cells may express receptors for homeostatic cytokines (IL-7 and IL-15) and can survive long-term in the absence of cognate antigen. Thus, although expression of KLRG1 may be associated with a decreasing potential for expansion, there are numerous observations indicating that these cells may be protective, and by way of their immediate effector capacity in fact could represent the most optimal type of vaccine-induced T-cell defence despite some limitations in proliferative capacity (Bachmann et al., 2005). An earlier study by the group of Rafi Ahmed investigating the responsiveness of mice undergoing repeated antigenic stimulation supports this view (Masopust et al., 2006). These authors found that increasing the number of antigenic challenges preferentially promoted the generation phenotypically similar memory cells that retained effector-like properties and showed preferential accumulation in non-lymphoid organs. Notably, neither the adenovirus primed CD8+ T cells nor those driven by repeated antigenic stimulation express the inhibitory receptor PD-1 typical of dysfunctional T cells (Barber et al., 2006; Bassett et al., 2011; Masopust et al., 2006).

3. Increasing the potency of adenovirus vectors

3.1 Improving antigen presentation

Even though adenovirus vectored vaccines stand among the most potent vaccine platforms for induction of CD8 T cell responses, it is apparent that better vaccines are needed still. Be that in magnitude of the response, breadth or phenotype of the induced cells. It is clear that simply providing more vaccine or administering adenovirus multiple times provide minimal benefit compared to low dose immunization, at least with potent antigens, and while awaiting a deeper understanding of non-hematopoietic antigen presentation, the goal is to do more with less (vaccine). Our group, and others in close pursuit, therefore set out to identify the mechanisms that would be rate limiting for adenovirus induced immune responses. We had prior experiences with enhancing the immune responses to DNA vaccines by covalently linking an ER exported minimal epitope to β-2 microglobulin as described (Uger et al., 1999; Uger & Barber, 1998), thereby presumably increasing the direct antigen presentation on DNA transduced cells (Bartholdy et al., 2003; Bartholdy et al., 2004). When the same antigen was cloned into an adenoviral vector and compared to full length LCMV glycoprotein, we saw an acceleration and augmentation of the response, and the transgene specific response which otherwise depended on CD4+ T cell help could now be induced in MHC class II deficient mice (Holst et al., 2007). We have since confirmed that the transgene works by loading the encoded antigen directly onto the MHC in a processing independent manner as TAP deficient cells transduced with adenoviral vectors expressing the β-2 microglobulin fused minimal epitope were fully competent in stimulating antigen specific T cells in vivo whereas an antigen expression system more potent in WT mice was not (Holst PJ and Bassi MR, unpublished).

3.2 Increasing the breadth of the CD8+ T cell response

We were surprised to find that the native LCMV glycoprotein induced a CD8+ T cell response which were severely limited in breadth and predominantly focused on the immunodominant GP33 epitope. In retrospect, the limited breadth of the induced response is perhaps not so surprising and tends to be a general draw-back of viral vectored vaccines. The vector backbone of adenoviruses, poxviruses and other systems encode many T cell epitopes which may compete with the transgene for the attention of the CD8+ T cells (Schirmbeck et al., 2008). In a search for adenovirus vaccine modifications which might lead to broader T cell responses, we decided to improve MHC class II restricted antigen presentation by covalently linking the encoded antigen to the MHC class II associated Invariant chain (Diebold et al., 2001; Holst et al., 2008; Rowe et al., 2006). Surprisingly, this strategy improved not only CD4+ T cell responses, but also the kinetics, breadth, magnitude and stability of the CD8+ T cell response via increased MHC class I presentation and independently of MHC class II (Holst et al., 2011). We have since then confirmed these findings with a variety of antigens and are able to conclude that the level of antigen presentation on the adenovirus transduced cell is a limiting factor with regard to the speed and breadth of CD8+ T cell responses (Hoegh-Petersen et al., 2009; Mikkelsen et al., 2011; Sorensen et al., 2009). Given the apparent dichotomy of fast hematopoietic and chronic non-hematopoietic antigen presentation in adenoviral vaccination, this is highly consistent with the hypothesis that the above described strategies work at least in part to increase the first wave of antigen presentation mediated by dendritic cells directly transduced by the vector (see figure 2). Remarkably, the CD8+ T cell response induced by adenoviral vaccination with this type of modified construct seem to have acquired a normal contraction phase and the CD8+ T cell response typically stabilizes at approximately 10% of the level of the peak response (see figure 1). Though augmentation of direct early presentation should lead to an accelerated response, it is unclear if this would also result in reduced late phase presentation thereby allowing the return to a nearly normal contraction pattern. One could speculate that increased MHC class I restricted antigen presentation, also in the tissue resident cells, would result in more efficient antigen elimination at these sites by the antigen-specific CD8+ T cells, but it is also possible that CD4+ T cells and MHC class II restricted antigen presentation by tissue resident cells could play a role. Thus, the more efficient early induction of CD4+ T cells by the MHC class II associated Invariant chain linked constructs combined with local production of interferon-γ, which could cause local MHC class II up-regulation and antigen presentation, might together set the stage for CD4+ T cell mediated antigen elimination.

3.3 Role of CD4+ T cell help

Interestingly, we also found that while ordinary adenovaccine primed CD8+ T cell responses were CD4+ T-cell help dependent, neither of the tethered constructs required CD4+ T cells for induction of a primary CD8+ T-cell response (Holst et al., 2007; Holst et al., 2011). However, as has previously been observed also with fully CD4+ T-cell helped CD8+ T cells, the functionality of the generated cells decreased faster in a CD4+ T-cell deficient environment (Sun et al., 2004). Still, however, we saw significant protection against a high-dose viral challenge in MHC class II deficient mice at 2 months post vaccination, which matched that found in wild type mice vaccinated with an ordinary adenovirus vaccine (Holst et al., 2007; Holst et al., 2011). This ability of our improved vaccine to induce an efficient acute and prolonged CD8+ T cell response in the absence of CD4+ T cells have clear implications as regards certain states of clinical immunodeficiency. Thus, in bone-marrow transplant recipients herpes virus infections represent a serious clinical problem. However, as the CD8+ T-cell population in these patients recovers faster than the CD4+ T cell population (Berger et al., 2008), this type of vaccine could be used to curtail such infections until the CD4+ T-cell population is restored.

Although several strategies can increase the immune response resulting from DNA vaccination there are not many strategies that have been published to augment the response to adenovirus vectored vaccines (reviewed in Holst et al. 2010 (Holst et al., 2010a)). Whether this reflects that very few strategies have actually been tested or that they have not worked efficiently is a matter of speculation, but it is tempting to conclude that virus vectored vaccines contains sufficient pathogen- associated molecular patterns to substitute for many a cytokine co-administered with the vaccine. Exceptions to the general rule has been antigen linked to the herpes viral tegument protein VP22 and calreticulin, which have been tested in Sindbis virus replicon particles (Cheng et al., 2002) and vaccinia vectors (Hsieh et al., 2004), respectively, and the herpes viral glycoprotein D (gD), which has been tested using an adenoviral vector. Both VP22 and calreticulin are suggested to work by increasing antigen presentations, but the herpes viral glycoprotein D was postulated to work by competitive inhibition of the interaction between the herpes virus entry mediator (HVEM) and the B and T lymphocyte attenuator (BTLA) (Lasaro et al., 2008). Although herpes viral gD fused to antigen was convincingly showed to interact with HVEM, there were no experiments performed in animals or cells deficient in HVEM or BTLA, nor was antigen presentation measured following use of this strategy. Thus whether or not HVEM-BTLA interaction is important in the immune response to adenoviral vectors remains to be determined (see (Holst et al., 2010a) for a detailed comment on this study). The MHC class II associated invariant chain linked antigen concept was also tested as a DNA vaccine, and found to increase CD8+ T cell responses working both alone and as a primer for an adenoviral boost. Moreover, the MHC class II associated Invariant chain linked antigen concept was also beneficial when applied in the booster supporting the conclusion that increased direct presentation benefits adenovirus induced CD8+ T cell responses after the initial priming (Grujic et al., 2009).

4. Adenovirus vectored vaccines compared to other vaccine technologies

4.1 Adenovirus induces unusually potent and protective CD8+ T cell responses

With regard to sheer potency of long term CD8+ T cell induction there are only a few reports challenging the supremacy of adenovirus vectors, and none of these have been verified in humans. In primates, adenoviral vectors have been tested side-by-side with MVA and DNA vectors and matched studies have been performed in humans (Bett et al., 2010; Casimiro et al., 2003; Shiver et al., 2002). These studies have unequivocally shown that adenoviral vectors induce superior frequencies of CD8+ T cells and, importantly, induce better T cell mediated protection against simian human immunodeficiency virus challenge (SHIV) in NHP's. However, other general findings include a low proliferative potential of induced T cells, effector memory rather than central memory phenotype of the induced T cells and a low frequency of IL-2 producing T cells (Tatsis et al., 2007a; Yang et al., 2006; Yang et al., 2007). Although several studies have addressed potency and immunogenicity of antigen presentation from various vectors, few direct comparisons exists between adenoviral vectors and other popular virus vectored vaccine candidates, most notably MVA and fowlpox vectors. A recent study has been made in mice comparing human adenovirus serotype 5, simian serotype C6, fowlpox vectors and MVA. These studies confirmed the tendencies reported above, but remarkably again demonstrated a superior protective efficacy of the adenoviral vector system. Thus, even though adenovirus vectors induce CD8+ T cells with functional and phenotypic properties most similar to those found in association with unresolved chronic infections, they still stand as superior vectors for T cell mediated protection against acute and chronic infections (Shiver et al., 2002; Sridhar et al., 2008). A paradox which has caused confusion, but in the opinion of these authors, a paradox which can be easily be appreciated if one considers the impact of the acute phase of an infection as a major determinant of the course of the chronic phase of an infection. Also, the negative result of the STEP trial regarding clinical protection against HIV may have attracted much too negative attention to the adenoviral vector system. Recent follow- up data of infected vaccinees revealed that the infecting HIV strains have accumulated mutations matching the most immunogenic epitopes of the vaccine, thus demonstrating that the adenovirus vectored vaccine has exerted an efficient selection pressure upon the infecting virus (Rolland et al., 2011). In conclusion, the vaccine induced T cells did work, but as the vaccine induced T-cell responses were rather narrowly targeted and raised against T-cell epitopes that can readily be mutated, the induced response simply was not sufficient to permanently control infection with a rapidly mutating virus like HIV. Some improvement strategies to the immunogenicity of the adenovirus vaccines have been discussed above (see the **"Increasing the potency of adenovirus vectors"** section above), whereas the most commonly applied strategy, prime-boost regimens will be discussed below.

4.2 Adenovirus induced antibody responses

Although the major focus of this review is on adenovirus induced T cell responses, it should be noted that the benefits of adenoviral vectors for induction of antibody responses is less clear. It is noteworthy that adenoviral vectors, despite their capacity for induction of high titers of antibodies, may fall short of MVA vectors when it comes to induction of cross-reacting antibodies against influenza and SIV. Thus, MVA vectors expressing the hemagglutinin antigen of influenza A H5N1/Vietnam/2004 provide efficient cross-clade protection against H5N1/Indonesia/2005 challenge in primates (Kreijtz et al., 2009), whereas similar adenovirus vectors appear less potent, and infectious virus may still be detectable after homologous challenge (Gao et al., 2006). Direct comparisons are lacking. Similarly, in the SHIV system, Robinson and colleagues have developed a DNA and MVA based vaccine which uses the large cloning capacity of the poxvirus vector to simultaneously encode gp41 and gag and thus produce virus-like particles. Highly avid antibodies to native gp41 appear to constitute a correlate of protection against peak viremia which transcends into improved control in the chronic phase of the infection (Zhao et al., 2009). Again, a similar strategy has not been tested with adenovirus vectors. Thus, there is suggestive evidence that MVA vectors are superior or at least as potent as adenovirus vectors with respect to induction of broadly reactive antibodies. Why adenovirus vectors induce superior CD8+ T cell responses, but only comparable antibody responses has not been systematically addressed. However, as vectors such as the MVA induce their associated immune response in considerable less time than do the adenoviral vectors, the former could be speculated to rely on the recruitment of more B cell precursors to reach the same levels as the adenovirus vectored vaccines and therefore induce more diverse responses.

5. Use of adenovirus vaccines in prime-boost regimens

5.1 Use of adenovirus in heterologous prime-boost regimens

Pre-clinically, adenovirus vectors have been used rather successful as boosters for DNA immunizations, and paradoxically as they potentially induce memory T cells with a restricted proliferative potential, also as primers for poxvirus booster immunizations. The use of DNA priming is logical and results in a broadening of the CD4+ T cell response, an increase in the IL-2 competence of the primed CD8+ T cells and improved protection after SIV challenge (Casimiro et al., 2005; Cox et al., 2008; Wu et al., 2005). Please note that although some animal studies point to an improved immunogenicity of DNA primed adenovirus immunizations (Grujic et al., 2009), this has not been verified in humans (Bett et al., 2010). Although DNA primed adenovirus immunization have shown some promise, it pales in comparison to the recent pre-clinical results obtained using adenoviruses of different serotypes (Liu et al., 2009) or adenovirus as primers for MVA vectors (Reyes-Sandoval et al., 2010). The use of such prime-boost regimens have improved the protective efficacy against SIV or rodent malaria compared to the use of either vector system alone, although it should be stressed that the reason for the improved protection is unclear. The heterologous adenovirus based immunization by Barouch and co-workers induced increased CD4+ T cell responses and CD8+ T cells of increased functionality, but the correlate of protection was with the breadth of the response (Liu et al., 2009). Similar phenotypic changes were seen in a rodent malaria model, yet here protection was correlated with the total numbers of IFN-γ producing CD8+ T cells (Reyes-Sandoval et al., 2010). As noted above, all these data strongly suggest that the T cells induced by adenoviral immunization are at least acutely protective. Notably, by documenting the ability of adenoviral vectors to prime for subsequent responses, these observations also questions the notion that adenovirus induced T cells necessarily have a limited proliferative capacity. Not only vaccines can boost adenovirus primed responses, also live LCMV infection in mice (Holst et al., 2011) or SIV in primates (Liu et al., 2009; Sun et al., 2008) cause massive post-exposure expansion of adenovirus primed T cells. In this context it is noteworthy that direct analysis of the adenovirus primed T cells' ability to proliferate have mostly been performed following what seems likely to be represent inoculation of unreasonably high doses of virus (see above for details), and the obtained results may therefore not be very relevant to a more real-life vaccine situation. An additional factor explaining the discrepancy may be that ex vivo analysis of proliferative capacity is typically performed on either blood or spleen cells, whereas an infection or an immunization can boost any T cell population present in the challenged animal. The phenotype and tissue localization of T cells responding with proliferation in response to a secondary immunization or challenge infection remains unknown, and the most relevant cells may not be present in blood or spleen in significant quantities.

5.2 Heterologous prime-boost regimens impact T cell quality

The study of Barouch and co-workers revealed an impact of the particular adenoviral serotype used for priming, on the phenotype and functionality of the ensuing T cell response, and suggested that special rare serotypes may have unique properties (Liu et al., 2008). However, as noted above, the heterologous prime-boost regimens in rodents using malaria antigens also reported an increased functionality of the induced CD8+ T cells (Reyes-Sandoval et al., 2010). An interesting observation in this regard was made when a triple sequential immunization was attempted using two different serotype of adenoviral vectors together with MVA. The third immunization induced further expansion of the CD8+ T cell response, increased their tissue homing and increased their cytokine producing competence (Tatsis et al., 2007b). Whereas expansion and increases in tissue homing capacity may be general phenomena following sequential immunization and has been seen in other systems as well as (Masopust et al., 2006), the increase in cytokine producing competence following the third immunization is harder to explain and has not been investigated. However, it is possible that the very strong response of transgene specific tissue homing CD8+ T cell may contribute to a rapid reduction of tissue localized vector, which would be in line with the notion that this pool of antigen contributes to induce CD8+ T cells of low cytokine producing competence.

6. Disease indications where the attributes of adenoviral vectored vaccines are especially useful

In principle adenoviral vectors would be useful wherever a strong and sustained antibody and/or CD8+ T cell response is readily inducible and contributing to protection. Acute infections such as avian influenza (Gao et al., 2006), Ebola (Richardson et al., 2009; Sullivan et al., 2003), foot-and-mouth disease virus (Pacheco et al., 2005) and rabies (Hu et al., 2006) are prime examples , but the list of published pre-clinical infections with high efficacy of adenovirus based vaccines essentially goes on and on. However, the more challenging vaccine targets are undoubtedly those involving infections with a propensity to become chronic such as HIV, HCV and the herpesviruses, or those where antibody inducing immunization may potentially exacerbate disease, such as dengue virus. These viruses have in common that sufficiently broad, high-titered and stable antibodies cannot readily be induced and that T cells therefore are needed to do the job. Accordingly, fairly solid pre-clinical data using adenoviral vectors have been obtained in the SIV model system (Liu et al., 2009) and the chimpanzee model of HCV infection (Folgori et al., 2006). However, the scientific community is still debating how to improve this further and develop clinically useful vaccines. In this review we would offer a different opinion from that of the majority regarding such diseases. Thus, while the focus have been on inducing immune responses capable of persisting during chronic infections, it is worth remembering that no actual intervention strategy succeeding in contributing to chronic virus control have done so without first reducing acute viral replication. An interesting case in this context is the SIV model for HIV infection. In this system, rapid application of highly active anti-retroviral therapy can lead to complete control of the virus and even protection against rechallenge (Lifson et al., 2001). This suggests that the rapidity of early virus control should be the goal for vaccine development. Another case supporting this suggestion is found in the MHV-68 model. In this system, a potent adenovirus vectored vaccine capable of reducing the splenic viral load after 14 days, was unable to impact the level of the latent infection. However, local immunization using intranasal application of the vaccine resulted in enhanced acute control at 7 days after infection as well as in improved control of the latent infection (Hoegh-Petersen et al., 2009). The lesson for vaccine development seems to be that increased efficacy can be expected against different disease targets by ensuring that CD8+ T cells are present and efficient at the site of virus entry/early virus replication and, furthermore, that these cells can rapidly acquire effector functions and reduce the viral load. Regarding the phenotype associated with acute control, adenovirus vaccines induce CD8+ T cells that for extended periods of time can exert immediate cytotoxic activity whereas immediate effector functions are quite limited in the less differentiated central memory T cells that seem to accumulate during controlled SIV or HIV infection. Also, regarding the ability to apply vaccines in manners that will induce local immunosurveillance at the likely site of virus entry or early replication, adenoviral vaccines have been found to be very useful. Thus, studies have suggested that local application can be used to augment mucosal CD8+ T cell memory (Belyakov et al., 2008; de Souza et al., 2007; Kaufman et al., 2010; Lemiale et al., 2007), and also that parenteral immunization can be used to induce T cell homing to mucosal sites (Haut et al., 2010; Kaufman et al., 2010; Lin et al., 2007; Tatsis et al., 2007b). The ability to induce local T cell responses is not a quality unique to adenovirus vectors and local immunity can also be obtained by mucosal application of pox-viral vectors (Corbett et al., 2008). Unfortunately, direct comparisons of vector systems for induction of mucosal immune responses seem to be lacking. While it may seem encouraging that parenteral immunization induces efficient T cell memory at mucosal sites, it should be noted that the assays performed to document mucosal homing are typically performed using tissue fractions or whole tissue homogenates. When we attempted a clean sampling of CD8+ T cells patrolling the mucosal surface of the lungs and airways by harvesting the bronchioalveolar lavage (BAL), only minimal frequencies of antigen specific cells could be detected after s.c. immunization whereas robust responses were seen after a single intranasal immunization. It seems possibly that there may be a difference between inducing the migration of T cells into a tissue with a large mucosal surface and to actually make the cells dedicated with respect to patrolling this surface for infected cells. In support of a compartmentalized CD8+ T cell memory at mucosal organs, immune responses in the mesenteric lymph nodes, which are frequently interpreted as a sign of induction of mucosal immunity in the gut, are efficiently induced following i.m. adenoviral immunization (Kaufman et al., 2010; Lin et al., 2007), whereas genuine mucosal immunization does not increase T cell frequencies in this site (Belyakov et al., 2008). Fortunately, concomitant subcutaneous and intranasal administration can induce T cell memory at both mucosal (BAL) (Hoegh-Petersen et al., 2009) and systemic (spleen) sites (these authors and Mette Hoegh-Petersen, unpublished).

7. Future perspectives

Apart from attempting to combat chronic infections prophylactically, the realization that adenovirus primes T cells for extended periods of time based on extra-nodal and perhaps even non-hematopoietic antigen presentation opens up an interesting avenue for further studies. Thus, as the understanding of extranodal priming increases, so will the ability to modulate it, for instance by co-encoding cytokines or inhibitors of immunomodulatory molecules. Adenovirus vectors could in this respect have unique qualities which could be exploited for therapeutic vaccines against cancer or chronic infection.

8. Acknowledgements

The authors wish to thank Grazyna Hahn Poulsen for making the layout of the figures.

9. References

Abbink P., Lemckert A.A., Ewald B.A., Lynch D.M., Denholtz M., Smits S., Holterman L., Damen I., Vogels R., Thorner A.R., O'Brien K.L., Carville A., Mansfield K.G., Goudsmit J., Havenga M.J. & Barouch D.H. (2007). Comparative seroprevalence and immunogenicity of six rare serotype recombinant adenovirus vaccine vectors from subgroups B and D. *J Virol* Vol. 81, No. 9: pp. 4654-4663.

Alkhatib G. & Briedis D.J. (1988). High-level eucaryotic in vivo expression of biologically active measles virus hemagglutinin by using an adenovirus type 5 helper-free vector system. *J Virol* Vol. 62, No. 8: pp. 2718-2727.

Antinozzi P.A., Berman H.K., O'Doherty R.M. & Newgard C.B. (1999). Metabolic engineering with recombinant adenoviruses. *Annu Rev Nutr* Vol. 19, No. 511-544.

Bachmann M.F., Wolint P., Schwarz K. & Oxenius A. (2005). Recall proliferation potential of memory CD8+ T cells and antiviral protection. *J Immunol* Vol. 175, No. 7: pp. 4677-4685.

Barber D.L., Wherry E.J., Masopust D., Zhu B., Allison J.P., Sharpe A.H., Freeman G.J. & Ahmed R. (2006). Restoring function in exhausted CD8 T cells during chronic viral infection. *Nature* Vol. 439, No. 7077: pp. 682-687.

Barefoot B., Thornburg N.J., Barouch D.H., Yu J.S., Sample C., Johnston R.E., Liao H.X., Kepler T.B., Haynes B.F. & Ramsburg E. (2008). Comparison of multiple vaccine vectors in a single heterologous prime-boost trial. *Vaccine* Vol. 26, No. 48: pp. 6108-6118.

Bartholdy C., Stryhn A., Christensen J.P. & Thomsen A.R. (2004). Single-epitope DNA vaccination prevents exhaustion and facilitates a broad antiviral CD8+ T cell response during chronic viral infection. *J Immunol* Vol. 173, No. 10: pp. 6284-6293.

Bartholdy C., Stryhn A., Hansen N.J., Buus S. & Thomsen A.R. (2003). Incomplete effector/memory differentiation of antigen-primed CD8+ T cells in gene gun DNA-vaccinated mice. *Eur J Immunol* Vol. 33, No. 7: pp. 1941-1948.

Bassett J.D., Yang T.C., Bernard D., Millar J.B., Swift S.L., McGray A.J., VanSeggelen H., Boudreau J.E., Finn J.D., Parsons R., Evelegh C., Damjanovic D., Grinshtein N., Divangahi M., Zhang L., Xing Z., Wan Y. & Bramson J.L. (2011). CD8+ T-cell expansion and maintenance after recombinant adenovirus immunization rely upon cooperation between hematopoietic and nonhematopoietic antigen-presenting cells. *Blood* Vol. 117, No. 4: pp. 1146-1155.

Belyakov I.M., Ahlers J.D., Nabel G.J., Moss B. & Berzofsky J.A. (2008). Generation of functionally active HIV-1 specific CD8+ CTL in intestinal mucosa following mucosal, systemic or mixed prime-boost immunization. *Virology* Vol. 381, No. 1: pp. 106-115.

Benlahrech A., Harris J., Meiser A., Papagatsias T., Hornig J., Hayes P., Lieber A., Athanasopoulos T., Bachy V., Csomor E., Daniels R., Fisher K., Gotch F., Seymour L., Logan K., Barbagallo R., Klavinskis L., Dickson G. & Patterson S. (2009). Adenovirus vector vaccination induces expansion of memory CD4 T cells with a mucosal homing phenotype that are readily susceptible to HIV-1. *Proc Natl Acad Sci U S A* Vol. 106, No. 47: pp. 19940-19945.

Berger M., Figari O., Bruno B., Raiola A., Dominietto A., Fiorone M., Podesta M., Tedone E., Pozzi S., Fagioli F., Madon E. & Bacigalupo A. (2008). Lymphocyte subsets recovery following allogeneic bone marrow transplantation (BMT): CD4+ cell count and transplant-related mortality. *Bone Marrow Transplant* Vol. 41, No. 1: pp. 55-62.

Bett A.J., Dubey S.A., Mehrotra D.V., Guan L., Long R., Anderson K., Collins K., Gaunt C., Fernandez R., Cole S., Meschino S., Tang A., Sun X., Gurunathan S., Tartaglia J., Robertson M.N., Shiver J.W. & Casimiro D.R. (2010). Comparison of T cell immune responses induced by vectored HIV vaccines in non-human primates and humans. *Vaccine* Vol. 28, No. 50: pp. 7881-7889.

Buchbinder S.P., Mehrotra D.V., Duerr A., Fitzgerald D.W., Mogg R., Li D., Gilbert P.B., Lama J.R., Marmor M., Del R.C., McElrath M.J., Casimiro D.R., Gottesdiener K.M., Chodakewitz J.A., Corey L. & Robertson M.N. (2008). Efficacy assessment of a cell-mediated immunity HIV-1 vaccine (the Step Study): a double-blind, randomised, placebo-controlled, test-of-concept trial. *Lancet* Vol. 372, No. 9653: pp. 1881-1893.

Casimiro D.R., Chen L., Fu T.M., Evans R.K., Caulfield M.J., Davies M.E., Tang A., Chen M., Huang L., Harris V., Freed D.C., Wilson K.A., Dubey S., Zhu D.M., Nawrocki D., Mach H., Troutman R., Isopi L., Williams D., Hurni W., Xu Z., Smith J.G., Wang S., Liu X., Guan L., Long R., Trigona W., Heidecker G.J., Perry H.C., Persaud N., Toner T.J., Su Q., Liang X., Youil R., Chastain M., Bett A.J., Volkin D.B., Emini E.A. & Shiver J.W. (2003). Comparative immunogenicity in rhesus monkeys of DNA plasmid, recombinant vaccinia virus, and replication-defective adenovirus vectors expressing a human immunodeficiency virus type 1 gag gene. *J Virol* Vol. 77, No. 11: pp. 6305-6313.

Casimiro D.R., Wang F., Schleif W.A., Liang X., Zhang Z.Q., Tobery T.W., Davies M.E., McDermott A.B., O'Connor D.H., Fridman A., Bagchi A., Tussey L.G., Bett A.J., Finnefrock A.C., Fu T.M., Tang A., Wilson K.A., Chen M., Perry H.C., Heidecker G.J., Freed D.C., Carella A., Punt K.S., Sykes K.J., Huang L., Ausensi V.I., Bachinsky M., Sadasivan-Nair U., Watkins D.I., Emini E.A. & Shiver J.W. (2005). Attenuation of simian immunodeficiency virus SIVmac239 infection by prophylactic immunization with dna and recombinant adenoviral vaccine vectors expressing Gag. *J Virol* Vol. 79, No. 24: pp. 15547-15555.

Chen H.H., Mack L.M., Kelly R., Ontell M., Kochanek S. & Clemens P.R. (1997). Persistence in muscle of an adenoviral vector that lacks all viral genes. *Proc Natl Acad Sci U S A* Vol. 94, No. 5: pp. 1645-1650.

Cheng W.F., Hung C.F., Hsu K.F., Chai C.Y., He L., Polo J.M., Slater L.A., Ling M. & Wu T.C. (2002). Cancer immunotherapy using Sindbis virus replicon particles encoding a VP22-antigen fusion. *Hum Gene Ther* Vol. 13, No. 4: pp. 553-568.

Coppieters K., Barral A.M., Juedes A., Wolfe T., Rodrigo E., Thery C., Amigorena S. & von Herrath M.G. (2009). No significant CTL cross-priming by dendritic cell-derived exosomes during murine lymphocytic choriomeningitis virus infection. *J Immunol* Vol. 182, No. 4: pp. 2213-2220.

Corbett M., Bogers W.M., Heeney J.L., Gerber S., Genin C., Didierlaurent A., Oostermeijer H., Dubbes R., Braskamp G., Lerondel S., Gomez C.E., Esteban M., Wagner R., Kondova I., Mooij P., Balla-Jhagjhoorsingh S., Beenhakker N., Koopman G., van der Burg S., Kraehenbuhl J.P. & Le P.A. (2008). Aerosol immunization with NYVAC and MVA vectored vaccines is safe, simple, and immunogenic. *Proc Natl Acad Sci U S A* Vol. 105, No. 6: pp. 2046-2051.

Cox K.S., Clair J.H., Prokop M.T., Sykes K.J., Dubey S.A., Shiver J.W., Robertson M.N. & Casimiro D.R. (2008). DNA gag/adenovirus type 5 (Ad5) gag and Ad5 gag/Ad5 gag vaccines induce distinct T-cell response profiles. *J Virol* Vol. 82, No. 16: pp. 8161-8171.

Cush S.S. & Flano E. (2011). KLRG1+NKG2A+ CD8 T Cells Mediate Protection and Participate in Memory Responses during {gamma}-Herpesvirus Infection. *J Immunol* Vol. 186, No. 7: pp. 4051-4058.

de Souza A.P., Haut L.H., Silva R., Ferreira S.I., Zanetti C.R., Ertl H.C. & Pinto A.R. (2007). Genital CD8+ T cell response to HIV-1 gag in mice immunized by mucosal routes with a recombinant simian adenovirus. *Vaccine* Vol. 25, No. 1: pp. 109-116.

Diebold S.S., Cotten M., Koch N. & Zenke M. (2001). MHC class II presentation of endogenously expressed antigens by transfected dendritic cells. *Gene Ther* Vol. 8, No. 6: pp. 487-493.

Dolan B.P., Gibbs K.D., Jr. & Ostrand-Rosenberg S. (2006). Dendritic cells cross-dressed with peptide MHC class I complexes prime CD8+ T cells. *J Immunol* Vol. 177, No. 9: pp. 6018-6024.

Finn J.D., Bassett J., Millar J.B., Grinshtein N., Yang T.C., Parsons R., Evelegh C., Wan Y., Parks R.J. & Bramson J.L. (2009). Persistence of transgene expression influences CD8+ T-cell expansion and maintenance following immunization with recombinant adenovirus. *J Virol* Vol. 83, No. 23: pp. 12027-12036.

Flatz L., Hegazy A.N., Bergthaler A., Verschoor A., Claus C., Fernandez M., Gattinoni L., Johnson S., Kreppel F., Kochanek S., Broek M., Radbruch A., Levy F., Lambert P.H., Siegrist C.A., Restifo N.P., Lohning M., Ochsenbein A.F., Nabel G.J. & Pinschewer D.D. (2010). Development of replication-defective lymphocytic choriomeningitis virus vectors for the induction of potent CD8+ T cell immunity. *Nat Med* Vol. 16, No. 3: pp. 339-345.

Flutter B., Edwards N., Fallah-Arani F., Henderson S., Chai J.G., Sivakumaran S., Ghorashian S., Bennett C.L., Freeman G.J., Sykes M. & Chakraverty R. (2010). Nonhematopoietic antigen blocks memory programming of alloreactive CD8+ T cells and drives their eventual exhaustion in mouse models of bone marrow transplantation. *J Clin Invest* Vol. 120, No. 11: pp. 3855-3868.

Folgori A., Capone S., Ruggeri L., Meola A., Sporeno E., Ercole B.B., Pezzanera M., Tafi R., Arcuri M., Fattori E., Lahm A., Luzzago A., Vitelli A., Colloca S., Cortese R. &

Nicosia A. (2006). A T-cell HCV vaccine eliciting effective immunity against heterologous virus challenge in chimpanzees. *Nat Med* Vol. 12, No. 2: pp. 190-197.

Gao W., Soloff A.C., Lu X., Montecalvo A., Nguyen D.C., Matsuoka Y., Robbins P.D., Swayne D.E., Donis R.O., Katz J.M., Barratt-Boyes S.M. & Gambotto A. (2006). Protection of mice and poultry from lethal H5N1 avian influenza virus through adenovirus-based immunization. *J Virol* Vol. 80, No. 4: pp. 1959-1964.

Grujic M., Holst P.J., Christensen J.P. & Thomsen A.R. (2009). Fusion of a viral antigen to invariant chain leads to augmented T-cell immunity and improved protection in gene-gun DNA-vaccinated mice. *J Gen Virol* Vol. 90, No. Pt 2: pp. 414-422.

Haut L.H., Lin S.W., Tatsis N., DiMenna L.J., Giles-Davis W., Pinto A.R. & Ertl H.C. (2010). Robust genital gag-specific CD8+ T-cell responses in mice upon intramuscular immunization with simian adenoviral vectors expressing HIV-1-gag. *Eur J Immunol* Vol. 40, No. 12: pp. 3426-3438.

Hoegh-Petersen M., Thomsen A.R., Christensen J.P. & Holst P.J. (2009). Mucosal immunization with recombinant adenoviral vectors expressing murine gammaherpesvirus-68 genes M2 and M3 can reduce latent viral load. *Vaccine* Vol. 27, No. 48: pp. 6723-6730.

Holst P.J., Bartholdy C., Stryhn A., Thomsen A.R. & Christensen J.P. (2007). Rapid and sustained CD4+ T-cell-independent immunity from adenovirus-encoded vaccine antigens. *J Gen Virol* Vol. 88, No. Pt 6: pp. 1708-1716.

Holst P.J., Bassi M.R., Thomsen A.R. & Christensen J.P. (2010a). DNA fusion gene vaccines. *Curr Opin Mol Ther* Vol. 12, No. 1: pp. 47-54.

Holst P.J., Christensen J.P. & Thomsen A.R. (2011). Vaccination against Lymphocytic Choriomeningitis Virus Infection in MHC Class II-Deficient Mice. *J Immunol* Vol. 186, No. 7: pp. 3997-4007.

Holst P.J., Orskov C., Thomsen A.R. & Christensen J.P. (2010b). Quality of the transgene-specific CD8+ T cell response induced by adenoviral vector immunization is critically influenced by virus dose and route of vaccination. *J Immunol* Vol. 184, No. 8: pp. 4431-4439.

Holst P.J., Sorensen M.R., Mandrup Jensen C.M., Orskov C., Thomsen A.R. & Christensen J.P. (2008). MHC class II-associated invariant chain linkage of antigen dramatically improves cell-mediated immunity induced by adenovirus vaccines. *J Immunol* Vol. 180, No. 5: pp. 3339-3346.

Hsieh C.J., Kim T.W., Hung C.F., Juang J., Moniz M., Boyd D.A., He L., Chen P.J., Chen C.H. & Wu T.C. (2004). Enhancement of vaccinia vaccine potency by linkage of tumor antigen gene to gene encoding calreticulin. *Vaccine* Vol. 22, No. 29-30: pp. 3993-4001.

Hu R., Zhang S., Fooks A.R., Yuan H., Liu Y., Li H., Tu C., Xia X. & Xiao Y. (2006). Prevention of rabies virus infection in dogs by a recombinant canine adenovirus type-2 encoding the rabies virus glycoprotein. *Microbes Infect* Vol. 8, No. 4: pp. 1090-1097.

Ibegbu C.C., Xu Y.X., Harris W., Maggio D., Miller J.D. & Kourtis A.P. (2005). Expression of killer cell lectin-like receptor G1 on antigen-specific human CD8+ T lymphocytes during active, latent, and resolved infection and its relation with CD57. *J Immunol* Vol. 174, No. 10: pp. 6088-6094.

Jimenez-Chillaron J.C., Newgard C.B. & Gomez-Foix A.M. (1999). Increased glucose disposal induced by adenovirus-mediated transfer of glucokinase to skeletal muscle in vivo. *FASEB J* Vol. 13, No. 15: pp. 2153-2160.

Kaufman D.R., Bivas-Benita M., Simmons N.L., Miller D. & Barouch D.H. (2010). Route of adenovirus-based HIV-1 vaccine delivery impacts the phenotype and trafficking of vaccine-elicited CD8+ T lymphocytes. *J Virol* Vol. 84, No. 12: pp. 5986-5996.

Kreijtz J.H., Suezer Y., de M.G., van den Brand J.M., van A.G., Schnierle B.S., Kuiken T., Fouchier R.A., Lower J., Osterhaus A.D., Sutter G. & Rimmelzwaan G.F. (2009). Recombinant modified vaccinia virus Ankara expressing the hemagglutinin gene confers protection against homologous and heterologous H5N1 influenza virus infections in macaques. *J Infect Dis* Vol. 199, No. 3: pp. 405-413.

Lasaro M.O., Tatsis N., Hensley S.E., Whitbeck J.C., Lin S.W., Rux J.J., Wherry E.J., Cohen G.H., Eisenberg R.J. & Ertl H.C. (2008). Targeting of antigen to the herpesvirus entry mediator augments primary adaptive immune responses. *Nat Med* Vol. 14, No. 2: pp. 205-212.

Lemiale F., Haddada H., Nabel G.J., Brough D.E., King C.R. & Gall J.G. (2007). Novel adenovirus vaccine vectors based on the enteric-tropic serotype 41. *Vaccine* Vol. 25, No. 11: pp. 2074-2084.

Lifson J.D., Rossio J.L., Piatak M., Jr., Parks T., Li L., Kiser R., Coalter V., Fisher B., Flynn B.M., Czajak S., Hirsch V.M., Reimann K.A., Schmitz J.E., Ghrayeb J., Bischofberger N., Nowak M.A., Desrosiers R.C. & Wodarz D. (2001). Role of CD8(+) lymphocytes in control of simian immunodeficiency virus infection and resistance to rechallenge after transient early antiretroviral treatment. *J Virol* Vol. 75, No. 21: pp. 10187-10199.

Lin S.W., Cun A.S., Harris-McCoy K. & Ertl H.C. (2007). Intramuscular rather than oral administration of replication-defective adenoviral vaccine vector induces specific CD8+ T cell responses in the gut. *Vaccine* Vol. 25, No. 12: pp. 2187-2193.

Lindsay R.W., Darrah P.A., Quinn K.M., Wille-Reece U., Mattei L.M., Iwasaki A., Kasturi S.P., Pulendran B., Gall J.G., Spies A.G. & Seder R.A. (2010). CD8+ T cell responses following replication-defective adenovirus serotype 5 immunization are dependent on CD11c+ dendritic cells but show redundancy in their requirement of TLR and nucleotide-binding oligomerization domain-like receptor signaling. *J Immunol* Vol. 185, No. 3: pp. 1513-1521.

Liu J., Ewald B.A., Lynch D.M., Denholtz M., Abbink P., Lemckert A.A., Carville A., Mansfield K.G., Havenga M.J., Goudsmit J. & Barouch D.H. (2008). Magnitude and phenotype of cellular immune responses elicited by recombinant adenovirus vectors and heterologous prime-boost regimens in rhesus monkeys. *J Virol* Vol. 82, No. 10: pp. 4844-4852.

Liu J., O'Brien K.L., Lynch D.M., Simmons N.L., La P.A., Riggs A.M., Abbink P., Coffey R.T., Grandpre L.E., Seaman M.S., Landucci G., Forthal D.N., Montefiori D.C., Carville A., Mansfield K.G., Havenga M.J., Pau M.G., Goudsmit J. & Barouch D.H. (2009). Immune control of an SIV challenge by a T-cell-based vaccine in rhesus monkeys. *Nature* Vol. 457, No. 7225: pp. 87-91.

Liu Z.X., Govindarajan S., Okamoto S. & Dennert G. (2001). Fas-mediated apoptosis causes elimination of virus-specific cytotoxic T cells in the virus-infected liver. *J Immunol* Vol. 166, No. 5: pp. 3035-3041.

Masopust D., Ha S.J., Vezys V. & Ahmed R. (2006). Stimulation history dictates memory CD8 T cell phenotype: implications for prime-boost vaccination. *J Immunol* Vol. 177, No. 2: pp. 831-839.

Mikkelsen M., Holst P.J., Bukh J., Thomsen A.R. & Christensen J.P. (2011). Enhanced and sustained CD8+ T cell responses with an adenoviral vector-based hepatitis C virus vaccine encoding NS3 linked to the MHC class II chaperone protein invariant chain. *J Immunol* Vol. 186, No. 4: pp. 2355-2364.

Moskophidis D., Lohler J. & Lehmann-Grube F. (1987). Antiviral antibody-producing cells in parenchymatous organs during persistent virus infection. *J Exp Med* Vol. 165, No. 3: pp. 705-719.

Moyron-Quiroz J.E., Rangel-Moreno J., Kusser K., Hartson L., Sprague F., Goodrich S., Woodland D.L., Lund F.E. & Randall T.D. (2004). Role of inducible bronchus associated lymphoid tissue (iBALT) in respiratory immunity. *Nat Med* Vol. 10, No. 9: pp. 927-934.

Okuyama T., Li X.K., Funeshima N., Fujino M., Sasaki K., Kita Y., Kosuga M., Takahashi M., Saito H., Suzuki S. & Yamada M. (1998). Fas-mediated apoptosis is involved in the elimination of gene-transduced hepatocytes with E1/E3-deleted adenoviral vectors. *J Gastroenterol Hepatol* Vol. 13 Suppl, No. S113-S118.

Pacheco J.M., Brum M.C., Moraes M.P., Golde W.T. & Grubman M.J. (2005). Rapid protection of cattle from direct challenge with foot-and-mouth disease virus (FMDV) by a single inoculation with an adenovirus-vectored FMDV subunit vaccine. *Virology* Vol. 337, No. 2: pp. 205-209.

Perreau M., Pantaleo G. & Kremer E.J. (2008). Activation of a dendritic cell-T cell axis by Ad5 immune complexes creates an improved environment for replication of HIV in T cells. *J Exp Med* Vol. 205, No. 12: pp. 2717-2725.

Prasad S.A., Norbury C.C., Chen W., Bennink J.R. & Yewdell J.W. (2001). Cutting edge: recombinant adenoviruses induce CD8 T cell responses to an inserted protein whose expression is limited to nonimmune cells. *J Immunol* Vol. 166, No. 8: pp. 4809-4812.

Reyes-Sandoval A., Berthoud T., Alder N., Siani L., Gilbert S.C., Nicosia A., Colloca S., Cortese R. & Hill A.V. (2010). Prime-boost immunization with adenoviral and modified vaccinia virus Ankara vectors enhances the durability and polyfunctionality of protective malaria CD8+ T-cell responses. *Infect Immun* Vol. 78, No. 1: pp. 145-153.

Richardson J.S., Yao M.K., Tran K.N., Croyle M.A., Strong J.E., Feldmann H. & Kobinger G.P. (2009). Enhanced protection against Ebola virus mediated by an improved adenovirus-based vaccine. *PLoS ONE* Vol. 4, No. 4: pp. e5308.

Rolland M., Tovanabutra S., Decamp A.C., Frahm N., Gilbert P.B., Sanders-Buell E., Heath L., Magaret C.A., Bose M., Bradfield A., O'Sullivan A., Crossler J., Jones T., Nau M., Wong K., Zhao H., Raugi D.N., Sorensen S., Stoddard J.N., Maust B.S., Deng W., Hural J., Dubey S., Michael N.L., Shiver J., Corey L., Li F., Self S.G., Kim J., Buchbinder S., Casimiro D.R., Robertson M.N., Duerr A., McElrath M.J., McCutchan F.E. & Mullins J.I. (2011). Genetic impact of vaccination on breakthrough HIV-1 sequences from the STEP trial. *Nat Med* Vol. 17, No. 3: pp. 366-371.

Rowe H.M., Lopes L., Ikeda Y., Bailey R., Barde I., Zenke M., Chain B.M. & Collins M.K. (2006). Immunization with a lentiviral vector stimulates both CD4 and CD8 T cell responses to an ovalbumin transgene. *Mol Ther* Vol. 13, No. 2: pp. 310-319.

Schirmbeck R., Reimann J., Kochanek S. & Kreppel F. (2008). The immunogenicity of adenovirus vectors limits the multispecificity of CD8 T-cell responses to vector-encoded transgenic antigens. *Mol Ther* Vol. 16, No. 9: pp. 1609-1616.

Shiver J.W., Fu T.M., Chen L., Casimiro D.R., Davies M.E., Evans R.K., Zhang Z.Q., Simon A.J., Trigona W.L., Dubey S.A., Huang L., Harris V.A., Long R.S., Liang X., Handt L., Schleif W.A., Zhu L., Freed D.C., Persaud N.V., Guan L., Punt K.S., Tang A., Chen M., Wilson K.A., Collins K.B., Heidecker G.J., Fernandez V.R., Perry H.C., Joyce J.G., Grimm K.M., Cook J.C., Keller P.M., Kresock D.S., Mach H., Troutman R.D., Isopi L.A., Williams D.M., Xu Z., Bohannon K.E., Volkin D.B., Montefiori D.C., Miura A., Krivulka G.R., Lifton M.A., Kuroda M.J., Schmitz J.E., Letvin N.L., Caulfield M.J., Bett A.J., Youil R., Kaslow D.C. & Emini E.A. (2002). Replication-incompetent adenoviral vaccine vector elicits effective anti-immunodeficiency-virus immunity. *Nature* Vol. 415, No. 6869: pp. 331-335.

Sorensen M.R., Holst P.J., Pircher H., Christensen J.P. & Thomsen A.R. (2009). Vaccination with an adenoviral vector encoding the tumor antigen directly linked to invariant chain induces potent CD4(+) T-cell-independent CD8(+) T-cell-mediated tumor control. *Eur J Immunol* Vol. 39, No. 10: pp. 2725-2736.

Sridhar S., Reyes-Sandoval A., Draper S.J., Moore A.C., Gilbert S.C., Gao G.P., Wilson J.M. & Hill A.V. (2008). Single-dose protection against Plasmodium berghei by a simian adenovirus vector using a human cytomegalovirus promoter containing intron A. *J Virol* Vol. 82, No. 8: pp. 3822-3833.

Sullivan N.J., Geisbert T.W., Geisbert J.B., Xu L., Yang Z.Y., Roederer M., Koup R.A., Jahrling P.B. & Nabel G.J. (2003). Accelerated vaccination for Ebola virus haemorrhagic fever in non-human primates. *Nature* Vol. 424, No. 6949: pp. 681-684.

Sun J.C., Williams M.A. & Bevan M.J. (2004). CD4+ T cells are required for the maintenance, not programming, of memory CD8+ T cells after acute infection. *Nat Immunol* Vol. 5, No. 9: pp. 927-933.

Sun Y., Santra S., Schmitz J.E., Roederer M. & Letvin N.L. (2008). Magnitude and quality of vaccine-elicited T-cell responses in the control of immunodeficiency virus replication in rhesus monkeys. *J Virol* Vol. 82, No. 17: pp. 8812-8819.

Tatsis N., Fitzgerald J.C., Reyes-Sandoval A., Harris-McCoy K.C., Hensley S.E., Zhou D., Lin S.W., Bian A., Xiang Z.Q., Iparraguirre A., Lopez-Camacho C., Wherry E.J. & Ertl H.C. (2007a). Adenoviral vectors persist in vivo and maintain activated CD8+ T cells: implications for their use as vaccines. *Blood* Vol. 110, No. 6: pp. 1916-1923.

Tatsis N., Lin S.W., Harris-McCoy K., Garber D.A., Feinberg M.B. & Ertl H.C. (2007b). Multiple immunizations with adenovirus and MVA vectors improve CD8+ T cell functionality and mucosal homing. *Virology* Vol. 367, No. 1: pp. 156-167.

Uger R.A. & Barber B.H. (1998). Creating CTL targets with epitope-linked beta 2-microglobulin constructs. *J Immunol* Vol. 160, No. 4: pp. 1598-1605.

Uger R.A., Chan S.M. & Barber B.H. (1999). Covalent linkage to beta2-microglobulin enhances the MHC stability and antigenicity of suboptimal CTL epitopes. *J Immunol* Vol. 162, No. 10: pp. 6024-6028.

Utsugi-Kobukai S., Fujimaki H., Hotta C., Nakazawa M. & Minami M. (2003). MHC class I-mediated exogenous antigen presentation by exosomes secreted from immature and mature bone marrow derived dendritic cells. *Immunol Lett* Vol. 89, No. 2-3: pp. 125-131.

Wu L., Kong W.P. & Nabel G.J. (2005). Enhanced breadth of CD4 T-cell immunity by DNA prime and adenovirus boost immunization to human immunodeficiency virus Env and Gag immunogens. *J Virol* Vol. 79, No. 13: pp. 8024-8031.

Yang T.C., Dayball K., Wan Y.H. & Bramson J. (2003). Detailed analysis of the CD8+ T-cell response following adenovirus vaccination. *J Virol* Vol. 77, No. 24: pp. 13407-13411.

Yang T.C., Millar J., Groves T., Grinshtein N., Parsons R., Takenaka S., Wan Y. & Bramson J.L. (2006). The CD8+ T cell population elicited by recombinant adenovirus displays a novel partially exhausted phenotype associated with prolonged antigen presentation that nonetheless provides long-term immunity. *J Immunol* Vol. 176, No. 1: pp. 200-210.

Yang T.C., Millar J.B., Grinshtein N., Bassett J., Finn J. & Bramson J.L. (2007). T-cell immunity generated by recombinant adenovirus vaccines. *Expert Rev Vaccines* Vol. 6, No. 3: pp. 347-356.

Zhao J., Lai L., Amara R.R., Montefiori D.C., Villinger F., Chennareddi L., Wyatt L.S., Moss B. & Robinson H.L. (2009). Preclinical studies of human immunodeficiency virus/AIDS vaccines: inverse correlation between avidity of anti-Env antibodies and peak postchallenge viremia. *J Virol* Vol. 83, No. 9: pp. 4102-4111.

Part 3

Adeno-associated-viral Vector

9

AAV Mediated β-Thalassemia Gene Therapy

Mengqun Tan[1,3] et al.*
[1]*Experimental Hematology Laboratory, Department of Physiology, XiangYa School of Medicine, Central South University, Changsha,*
[3]*Xiangya Biological Medicine Institute, Shenzhen,*
China

1. Introduction

β-thalassemia is one of the most common monogenic disease due to mutation or deletion in the β-globin gene on chromosome 11, inherited in an autosomal recessive fashion, with a global estimated annual birth incidence of 40,000/year[1]. The disease is particularly prevalent among Mediterranean peoples, Middle Eastern and Southeast Asians [1].

The severity of the disease depends on the production of functional β-globin chain. Mutations of β-globin gene cause reduced β-chain synthesis (β^{+}) lead to β thalassemia minor or intermedia, while mutations cause no β-chain synthesis (β^{o}) usually resulted in β-thalassemia major or Cooley's anemia[2]. Lacking of β-chain causes ineffective production of oxygen-carrying protein haemoglobin, therefore results in anemia. The relative excess of α-chains bind to the red blood cell membrane, undermine membrane, even form toxic aggregates, which aggravates anemia of patients. According to statistics, there are an estimated 80 million carriers of mutation of β-globin gene in the world[3]. The severe thalassemia is characterized by markedly ineffective erythropoiesis and severe anemia.

The treatment for β-thalassemia major usually includes lifelong blood transfusion and allogeneic hematopoietic transplantation[4]. Chronic blood transfusion often causes iron overload, accumulated iron produces tissue damage in multiple organs, so that iron chelating treatment is required to prevent iron overload damage to the internal organs in patients. To most of patients receiving the treatment, it is an expensive and inconvenience therapy for maintaining a long life.

Bone marrow transplantation is the other effective therapy, which can eliminate a patient's dependence on blood transfusions[5,6]. However, it is difficult to find the matching donors for the most of patients, which is only available for a minority of patients.

Gene therapy is one potential novel therapeutic avenue for the treatment of inherited monogenic disorder. It is a technology for correcting defective genes by introducing of the normal genes directly into patient's cells. This strategy mainly focuses on diseases caused

---

* Xiaojuan Sun[2], Zhenqin Liu[1,3], Liujian Song[1,3], Jing Tian[1,3], Xiaolin Yin[4] and Xinhua Zhang[4]
1 *Experimental Hematology Laboratory, Department of Physiology, XiangYa School of Medicine, Central South University, Changsha, China,*
2 *Central Laboratory,the First Affiliated Hospital of ShenZhen University,ShenZhen, China,*
3 *Xiangya Biological Medicine Institute, Shenzhen, China,*
4 *Department of Hematology, 303rd Hospital of People's Liberation Army, Nanning, Guangxi, China.*

by single-gene defects, such as β-thalassemia. For patients lacking a suitable bone marrow (BM) donor, gene therapy is not limited by the histocompatibility barrier and does not require immunosuppression.

The general strategy for β-thalassemia gene therapy is to obtain hematopoietic stem cell (HSC) from patient's bone marrow first, then, deliver a normal β-globin gene to patient's HSC by recombinant viral vector *in vitro*, the transfected cells will be transplanted into patients, the exogenous normal β-globin gene would be expressed in erythroid lineage cells under the regulation of the promoter, the ratio of β-chain to α-chain in red cells will be corrected in eripheralcirculation system eventually[7] (Fig1.).

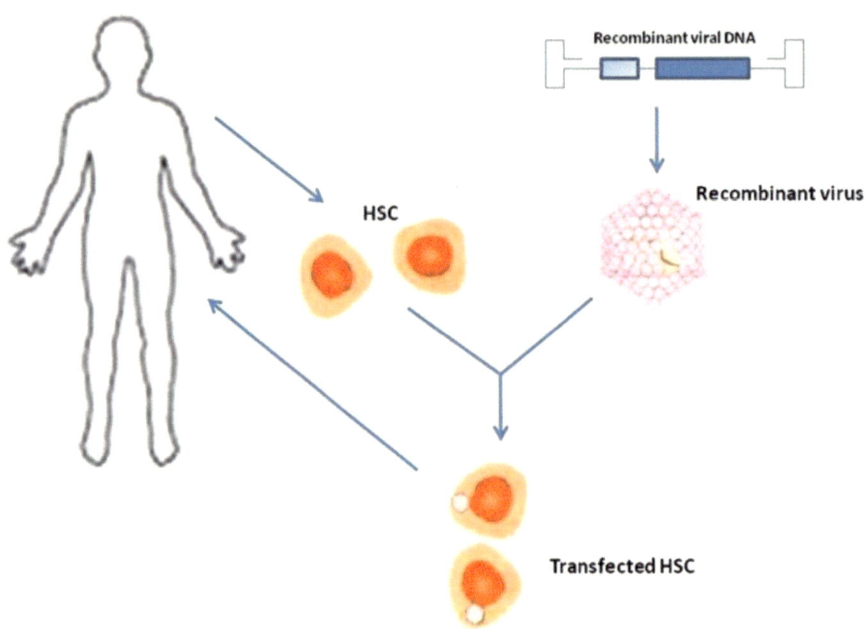

Fig. 1. The general strategy for β-thalassemia gene therapy.

To get a persistent expression of β-globin gene, $CD34^+$ cells are usually selected to be the target of gene transfer and transplantation. CD34 is considered as a maker for hematopoietic cells which possess self-renew and multiple lineage differentiation potentials, covering not only stem cells but also earlier multipotent progenitors and later lineage-restricted progenitors[8]. The success of transfecting exogenous β-globin gene into $CD34^+$ cells is the precondition of β-thalassemia gene therapy, which ensures the long term expression of the β-globin gene due to $CD34^+$ cells keeping differentiation into erythroid lineage cells, the erythroid lineage-specific expression of β-globin gene will be induced and regulated in these cells[9].

Human β-globin locus is composed of five genes which includes β, δ, $^A\gamma$, $^G\gamma$, and ε globin gene, located on a short region of chromosome 11, arranged as the sequence of 5' –ε- $^G\gamma$- $^A\gamma$- δ- β - 3'. Expression of all of these genes is controlled by single locus control region (LCR), and forms of hemoglobin expressed change during development. Genes are expressed in the order in which they are arranged in the cluster[10](Fig.2).

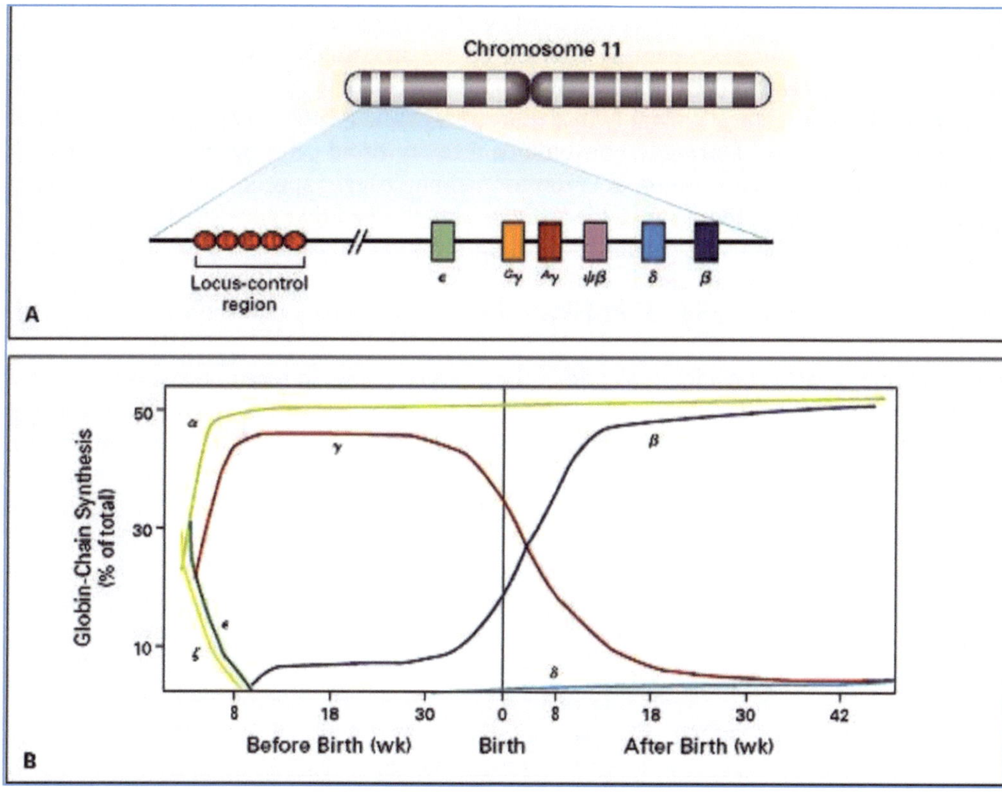

From Olivieri NF. The β-thalassemias. The N Engl J Med，1999，341:99-109.

Fig. 2. The β-Globin Gene Cluster on the Short Arm of Chromosome 11. **A**, the β -globin-like genes are arranged in the order in which they are expressed during development. **B**, shows the timing of the normal developmental switching of human hemoglobin.

2. Gene therapy for β-thalassemia

As a classic gene model for human genetics,β-globin gene has been extensively studied in the fields of gene structure, gene evolution, gene transcription and regulation. Gene therapy for β-thalassemia was started in 1980'. The retrovirus is the earliest and the most frequently used vector. It was reported in 1988 that the retrovirus (RV) containing β-globin gene successfully transfected HSC, although the erythroid lineage-specific expression of β-globin gene was low, only 1% of normal expression level[11]. It is generally considered in current studies that there is a therapeutic meaning only after the expression of exogenous β-globin gene reaches 10-20% of normal endogenous expression level. The discovering of the locus control region (LCR) in the range of 20 kb upstream of ε-gene greatly improved the erythroid lineage-specific expression of β-globin. LCR is composed of a series of hypersensitivities (HS) including HS1-HS5[12]. Sadelain et al. tried different HS combinations, reconstructed the RV vectors, got increased expression of β-globin gene, as high as 5%of normal β-globin gene expression level in mice[13]. But 4 months later, the expression of β-globin gene cannot be detected, suggested the gene silencing appeared. Gene silencing is a phenomenon that the specific gene is not expressed *in vivo* for a variety of reasons.

Studies show that the RV has the characteristics of random integrate into the host genome, while expression of β-globin gene is affected by the integrated position, which is called position effect variegation (PEV)[14]. The possible reason
for both of PEV and gene silencing is that transduced gene located in other regions outside of a normal gene locus. During the development of erythroid cells, over expressed mRNA from abnormal integrated position in chromosome may trigger specific mRNA degradation to prevent expression of the gene. Other studies also showed that gene silencing caused by RV is relative with the DNA sequences of long terminal repeats (LTR) and frame of RV virus[15].
The transduction efficiency of RV in HSC is low due to retrovirus vector only can infect dividing cells, but most of the HSCs are in quiescent stage, lacking of receptors for RV coat in HSC surface is also considered as one of the main reasons. In recent years, it was found that the random integration features of RV creates the potential risk of activating oncogenes or inactivating tumor suppressor genes, so application of RV in clinic is relatively limited[16].
The insufficiency of RV prompts people to try to develop new viral vectors for β-thalassemia gene therapy, such as lentivirus (LV), adeno associated virus (AAV),et al. The well-known lentivirus is human immunodeficiency virus－I (HIV－1). Although LV belongs to retroviridae, it can effectively infect non-dividing cells. May et al. firstly obtained steady expression of β-globin gene in β-thalassemia mice by transducing HSCs with LV containing large fragment of LCR and β-globin gene, the expression of β-globin gene reached 10-20% of normal level, and lasted for more than 15 weeks without PEV effect, which showed preferable therapeutic action[17]. It was reported recently that a severe transfusion dependent thalassemia patient who accept β-globin gene therapy through lentivirus became transfusion independent for 21 months[18]. However, it is also noticeable that whether recombinant HIV-1 vector lost the pathogenicity completely so there will be no risk for patients to gain acquired immune deficiency syndrome (AIDS). Therefore, the safety of vector still need be monitored and valued in a long term through more experiments in vivo[19].

3. AAV mediated β-thalassemia gene therapy

Adeno-associated virus (AAV) is often found in cells that are simultaneously infected with adenovirus (Ad). However, unlike Ad, AAV does not stimulate inflammation in the host; causes a very mild immune response has a wide range of host of human and non-human cells, which can be dividing and non-dividing cells; wild AAV inserts preferentially at a specific site on human chromosome 19. AAV is not known to cause direct disease in humans and considered as the safest viral vector so far. In the absence of helper virus, recombinant AAV will stably integrate into the host cell genome, mediating the long and stable expression of the transgene. The main deficiency of AAV is the small packing capacity, only 4.5 kb[20].
AAV is a small (20 nm) replication-defective, nonenveloped virus, belongs to the genus Dependovirus, family Parvoviridae. The genome of AAV is built of single-stranded deoxyribonucleic acid (ssDNA), comprises two open reading frames (ORFs), *rep* and *cap*, flanked by inverted terminal repeats (ITRs) at both ends of DNA strand. The *rep* gene encodes 4 kinds of *Rep* proteins required for the AAV replication and rescue: *Rep* 78, Rep68, Rep52, Rep40. And the *cap* gene contains nucleotide sequences of capsid proteins: VP1, VP2 and VP3, which interact together to form a capsid of an icosahedral symmetry. The ITR

sequences comprise 145 bases each, are required in cis for efficient virus replication, integration, rescue, and encapsidation[21,22](Fig.3).

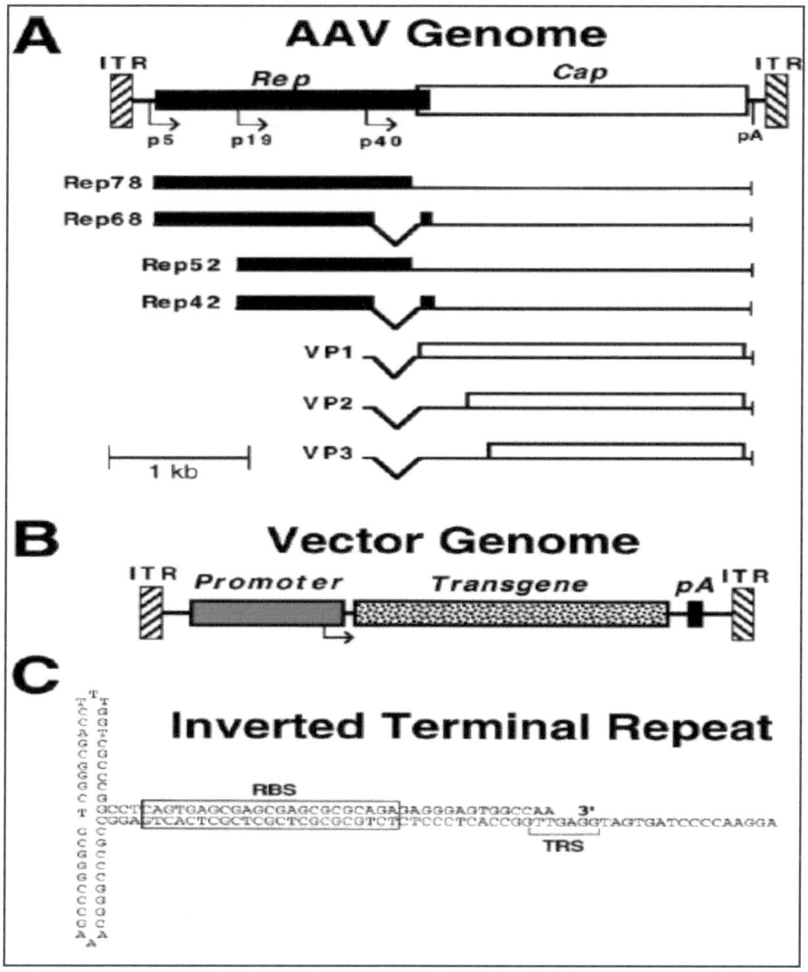

From Blood, Vol. 94 No. 3 (August 1), 1999: pp. 864-874. Adeno-Associated Virus Vectors and Hematology .

Fig. 3. Structure of wild-type and vector AAV genomes. **A,** Map of the wild-type AAV genome, including *Rep* (solid) and *Cap* (open) reading frames, promoters (p5, p19, and p40), polyadenylation site (pA), and inverted terminal repeats (ITR). The viral transcripts encoding the different *Rep* and *Cap* (VP1-3) proteins are shown below the genome. The smaller *Rep* proteins, VP2 and VP3, are translated from internal initiation sites. **B,** Map of a typical AAV vector, showing replacement of the viral *Rep* and *Cap* genes with a transgene cassette (promoter, transgene cDNA, and polyadenylation site). **C,** Secondary structure of the AAV ITR, with the locations of the *Rep* binding site (RBS) and terminal resolution site (TRS) indicated.

There have been 11 AAV serotypes identified, of which serotype 2 (AAV2) has been the most extensively examined so far[23]. AAV2 presents natural tropism towards skeletal muscles, neurons, vascular smooth muscle cells and hepatocytes[24]. Currently, the application of AAV serotype 2 in hemophilia B gene therapy gets a promising development[25]. AAV2 is also studied in gene therapy for pulmonary cystic fibrosis, tumor and β-thalassemia. Although AAV2 is the most popular serotype in various AAV studies, it has been shown that other serotypes can be more effective as gene delivery vectors for specific tissue. Preliminary studies have demonstrated other AAV serotypes display different tissue tropisms[26]. For instance, AAV6 has a higher efficiency in infecting airway epithelial cells compare to other serotypes[27], AAV8 presents very high transduction rate of hepatocytes[28], AAV1 and 5 were shown to be very efficient in gene delivery to vascular endothelial cells[29]. The main reason causing the difference is there are distinctions among the capsid proteins of AAV serotypes, while the primary factor for virus entering into cells is the binding of capsid proteins with specific cell receptors. For example, the receptors that mediate AAV2 entering into cells are [30], fibroblast growth factor receptor and the integrin $\alpha V\beta 5$[31,32]. So transduction efficiency of AAV serotypes is affected by distribution of specific AAV receptors in various tissues.

In 1994, Srivastava et al. first reported successful transduction of $CD34^+$ human primitive hematopoietic cells by recombinant AAV2 vectors at a relatively low vector:cell ratio of 1,000[33], indicated the potential of AAV2 in β-thalassemia gene therapy. Subsequently, AAV2 mediated transduction of $CD34^+$ cell were reported by a number of investigators [34-36]. High transduction efficiency of AAV2-mediated transgene expression in HSCs was found when the AAV2 vector particle:cell exceeded 10^6 by some groups [35,36]. A few of groups concluded that human $CD34^+$ cells were impervious to transduction by recombinant AAV2 vectors, and the transgene expression observed by others was due to 'pseudo-transduction' mediated by contaminants in the vector stocks[37], which causes people focus more on the generation of rAAV.

The helper virus or plasmid is required in production of recombinant AAV (rAAV) due to the AAV's replication deficiency characteristic. The traditional rAAV production system involves transfecting HEK 293 cells with a recombinant AAV vector plasmid and an AAV helper plasmid in the presence of a helper virus function[38,39]. The vector plasmid contains AAV ITRs and a transgene cassette. The helper plasmid contains the AAV *rep* and *cap* gene, but not ITRs. Ad is the most used helper virus, which provides adequate function in helping the replication of the recombinant AAV. However, Ad contamination is liable to occur in the latter procedures of purify of AAV. Thus, helper plasmid containing VA、E2a and E4 gene of Ad genome is developed and used in many studies[40-42].

In our study, we constructed rAAV plasmid (pMT-2) containing genomic sequences of human β-globin gene and mini-cassette of locus control region (LCR) element, as described previously. The plasmid pAAV2-RC contains AAV2 *rep* and *cap* genes and plasmid pHelpers contains adenovirus-derived genes (i.e. the E2A, E4, and VARNA genes. The pMT-2 together with pAAV2-RC and pHelper were cotransfected into HEK 293 cells to generate rAAV2-β-globin virions. The packaged rAAV2 virions were purified using a single-step gravity-flow column[43]. The purity of recombinant virions was evaluated by sodium dodecyl sulfate- polyacrylamide gel electrophoresis (SDS-PAGE), and the titer of purified viral stock was determined by quantitative DNA dot-blots. The titer of rAAV2-β-globin was near 1.3×10^{10} virus particles/ml, as determined by quantitative DNA slot blots .SDS-PAGE analysis revealed that rAAV2-β-globin contained VP1, VP2, and VP3 proteins at a ratio of approximately 1:1:10, suggesting high purity of rAAV2-β-globin.

To investigate the function of rAAV2-β-globin in β- thalassemia gene therapy, we first detected rAAV2 mediated transduction and β-globin gene expression in human fetal liver hematopoietic cells from aborted fetus, as the expression of β -globin gene in early fetal has not been initiated. The results showed that rAAV2 efficiently transduced human fetal liver hematopoietic cells, and mediated expression of human β-globin gene in vivo, the detection of expression of β -globin gene was stopped at 2 weeks post transplanted considering the activation of endogenous β –globin gene. Following that, we investigated whether rAAV2 could mediate the expression of normal β-globin gene in human hematopoietic cells from β-thalassemia patients. We found that rAAV2-β-globin transduced human fetal hematopoietic cells, as determined by allele-specific PCR analysis. Furthermore, β-globin transgene expression was detected in human hematopoietic cells up to 70 days post-transplantation in the recipient mice. High pressure liquid chromatography (HPLC) analysis showed that human β-globin expression level increased significantly compared with control, as indicated by a 1.2–2.8 fold increase in the ratio of β/α globin chain.[44,45] These novel data demonstrate that rAAV2 can transduce and mediate normal β-globin gene expression in fetal hematopoietic cells from β-thalassemia patients. Our findings further support the potential use of rAAV-based gene therapy in treatment of human β-thalassemia, How to improve the transfection efficiency of AAV mediated HSC transduction, however is still an important issue.

Recent article reported that mutation of tyrosine residues on AAV2 capsid greatly enhanced transduction efficiency of AAV2 in HSC. They generated novel AAV vectors by mutating 7 tyrosine residues on AAV2 capsid to phenylalanine, respectively, named Y252,Y272,Y444,Y500,Y700,Y704 and Y730. It was showed that the transduction efficiency of Y444F was 8-11 times higher than wt AAV2, next followed by Y500F and Y730F. Furthermore, the combination of mutations Y444 + Y500F+Y730F showed even more increased transduction efficiency (4 times) compare to Y444F. The similar effect also was observed when the tyrosine residues on AAV6 capsid was mutated to phenylalanine. They discovered that increased efficiency is relative with phosphorylation of tyrosine residues on AAV capsid. Tyrosine residues exposed on AAV capsid surface could be phosphorylated by epidermal growth factor receptor protein tyrosine kinase (EGFR-PTK) on cell surface, which has no effect on the steps of AAV entering into cells.[46,47] However, phosphorylation of tyrosine residues on AAV capsid consequently triggered degradation of ubiquitin and proteasomal when AAV was present in cell plasma, which further caused the AAV degradation. The degradation of AAV is successful avoided by mutation of tyrosine residues on AAV2 capsid to phenylalanine, thus improved transduction efficiency of AAV. Base on these encouraging results, we are trying to improve AAV transduction efficiency in HSC by mutating the single or combination of tyrosine residues on AAV capsid after analysis of sequence of AAV capsid protein, in order to facilitate the use of AAV in transduction of hematopoietic stem cells, and provide an effective therapeutic way for β-thalassemia gene therapy.

4. Acknowledgments

This work was supported by grants from China National Nature Science Fundation (30971299;30470743;30170390) to Mengqun Tan. We thank Drs. Arun Srivastava and Keyun Qing for their helpful reading and suggestion

5. References

[1] Cao A, Galanello R: Beta-thalassemia. *Genet Med 2010*; 12: 61-76.
[2] Winichagoon P, Fucharoen S, Chen P, Wasi P: Genetic factors affecting clinical severity in beta-thalassemia syndromes. *J Pediatr Hematol Oncol* 2000; 22: 573-580.
[3] Weatherall DJ, Clegg JB: Thalassemia--a global public health problem. *Nat Med* 1996; 2: 847-849.
[4] Olivieri NF, Nathan DG, MacMillan JH *et al*: Survival in medically treated patients with homozygous beta-thalassemia. *N Engl J Med* 1994; 331: 574-578.
[5] Gaziev J, Sodani P, Polchi P, Andreani M, Lucarelli G: Bone marrow transplantation in adults with thalassemia: Treatment and long-term follow-up. *Ann N Y Acad Sci* 2005; 1054: 196-205.
[6] Angelucci E: Hematopoietic stem cell transplantation in thalassemia. *Hematology Am Soc Hematol Educ Program 2010*; 2010; 456-462.
[7] Roselli EA, Mezzadra R, Frittoli MC *et al*: Correction of beta-thalassemia major by gene transfer in haematopoietic progenitors of pediatric patients. *EMBO Mol Med 2010*; 2: 315-328.
[8] Collins RH, Jr.: CD34+ selected cells in clinical transplantation. *Stem Cells* 1994; 12: 577-585.
[9] Persons DA: Hematopoietic stem cell gene transfer for the treatment of hemoglobin disorders. *Hematology Am Soc Hematol Educ Program* 2009; 690-697.
[10] Mahajan MC, Karmakar S, Weissman SM: Control of beta globin genes. *J Cell Biochem* 2007; 102: 801-810.
[11] Karlsson S, Bodine DM, Perry L, Papayannopoulou T, Nienhuis AW: Expression of the human beta-globin gene following retroviral-mediated transfer into multipotential hematopoietic progenitors of mice. *Proc Natl Acad Sci U S A* 1988; 85: 6062-6066.
[12] Leboulch P, Huang GM, Humphries RK *et al*: Mutagenesis of retroviral vectors transducing human beta-globin gene and beta-globin locus control region derivatives results in stable transmission of an active transcriptional structure. *EMBO J* 1994; 13: 3065-3076.
[13] Burgess-Beusse B, Farrell C, Gaszner M *et al*: The insulation of genes from external enhancers and silencing chromatin. *Proc Natl Acad Sci U S A* 2002; 99 Suppl 4: 16433-16437.
[14] Arumugam P, Malik P: Genetic therapy for beta-thalassemia: from the bench to the bedside. *Hematology Am Soc Hematol Educ Program 2010*; 2010: 445-450.
[15] Festenstein R, Tolaini M, Corbella P *et al*: Locus control region function and heterochromatin-induced position effect variegation. *Science* 1996; 271: 1123-1125.
[16] Brenner S, Malech HL: Current developments in the design of onco-retrovirus and lentivirus vector systems for hematopoietic cell gene therapy. *Biochim Biophys Acta* 2003; 1640: 1-24.
[17] May C, Rivella S, Callegari J *et al*: Therapeutic haemoglobin synthesis in beta-thalassaemic mice expressing lentivirus-encoded human beta-globin. *Nature* 2000; 406: 82-86.
[18] Cavazzana-Calvo M, Payen E, Negre O *et al*: Transfusion independence and HMGA2 activation after gene therapy of human beta-thalassaemia. *Nature 2010*; 467: 318-322.

[19] Yannaki E, Emery DW, Stamatoyannopoulos G: Gene therapy for beta-thalassaemia: the continuing challenge. *Expert Rev Mol Med 2010*; 12: e31.
[20] Grimm D, Kay MA: From virus evolution to vector revolution: use of naturally occurring serotypes of adeno-associated virus (AAV) as novel vectors for human gene therapy. *Curr Gene Ther* 2003; 3: 281-304.
[21] Carter BJ: Adeno-associated virus vectors. *Curr Opin Biotechnol* 1992; 3: 533-539.
[22] Flotte TR, Carter BJ: Adeno-associated virus vectors for gene therapy. *Gene Ther* 1995; 2: 357-362.
[23] Liu J, Saghizadeh M, Tuli SS *et al*: Different tropism of adenoviruses and adeno-associated viruses to corneal cells: implications for corneal gene therapy. *Mol Vis* 2008; 14: 2087-2096.
[24] Kwon I, Schaffer DV: Designer gene delivery vectors: molecular engineering and evolution of adeno-associated viral vectors for enhanced gene transfer. *Pharm Res* 2008; 25: 489-499.
[25] Couto LB: Preclinical gene therapy studies for hemophilia using adeno-associated virus (AAV) vectors. *Semin Thromb Hemost* 2004; 30: 161-171.
[26] Van Vliet KM, Blouin V, Brument N, Agbandje-McKenna M, Snyder RO: The role of the adeno-associated virus capsid in gene transfer. *Methods Mol Biol* 2008; 437: 51-91.
[27] Halbert CL, Allen JM, Miller AD: Adeno-associated virus type 6 (AAV6) vectors mediate efficient transduction of airway epithelial cells in mouse lungs compared to that of AAV2 vectors. *J Virol* 2001; 75: 6615-6624.
[28] Ho KJ, Bass CE, Kroemer AH, Ma C, Terwilliger E, Karp SJ: Optimized adeno-associated virus 8 produces hepatocyte-specific Cre-mediated recombination without toxicity or affecting liver regeneration. *Am J Physiol Gastrointest Liver Physiol* 2008; 295: G412-419.
[29] Sen S, Conroy S, Hynes SO *et al*: Gene delivery to the vasculature mediated by low-titre adeno-associated virus serotypes 1 and 5. *J Gene Med* 2008; 10: 143-151.
[30] Opie SR, Warrington KH, Jr., Agbandje-McKenna M, Zolotukhin S, Muzyczka N: Identification of amino acid residues in the capsid proteins of adeno-associated virus type 2 that contribute to heparan sulfate proteoglycan binding. *J Virol* 2003; 77: 6995-7006.
[31] Belur LR, Kaemmerer WF, McIvor RS, Low WC: Adeno-associated virus type 2 vectors: transduction and long-term expression in cerebellar Purkinje cells in vivo is mediated by the fibroblast growth factor receptor 1 : bFGFR-1 mediates AAV2 transduction of Purkinje cells. *Arch Virol* 2008; 153: 2107-2110.
[32] Asokan A, Hamra JB, Govindasamy L, Agbandje-McKenna M, Samulski RJ: Adeno-associated virus type 2 contains an integrin alpha5beta1 binding domain essential for viral cell entry. *J Virol* 2006; 80: 8961-8969.
[33] Zhou SZ, Cooper S, Kang LY *et al*: Adeno-associated virus 2-mediated high efficiency gene transfer into immature and mature subsets of hematopoietic progenitor cells in human umbilical cord blood. *J Exp Med* 1994; 179: 1867-1875.
[34] Nathwani AC, Hanawa H, Vandergriff J, Kelly P, Vanin EF, Nienhuis AW: Efficient gene transfer into human cord blood CD34+ cells and the CD34+CD38- subset using highly purified recombinant adeno-associated viral vector preparations that are free of helper virus and wild-type AAV. *Gene Ther* 2000; 7: 183-195.

[35] Hargrove PW, Vanin EF, Kurtzman GJ, Nienhuis AW: High-level globin gene expression mediated by a recombinant adeno-associated virus genome that contains the 3' gamma globin gene regulatory element and integrates as tandem copies in erythroid cells. *Blood* 1997; 89: 2167-2175.

[36] Malik P, McQuiston SA, Yu XJ *et al*: Recombinant adeno-associated virus mediates a high level of gene transfer but less efficient integration in the K562 human hematopoietic cell line. *J Virol* 1997; 71: 1776-1783.

[37] Alexander IE, Russell DW, Miller AD: Transfer of contaminants in adeno-associated virus vector stocks can mimic transduction and lead to artifactual results. *Hum Gene Ther* 1997; 8: 1911-1920.

[38] Rolling F: Generation of recombinant adeno-associated virus. *Methods Mol Med* 2001; 47: 157-170.

[39] Zhang X, Li CY: Generation of recombinant adeno-associated virus vectors by a complete adenovirus-mediated approach. *Mol Ther* 2001; 3: 787-792.

[40] Matsushita T, Elliger S, Elliger C *et al*: Adeno-associated virus vectors can be efficiently produced without helper virus. *Gene Ther* 1998; 5: 938-945.

[41] Matsushita T, Okada T, Inaba T, Mizukami H, Ozawa K, Colosi P: The adenovirus E1A and E1B19K genes provide a helper function for transfection-based adeno-associated virus vector production. *J Gen Virol* 2004; 85: 2209-2214.

[42] Qiao C, Li J, Skold A, Zhang X, Xiao X: Feasibility of generating adeno-associated virus packaging cell lines containing inducible adenovirus helper genes. *J Virol* 2002; 76: 1904-1913.

[43] Auricchio A, Hildinger M, O'Connor E, Gao GP, Wilson JM: Isolation of highly infectious and pure adeno-associated virus type 2 vectors with a single-step gravity-flow column. *Hum Gene Ther* 2001; 12: 71-76.

[44] Sun Xj, Tian J, Tan MQ* Adeno-associated virus serotype 2 mediated transduction and expression of the human – β globin gene in human early fetal liver hematopoietic cells.Progress in Biochemistry and Biophysics 2007,34(5):525-532

[45] Jing Tian, Feng Wang, Jin-Feng Xue Fei Zhao, Liu-Jiang Song, Meng-Qun Tan Recombinant AAV2-mediated β-globin expression in human fetal hematopoietic cells from the aborted fetuses with β-thalassemia major International Journal of Hematology(This paper in the March 22,2011has been accepted ,No. IJHM-D-10-00214R4)

[46] Mengxin Li, Giridhara R. Jayandharan, Baozheng Li, *et al.* High-Efficiency Transduction of Fibroblasts and Mesenchymal Stem Cells by Tyrosine-Mutant AAV2 Vectors for Their Potential Use in Cellular Therapy. Human gene therapy. 2010; 21:1527–1543.

[47] M. Ariel Kauss, Laura J. Smith, Li Zhong, *et al.* Enhanced Long-Term Transduction and Multilineage Engraftment of Human Hematopoietic Stem Cells Transduced with Tyrosine-Modified Recombinant Adeno-Associated Virus Serotype 2. Human gene therapy. 2010; 21:1129–1136

10

Comparison of AAV Serotypes for Gene Delivery to Dopaminergic Neurons in the Substantia Nigra

J.A. Korecka[1], M. Schouten[1], R. Eggers[1], A. Ulusoy[2], K. Bossers[1] and J. Verhaagen[1]
[1]*Netherlands Institute for Neuroscience, Institute of the Royal Netherlands Academy of Arts and Sciences, Amsterdam,*
[2]*German Center for Neurodegenerative Diseases, Bonn,*
[1]*Netherlands*
[2]*Germany*

1. Introduction

Targeted viral vector-mediated gene transfer to specific population of neurons in the central nervous system (CNS) is a relatively novel, but fast developing approach to study gene function in a number of neurodegenerative diseases (reviewed in Korecka, Verhaagen, & Hol, 2007; Manfredsson & Mandel, 2010). Moreover, several early phase clinical trials based on viral vector-mediated therapeutic gene transfer have been completed or are underway for neurological disorders (Kaplitt et al., 2007; reviewed in Korecka et al., 2007; Marks, Jr. et al., 2010; Muramatsu et al., 2010; Tuszynski et al., 2005). Gene therapy is especially attractive for diseases where neuronal degeneration is largely restricted to a single neuronal population in a specific anatomical area. Parkinson disease (PD) is a neurodegenerative disease mainly characterized by a progressive degeneration of dopaminergic (DAergic) neurons in the Substantia Nigra (SN) (Dauer & Przedborski, 2003). It would be desirable to direct transgene expression to the dopaminergic neurons in animal models for neurodegenerative diseases, allowing for a range of investigations into the function of that gene in normal, adult DAergic neurons or following neurotoxic insult.

Lentiviral vectors (LV) and adeno-associated viral vectors (AAV) are increasingly regarded as the two most useful gene therapy vectors for the CNS. Both vectors have been successfully used to express a foreign gene in a variety of brain regions and neuronal cell types (Lim, Airavaara, & Harvey, 2010; Manfredsson & Mandel, 2010; Papale, Cerovic, & Brambilla, 2009; Schneider, Zufferey, & Aebischer, 2008). LV vectors have been shown to direct long-lasting expression of a number of transgenes in the brain (Lundberg et al., 2008) including in neurons in the rat SN (Deglon et al., 2000). AAV vectors are considered to be the most appealing vectors for transgene expression in the CNS, due to their efficient neuronal transduction, their capacity to direct long-term transgene expression and their safety profile (Kaplitt et al., 2007; Mandel et al., 2006; McCown, 2005). The early AAV vectors were based on AAV serotype 2 (Kaplitt et al., 1994; Peel & Klein, 2000), but subsequent vectors have been generated with novel serotypes that differ in their tissue and cellular tropism (Wu, Asokan, & Samulski, 2006).

So far, three studies engaged in exploring the possibility of AAV transgene expression in the mouse SN. In two studies only AAV vectors based on serotype 2 were used inducing either alpha-synuclein (St Martin et al., 2007) or dual leucine zipper kinase (Chen et al., 2008) expression in the DAergic neurons of the mouse SN. In the third study AAV serotypes 1, 2, 5, 7 and 8 were injected into the mouse SN and compared for their tropism for DAergic neurons (Taymans et al., 2007). Although, AAV1 and 5 displayed the most promising transduction rates, this data was qualitatively assessed. In contrast, the rat dopaminergic system has been studied much more extensively with five studies investigating the performance of various AAV serotypes tropism. These studies compared the levels of GFP expression in the rat SN after injection of AAV vector serotype 1, 2 and 5 (Burger et al., 2004; Paterna, Feldon, & Bueler, 2004), AAV8 (Klein et al., 2006; McFarland, Lee, Hyman, & McLean, 2009), and AAV9 and 10 (Klein, Dayton, Tatom, Diaczynsky, & Salvatore, 2008). A general conclusion for all these studies establishes AAV2 as the lowest transducing vector of dopaminergic neurons in the rat SN. Finally and most recently, one AAV serotype study has been performed in primate CNS, where AAV1 to 6 viral vectors were injected into the SN (Markakis et al., 2010). In the primate AAV5 displays the most promising transduction of neurons in this area.

In the following study, we have compared multiple AAV serotypes for transduction of mouse and rat mesencephalic DAergic neurons. AAV vectors were developed to contain either a cytomegalovirus (CMV) promoter or the human synapsin 1 (SYN) promoter. We demonstrate that the synapsin promoter leads to higher nigral transduction compared to the CMV promoter in mice. Additionally we also show that in our setting, AAV serotype 5 and 7 give the highest transduction rate of DAergic neurons in the mouse SN, where as rat SN can be equally well transduced with all serotypes tested. We compare our study with the published data and underline the differences in the methodology and outcome measures.

2. Methods

2.1 AAV constructs and production

Lentiviral vectors were produced as described before (Hendriks, Eggers, Verhaagen, & Boer, 2007). Two plasmids, designated pTRCGw and pTRUF20B-SEW, were used for the production of AAV. The pTRCGW plasmid contained inverted terminal repeats of AAV2 flanking a cytomegalovirus (CMV) promoter driving expression of GFP, a woodchuck hepatitis virus posttranscriptional regulatory element (WPRE), and a polyadenylation signal (Ruitenberg, Eggers, Boer, & Verhaagen, 2002). The second plasmid, designated pTRUF20B-SEW, was a generous gift from Prof. Deniz Kirik (Lund University, Sweden). This plasmid also contained two inverted terminal repeats of AAV2 flanking a human synapsin 1 (SYN) promoter driving expression of GFP, a WPRE, and a polyadenylation signal. For the production of different serotypes helper plasmids were used provided by J.A. Kleinschmidt (AAV1 to 6) (Grimm, Kay, & Kleinschmidt, 2003) and J.M. Wilson (AAV7 and 8) (Gao et al., 2002). For each serotype eight 15 cm petridishes containing $1x10^7$ HEK293T cells were transfected with the use of polyethylenimine (PEI, MW25000; Polysciences Inc., Warrington, PA, USA). Cells were grown in Dulbecco's modified Eagle's medium (DMEM) containing 10% fetal calf serum (FCS) and 1% penicillin/streptomycin (GIBCO-Invitrogen Corp, New York, NY, USA). pTRCGW or pTRUF20B-SEW AAV plasmids were cotransfected with packaging plasmids in different ratios as follows: AAV1 to 6 in a ratio of AAV plasmid over capsid plasmid 1:3 with a total amount of 50µg of DNA per plate, and AAV7 and 8 in a ratio of 1:2:2 of AAV plasmid over helper plasmid pAdΔF6 and capsid plasmid with total amount of 62.5µg of DNA per plate. Two days after the transfection cells were harvested in D-phosphate buffered saline (PBS) (Gibco) containing 10µg/ml DNAseI (Roche Diagnostics GmbH, Mannheim, Germany) and incubated for 1 hour at 37°C. Cells were lysed by three freeze-thaw cycles, spun down 30 min at 4000rpm and crude lysate was collected. Virus was purified by the iodixanol gradient ultra-centrifugation method (Hermens et al., 1999; Zolotukhin et al., 1999), diluted in D-PBS/5% sucrose and concentrated using Amicon 100kDA MWCO Ultra-15 device (Millipore, Billerica, MA, USA). All AAV vectors were stored at -80°C until use. Titers were determined by repeated quantitative PCR for viral genomic copies extracted from DNAse-treated viral particles using WPRE directed primers (forward: CAGGTGTATTGCCACAAGACAAA and reverse: TGCACAGGTGAAGACCAAGCAA). Table 1 provides an overview of all viral stocks and their titers used in this study.

Serotype	Titer (GCs/ml)	Injection coordinates in mice	Injection coordinates in rats
LV-CMV	9.0x10^9	AP -2.8, L -1.3, VD -4.2	
AAV1-CMV	6.6x10^12	AP -2.8, L -1.3, VD -4.1	
AAV2-CMV	1.0x10^12	AP -2.8, L -1.3, VD -4.1	
AAV5-CMV	7.1x10^11	AP -2.8, L -1.3, VD -4.1	
AAV6-CMV	1.5x10^12	AP -2.8, L -1.3, VD -4.1	
AAV7-CMV	3.2x10^12	AP -2.8, L -1.3, VD -4.2	
AAV8-CMV	9.9x10^11	AP -2.8, L -1.3, VD -4.1	
AAV5-SYN***	1.2x10^13	AP -2.8, L -1.3, VD -4.3	AP -5.2, L -2.0, VD -7.2
AAV6-SYN	3.7x10^12	AP -2.8, L -1.3, VD -4.3	AP -5.2, L -2.0, VD -7.2
AAV7-SYN	3.0x10^12	AP -2.8, L -1.3, VD -4.3	AP -5.2, L -2.0, VD -7.2
AAV8-SYN	1.4x10^12	AP -2.8, L -1.3, VD -4.3	AP -5.2, L -2.0, VD -7.2

Table 1. Viral vectors, titers and injection coordinates. All AAV batches have a similar range of titer with an exception of AAV5-SYN, which has a significantly higher titer than the other AAV-SYN viruses (after multiple testing, $P<0.001$, one way ANOVA). The injection coordinates are indicated for mice and rats respectively. Abbreviations: CMV-cytomegalovirus, SYN-synapsin, GCs/ml- genomic copies per milliliter, AP- Anterior Posterior, L- lateral, and VD- Ventral Dorsal distances from bregma.

2.2 Experimental animals and surgical procedures

A total of 43 male C57BL/6 mice weighing 20-25g and 16 female Sprague-Dawley rats weighing 200-250g were used (Harlan, Zeist, The Netherlands). Animals were housed with food and water *ad libitum*, with 12 hour light and dark cycles. All the experimental procedures and postoperative care was carried out in accordance with the local animal experimental ethical committee.

The viral injections were carried out with the use of glass capillaries (0.78/1.0mm internal/external diameter; Harvard Apparatus, Holliston, MA, USA) with an 80µm tip. These glass capillaries were connected to Portex polyethylene tubing in turn connected to a Hamilton syringe fixed in a micro-infusion pump (PHD2000, Harvard Apparatus). The system was filled with water and a target volume of 1µl and an infusion rate of 0.2µl/min

was set for mice injections and target volume of 2µl and an infusion rate of 0.4 µl/min for rats. The glass needles were mounted on a stereotactic device (David Kopf Instruments, Tujunga, CA, USA). A total of 1.1µl of virus was loaded for mice and 2.3 µl for rats for each injection separately.
Mice were intraperitoneally (IP) injected with FFM mix made of Hypnorm (0.1 mg/kg Fentanyl citrate/ 3.3 mg/kg Fluanisone HCl, Janssen Pharmaceuticals) and Dormicum (8.3 mg/kg Midazolam, Roche) and placed into a stereotactic device where they were fixed and the skull was exposed. The skull was leveled based on the heights of bregma, lambda and two additional and very crucial lateral measurements of 2.0 mm from bregma. The injection coordinates were calculated from bregma with anterior posterior (AP) being -2.8 mm and lateral (L) -1.3 mm. Ventral dorsal (VD) coordinate was measured from the dura of either -4.1, -4.2 or -4.3 mm depending on the viral injection (see table 1). Subsequently, the needle was lowered into the brain 0.1 mm below the VD coordinate and retracted back up to the correct level. After the infusion, the needle was left in place for 5min before retraction.
Rats were anesthetized by intramuscular injection of 0.08ml/100g of Hypnorm and mounted in the stereotact. The skull level was controlled by measurement of bregma and lambda. 2µl of each AAV virus was injected at the following coordinates with VD being measured from dura: AP -5.2, L -2.0, and VD 7.2 (Ulusoy, Sahin, Bjorklund, Aebischer, & Kirik, 2009).
All of the animals recovered on a heating pad at 37°C and were allowed to survive for 4 weeks post surgery after which they were sacrificed by an IP overdose with Pentobarbital (50mg/µl) and transcardially perfused with 0.9% saline followed by 4% paraformaldehyde (PFA, Sigma-Aldrich Co., St. Louis, MO, USA) in PBS pH 7.4. The brains were further post-fixed overnight and 4 series of 30µm thick coronal sections were cut on a vibratome. The sections were stored free-floating at 4°C in 1% PFA in PBS pH 7.6.

2.3 Immunohistochemistry and histological quantification

All immunohistochemical (IHC) stainings were performed on free-floating sections. Prior to the staining, one series of sections was pre-blocked in 1x tris buffered saline (TBS) (Sigma) with 2.5% fetal calf serum (FCS) and 0.2% Triton-X (Sigma) for 1 hour at room temperature. Sections were then incubated with anti-tyrosine hydroxilase (TH) rabbit polyclonal antibody (Institute Jacques Boy SA, Reims, France) at 1:1000 dilution in blocking buffer and anti-GFP (Millipore) chicken monoclonal antibody at 1:1000 for 1 hour at room temperature followed by overnight incubation at 4°C. Secondary goat anti-rabbit antibody Alexa 594 (1:400, Invitrogen, Carlsbad, CA, USA) was used for the detection of the TH antibody and donkey anti-chicken Alexa 488 (1:400, Invitrogen) for the detection of the GFP antibody. These antibodies were incubated for 1 hour at room temperature. Sections were then mounted on chrome-aluin and gelatin coated glass slides.
Images were acquired with an Axioplan microscope (Zeiss, Sliedrecht, The Netherlands). Images for quantification of the transduced neurons of the SN were taken at 10x magnification for mice and 5x magnification for rats with fixed exposure times for both TH and GFP signal. The sections of the striatum area were photographed at 2.5x magnification also with fixed exposure times for both TH and GFP fluorescent signal.
ImagePro Plus Fluorviewer software (Media cybernetics, Bethesda, MD, USA) was used for the SN transduction quantification. All TH-positive neurons were manually counted in a single-blinded setup. Furthermore, TH and GFP colocalization was assessed using cellular morphology and fluorescent intensity parameters. For each section the percentage of GFP-

positive and TH-positive cells was determined, and all values from all of the sections were averaged to give the total percentage of colocalized cells in the whole structure. In the AAV-SYN comparison study one animal in AAV8 group, which the injection had missed the SN structure, was excluded from further statistics unless specified. Caudate quantification was performed with the use of ImagePro Plus Measure Threshold macro. The striatal areas in both hemispheres were outlined based on the TH expression in the striatal fibers. The average GFP background signal measured in cortex areas in both hemispheres was subtracted from each ipsilateral striatum signal. Next, the recalculated intensity from the non-injected striatum was subtracted from the injected side. Finally, this average intensity value in the injected striatum was multiplied by the size of the area resulting in total GFP intensity of the measured area.

3. All AAV serotype vectors with the CMV promoter direct poor transgene expression in DAergic neurons of the mouse SN

Vectors based on AAV serotypes 1, 2, 5, 7, 8 and LV that contained the CMV-GFP expression cassette were injected into the mouse SN. Four weeks after the injection, the number of TH-positive neurons expressing GFP was quantified. All AAV serotypes and the LV vector showed very low numbers of transduced TH-positive neurons (Figure 1B). AAV7 directs the highest transduction rate with 8% of the TH-positive SN cells expressing GFP. Most of the serotypes, with the exception of AAV2, showed high rates of cellular transduction in and around the SN, but the transduced neurons were TH-negative (Figure 1A). AAV1 and LV also transduced glial cells particularly in the area directly surrounding the injection site (data not shown). Glial transduction has not been observed with any other AAV serotypes.
Three groups have reported on AAV-mediated gene transfer to the mouse SN (Chen et al., 2008; St Martin et al., 2007; Taymans et al., 2007). Experimental details, including the serotype and promoter used in these studies are summarized in Table 2.

Study	Viral vector used	Analysis parameters	Used promoter
Taymans et al., 2007	AAV1, 2, 5, 7 and 8	GFP expression in the SN & the striatum	CMV
St Martin et al., 2007	AAV2	GFP and TH colocalization in the SN	CBA
Chen et al., 2008	AAV2	GFP and TH colocalization in the SN	CBA

Table 2. Summary of literature reports using AAV vectors for gene transfer in mouse SN.

A comparative analysis of AAV1, 2, 5, 7 and 8 showed efficient transduction of cells in the SN area (Taymans et al., 2007). AAV 1 and 5 showed robust GFP expression in the fibers of the striatum. In contrast AAV7 and 8 directed only low GFP levels in this projection area of the SN DAergic neurons. Additionally, a few GFP positive cells were observed in the striatum in all of the serotypes. Consistent with our observations, AAV2 showed poor transgene expression in the SN. The efficiency of AAV-CMV driven GFP expression was assessed qualitatively and no specification of the DAergic lineage of the transduced cells was performed. We have also found high numbers of GFP expressing cells with AAV-CMV vectors in and around the SN, however, quantification of the TH-positive GFP-labeled cells revealed very low numbers of GFP expressing DAergic neurons in the SN (Figure 1).

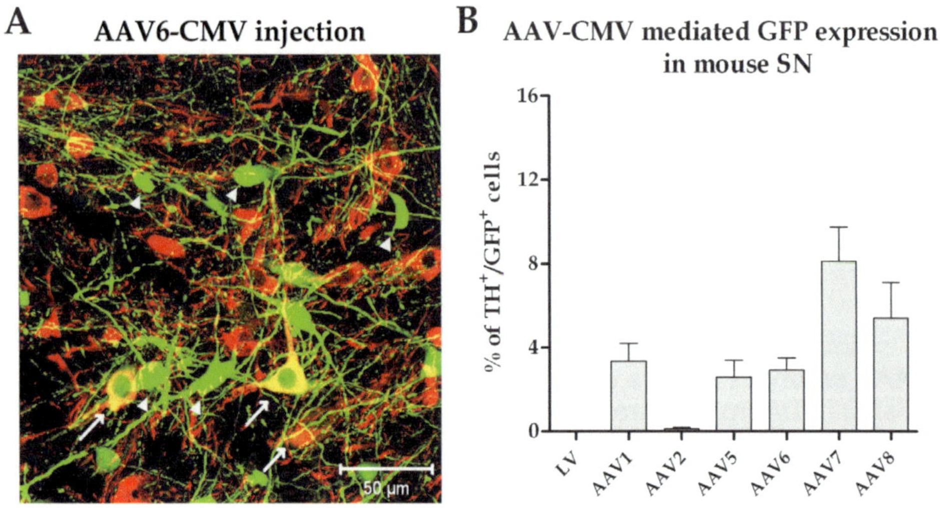

Fig. 1. AAV-CMV-mediated GFP expression in the mouse Substantia Nigra. **A.** Confocal Z-stack image of an immunohistochemical staining of the mouse SN showing GFP transgene expression in a small number of dopaminergic neurons identified by TH staining (arrows indicate the double labeled cells) but also in non-dopaminergic neurons (arrowheads) after AAV6-CMV injection. TH neurons are shown in red, GFP is shown in green. The scale bar indicates 50µm. **B.** Quantification of transduced DAergic neurons in the mouse SN (n=3) using LV-CMV-GFP and AAV-CMV-GFP viral vectors. The bars represent the percentage of TH positive neurons in the SN expressing GFP. AAV7 shows the highest transduction of 8% of DAergic neurons in the SN. Error bars indicate the SEM.

The other two studies, performing AAV mediated gene transfer in mouse SN used only serotype 2. In the first study, injection of AAV2 into the SN showed between 10 and 80% of TH-positive neurons that express GFP in individual sections (St Martin et al., 2007). In the second study AAV2 was injected into the posterior SN, which resulted in transduction of 71.1±6.0% of TH-positive neurons (Chen et al., 2008). The number of GFP transduced cells in both of these studies is much higher compared to our study, where AAV2-CMV led to the lowest transduction rate of SN neurons. Although both studies used slightly different injection coordinates than we did, it is unlikely that this caused significant differences in AAV2 transduction efficiencies. The most likely explanation for this difference is the use of the chicken β-actin (CBA) promoter, a promoter known to drive stronger and more persistent expression in several population of neurons (Fitzsimons, Bland, & During, 2002). Unfortunately there were no other serotypes used in these studies.

4. AAV vectors that harbor the synapsin promoter direct high-level transgene expression in dopaminergic neurons of the mouse SN

Based on our results and the available literature, the CMV promoter appears to direct less efficient transgene expression in different cell types, including striatal neurons (Jakobsson, Ericson, Jansson, Bjork, & Lundberg, 2003), cochlea cells (Liu et al., 2007), human embryonic stem cells (Orban et al., 2009) and finally rat SN neurons (Paterna, Moccetti, Mura, Feldon, & Bueler, 2000; Wang et al., 2005). Therefore we conclude that the CMV promoter leads to a

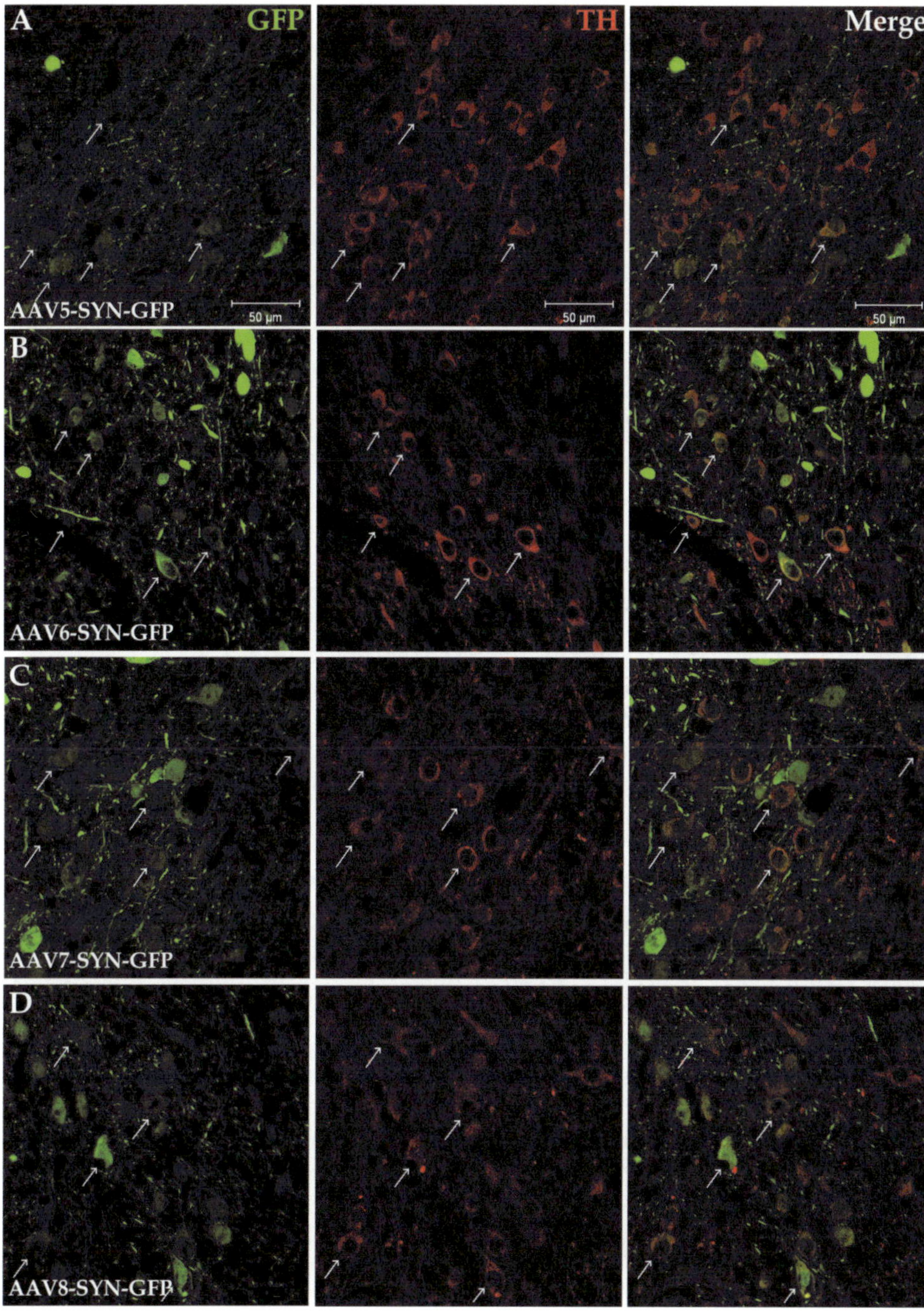

Fig. 2. GFP expression in AAV-SYN injected mouse SN. GFP stained (green) and TH stained (red) neurons are visualized in confocal images. Arrows point to examples of GFP positive and TH positive cells in all viral serotypes. **A.** AAV5-SYN-GFP; **B.** AAV6-SYN-GFP; **C.** AAV7-SYN-GFP; and **D.** AAV8-SYN-GFP. The scale of 50µm is represented by a bar in panel A.

limited transduction in the mouse SN and may not be suitable to drive viral vector-mediated transgene expression in the DAergic neurons of the mouse SN. The human synapsin 1 promoter, on the other hand, has been shown to be an excellent neuron specific promoter in co-cultured primary hippocampal neurons isolated from embryonic brain (Kugler, Lingor, Scholl, Zolotukhin, & Bahr, 2003), in primary dorsal root ganglion cultures (Sims et al., 2008) and *in vivo* following injection of an adenoviral vector in rat brain, including the SN (Hermening, Kugler, Bahr, & Isenmann, 2006; Kugler, Kilic, & Bahr, 2003; Kugler et al., 2003). We therefore produced 4 AAV vectors (AAV5, 6, 7 and 8) that harbored a GFP reporter gene under the human synapsin 1 promoter. The performance of these AAV vectors was tested in mice and rats after injection in the SN.

4.1 AAV-synapsin-GFP drives transgene expression in tyrosine hydroxylase positive neurons

Vectors based on AAV serotypes 5, 6, 7 and 8 that contained a SYN-GFP expression cassette were injected in the SN in the same fashion as the AAV-CMV-GFP viral vectors. All serotypes directed GFP expression in neurons throughout the midbrain, including the SN. AAV7 injected mice showed the most widespread viral transduction with GFP-positive neurons in multiple midbrain areas (data not shown).

Subsequently, we specifically investigated the transduction efficiency of DAergic neurons of the SN. Immunohistochemical staining showed that all serotypes transduce TH positive neurons in the mouse SN (Figure 2). Interestingly, the level of GFP expression in the individual TH positive cells appears to be lower than in other TH-negative neurons in the SN area. This was also observed following transduction with AAV-CMV vectors. In addition, large numbers of GFP positive fibers were observed in the SN. Based on cellular morphology, no other cell types expressed GFP. This indicates that the AAV-SYN-GFP construct drives neuron-specific expression.

4.2 AAV5 and AAV7 mediate the highest transduction of TH positive neurons in the mouse SN

Quantification of the number of TH-positive and GFP-positive neurons in the SN demonstrated a much higher proportion of double labeled neurons with all AAV-SYN vectors compared to the AAV-CMV vectors. AAV5 and AAV7 lead to significantly higher percentage of the GFP labeled DAergic neurons compared to AAV6 and AAV8. These two serotypes directed GFP expression in 76-80%of TH-positive neurons (Figure 3A). The homogeneous distribution of the TH and GFP-positive neurons from the posterior to the anterior side of the SN corroborates the superiority of AAV5 and AAV7 compared to AAV6 and AAV8 at each anatomical level (figure 3B, for more details see supplementary figure 1).

In conclusion, AAV5-SYN and AAV7-SYN are the most effective vectors for transduction of DAergic neurons in mouse SN. Interestingly, even though AAV5 had a significantly higher titer in comparison to AAV7, it transduces a comparable number of DAergic neurons throughout the SN. In contrast, AAV8 injected animals, apart from a relatively low total percentage of TH and GFP-positive neurons, display a decrease in the number of these neurons in the anterior portion of the SN. AAV6 shows quite poor transduction efficiency throughout the SN. This is in accordance with the relative low overall percentage of TH-positive neurons that express GFP (Figure 3A).

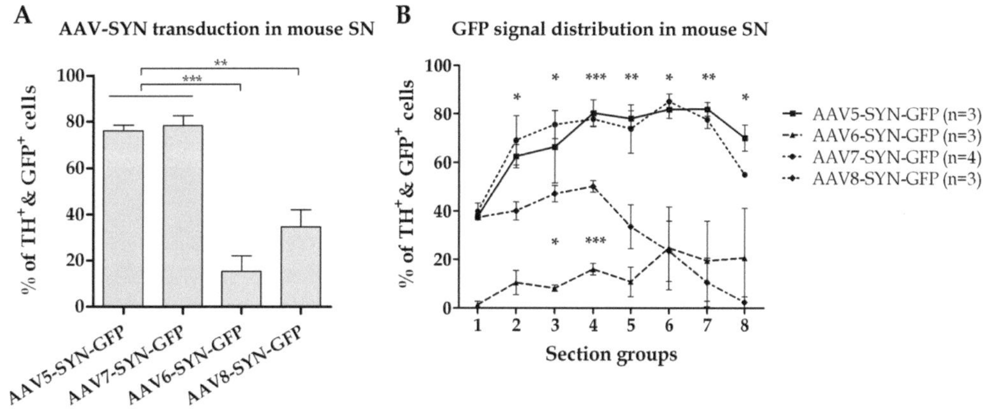

Fig. 3. AAV-SYN-GFP transduction of mouse SN. **A.** Quantification of TH positive (TH+) and GFP positive (GFP+) neurons in mouse SN transduced with different AAV serotypes. In the AAV5 and AAV7 groups, almost 80% of TH+ neurons express GFP, which is significantly higher than the AAV6 group where < 20% of the DAergic neurons are GFP positive (P<0.001), and the AAV8 group where 35% of the DAergic neurons express GFP (P<0.01). **B.** Quantification of GFP expressing TH+ cells per serotype in SN serial sections arranged according to the Allan Brain Atlas TH in situ hybridization (Lein et al., 2007) with 1 being most posterior and 8 being the most anterior part of the SN (supplementary figure 1). Throughout the groups there was no statistical significant difference between AAV5 and AAV7, however in section groups 2, 4, 5, 6 and 7 AAV7 showed significantly higher average of GFP+/TH+ cells than the other two serotypes (* $P < 0.05$, ** $P < 0.01$, *** $P < 0.001$), where as in section 3 only comparing to AAV6 ($P < 0.01$). AAV5 showed a significantly higher GFP expression in comparison to AAV6 and AAV8 serotypes in section groups 4, 5, 6, 7 and 8 and in section 2 and 3 to AAV6 only. AAV8 shows significantly higher GFP expression to AAV6 in group 3 and 4 (* $P < 0.05$, ** $P < 0.01$, *** $P < 0.001$).

4.3 AAV7 shows the most GFP positive fibers ascending through the nigrostriatal tract

The DAergic neurons of the substantia nigra anatomically project to the striatum creating the nigral-striatal pathway. Accordingly, when the DAergic neurons in the substantia nigra are transduced their fibers in the striatum are expected to be GFP positive. To investigate this relationship, we have quantified the intensity of GFP fluorescent signal in the mouse striatum and compared this to the effectiveness of the AAV serotypes to target the DAergic neurons in the SN (Figure 4). While AAV5-SYN-GFP and AAV7-SYN-GFP display a high fluorescence intensity of GFP, AAV6-SYN-GFP and AAV8-SYN-GFP show a low level of GFP expression in the striatum. Furthermore, AAV7-SYN directs significantly higher levels of GFP expression in the striatum compared to AAV5-SYN (Figure 4 E). Moreover, we have found a significant correlation between the transduction efficiency of the SN and the labeling intensity of the fibers in the striatum (Figure 4F). This corroborates the superiority of the AAV7 and AAV5 serotypes in transducing DAergic neurons in the mouse SN.

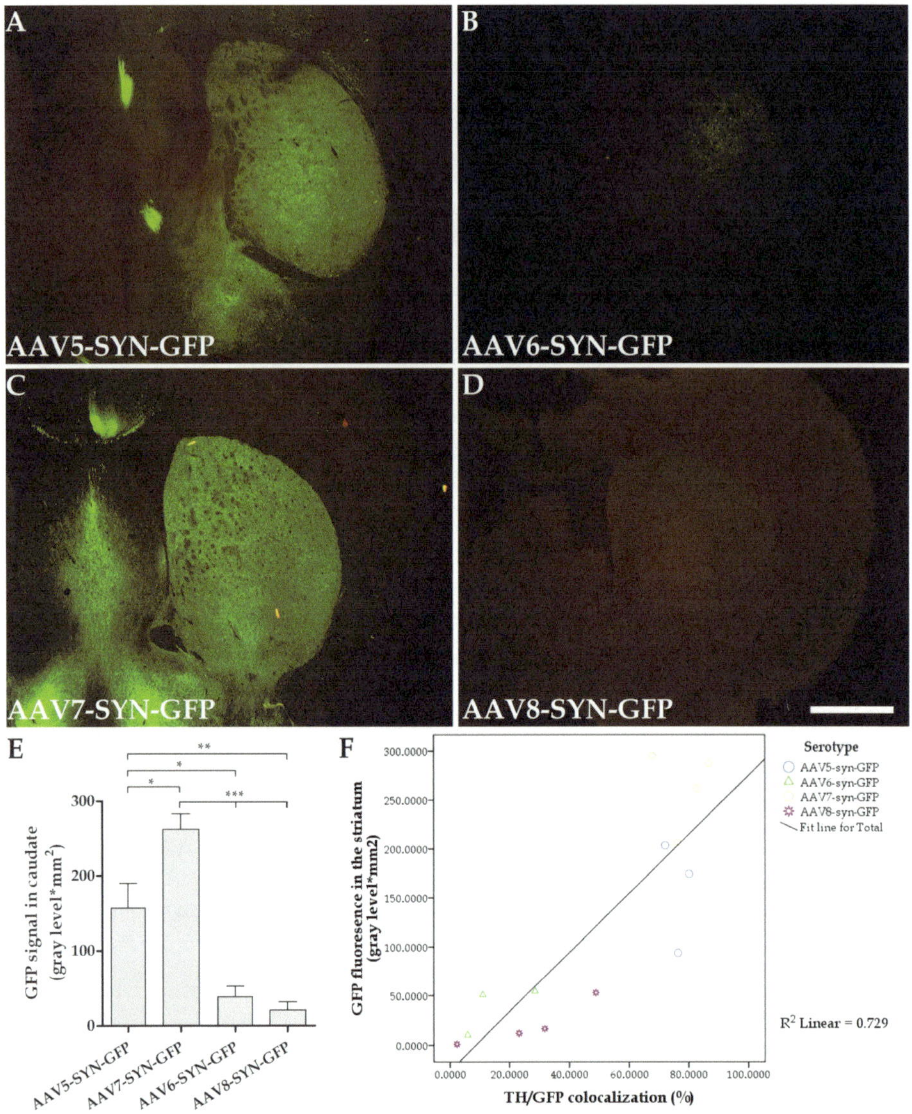

Fig. 4. GFP expression in the mouse striatum after SN AAV transduction. **A-D.** Mouse striatal sections stained with anti-TH (red) and-GFP (green) antibody transduced with different AAV serotype. The scale bar represents 1mm. **E.** Quantification of GFP fluorescent intensity in all AAV-SYN serotypes. Each striatal section was measured for GFP intensity and corrected for the measured area (gray level*mm^2). Statistical analysis indicates AAV7-SYN-GFP result in the highest GFP expression in the striatum, with AAV5 inducing the second best expression (*$P<0.05$, **$P< 0.01$ and ***$P<0.001$). **F.** The percentage of TH+ neurons expressing GFP in the SN and the level of GFP fluorescence in the striatum are significantly correlated (Pearson correlation, $R^2=0.729$, $P<0.001$). Each individual animal belonging to a specific AAV serotype injection group is depicted by different marker described in the figure legend. Animal with missed injection in AAV8-SYN group (as described in Methods section) was also included in this analysis.

Taken together, these observations demonstrate that AAV7-SYN is the best vector for the transduction of TH-positive neurons of mouse SN among the tested serotypes regarding the specificity and the transduction rate. Although both AAV5 and AAV7 effectively transduced large numbers of TH-positive neurons in the SN, AAV7 showed significantly higher GFP expression in the striatum. Injection of AAV7-SYN also resulted in a substantial transduction of other neurons in the midbrain. This indicates that AAV7 spreads further than other serotypes and/or has a more ubiquitous neuronal tropism in the mouse brain. It would be worthwhile to investigate whether it is possible to more specifically target only DAergic neurons in the SN by e.g. lowering the volume of the viral vector solution that is injected into the SN. Finally, we have not seen any signs of toxicity following the injection of high titer AAV vectors in the mouse brain.

5. All AAV-vectors harboring the synapsin promoter direct similar level of transgene expression in the rat SN and the striatum

5.1 All AAV-synapsin serotypes show similar GFP expression throughout the rat SN

Female Sprague-Dawley rats were injected with AAV-SYN-GFP viral vectors 5, 6, 7 and 8 into the SN. The viral stocks used were the same as in mouse SN injections. To estimate the transduction efficiency, the TH-positive and GFP-positive neurons of the SN were quantified in the same fashion as described in the mouse study. All AAV serotypes showed similar numbers of GFP-positive neurons in the rat SN (Figure 5A) with no significant

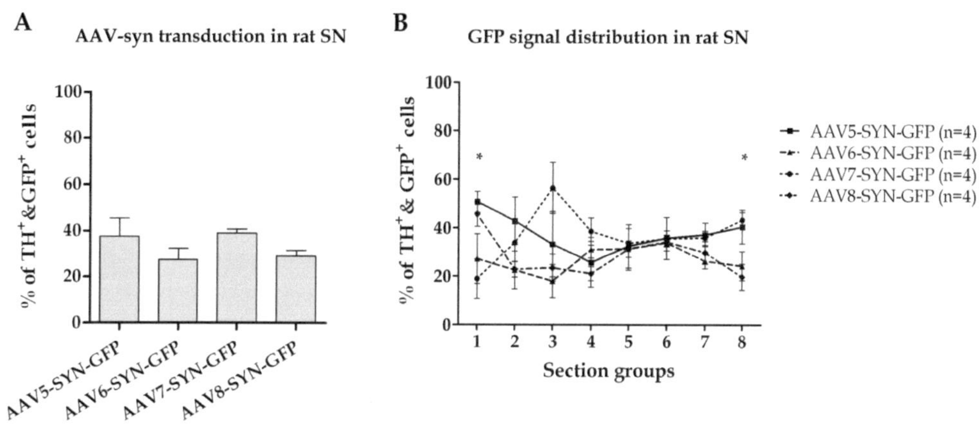

Fig. 5. AAV-SYN-GFP transduction of rat SN. **A.** Quantification of TH positive (TH+) and GFP positive (GFP+) neurons in rat SN transduced by different AAV serotypes. All serotypes showed similar GFP expression in about 30-40%of DAergic neurons. **B.** Quantification of GFP expressing TH-positive cells per serotype in the SN serial sections arranged in posterior-distal direction accordingly to the 'The rat brain atlas' by Paxinos and Watson (2007) (arrangement was based on the stereotact anatomical slides and adjacent Acetylcholinesterase (AChE) stainings with 1 being most posterior area and 8 being the most anterior area of the SN (supplementary figure 2)). All of the serotypes show similar GFP distribution within the SN structure with two exceptions: section 1 shows AAV5 expressing significantly higher amount of GFP + in TH+ cells comparing to AAV7 (* $P < 0.05$) and section 8 where AAV7 has greater amount of GFP+ DAergic cells than AAV8 (* $P < 0.05$).

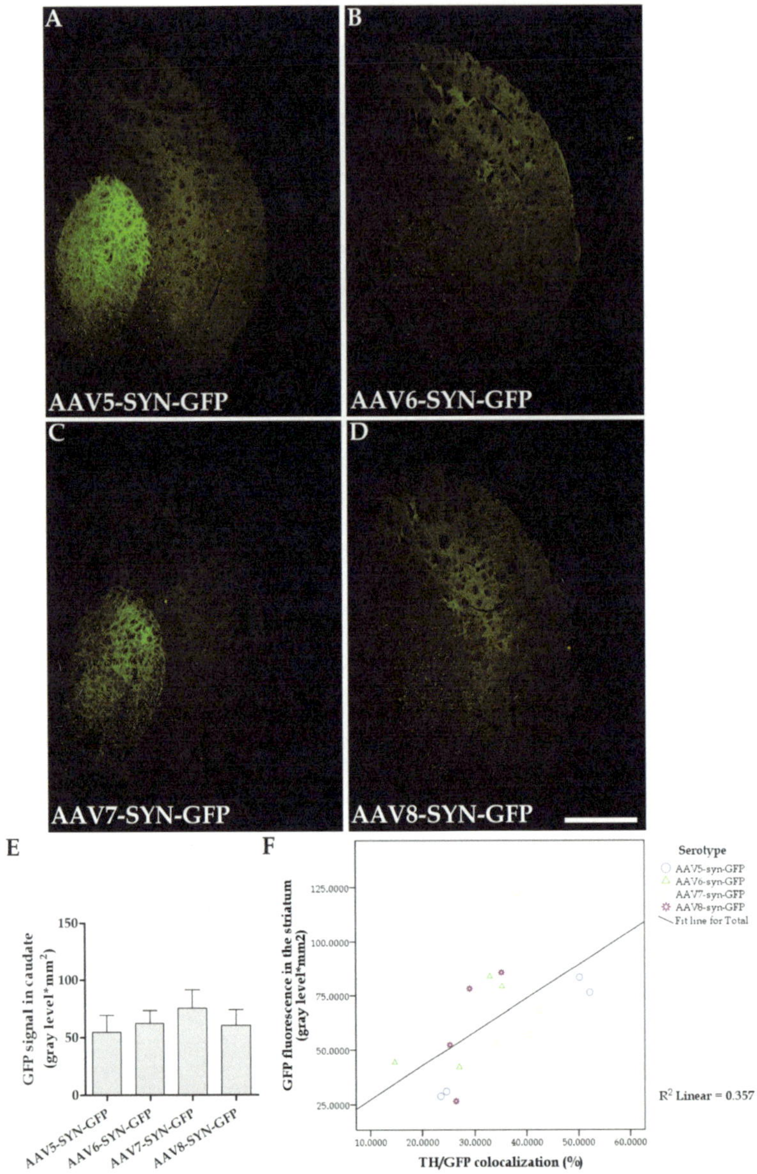

Fig. 6. GFP expression in the rat striatum after SN AAV injection. **A-D.** Rat striatal sections stained with anti-TH (red) and-GFP (green) antibodies. The scale bar represents 1mm. **E.** GFP fluorescent intensity quantification in the striatum for all AAV-SYN serotypes. Whole striatum was cut, stained and each section was measured for GFP intensity and corrected for the measured area (gray level*mm^2). Statistical analysis shows no differences in GFP expression levels between the different AAV serotypes. **F.** The percentage of TH+ neurons expressing GFP in the SN and the level of the GFP fluorescence in the striatum are significantly correlated (Pearson correlation R^2=0.357, P<0.05). Each individual animal belonging to a specific AAV serotype injection group is depicted by different marker described in the figure legend.

differences between the serotypes. For AAV5 and AAV7 the proportion of transduced TH-positive neurons is lower in the rat SN compared to the mouse SN. AAV6 directed transgene expression in a higher proportion of DAergic neurons in the rat SN (27%) than in mouse SN (16%), whereas AAV8 shows slightly higher number of GFP-positive neurons in the mouse SN (36%). These results suggest differential AAV tropism for DAergic neurons in rats comparing to mice.

Analysis of the distribution of the GFP-positive neurons within the SN also shows no major differences between the AAV serotypes (Figure 5B) except for two anatomical levels where AAV5 shows significantly higher amount of TH-positive and GFP-positive cells when compared to AAV7 in section 1, and AAV7 shows more GFP-positive DAergic neurons when compared to AAV8 in section 8. Although significant, these differences are not prominent enough to allow us to speculate on either of the serotype superiority in transducing rat DAergic neurons.

5.3 All AAV-SYN serotypes show GFP expression in the fibers of the rat striatum

As in the mouse study, we have quantified the intensity of GFP signal in the rat striatum to compare the effectiveness of AAV serotype transduction of the rat SN anatomical projection (Figure 6). All AAV serotypes showed similar, relatively high levels of GFP expression in the striatum (Figure 6E). A correlation analysis revealed a significant correlation between the numbers of TH and GFP-positive neurons and the levels of GFP expression in striatum (Figure 4F). This further supports that all AAV serotypes are equally effective in targeting rat substantia nigra DAergic neurons. In addition, we have observed a transduction of the globus pallidus fibers by AAV5 and AAV7 serotypes. This may suggest more spread of these viral vectors in the rat brain.

5.4 AAV7 viral vector injection decreases the amount of TH-positive cells in the rat SN

We observed a > 50% decrease of number of TH-positive neurons in rat SN after AAV7 injection when compared to the non injected contra-lateral side of the structure (Figure 7). We also studied the expression of vesicular monoamine transporter-2 (VMAT2), another DAergic phenotype marker, and found its protein levels also strongly decreased in the injected SN (data not shown). Interestingly, the number of TH-positive and GFP-positive neurons in the SN is not less than in the other serotypes (Figure 5) as well as the intensity of GFP-positive fibers in the striatum (Figure 6).

6. Discussion and concluding remarks

Targeted gene delivery to mesencephalic DAergic neurons can be a very valuable approach to study the molecular mechanisms that underlie the development and progression of PD. Gene delivery to DAergic neurons has also a potential to evolve into a new therapeutic strategy for PD. In this study we have compared the capacity of multiple AAV serotypes to deliver a reporter gene to DAergic neurons in the adult mouse and rat SN. We have quantified the transduction efficiency of AAV vectors harboring two different promoters: the CMV and human synapsin 1 (SYN) promoter. We have demonstrated that following stereotactic injection of vectors containing the SYN promoter, a large number of DAergic neurons express GFP in the mouse as well as the rat SN. AAV7 is the most effective serotype for transduction of mouse SN DAergic neurons. AAV5 also displayed high transduction efficiency for TH-positive neurons, but the GFP expression levels in the striatum were consistently lower when compared to AAV7. In the rat, all AAV-SYN vectors efficiently transduced DAergic neurons in the SN. AAV vectors containing the CMV promoter directed expression only in a small proportion of TH-positive SN neurons in mice, thereby demonstrating superiority of the synapsin promoter in this specific neuronal subtype. Collectively, these observations are useful for future experiments that aim to study the function of specific genes in the mesencephalic DAergic system.

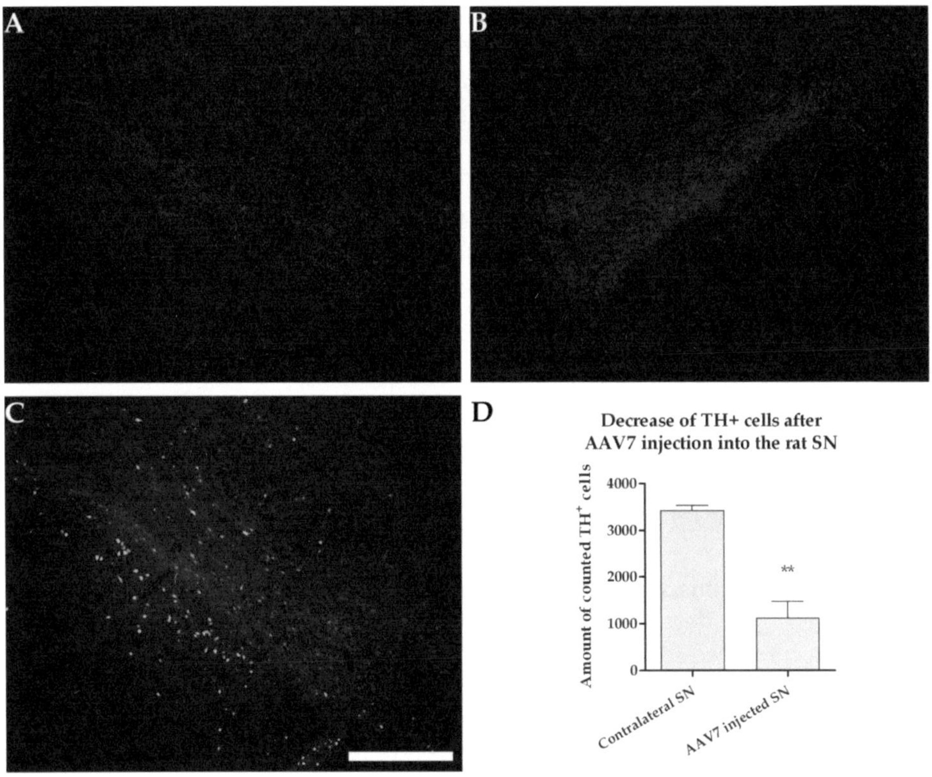

Fig. 7. AAV7 decrease of TH immunohistochemical signal in rat SN. All of the images were obtained from the same brain section. **A.** and **C.** Rat SN injected with AAV7-SYN-GFP **B.** Contra-lateral non injected side of the rat SN. Section was stained for TH (red), a nuclear marker Hoechst (blue) and GFP (green). The scale bar in panel C represents 0.5mm. **D.** Quantification of the TH positive neurons in the rat SN after AAV7 transduction. TH positive neurons were counted in both the AAV7 injected side of the SN and the contra-lateral side in each section. One way ANOVA indicated a significant decrease of TH+ neurons in the AAV7 injected SN (** $P < 0.01$).

So far, one study has compared five AAV serotypes (AAV 1, 2, 5, 7 and 8) for gene delivery to the mouse SN (Taymans et al., 2007). All vectors, except for AAV2, showed positive transduction of the SN area, with AAV1 and AAV5 implicating to direct highest levels of GFP in the striatal fibers. This study did not show quantifications of the numbers of GFP and TH-positive neurons and GFP expression in striatal fibers, and can therefore not be directly compared to our study.

For the rat SN, the four tested AAV serotypes directed equally efficient transduction in DAergic neurons. In comparison, AAV5 and AAV8 appear to display the most consistent transduction efficiencies in the literature (Klein et al., 2006; McFarland et al., 2009; Paterna et al., 2004). Additionally, AAV9 and AAV10 have also been tested and indicated to have higher tau expression in the SN area and higher TH neuronal loss evoked by tau expression comparing to AAV2 and AAV8 (Klein et al., 2008). These observations in combination with our results indicate that multiple AAV serotypes share relatively high tropism for DAergic neurons of the rat SN.

In the mouse SN, AAV vectors with the SYN promoter were superior to the AAV vectors containing the CMV promoter. In contrast, in the rat, a range of promoters have been used very successfully to direct the transgene expression in the DAergic neurons of the SN via an AAV vector including the CMV (McFarland et al., 2009), CBA (Burger et al., 2004; Klein et al., 2006; Paterna et al., 2004; Ulusoy et al., 2009), CMV/CBA hybrid (Klein et al., 2008) and PDGV (Paterna et al., 2000)) promoters. This suggests that for experiments in the rat the choice of the promoter is not as critical as it appears to be for the mouse.

Following AAV7-SYN-GFP injection, a dramatic decline in TH and VMAT2 expression occurred in the DAergic neurons in the rat SN. Klein et al. also observed a decrease in the number of TH-positive cells following high titer AAV8-GFP application, but not after AAV8-empty vector. Moreover, following the application of lower AAV8-GFP viral titer, no decrease of TH signal was noted. Therefore the authors suggest that the high concentrations of GFP can be neurotoxic to the DAergic neurons of the rat SN (Klein et al., 2006). Ulusoy et al. also reported a neurotoxic effect of high titer AAV5-GFP viral vectors. In this study not only TH was diminished, but also the expression of VMAT2. In subsequent experiments with low titer AAV5-GFP injections this effect was not seen anymore (Ulusoy et al., 2009). We speculate that in our case, the high tropism of AAV7 for DAergic neurons induces more GFP expression, and as a consequence causes DAergic neurotoxicity. We do not see this effect on TH expression in mice SN after the AAV7 injection.

As presented here, the specifications of the delivery vehicle can be crucial for successful and accurate cellular transduction. We have demonstrated that targeting SN in the mouse is difficult and could only be successfully achieved in our set up with AAV serotypes 7 and 5 harboring the SYN promoter. In contrast targeting rat SN can be efficiently achieved by multiple AAV viral vectors. It is therefore necessary to determine the vector potential for each animal species before pursuing genetic manipulation in the DAergic system. This can also be valid for human clinical PD gene therapy studies. So far AAV2 has been the only vector injected into the human brain as a delivery vehicle for PD gene therapy (Kaplitt et al., 2007; Marks, Jr. et al., 2010; Muramatsu et al., 2010). As discussed before, AAV2 seams to be the least efficient vector in the transduction of DAergic neurons in the rodent brain. Understandably human serotype studies are not possible, but primate studies may shed more light on the transduction efficiency of different delivery vehicles and can improve the efficiency of the gene therapies dramatically. One such study has recently indicated AAV5 to be the most efficient in transducing neurons in the area of SN but also glial cells, whereas glial transduction by AAV5 is not observed in the rodent brain (Markakis et al., 2010). This clearly illustrates the differences between viral vector transduction preferences between animal species.

Another major concern at the moment in the field of gene therapy is the specification of the target area. Two of the above mentioned clinical studies have targeted the putamen of PD patients (Marks, Jr. et al., 2010; Muramatsu et al., 2010) and one the subthalamic nucleus (Kaplitt et al., 2007). Depending on the function of the target gene, the location of the target area is crucial for successful therapeutic application. It is therefore rational to apply gene therapy for dopamine synthesis enzymes such as AADC to the putamen to increase the dopamine production at that area to alleviate the motor-related clinical symptoms (Muramatsu et al., 2010). On the other hand, it may not be as beneficial to induce an expression of a neurotrophic factor in the area not significantly affected by neuronal death (Marks, Jr. et al., 2010). It was therefore extensively discussed and suggested for the future to target the SN DAergic neurons when applying pro-survival and regenerative therapeutic agents (Benabid, 2010; Marks, Jr. et al., 2010). Concluding, it is therefore necessary to apply the right vectors in the specific animal species and target the appropriate area of interest, depending on the function of the expression gene, for the most effective targeted gene delivery.

7. Acknowledgements

The work presented in this paper was funded by Top Institute Pharma, Leiden, The Netherlands, project T5-207

8. Supplementary figures

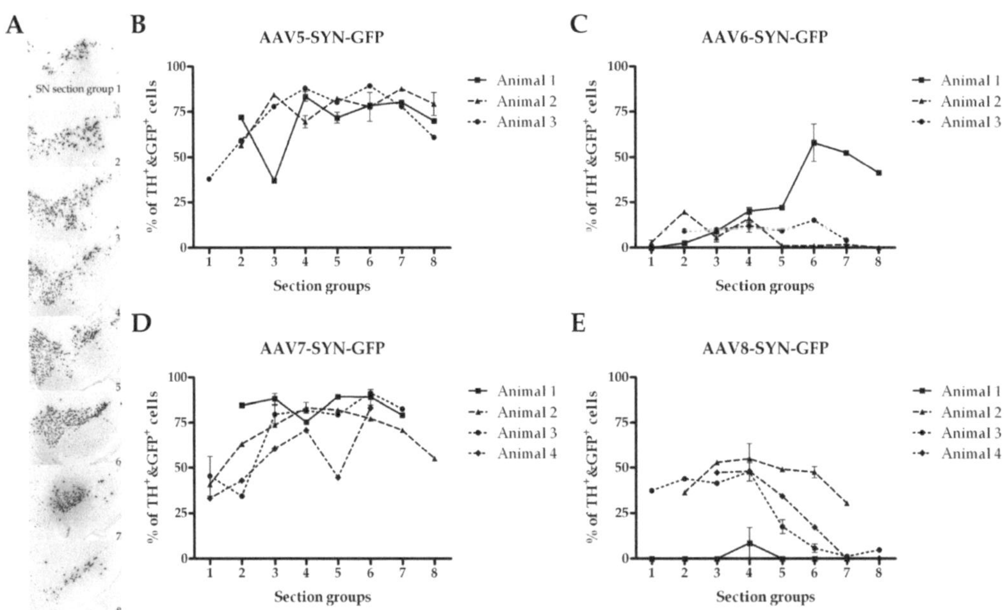

Supplementary Fig. 1. Quantitative overview of AAV-SYN-GFP transduction throughout the mouse SN in 4 different viral serotypes. **A.** The sorting of SN anatomical areas through section groups 1-8 is based on a TH in situ hybridization presented by the Allen Brain Atlas (Lein et al., 2007). Section group 1 is the most posterior group and section group 8 the most anterior. **B-E.** Quantification of SN AAV transduction throughout the structure in 4 different viral serotypes in individual animals. Values represent mean of all quantified sections belonging to the sorted section group and their SEM.

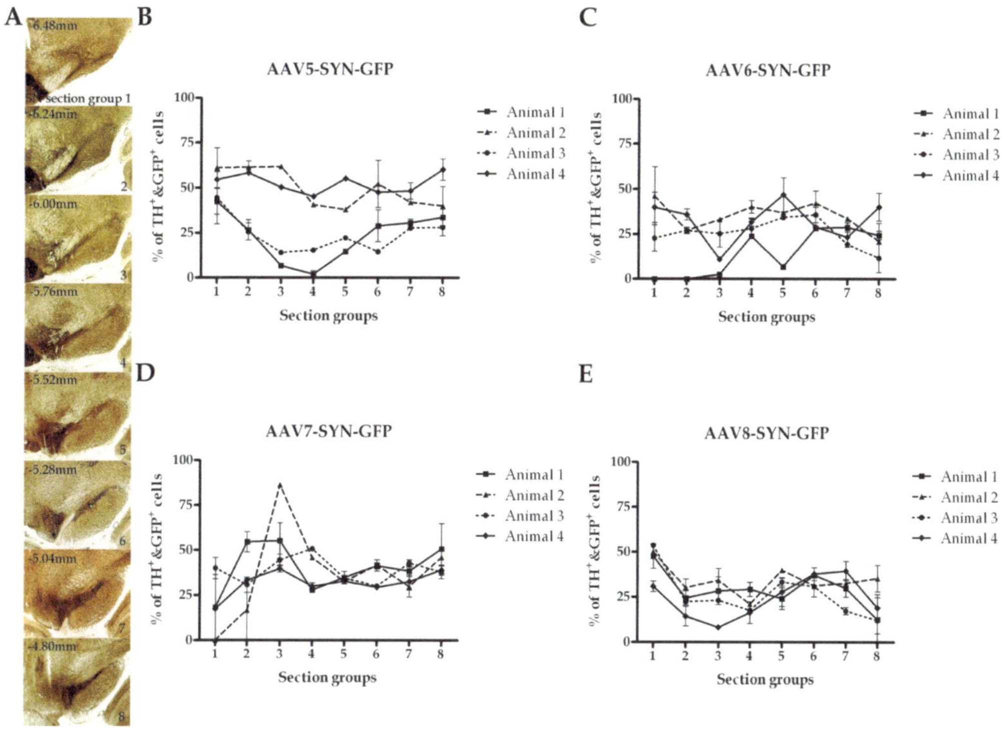

Supplementary Fig. 2. Quantitative overview of AAV-SYN-GFP transduction throughout the rat SN in 4 different viral serotypes. **A.** The sorting of SN anatomical areas through section groups 1-8 is based on the anatomical AChE stainings presented by 'The rat brain atlas' by Paxinos and Watson (2007). Section group 1 is the most posterior group and section group 8 the most anterior with indicated distances from the bregma. **B-E.** Quantification of SN AAV transduction throughout the structure in 4 different viral serotypes in individual animals. Values represent mean of all quantified sections belonging to the sorted section group and their SEM.

9. References

Benabid, A. L. (2010). Gene therapy for Parkinson's disease: do we have the cure? *Lancet Neurol., 9,* 1142-1143.

Burger, C., Gorbatyuk, O. S., Velardo, M. J., Peden, C. S., Williams, P., Zolotukhin, S. et al. (2004). Recombinant AAV viral vectors pseudotyped with viral capsids from serotypes 1, 2, and 5 display differential efficiency and cell tropism after delivery to different regions of the central nervous system. *Mol.Ther., 10,* 302-317.

Chen, X., Rzhetskaya, M., Kareva, T., Bland, R., During, M. J., Tank, A. W. et al. (2008). Antiapoptotic and trophic effects of dominant-negative forms of dual leucine zipper kinase in dopamine neurons of the substantia nigra in vivo. *J.Neurosci., 28,* 672-680.

Dauer, W. & Przedborski, S. (2003). Parkinson's disease: mechanisms and models. *Neuron, 39,* 889-909.

Deglon, N., Tseng, J. L., Bensadoun, J. C., Zurn, A. D., Arsenijevic, Y., Pereira de, A. L. et al. (2000). Self-inactivating lentiviral vectors with enhanced transgene expression as potential gene transfer system in Parkinson's disease. *Hum.Gene Ther., 11,* 179-190.

Fitzsimons, H. L., Bland, R. J., & During, M. J. (2002). Promoters and regulatory elements that improve adeno-associated virus transgene expression in the brain. *Methods, 28,* 227-236.

Gao, G. P., Alvira, M. R., Wang, L., Calcedo, R., Johnston, J., & Wilson, J. M. (2002). Novel adeno-associated viruses from rhesus monkeys as vectors for human gene therapy. *Proc.Natl.Acad.Sci.U.S.A, 99,* 11854-11859.

Grimm, D., Kay, M. A., & Kleinschmidt, J. A. (2003). Helper virus-free, optically controllable, and two-plasmid-based production of adeno-associated virus vectors of serotypes 1 to 6. *Mol.Ther., 7,* 839-850.

Hendriks, W. T., Eggers, R., Verhaagen, J., & Boer, G. J. (2007). Gene transfer to the spinal cord neural scar with lentiviral vectors: predominant transgene expression in astrocytes but not in meningeal cells. *J.Neurosci.Res., 85,* 3041-3052.

Hermening, S., Kugler, S., Bahr, M., & Isenmann, S. (2006). Improved high-capacity adenoviral vectors for high-level neuron-restricted gene transfer to the CNS. *J.Virol.Methods, 136,* 30-37.

Hermens, W. T., ter, B. O., Dijkhuizen, P. A., Sonnemans, M. A., Grimm, D., Kleinschmidt, J. A. et al. (1999). Purification of recombinant adeno-associated virus by iodixanol gradient ultracentrifugation allows rapid and reproducible preparation of vector stocks for gene transfer in the nervous system. *Hum.Gene Ther., 10,* 1885-1891.

Jakobsson, J., Ericson, C., Jansson, M., Bjork, E., & Lundberg, C. (2003). Targeted transgene expression in rat brain using lentiviral vectors. *J.Neurosci.Res., 73,* 876-885.

Kaplitt, M. G., Feigin, A., Tang, C., Fitzsimons, H. L., Mattis, P., Lawlor, P. A. et al. (2007). Safety and tolerability of gene therapy with an adeno-associated virus (AAV) borne GAD gene for Parkinson's disease: an open label, phase I trial. *Lancet, 369,* 2097-2105.

Kaplitt, M. G., Leone, P., Samulski, R. J., Xiao, X., Pfaff, D. W., O'Malley, K. L. et al. (1994). Long-term gene expression and phenotypic correction using adeno-associated virus vectors in the mammalian brain. *Nat.Genet., 8,* 148-154.

Klein, R. L., Dayton, R. D., Leidenheimer, N. J., Jansen, K., Golde, T. E., & Zweig, R. M. (2006). Efficient neuronal gene transfer with AAV8 leads to neurotoxic levels of tau or green fluorescent proteins. *Mol.Ther., 13,* 517-527.

Klein, R. L., Dayton, R. D., Tatom, J. B., Diaczynsky, C. G., & Salvatore, M. F. (2008). Tau expression levels from various adeno-associated virus vector serotypes produce graded neurodegenerative disease states. *Eur.J.Neurosci., 27,* 1615-1625.

Korecka, J. A., Verhaagen, J., & Hol, E. M. (2007). Cell-replacement and gene-therapy strategies for Parkinson's and Alzheimer's disease. *Regen.Med., 2,* 425-446.

Kugler, S., Kilic, E., & Bahr, M. (2003). Human synapsin 1 gene promoter confers highly neuron-specific long-term transgene expression from an adenoviral vector in the adult rat brain depending on the transduced area. *Gene Ther., 10,* 337-347.

Kugler, S., Lingor, P., Scholl, U., Zolotukhin, S., & Bahr, M. (2003). Differential transgene expression in brain cells in vivo and in vitro from AAV-2 vectors with small transcriptional control units. *Virology, 311,* 89-95.

Lein, E. S., Hawrylycz, M. J., Ao, N., Ayres, M., Bensinger, A., Bernard, A. et al. (2007). Genome-wide atlas of gene expression in the adult mouse brain. *Nature, 445,* 168-176.

Lim, S. T., Airavaara, M., & Harvey, B. K. (2010). Viral vectors for neurotrophic factor delivery: a gene therapy approach for neurodegenerative diseases of the CNS. *Pharmacol.Res., 61,* 14-26.

Liu, Y., Okada, T., Nomoto, T., Ke, X., Kume, A., Ozawa, K. et al. (2007). Promoter effects of adeno-associated viral vector for transgene expression in the cochlea in vivo. *Exp.Mol.Med., 39,* 170-175.

Lundberg, C., Bjorklund, T., Carlsson, T., Jakobsson, J., Hantraye, P., Deglon, N. et al. (2008). Applications of lentiviral vectors for biology and gene therapy of neurological disorders. *Curr.Gene Ther., 8,* 461-473.

Mandel, R. J., Manfredsson, F. P., Foust, K. D., Rising, A., Reimsnider, S., Nash, K. et al. (2006). Recombinant adeno-associated viral vectors as therapeutic agents to treat neurological disorders. *Mol.Ther., 13,* 463-483.

Manfredsson, F. P. & Mandel, R. J. (2010). Development of gene therapy for neurological disorders. *Discov.Med., 9,* 204-211.

Markakis, E. A., Vives, K. P., Bober, J., Leichtle, S., Leranth, C., Beecham, J. et al. (2010). Comparative transduction efficiency of AAV vector serotypes 1-6 in the substantia nigra and striatum of the primate brain. *Mol.Ther., 18,* 588-593.

Marks, W. J., Jr., Bartus, R. T., Siffert, J., Davis, C. S., Lozano, A., Boulis, N. et al. (2010). Gene delivery of AAV2-neurturin for Parkinson's disease: a double-blind, randomised, controlled trial. *Lancet Neurol., 9,* 1164-1172.

McCown, T. J. (2005). Adeno-associated virus (AAV) vectors in the CNS. *Curr.Gene Ther., 5,* 333-338.

McFarland, N. R., Lee, J. S., Hyman, B. T., & McLean, P. J. (2009). Comparison of transduction efficiency of recombinant AAV serotypes 1, 2, 5, and 8 in the rat nigrostriatal system. *J.Neurochem., 109,* 838-845.

Muramatsu, S., Fujimoto, K., Kato, S., Mizukami, H., Asari, S., Ikeguchi, K. et al. (2010). A phase I study of aromatic L-amino acid decarboxylase gene therapy for Parkinson's disease. *Mol.Ther., 18,* 1731-1735.

Orban, T. I., Apati, A., Nemeth, A., Varga, N., Krizsik, V., Schamberger, A. et al. (2009). Applying a "double-feature" promoter to identify cardiomyocytes differentiated from human embryonic stem cells following transposon-based gene delivery. *Stem Cells, 27,* 1077-1087.

Papale, A., Cerovic, M., & Brambilla, R. (2009). Viral vector approaches to modify gene expression in the brain. *J.Neurosci.Methods, 185,* 1-14.

Paterna, J. C., Feldon, J., & Bueler, H. (2004). Transduction profiles of recombinant adeno-associated virus vectors derived from serotypes 2 and 5 in the nigrostriatal system of rats. *J.Virol., 78,* 6808-6817.

Paterna, J. C., Moccetti, T., Mura, A., Feldon, J., & Bueler, H. (2000). Influence of promoter and WHV post-transcriptional regulatory element on AAV-mediated transgene expression in the rat brain. *Gene Ther., 7,* 1304-1311.

Peel, A. L. & Klein, R. L. (2000). Adeno-associated virus vectors: activity and applications in the CNS. *J.Neurosci.Methods, 98,* 95-104.

Ruitenberg, M. J., Eggers, R., Boer, G. J., & Verhaagen, J. (2002). Adeno-associated viral vectors as agents for gene delivery: application in disorders and trauma of the central nervous system. *Methods, 28,* 182-194.

Schneider, B., Zufferey, R., & Aebischer, P. (2008). Viral vectors, animal models and new therapies for Parkinson's disease. *Parkinsonism.Relat Disord., 14 Suppl 2,* S169-S171.

Sims, K., Ahmed, Z., Gonzalez, A. M., Read, M. L., Cooper-Charles, L., Berry, M. et al. (2008). Targeting adenoviral transgene expression to neurons. *Mol.Cell Neurosci., 39,* 411-417.

St Martin, J. L., Klucken, J., Outeiro, T. F., Nguyen, P., Keller-McGandy, C., Cantuti-Castelvetri, I. et al. (2007). Dopaminergic neuron loss and up-regulation of chaperone protein mRNA induced by targeted over-expression of alpha-synuclein in mouse substantia nigra. *J.Neurochem., 100,* 1449-1457.

Taymans, J. M., Vandenberghe, L. H., Haute, C. V., Thiry, I., Deroose, C. M., Mortelmans, L. et al. (2007). Comparative analysis of adeno-associated viral vector serotypes 1, 2, 5, 7, and 8 in mouse brain. *Hum.Gene Ther., 18,* 195-206.

Tuszynski, M. H., Thal, L., Pay, M., Salmon, D. P., HS, U., Bakay, R. et al. (2005). A phase 1 clinical trial of nerve growth factor gene therapy for Alzheimer disease. *Nat.Med., 11,* 551-555.

Ulusoy, A., Sahin, G., Bjorklund, T., Aebischer, P., & Kirik, D. (2009). Dose optimization for long-term rAAV-mediated RNA interference in the nigrostriatal projection neurons. *Mol.Ther., 17,* 1574-1584.

Wang, C. Y., Guo, H. Y., Lim, T. M., Ng, Y. K., Neo, H. P., Hwang, P. Y. et al. (2005). Improved neuronal transgene expression from an AAV-2 vector with a hybrid CMV enhancer/PDGF-beta promoter. *J.Gene Med., 7,* 945-955.

Wu, Z., Asokan, A., & Samulski, R. J. (2006). Adeno-associated virus serotypes: vector toolkit for human gene therapy. *Mol.Ther., 14,* 316-327.

Zolotukhin, S., Byrne, B. J., Mason, E., Zolotukhin, I., Potter, M., Chesnut, K. et al. (1999). Recombinant adeno-associated virus purification using novel methods improves infectious titer and yield. *Gene Ther., 6,* 973-985.

11

Progress and Challenges in AAV-Mediated Gene Therapy for Duchenne Muscular Dystrophy

Takashi Okada and Shin'ichi Takeda
National Institute of Neuroscience, National Center of Neurology and Psychiatry
Japan

1. Introduction

Duchenne muscular dystrophy (DMD) is the most common form of childhood muscular dystrophy. DMD is an X-linked recessive disorder with an incidence of one in 3500 live male births (Emery, 1991). DMD causes progressive degeneration and regeneration of skeletal and cardiac muscles due to mutations in the *dystrophin* gene, which encodes a 427-kDa subsarcolemmal cytoskeletal protein (Hoffman et al., 1987). DMD is associated with severe, progressive muscle weakness and typically leads to death between the ages of 20 and 35 years. Due to recent advances in respiratory care, much attention is now focused on treating the cardiac conditions suffered by DMD patients.

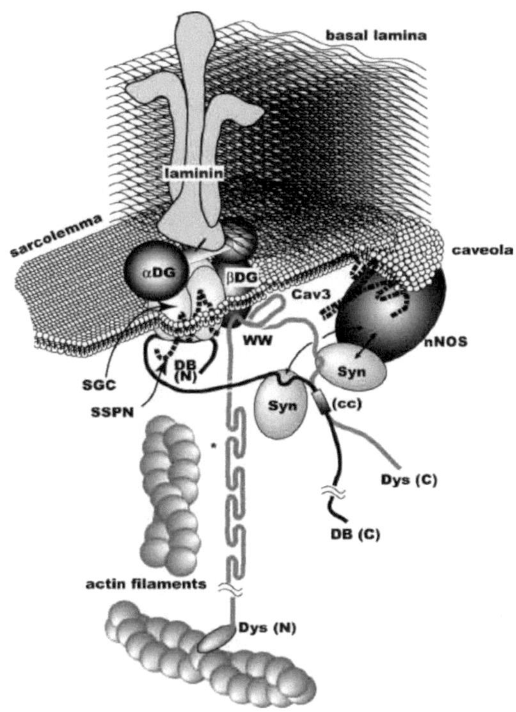

Fig. 1. Dystrophin-glycoprotein complex.

Molecular structure of the dystrophin-glycoprotein complex and related proteins superimposed on the sarcolemma and subsarcolemmal actin network (redrawn from Yoshida *et al.* (Yoshida et al., 2000), with modifications). cc, coiled-coil motif on dystrophin (Dys) and dystrobrevin (DB); SGC, sarcoglycan complex; SSPN, sarcospan; Syn, syntrophin; Cav3, caveolin-3; N and C, the N and C termini, respectively; G, G-domain of laminin; asterisk indicates the actin-binding site on the dystrophin rod domain; WW, WW domain.

The approximately 2.5-megabase *dystrophin* gene is the largest gene identified to date, and because of its size, it is susceptible to a high sporadic mutation rate. Absence of dystrophin and the dystrophin-glycoprotein complex (DGC) from the sarcolemma leads to severe muscle wasting (Figure 1). Whereas DMD is characterized by the absence of functional protein, Becker muscular dystrophy, which is commonly caused by in-frame deletions of the *dystrophin* gene, results in the synthesis of a partially functional protein.

2. Gene-replacement strategies using virus vectors

2.1 Choice of vector

Successful therapy for DMD requires the restoration of dystrophin protein in skeletal and cardiac muscles. While various viral vectors have been considered for the delivery of genes to muscle fibers, the adeno-associated virus (AAV)-based vector is emerging as the gene transfer vehicle with the most potential for use in DMD gene therapies. The advantages of the AAV vector include the lack of disease associated with a wild-type virus, the ability to transduce non-dividing cells, and the long-term expression of the delivered transgenes (Okada et al., 2002). Serotypes 1, 6, 8 and 9 of recombinant AAV (rAAV) exhibit a potent tropism for striated muscles (Inagaki et al., 2006). Since a 5-kb genome is considered to be the upper limit for a single AAV virion, a series of rod-truncated micro-dystrophin genes is used in this treatment (Yuasa et al., 1998).

Due to ingenious cloning and preparation techniques, adenovirus vectors are efficient delivery systems of episomal DNA into eukaryotic cell nuclei (Okada et al., 1998). The utility of adenovirus vectors has been increased by capsid modifications that alter tropism, and by the generation of hybrid vectors that promote chromosomal insertion (Okada et al., 2004). Also, gutted adenovirus vectors devoid of all adenoviral genes allow for the insertion of large transgenes, and trigger fewer cytotoxic and immunogenic effects than do those only deleted in the E1 regions (from bases 343 to 2270) (Hammerschmidt, 1999). Human artificial chromosomes (HACs) have the capacity to deliver a large gene (roughly 6-10 megabases) into host cells without integrating the gene into the host genome, thereby preventing the possibility of insertional mutagenesis and genomic instability (Hoshiya et al., 2008).

A goal in clinical gene therapy is to develop gene transfer vehicles that can integrate exogenous therapeutic genes at specific chromosomal loci, so that insertional oncogenesis is prevented. AAV can insert its genome into a specific locus, designated AAVS1, on chromosome 19 of the human genome (Kotin et al., 1992). The AAV Rep78/68 proteins and the Rep78/68-binding sequences are the trans- and cis-acting elements needed for this reaction. A dual high-capacity adenovirus-AAV hybrid vector with full-length human dystrophin-coding sequences flanked by AAV integration-enhancing elements was tested for targeted integration (Goncalves et al., 2005).

Gene correction is a process whereby sequence alterations in genes can be corrected by homologous recombination-mediated gene conversion between the recipient target locus and a donor construct encoding the correct sequence (Klug, 2005). The introduction of a corrective sequence together with a site-specific nuclease to induce a double-stranded break (DSB) at sites responsible for monogenic disorders would activate gene correction. Pairs of designated zinc-finger protein with tandem DNA binding sites fused to the cleavage domain of the Fok1 protein were introduced into model systems or cell lines and produced corrections in 10–30% of cases tested (Porteus and Baltimore, 2003).

2.2 Modification of the dystrophin gene and promoter

Due to the large deletion in its genome, the gutted adenovirus vector can package 14-kb of full-length *dystrophin* cDNA. Multiple proximal muscles of seven-day-old utrophin/dystrophin double knockout mice (*dko* mice), which typically show symptoms similar to human DMD, were effectively transduced with the gutted adenovirus bearing full-length murine *dystrophin* cDNA (Kawano et al., 2008). However, further improvements are needed to regulate the virus-associated host immune response before clinical trials can be performed.

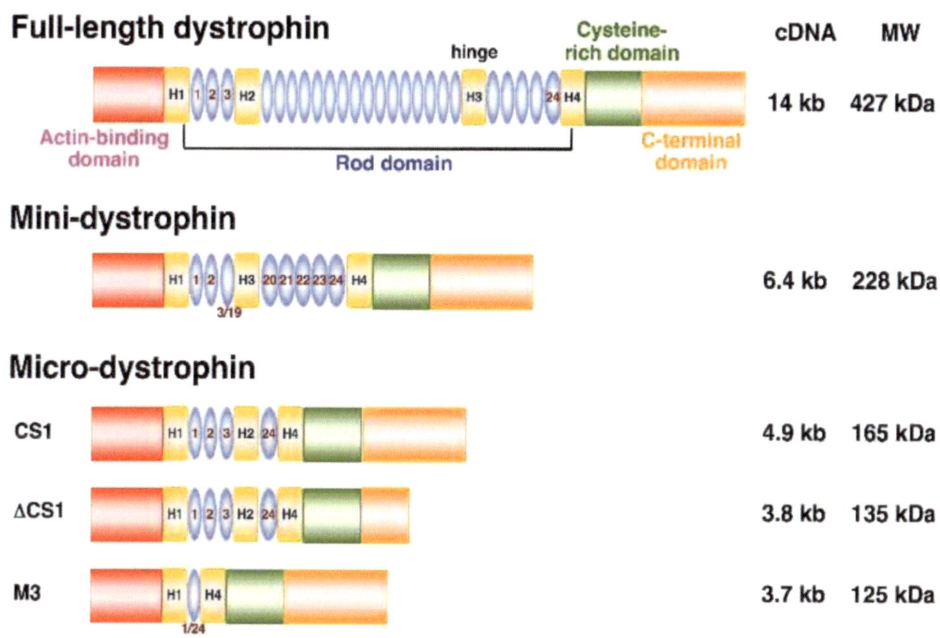

Fig. 2. Structures of full-length and truncated dystrophin.

Helper-dependent adenovirus vector can package 14-kb of full-length dystrophin cDNA because of the large-sized deletion in its genome. A mini-dystrophin is cloned from a patient with Becker muscular dystrophy, which is caused by in-frame deletions resulting in the synthesis of partially functional protein. A series of truncated micro-dystrophin cDNAs harboring only four rod repeats with hinge 1, 2, and 4 (CS1); the same components, except that the C-terminal domain is deleted (delta CS1); or one rod repeat with hinge 1 and 4 (M3), are constructed to be packaged in the AAV vector.

A series of truncated *dystrophin* cDNAs containing rod repeats with hinge 1, 2, and 4 were constructed (Figure 2) (Yuasa et al., 1998). Although AAV vectors are too small to package the full-length *dystrophin* cDNA, AAV vector-mediated gene therapy using a rod-truncated *dystrophin* gene provides a promising approach (Wang et al., 2000). The structure and, particularly, the length of the rod are crucial for the function of micro-dystrophin (Sakamoto et al., 2002). An AAV type 2 vector expressing micro-dystrophin (DeltaCS1) under the control of a muscle-specific MCK promoter was injected into the tibialis anterior (TA) muscles of dystrophin-deficient *mdx* mice (Yoshimura et al., 2004), and resulted in extensive and long-term expression of micro-dystrophin that exhibited improved force generation.

The impact of codon usage optimization on micro-dystrophin expression and function in the *mdx* mouse was assessed to compare the function of two different configurations of codon-optimized *micro-dystrophin* genes under the control of a muscle-restrictive promoter (Spc5-12) (Foster et al., 2008). Codon optimization of micro-dystrophin significantly increased micro-dystrophin mRNA and protein levels after intramuscular and systemic administration of plasmid DNA or rAAV8. By randomly assembling myogenic regulatory elements into synthetic promoter recombinant libraries, several artificial promoters were isolated whose transcriptional potencies greatly exceed those of natural myogenic and viral gene promoters (Li et al., 1999).

2.3 Use of surrogate genes

An approach using a surrogate gene would bypass the potential immune responses associated with the delivery of exogenous dystrophin. Methods to increase expression of utrophin, a dystrophin paralog, show promise as a treatment for DMD. rAAV6 harboring a murine codon-optimized micro-utrophin transgene was intravenously administered into adult *dko* mice to alleviate the pathophysiological abnormalities (Odom et al., 2008). The paralogous gene efficiently acted as a surrogate for *dystrophin*. Myostatin is extensively documented as being a negative regulator of muscle growth. Systemic gene delivery of myostatin propeptide, a natural inhibitor of myostatin, enhanced body-wide skeletal muscle growth in both normal and *mdx* mice (Qiao et al., 2008). The delivery of various growth factors, such as insulin-like growth factor-I (IGF-I), has been successful in promoting skeletal muscle regeneration after injury (Schertzer and Lynch, 2006).

Matrix metalloproteinases (MMPs) are key regulatory molecules in the formation, remodeling and degradation of all extracellular matrix (ECM) components in pathological processes. MMP-9 is involved predominantly in the inflammatory process during muscle degeneration (Fukushima et al., 2007). In contrast, MMP-2 is associated with ECM remodeling during muscle regeneration and fiber growth.

3. AAV-mediated transduction of animal models

3.1 Vector production

When adenovirus helper plasmid is co-transfected into human embryonic kidney 293 cells along with a vector plasmid encoding the AAV vector and an AAV packaging plasmid harboring *rep-cap* genes, the AAV vector is produced as efficiently as when using adenovirus infection. A large-scale transduction method to produce AAV vectors with an active gassing system makes use of large culture vessels for labor- and cost-effective transfection in a closed system. Samples containing vector particles are further purified with a two-tier CsCl gradient or dual ion-exchange chromatography to obtain highly purified vector particles.

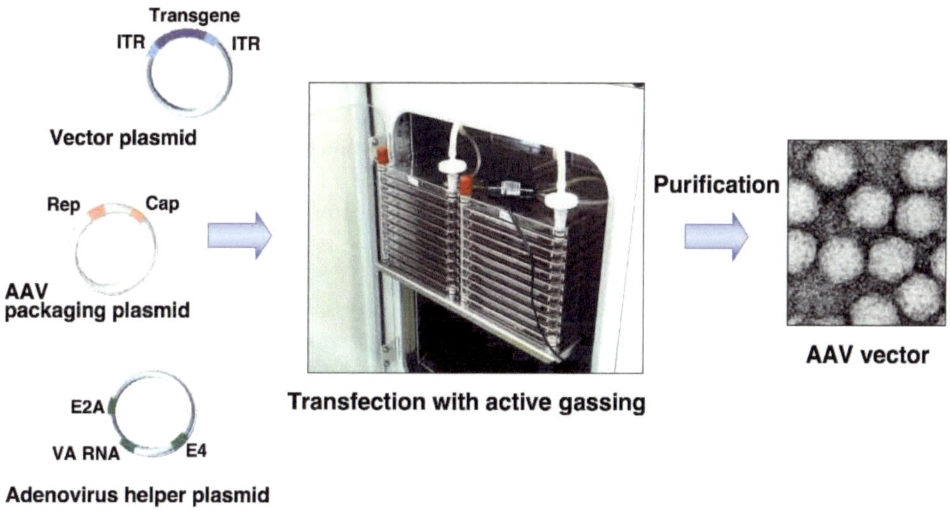

Fig. 3. A scalable triple plasmid transfection system using active gassing.

To gain acceptance as a medical treatment with a dose of over $1x10^{13}$ genome copies (g.c.)/kg body weight, AAV vectors require a scalable and economical production method. A production protocol of AAV vectors in the absence of a helper virus (Matsushita et al., 1998) is widely employed for triple plasmid transduction of human embryonic kidney 293 cells (Okada et al., 2002). The adenovirus regions that mediate AAV vector replication (namely, the VA, E2A and E4 regions) were assembled into a helper plasmid. When this helper plasmid is co-transfected into human embryonic kidney 293 cells along with plasmids encoding the AAV vector genome and *rep-cap* genes, the AAV vector is produced as efficiently as when using adenovirus infection (Figure 3). Importantly, contamination of most adenovirus proteins can be avoided in AAV vector stock made by this helper virus-free method. Samples containing vector particles are further purified with a two-tier CsCl gradient or dual ion-exchange chromatography to obtain highly purified vector particles (Okada et al., 2002).

Despite improvements in vector production, including the development of packaging cell lines expressing Rep/Cap, and of methods that induce the expression and regulation of Rep/Cap (Okada et al., 2001), maintaining such cell lines remains difficult, as the early expression of Rep proteins is toxic to cells. A scalable method, using active gassing and large culture vessels, was developed to transfect rAAV in a closed system, in a labor- and cost-effective manner (Okada et al., 2005). This vector production system achieved a yield of more than $5x10^{13}$ g.c./flask by improving gas exchange to maintain the physiological pH in the culture medium. Recent developments in ion-exchange chromatography also suggest that vector production using transduction culture supernatant would be compatible with current good manufacturing practice and production on an industrial scale (Okada et al., 2009). Moreover, AAV vector production in insect cells would be compatible with current good manufacturing practice production on an industrial scale (Cecchini et al., 2008).

3.2 Animal models for the gene transduction study

Dystrophin-deficient canine X-linked muscular dystrophy was found in a golden retriever with a 3′ splice-site point mutation in intron 6 (Valentine et al., 1988). The clinical and pathological characteristics of dystrophic dogs are more similar to those of DMD patients than are those of *mdx* mice. A beagle-based model of canine X-linked muscular dystrophy, which is smaller and easier to handle than the golden retriever-based muscular dystrophy dog (GRMD) model, has been established in Japan, and is referred to as $CXMD_J$ (Shimatsu et al., 2005). The limb and temporal muscles of $CXMD_J$ are affected by two-month-old, which is the age corresponding to the second peak of serum creatine kinase.

Interestingly, we found extensive lymphocyte-mediated immune responses to rAAV2-*lacZ* after direct intramuscular injection into $CXMD_J$ dogs, despite successful delivery of the same viral construct into mouse skeletal muscle (Yuasa et al., 2007). In contrast to rAAV2, rAAV8-mediated transduction of canine skeletal muscles produced significantly higher transgene expression with less lymphocyte proliferation than rAAV2 (Ohshima et al., 2008).

It is increasingly important to develop strategies to treat DMD that consider the effect on cardiac muscle. The pathology of the conduction system in $CXMD_J$ was analyzed to establish the therapeutic target for DMD (Urasawa et al., 2008). Although dystrophic changes of the ventricular myocardium were not evident at the age of 1 to 13 months, Purkinje fibers showed remarkable vacuolar degeneration when dogs were as young as four-months-old. Furthermore, degeneration of Purkinje fibers was coincident with overexpression of Dp71 at the sarcolemma. The degeneration of Purkinje fibers could be associated with the distinct deep Q waves present in ECGs and the fatal arrhythmias seen in cases of dystrophin deficiency (Urasawa et al., 2008).

3.3 Immunological Issues of rAAV

Neo-antigens introduced by AAV vectors evoke significant immune reactions in DMD muscle, since increased permeability of sarcolemma allows leakage of the transgene products from the dystrophin-deficient muscle fibers (Yuasa et al., 2002). rAAV2 transfer into skeletal muscles of normal dogs resulted in low and transient expression, together with intense cellular infiltration, and the marked activation of cellular and humoral immune responses (Yuasa et al., 2007). Furthermore, an *in vitro* interferon-gamma release assay showed that canine splenocytes respond to immunogens or mitogens more strongly than do murine splenocytes. In fact, co-administration of immunosuppressants, cyclosporine (CSP) and mycophenolate mofetil (MMF) improved rAAV2 transduction. The AAV2 capsids can induce a cellular immune response via MHC class I antigen presentation with a cross-presentation pathway, and rAAV2 has also been proposed to have an effect on human dendritic cells (DCs). In contrast, other serotypes, such as rAAV8, induced T-cell activation to a lesser degree (Ohshima et al., 2008). Immunohistochemical analysis revealed that the rAAV2-injected muscles showed higher rates of infiltration of $CD4^+$ and $CD8^+$ T lymphocytes in the endomysium than the rAAV8-injected muscles (Ohshima et al., 2008).

Resident antigen-presenting cells, such as DCs, myoblasts, myotubes and regenerating immature myofibers, might play a role in the immune response. A recent study also showed that mRNA levels of MyD88 and co-stimulating factors, such as CD80, CD86 and type I interferon, are elevated in both rAAV2- and rAAV8-transduced dog DCs *in vitro* (Ohshima et al., 2008). A brief course of immunosuppression with a combination of anti-thymocyte globulin (ATG), CSP and MMF was effective in permitting AAV6-mediated, long-term and robust expression of a canine micro-dystrophin in the skeletal muscle of a dog DMD model (Wang et al., 2007).

3.4 Intravascular vector administration by limb perfusion

Although recent studies suggest that vectors based on AAV are capable of body-wide transduction in rodents, translating this finding into large animals remains a challenge. Intravascular delivery can be performed as a form of limb perfusion, which might bypass the immune activation of DCs in the injected muscle (Ohshima et al., 2008). We performed limb perfusion-assisted intravenous administration of rAAV8-lacZ into the hind limb of normal dogs and rAAV8-micro-dystrophin into the hind limb of $CXMD_J$ dogs (Figure 4) (Ohshima et al., 2008). Administration of rAAV8-micro-dystrophin by limb perfusion produced extensive transgene expression in the distal limb muscles of $CXMD_J$ dogs without obvious immune responses for as long as eight weeks after injection.

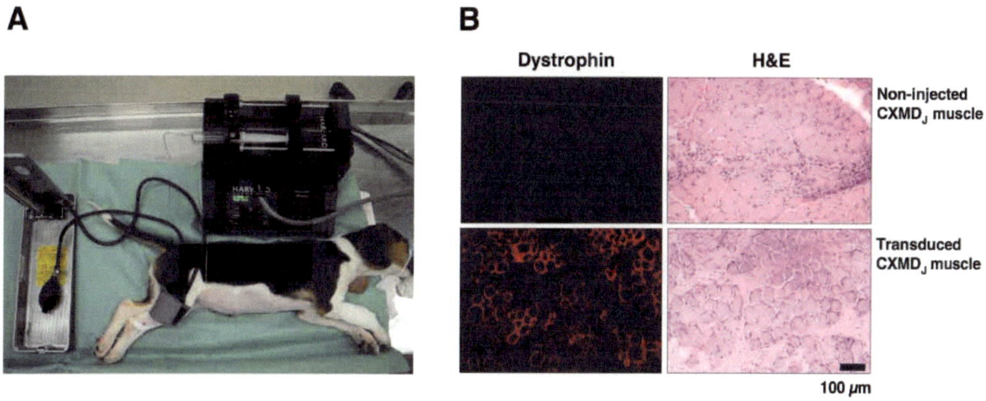

Fig. 4. Intravascular vector administration by limb perfusion.

(A) A blood pressure cuff is applied just above the knee of an anesthetized $CXMD_J$ dog. A 24-gauge intravenous catheter is inserted into the lateral saphenous vein, connected to a three-way stopcock, and flushed with saline. With a blood pressure cuff inflated to over 300 mmHg, saline (2.6 ml/kg) containing papaverine (0.44 mg/kg, Sigma-Aldrich, St. Louis, MO) and heparin (16 U/kg) is injected by hand over a 10 second period. The three-way stopcock is connected to a syringe containing rAAV8 expressing micro-dystrophin (1×10^{14} vg/kg, 3.8 ml/kg). The syringe is placed in a PHD 2000 syringe pump (Harvard Apparatus, Edenbridge, UK). Five minutes after the papaverine/heparin injection, rAAV8 is injected at a rate of 0.6 ml/sec. (B) Administration of rAAV8-micro-dystrophin by limb perfusion produces extensive transgene expression in the distal limb muscles of $CXMD_J$ dogs without obvious immune responses at four weeks after injection.

3.5 Global muscle therapies

In comparison with fully dystrophin-deficient animals, targeted transgenic repair of skeletal muscle, but not cardiac muscle, paradoxically elicits a five-fold increase in cardiac injury and dilated cardiomyopathy (Townsend et al., 2008). Because the dystrophin-deficient heart is highly sensitive to increased stress, increased activity by the repaired skeletal muscle provides the stimulus for heightened cardiac injury and heart remodeling. In contrast, a single intravenous injection of AAV9 vector expressing micro-dystrophin efficiently transduces the entire heart in neonatal *mdx* mice, thereby ameliorating cardiomyopathy (Bostick et al., 2008).

Since a number of muscular dystrophy patients can be identified through newborn screening, neonatal transduction may lead to an effective early intervention in DMD patients. After a single intravenous injection, robust skeletal muscle transduction with AAV9 vector throughout the body was observed in neonatal dogs (Yue et al., 2008). Systemic transduction was achieved in the absence of pharmacological intervention or immune suppression and lasted for at least six months, whereas cardiac muscle was barely transduced in the dogs.

4. Safety and potential impact of clinical trials

The initial clinical studies lay the foundation for future studies, providing important information about vector dose, viral serotype selection, and immunogenicity in humans. The first virus-mediated gene transfer for muscle disease was carried out for limb-girdle muscular dystrophy type 2D using rAAV1. The study, consisting of intramuscular injection of virus into a single muscle, was discharged to establish the safety of this procedure in phase I clinical trials (Rodino-Klapac et al., 2007). The first clinical gene therapy trial for DMD began in March 2006 (Mendell et al., 2010). This was a Phase I/IIa study in which an AAV vector was used to deliver micro-dystrophin to the biceps of boys with DMD. The study was conducted on six boys with DMD, each of whom was transduced with mini-dystrophin genes in a muscle of one arm in the absence of serious adverse events. Interestingly, dystrophin-specific T cells were detected after treatment, providing evidence of transgene expression. The potential for T-cell immunity to self and nonself dystrophin epitopes should be considered in designing and monitoring experimental therapies for this disease.

While low immunogenicity was considered a major strength supporting the use of rAAV in clinical trials, a number of observations have recently provided a more balanced view of this procedure (Manno et al., 2006). An obvious barrier to AAV transduction is the presence of circulating neutralizing antibodies that prevent the virion from binding to its cellular receptor (Scallan et al., 2006). This potential threat can be reduced by prescreening patients for AAV serotype-specific neutralizing antibodies or by performing procedures such as plasmapheresis before gene transfer. Another challenge recently revealed is the development of a cell-mediated cytotoxic T-cell (CTL) response to AAV capsid peptides. In the human factor IX gene therapy trial in which rAAV was delivered to the liver, only short-term transgene expression was achieved and levels of therapeutic protein declined to baseline levels 10 weeks after vector infusion (Manno et al., 2006). This was accompanied by elevation of serum transaminase levels and a CTL response toward specific AAV capsid peptides. To overcome this response, transient immunosuppression may be required until AAV capsids are completely cleared. Additional findings suggest that T-cell activation requires AAV2 capsid binding to the heparan sulfate proteoglycan (HSPG) receptor, which would permit virion shuttling into a DC pathway, as cross-presentation (Vandenberghe et al., 2006). Exposure to vectors from other AAV clades, such as AAV8, did not activate capsid-specific T-cells.

5. Challenges and limitations of related strategies

5.1 Design of read-through drugs

To suppress premature stop codon mutations, treatments involving aminoglycosides and other agents have been attempted. PTC124, a novel drug capable of suppressing premature termination and selectively inducing ribosomal read-through of premature, but not normal, termination codons, was recently identified using nonsense-containing reporters (Welch et al., 2007). The selectivity of PTC124 for premature termination codons, its oral bioavailability and its pharmacological properties indicate that this drug may have broad clinical potential for the treatment of a large group of genetic disorders with limited or no therapeutic options.

5.2 Modification of mRNA splicing

By inducing the skipping of specific exons during mRNA splicing, antisense compounds against exonic and intronic splicing regulatory sequences were shown to correct the open reading frame of the DMD gene and thus to restore truncated yet functional dystrophin expression *in vitro* (Takeshima et al., 1995). Intravenous infusion of an antisense phosphorothioate oligonucleotide created an in-frame *dystrophin* mRNA via exon skipping in a 10-year-old DMD patient possessing an out-of-frame exon 20 deletion of the *dystrophin* gene (Takeshima et al., 2006). Moreover, the adverse-event profile and local dystrophin-restoring effect of a single intramuscular injection of an antisense 2'-O-methyl phosphorothioate oligonucleotide, PRO051, in patients with DMD were explored (van Deutekom et al., 2007). Four patients received a dose of 0.8 mg of PRO051 in the TA muscle. Each patient showed specific skipping of exon 51 of dystrophin in 64 to 97% of myofibers, without clinically apparent adverse side effects.

The efficacy and toxicity of intravenous injection of stable morpholino phosphorodiamidate (morpholino)-induced exon skipping were tested using $CXMD_J$ dogs, and widespread rescue of dystrophin expression to therapeutic levels was observed (Yokota et al., 2009). Furthermore, a morpholino oligomer with a designed cell-penetrating peptide can efficiently target a mutated *dystrophin* exon in cardiac muscles (Wu et al., 2008).

Long-term benefits can be obtained through the use of viral vectors expressing antisense sequences against regions within *dystrophin* gene. The sustained production of dystrophin at physiological levels in entire groups of muscles as well as the correction of muscular dystrophy were achieved by treatment with exon-skipping AAV1-U7 (Goyenvalle et al., 2004).

5.3 *Ex vivo* gene therapy

Transplantation of genetically corrected autologous myogenic cells is a possible treatment for DMD. Freshly isolated satellite cells transduced with lentiviral vectors expressing micro-dystrophin were transplanted into the TA muscles of *mdx* mice, and these cells efficiently contributed to the regeneration of muscles with micro-dystrophin expression at the sarcolemma (Ikemoto et al., 2007). Mesoangioblasts are vessel-associated stem cells and might be candidates for future stem cell therapy for DMD (Sampaolesi et al., 2006). Intra-arterial delivery of wild-type canine mesoangioblasts resulted in the extensive recovery of *dystrophin* expression, normal muscle morphology and function in the GRMD. Multipotent mesenchymal stromal cells (MSCs) are less immunogenic and have the potential to differentiate and display a myogenic phenotype (Dezawa et al., 2005).

6. Future perspectives

6.1 Pharmacological Intervention

The use of a histone deacetylase (HDAC) inhibitor would likely enhance the utility of rAAV-mediated transduction strategies in the clinic (Okada et al., 2006). In contrast to adenovirus-mediated transduction, the improved transduction with rAAV induced by the HDAC inhibitor is due to enhanced transgene expression rather than to increased viral entry. The enhanced transduction was proposed to be related to the histone-associated chromatin form of the rAAV concatemer in transduced cells. Since various HDAC inhibitors are currently being tested in clinical trials for many diseases, the use of such agents in rAAV-mediated DMD gene therapy is theoretically and practically reasonable.

6.2 Capsid modification

A DNA shuffling-based approach for developing cell type-specific vectors is an intriguing possibility to achieve altered tropism. Capsid genomes of AAV serotypes 1-9 were randomly reassembled using PCR to generate a chimeric capsid library (Li et al., 2008). A single infectious clone (chimeric-1829) containing genome fragments from AAV1, 2, 8, and 9 was isolated from an integrin minus hamster melanoma cell line previously shown to have low permissiveness to AAV.

7. Conclusion

DMD remains an untreatable genetic disease that severely limits motility and life expectancy in affected children. The systemic delivery of rAAV to transduce truncated dystrophin is predicted to ameliorate the symptoms of DMD patients in the future. To translate gene transduction technologies into clinical practice, development of an effective delivery system with improved vector constructs as well as efficient immunological modulation must be established. A novel protocol that considers all of these issues would help improve the therapeutic benefits of DMD gene therapy.

8. Acknowledgment

This work was supported by the Grant for Research on Nervous and Mental Disorders, Health Science Research Grants for Research on the Human Genome and Gene Therapy; and the Grant for Research on Brain Science from the Ministry of Health, Labor and Welfare of Japan. This work was also supported by Grants-in-Aid for Scientific Research from the Ministry of Education, Culture, Sports, Science and Technology (MEXT). We would like to thank Dr. James M. Wilson for providing p5E18-VD2/8.

9. References

Bostick, B.; Yue, Y.; Lai, Y.; Long, C.; Li, D. & Duan, D. (2008). Adeno-associated virus serotype-9 microdystrophin gene therapy ameliorates electrocardiographic abnormalities in mdx mice. *Hum Gene Ther*, Vol.19, No.8, pp. 851-856, ISSN 1043-0342

Cecchini, S.; Negrete, A. & Kotin, R.M. (2008). Toward exascale production of recombinant adeno-associated virus for gene transfer applications. *Gene Ther*, Vol.15, No.11, pp. 823-830, ISSN 0969-7128

Dezawa, M.; Ishikawa, H.; Itokazu, Y.; Yoshihara, T.; Hoshino, M.; Takeda, S.; Ide, C. & Nabeshima, Y. (2005). Bone marrow stromal cells generate muscle cells and repair muscle degeneration. *Science*, Vol.309, No.5732, pp. 314-317, ISSN 0193-4511

Emery, A.E. (1991). Population frequencies of inherited neuromuscular diseases--a world survey. *Neuromuscul Disord*, Vol.1, No.1, pp. 19-29, ISSN 0960-8966

Foster, H.; Sharp, P.S.; Athanasopoulos, T.; Trollet, C.; Graham, I.R.; Foster, K.; Wells, D.J. & Dickson, G. (2008). Codon and mRNA sequence optimization of microdystrophin transgenes improves expression and physiological outcome in dystrophic mdx mice following AAV2/8 gene transfer. *Mol Ther*, Vol.16, No.11, pp. 1825-1832, ISSN 1525-0016

Fukushima, K.; Nakamura, A.; Ueda, H.; Yuasa, K.; Yoshida, K.; Takeda, S. & Ikeda, S. (2007). Activation and localization of matrix metalloproteinase-2 and -9 in the skeletal muscle of the muscular dystrophy dog (CXMDJ). *BMC Musculoskelet Disord*, Vol.8, pp. 54, ISSN 1471-2474

Goncalves, M.A.; Van Nierop, G.P.; Tijssen, M.R.; Lefesvre, P.; Knaan-Shanzer, S.; Van Der Velde, I.; Van Bekkum, D.W.; Valerio, D. & De Vries, A.A. (2005). Transfer of the full-length dystrophin-coding sequence into muscle cells by a dual high-capacity hybrid viral vector with site-specific integration ability. *J Virol*, Vol.79, No.5, pp. 3146-3162, ISSN 1098-5514

Goyenvalle, A.; Vulin, A.; Fougerousse, F.; Leturcq, F.; Kaplan, J.C.; Garcia, L. & Danos, O. (2004). Rescue of dystrophic muscle through U7 snRNA-mediated exon skipping. *Science*, Vol.306, No.5702, pp. 1796-1799, ISSN 0193-4511

Hammerschmidt, D.E. (1999). Development of a gutless vector. *J Lab Clin Med*, Vol.134, No.3, pp. C3, ISSN 0022-2143

Hoffman, E.P.; Brown, R.H., Jr. & Kunkel, L.M. (1987). Dystrophin: the protein product of the Duchenne muscular dystrophy locus. *Cell*, Vol.51, No.6, pp. 919-928, 0092-8674

Hoshiya, H.; Kazuki, Y.; Abe, S.; Takiguchi, M.; Kajitani, N.; Watanabe, Y.; Yoshino, T.; Shirayoshi, Y.; Higaki, K.; Messina, G.; Cossu, G. & Oshimura, M. (2008). A highly Stable and Nonintegrated Human Artificial Chromosome (HAC) Containing the 2.4 Mb Entire Human Dystrophin Gene. *Mol Ther*, pp. 309-317, ISSN 1525-0016

Ikemoto, M.; Fukada, S.; Uezumi, A.; Masuda, S.; Miyoshi, H.; Yamamoto, H.; Wada, M.R.; Masubuchi, N.; Miyagoe-Suzuki, Y. & Takeda, S. (2007). Autologous transplantation of SM/C-2.6(+) satellite cells transduced with micro-dystrophin CS1 cDNA by lentiviral vector into mdx mice. *Mol Ther*, Vol.15, No.12, pp. 2178-2185, ISSN 1525-0016

Inagaki, K.; Fuess, S.; Storm, T.A.; Gibson, G.A.; Mctiernan, C.F.; Kay, M.A. & Nakai, H. (2006). Robust systemic transduction with AAV9 vectors in mice: efficient global cardiac gene transfer superior to that of AAV8. *Mol Ther*, Vol.14, No.1, pp. 45-53, ISSN 1525-0016

Kawano, R.; Ishizaki, M.; Maeda, Y.; Uchida, Y.; Kimura, E. & Uchino, M. (2008). Transduction of full-length dystrophin to multiple skeletal muscles improves motor performance and life span in utrophin/dystrophin double knockout mice. *Mol Ther*, Vol.16, No.5, pp. 825-831, ISSN 1525-0016

Klug, A. (2005). Towards therapeutic applications of engineered zinc finger proteins. *FEBS Lett*, Vol.579, No.4, pp. 892-894, ISSN 0014-5793

Kotin, R.M.; Linden, R.M. & Berns, K.I. (1992). Characterization of a preferred site on human chromosome 19q for integration of adeno-associated virus DNA by non-homologous recombination. *Embo J*, Vol.11, No.13, pp. 5071-5078, ISSN 0261-4189

Li, W.; Asokan, A.; Wu, Z.; Van Dyke, T.; Diprimio, N.; Johnson, J.S.; Govindaswamy, L.; Agbandje-Mckenna, M.; Leichtle, S.; Redmond, D.E., Jr.; Mccown, T.J.; Petermann, K.B.; Sharpless, N.E. & Samulski, R.J. (2008). Engineering and selection of shuffled AAV genomes: a new strategy for producing targeted biological nanoparticles. *Mol Ther*, Vol.16, No.7, pp. 1252-1260, ISSN 1525-0016

Li, X.; Eastman, E.M.; Schwartz, R.J. & Draghia-Akli, R. (1999). Synthetic muscle promoters: activities exceeding naturally occurring regulatory sequences. *Nat Biotechnol*, Vol.17, No.3, pp. 241-245, ISSN 1087-0156

Manno, C.S.; Pierce, G.F.; Arruda, V.R.; Glader, B.; Ragni, M.; Rasko, J.J.; Ozelo, M.C.; Hoots, K.; Blatt, P.; Konkle, B.; Dake, M.; Kaye, R.; Razavi, M.; Zajko, A.; Zehnder, J.; Rustagi, P.K.; Nakai, H.; Chew, A.; Leonard, D.; Wright, J.F.; Lessard, R.R.; Sommer, J.M.; Tigges, M.; Sabatino, D.; Luk, A.; Jiang, H.; Mingozzi, F.; Couto, L.; Ertl, H.C.; High, K.A. & Kay, M.A. (2006). Successful transduction of liver in hemophilia by AAV-Factor IX and limitations imposed by the host immune response. *Nat Med*, Vol.12, No.3, pp. 342-347, ISSN 1078-8956

Matsushita, T.; Elliger, S.; Elliger, C.; Podsakoff, G.; Villarreal, L.; Kurtzman, G.J.; Iwaki, Y. & Colosi, P. (1998). Adeno-associated virus vectors can be efficiently produced without helper virus. *Gene Ther*, Vol.5, No.7, pp. 938-945, ISSN 0969-7128

Mendell, J.R.; Campbell, K.; Rodino-Klapac, L.; Sahenk, Z.; Shilling, C.; Lewis, S.; Bowles, D.; Gray, S.; Li, C.; Galloway, G.; Malik, V.; Coley, B.; Clark, K.R.; Li, J.; Xiao, X.; Samulski, J.; Mcphee, S.W.; Samulski, R.J. & Walker, C.M. (2010). Dystrophin immunity in Duchenne's muscular dystrophy. *N Engl J Med*, Vol.363, No.15, pp. 1429-1437, ISSN 0028-4793

Odom, G.L.; Gregorevic, P.; Allen, J.M.; Finn, E. & Chamberlain, J.S. (2008). Microutrophin delivery through rAAV6 increases lifespan and improves muscle function in dystrophic dystrophin/utrophin-deficient mice. *Mol Ther*, Vol.16, No.9, pp. 1539-1545, ISSN 1525-0016

Ohshima, S.; Shin, J.H.; Yuasa, K.; Nishiyama, A.; Kira, J.; Okada, T. & Takeda, S. (2008). Transduction Efficiency and Immune Response Associated With the Administration of AAV8 Vector Into Dog Skeletal Muscle. Mol Ther, pp. 73-91, ISSN 1525-0016

Okada, T.; Caplen, N.J.; Ramsey, W.J.; Onodera, M.; Shimazaki, K.; Nomoto, T.; Ajalli, R.; Wildner, O.; Morris, J.; Kume, A.; Hamada, H.; Blaese, R.M. & Ozawa, K. (2004). In situ generation of pseudotyped retroviral progeny by adenovirus-mediated transduction of tumor cells enhances the killing effect of HSV-tk suicide gene therapy in vitro and in vivo. *J Gene Med*, Vol.6, No.3, pp. 288-299, ISSN 1521-2254

Okada, T.; Mizukami, H.; Urabe, M.; Nomoto, T.; Matsushita, T.; Hanazono, Y.; Kume, A.; Tobita, K. & Ozawa, K. (2001). Development and characterization of an antisense-mediated prepackaging cell line for adeno-associated virus vector production. *Biochem Biophys Res Commun*, Vol.288, No.1, pp. 62-68., ISSN 1090-2104

Okada, T.; Nomoto, T.; Yoshioka, T.; Nonaka-Sarukawa, M.; Ito, T.; Ogura, T.; Iwata-Okada, M.; Uchibori, R.; Shimazaki, K.; Mizukami, H.; Kume, A. & Ozawa, K. (2005). Large-scale production of recombinant viruses by use of a large culture vessel with active gassing. *Hum Gene Ther*, Vol.16, No.10, pp. 1212-1218, ISSN 1043-0342

Okada, T.; Nonaka-Sarukawa, M.; Uchibori, R.; Kinoshita, K.; Hayashita-Kinoh, H.; Nitahara-Kasahara, Y.; Takeda, S. & Ozawa, K. (2009). Scalable purification of adeno-associated virus serotype 1 (AAV1) and AAV8 vectors, using dualion-exchange adsorptive membranes. *Hum Gene Ther*, Vol.20, No.9, pp. 1013-1021, ISSN 1043-0342

Okada, T.; Ramsey, J.; Munir, J.; Wildner, O. & Blaese, M. (1998). Efficient directional cloning of recombinant adenovirus vectors using DNA-protein complex. *Nucleic Acids Res.*, Vol.26, No.8, pp. 1947-1950, ISSN 0305-1048

Okada, T.; Shimazaki, K.; Nomoto, T.; Matsushita, T.; Mizukami, H.; Urabe, M.; Hanazono, Y.; Kume, A.; Tobita, K.; Ozawa, K. & Kawai, N. (2002). Adeno-associated viral vector-mediated gene therapy of ischemia-induced neuronal death. *Methods Enzymol*, Vol.346, pp. 378-393., ISSN 0076-6879

Okada, T.; Uchibori, R.; Iwata-Okada, M.; Takahashi, M.; Nomoto, T.; Nonaka-Sarukawa, M.; Ito, T.; Liu, Y.; Mizukami, H.; Kume, A.; Kobayashi, E. & Ozawa, K. (2006). A histone deacetylase inhibitor enhances recombinant adeno-associated virus-mediated gene expression in tumor cells. *Mol Ther*, Vol.13, No.4, pp. 738-746, ISSN 1525-0016

Porteus, M.H. & Baltimore, D. (2003). Chimeric nucleases stimulate gene targeting in human cells. *Science*, Vol.300, No.5620, pp. 763, ISSN 0193-4511

Qiao, C.; Li, J.; Jiang, J.; Zhu, X.; Wang, B.; Li, J. & Xiao, X. (2008). Myostatin propeptide gene delivery by adeno-associated virus serotype 8 vectors enhances muscle growth and ameliorates dystrophic phenotypes in mdx mice. *Hum Gene Ther*, Vol.19, No.3, pp. 241-254, ISSN 1043-0342

Rodino-Klapac, L.R.; Chicoine, L.G.; Kaspar, B.K. & Mendell, J.R. (2007). Gene therapy for duchenne muscular dystrophy: expectations and challenges. *Arch Neurol*, Vol.64, No.9, pp. 1236-1241, ISSN 0003-9942

Sakamoto, M.; Yuasa, K.; Yoshimura, M.; Yokota, T.; Ikemoto, T.; Suzuki, M.; Dickson, G.; Miyagoe-Suzuki, Y. & Takeda, S. (2002). Micro-dystrophin cDNA ameliorates dystrophic phenotypes when introduced into mdx mice as a transgene. *Biochem Biophys Res Commun*, Vol.293, No.4, pp. 1265-1272, ISSN 1090-2104

Sampaolesi, M.; Blot, S.; D'antona, G.; Granger, N.; Tonlorenzi, R.; Innocenzi, A.; Mognol, P.; Thibaud, J.L.; Galvez, B.G.; Barthelemy, I.; Perani, L.; Mantero, S.; Guttinger, M.; Pansarasa, O.; Rinaldi, C.; Cusella De Angelis, M.G.; Torrente, Y.; Bordignon, C.; Bottinelli, R. & Cossu, G. (2006). Mesoangioblast stem cells ameliorate muscle function in dystrophic dogs. *Nature*, Vol.444, No.7119, pp. 574-579, ISSN 0028-0836

Scallan, C.D.; Jiang, H.; Liu, T.; Patarroyo-White, S.; Sommer, J.M.; Zhou, S.; Couto, L.B. & Pierce, G.F. (2006). Human immunoglobulin inhibits liver transduction by AAV vectors at low AAV2 neutralizing titers in SCID mice. *Blood*, Vol.107, No.5, pp. 1810-1817, ISSN 0006-4971

Schertzer, J.D. & Lynch, G.S. (2006). Comparative evaluation of IGF-I gene transfer and IGF-I protein administration for enhancing skeletal muscle regeneration after injury. *Gene Ther*, Vol.13, No.23, pp. 1657-1664, ISSN 0969-7128

Shimatsu, Y.; Yoshimura, M.; Yuasa, K.; Urasawa, N.; Tomohiro, M.; Nakura, M.; Tanigawa, M.; Nakamura, A. & Takeda, S. (2005). Major clinical and histopathological characteristics of canine X-linked muscular dystrophy in Japan, CXMDJ. *Acta Myol*, Vol.24, No.2, pp. 145-154, ISSN 1128-2460

Takeshima, Y.; Nishio, H.; Sakamoto, H.; Nakamura, H. & Matsuo, M. (1995). Modulation of in vitro splicing of the upstream intron by modifying an intra-exon sequence which is deleted from the dystrophin gene in dystrophin Kobe. *J Clin Invest*, Vol.95, No.2, pp. 515-520, ISSN 0021-9738

Takeshima, Y.; Yagi, M.; Wada, H.; Ishibashi, K.; Nishiyama, A.; Kakumoto, M.; Sakaeda, T.; Saura, R.; Okumura, K. & Matsuo, M. (2006). Intravenous infusion of an antisense oligonucleotide results in exon skipping in muscle dystrophin mRNA of Duchenne muscular dystrophy. *Pediatr Res*, Vol.59, No.5, pp. 690-694, ISSN 0031-3998

Townsend, D.; Yasuda, S.; Li, S.; Chamberlain, J.S. & Metzger, J.M. (2008). Emergent dilated cardiomyopathy caused by targeted repair of dystrophic skeletal muscle. *Mol Ther*, Vol.16, No.5, pp. 832-835, ISSN 1525-0016

Urasawa, N.; Wada, M.R.; Machida, N.; Yuasa, K.; Shimatsu, Y.; Wakao, Y.; Yuasa, S.; Sano, T.; Nonaka, I.; Nakamura, A. & Takeda, S. (2008). Selective vacuolar degeneration in dystrophin-deficient canine Purkinje fibers despite preservation of dystrophin-associated proteins with overexpression of Dp71. *Circulation*, Vol.117, No.19, pp. 2437-2448, ISSN 0009-7322

Valentine, B.A.; Cooper, B.J.; De Lahunta, A.; O'quinn, R. & Blue, J.T. (1988). Canine X-linked muscular dystrophy. An animal model of Duchenne muscular dystrophy: clinical studies. *J Neurol Sci*, Vol.88, No.1-3, pp. 69-81, ISSN 1878-5883

Van Deutekom, J.C.; Janson, A.A.; Ginjaar, I.B.; Frankhuizen, W.S.; Aartsma-Rus, A.; Bremmer-Bout, M.; Den Dunnen, J.T.; Koop, K.; Van Der Kooi, A.J.; Goemans, N.M.; De Kimpe, S.J.; Ekhart, P.F.; Venneker, E.H.; Platenburg, G.J.; Verschuuren, J.J. & Van Ommen, G.J. (2007). Local dystrophin restoration with antisense oligonucleotide PRO051. *N Engl J Med*, Vol.357, No.26, pp. 2677-2686, ISSN 0028-4793

Vandenberghe, L.H.; Wang, L.; Somanathan, S.; Zhi, Y.; Figueredo, J.; Calcedo, R.; Sanmiguel, J.; Desai, R.A.; Chen, C.S.; Johnston, J.; Grant, R.L.; Gao, G. & Wilson, J.M. (2006). Heparin binding directs activation of T cells against adeno-associated virus serotype 2 capsid. *Nat Med*, Vol.12, No.8, pp. 967-971, ISSN 1078-8956

Wang, B.; Li, J. & Xiao, X. (2000). Adeno-associated virus vector carrying human minidystrophin genes effectively ameliorates muscular dystrophy in mdx mouse model. *Proc Natl Acad Sci U S A*, Vol.97, No.25, pp. 13714-13719, ISSN 0027-8424

Wang, Z.; Kuhr, C.S.; Allen, J.M.; Blankinship, M.; Gregorevic, P.; Chamberlain, J.S.; Tapscott, S.J. & Storb, R. (2007). Sustained AAV-mediated Dystrophin Expression in a Canine Model of Duchenne Muscular Dystrophy with a Brief Course of Immunosuppression. *Mol Ther*, Vol.15, No.6, pp. 1160-1166, ISSN 1525-0016

Welch, E.M.; Barton, E.R.; Zhuo, J.; Tomizawa, Y.; Friesen, W.J.; Trifillis, P.; Paushkin, S.; Patel, M.; Trotta, C.R.; Hwang, S.; Wilde, R.G.; Karp, G.; Takasugi, J.; Chen, G.; Jones, S.; Ren, H.; Moon, Y.C.; Corson, D.; Turpoff, A.A.; Campbell, J.A.; Conn, M.M.; Khan, A.; Almstead, N.G.; Hedrick, J.; Mollin, A.; Risher, N.; Weetall, M.; Yeh, S.; Branstrom, A.A.; Colacino, J.M.; Babiak, J.; Ju, W.D.; Hirawat, S.; Northcutt, V.J.; Miller, L.L.; Spatrick, P.; He, F.; Kawana, M.; Feng, H.; Jacobson, A.; Peltz, S.W. & Sweeney, H.L. (2007). PTC124 targets genetic disorders caused by nonsense mutations. *Nature*, Vol.447, No.7140, pp. 87-91, ISSN 0028-0836

Wu, B.; Moulton, H.M.; Iversen, P.L.; Jiang, J.; Li, J.; Li, J.; Spurney, C.F.; Sali, A.; Guerron, A.D.; Nagaraju, K.; Doran, T.; Lu, P.; Xiao, X. & Lu, Q.L. (2008). Effective rescue of dystrophin improves cardiac function in dystrophin-deficient mice by a modified morpholino oligomer. *Proc Natl Acad Sci U S A*, Vol.105, No.39, pp. 14814-14819, ISSN 0027-8424

Yokota, T.; Lu, Q.; Partridge, T.; Kobayashi, M.; Nakamura, A.; Takeda, S. & Hoffman, E.P. (2009). Efficacy of systemic morpholino exon-skipping in Duchenne dystrophy dogs. *Annals Neurol*, pp. 667-676, ISSN 0364-5134

Yoshida, M.; Hama, H.; Ishikawa-Sakurai, M.; Imamura, M.; Mizuno, Y.; Araishi, K.; Wakabayashi-Takai, E.; Noguchi, S.; Sasaoka, T. & Ozawa, E. (2000). Biochemical evidence for association of dystrobrevin with the sarcoglycan-sarcospan complex as a basis for understanding sarcoglycanopathy. *Hum Mol Genet*, Vol.9, No.7, pp. 1033-1040, ISSN 0964-6906

Yoshimura, M.; Sakamoto, M.; Ikemoto, M.; Mochizuki, Y.; Yuasa, K.; Miyagoe-Suzuki, Y. & Takeda, S. (2004). AAV vector-mediated microdystrophin expression in a relatively small percentage of mdx myofibers improved the mdx phenotype. *Mol Ther*, Vol.10, No.5, pp. 821-828, ISSN 1525-0016

Yuasa, K.; Miyagoe, Y.; Yamamoto, K.; Nabeshima, Y.; Dickson, G. & Takeda, S. (1998). Effective restoration of dystrophin-associated proteins in vivo by adenovirus-mediated transfer of truncated dystrophin cDNAs. *FEBS Lett*, Vol.425, No.2, pp. 329-336, ISSN 0014-5793

Yuasa, K.; Sakamoto, M.; Miyagoe-Suzuki, Y.; Tanouchi, A.; Yamamoto, H.; Li, J.; Chamberlain, J.S.; Xiao, X. & Takeda, S. (2002). Adeno-associated virus vector-mediated gene transfer into dystrophin-deficient skeletal muscles evokes enhanced immune response against the transgene product. *Gene Ther*, Vol.9, No.23, pp. 1576-1588, ISSN 0969-7128

Yuasa, K.; Yoshimura, M.; Urasawa, N.; Ohshima, S.; Howell, J.M.; Nakamura, A.; Hijikata, T.; Miyagoe-Suzuki, Y. & Takeda, S. (2007). Injection of a recombinant AAV serotype 2 into canine skeletal muscles evokes strong immune responses against transgene products. *Gene Ther*, Vol.14, No.17, pp. 1249-1260, ISSN 0969-7128

Yue, Y.; Ghosh, A.; Long, C.; Bostick, B.; Smith, B.F.; Kornegay, J.N. & Duan, D. (2008). A single intravenous injection of adeno-associated virus serotype-9 leads to whole body skeletal muscle transduction in dogs. *Mol Ther*, Vol.16, No.12, pp. 1944-1952, ISSN 1525-0016

12

Viral Vectors as Tools to Investigate the Role of Dysregulated Proteins in Nervous System Pathologies: The Case of Acquired Motor Neuropathies

Carmen R. Sunico and Bernardo Moreno-López
Grupo de NeuroDegeneración y NeuroReparación (GRUNEDERE), Universidad de Cádiz Spain

1. Introduction

Gene therapy involves the insertion, removal or alteration of genes within cells and tissues of a living organism. Although it emerged as a tool to correct hereditary diseases due to a non-functional or missing protein, gene therapy also constitutes an experimental tool to investigate gene function. Since the 1960s, most gene therapy studies are aimed at cancer and hereditary diseases. As a research tool, the most traditional form of gene therapy involves the insertion of a functional gene at a specific location in the host genome in order to replace a mutated or missing gene. This is accomplished by isolating and amplifying the gene of interest, generating a construct containing the necessary elements for the right expression, and inserting this construct into the host organism. Another current approach to the study of gene function involves the genetic engineering of knock-out animals (generally mice), in which a specific gene is turned off through a targeted mutation. The resulting phenotype of a knock-out mouse may provide valuable information regarding the function of the missing gene. However, in some cases the targeted gene is necessary for the embryonic development, in which case the knock-out of that gene is not feasible. Alternatively, individual development may be directed towards compensating for that knock-down gene, in which case the phenotype would not provide much relevant information. Another research tool to study gene function is to create a transgenic organism, which can be a microbe, a plant, a fruit fly, a mouse, a zebrafish, a worm … in which foreign, recombinant DNA (i.e., a transgene) is transferred directly into embryos to result in modified or novel genes. The resulting phenotype can provide valuable information about the role of genes in development, physiology, and disease. Although a transgene integrates in the host cell in a chromosomal location different from the endogenous site, the pattern of expression usually mimics that of the endogenous gene. Transgenic organisms are broadly used for agriculture, production of pharmaceutical drugs and proteins such as insulin, biomedical research, and gene therapy in experimental medicine.

Recent developments have provided us with different kinds of vectors to deliver, remove or modify genes within individual cells and tissues, bypassing undesirable effects of broad knock-down or transgene expression. Basically, vectors used in gene therapy for release of specific genes can be viral or non-viral. Non-viral vectors include naked DNA, oligonucleotides, dendrimers, lipoplexes, and polyplexes, as well as nanoengineered, organically modified silicates. However, whereas artificial DNA transfer methods have very low efficiency and are not useful for some types of cells, natural selection and evolution have led viruses to naturally develop specialized molecular mechanisms to efficiently transport their genomes into the cells that they infect. Delivery of genetic material by a virus is called transduction, and the infected cells are termed as transduced. Actually, the earliest DNA transfer method for bacteria was bacteriophages, which are still commonly used in experimentation. For mammalian cells, the first viral vectors were based on the monkey tumor virus SV40, in which some viral genes can be replaced by foreign genes. Nonetheless, the advantages of viruses like SV40 are limited because only a few genes can be inserted into their genome before the length of the DNA molecule becomes too large to be packed into the viral coat.

Additionally, the genetic material of SV40 is usually degraded after it infects the cells. Therefore, viral vectors experimentally designed for gene therapy are usually created from pathogenic viruses, whose infectivity is much more effective, but they are modified to minimize the biohazard. Modifications usually involve the elimination of part of the viral machinery necessary for their replication, so that the virus can efficiently infect the cells but lacks the necessary proteins for the production of new virions. Experimentally modified viral vectors also have low toxicity, which means minimal unwanted effects on the physiology and viability of the transduced cells. Additionally, lytic viruses, which kill the cells after replicating into them to propagate the infection, cannot be used as vectors. Thus, a limited number of nonlytic viruses modified from the *retrovirus, adenovirus (AVV),* and *adeno-associated virus* groups can be used in gene therapy to stably introduce a gene into a cell. Retroviruses insert the genetic material in the form of a RNA molecule, which will produce a DNA copy by the action of the enzyme reverse transcriptase. This viral DNA is efficiently inserted into the host genome as a provirus, where it permanently replicates together with host DNA at each cell division. However, most retroviruses can only infect dividing cells. *Lentiviruses* (LVVs, like HIV) are a subtype of retroviruses. AVVs and adeno-associated viruses insert their genome in the form of a DNA molecule. Adeno-associated viruses, so named because they need the help of an adenovirus for replication, are small viruses whose genome consists of a single stranded DNA molecule. Once the adeno-associated virus enters the nucleus, their single-stranded DNA becomes double-stranded and integrates into the host genome, like retroviruses. However, AVVs enter the nucleus but do not replicate, remaining as extrachromosomal double-stranded DNA molecules. As many differentiated cells in the brain and other tissues lack the capability to divide, LVVs, AVVs, and adeno-associated viruses are acquiring increasing popularity in gene therapy applications because they can transduce non-dividing cells.

Currently, gene therapy is mainly being focused on the study of genetic disorders such as cancer, diabetes mellitus, cardiovascular diseases and nervous system pathologies, among others. More specifically, regarding the applications in the nervous system, this chapter will highlight the potential of viral vectors as tools for the investigation of the role of altered proteins in neuropathological processes and review our recently published findings (Sunico et al., 2008; 2010; Sunico & Moreno-López, 2010; Montero et al., 2010) in the context of the existing literature. Briefly, we have used AVVs and LVVs to study the function of 2 dysregulated proteins in pathological events occurring at the peripheral (nerve) and central (motoneuron) levels after the severe crushing of a motor nerve in adult rats. The use of AVVs is proposed as a feasible gene therapy strategy for the enhancement of peripheral nerve regeneration in acquired peripheral neuropathies. Additionally, our outcomes support the promising benefits of gene therapy for the delivery of diverse genetic elements into specific populations of brain cells to treat several neurodegenerative disorders.

2. The case of acquired motor neuropathies: an useful experimental model to analyze protein dysregulation in neuropathological conditions

Most neurodegenerative disorders and prion diseases have common cellular and molecular mechanisms, including dysregulation of protein expression, function and/or aggregation. Alteration in the expression level of nitric oxide (NO) synthase (NOS) is a hallmark of Alzheimer (AD), Parkinson (PD), and Huntington diseases (HD), amyotrophic lateral sclerosis (ALS), multiple sclerosis (MS), and HIV dementia in humans and/or in animal models, as well as after peripheral and central traumatic lesions of the nervous system (Montero et al., 2010; Moreno-López et al., 2011). Subsequently, dysregulation of protein expression and/or function is a key event in a broad spectrum of neuropathological states. Unmasking the role of imbalanced proteins in anatomo-functional alterations of neurons in neurodegenerative disorders deserves attention. Our research has shown that viral vectors may be useful tools to explore the role of altered proteins in neuropathological processes. Using AVVs and LVVs, we studied the role of 2 NOS isoforms in pathological events occurring at the peripheral nerve and at the motoneuron after XIIth nerve crushing in adult rats.

NO is a short-lived, bioactive free radical which, as a gaseous molecule, freely crosses plasma membrane. NO and L-citrulline are the products of hydroxylation of a guanidine nitrogen of L-arginine and subsequent oxidization of the N^{ω}-hydroxy-L-arginine intermediate by NOS, a heme-containing enzyme that utilizes tetrahydrobiopterin (H_4B) as a redox cofactor. Electron transfer reactions carried out by NOS are regulated by a Ca^{2+}-binding protein (calmodulin). NOS also needs NADPH as an electron donor and requires molecular oxygen to carry out the reaction. In their active form, the known NOS enzymes form dimers in which each NOS monomer is associated with a calmodulin molecule. Three major isoforms of NOS have been identified, coded by different genes and differing in localization, regulation, catalytic properties, and inhibitor sensitivity. The nNOS isoform was the first to be purified and cloned (also known as NOS-I) and is predominantly found in the neuronal tissue. Through their specialized postsynaptic density-95/disks large/zona occludens-1 domains, nNOS can physically associate with postsynaptic density protein-95 (PSD-95). In turn, PSD-95 binds to motifs in the C-terminus of NMDA receptor NR2 subunits. These molecular interactions may provide the mechanistic basis for a functional coupling between Ca^{2+} influx through NMDA receptors and NO production. The iNOS isoform (also known as NOS-II) is inducible in a wide range of cells and tissues, including activated macrophages and, astroglia and microglia in the pathological CNS. This isotype is Ca^{2+}-independent and always catalytically active when expressed. However, iNOS is not the only isoform induced in pathological conditions. Finally, eNOS (or NOS-III) is the primary isoform found in vascular endothelial cells (Moreno-López et al., 2011).

Injured nerve fibers in the peripheral nervous system maintain the capacity to regenerate even over long distances in adult mammals. However, after nerve transection, stumps of damaged nerves must be surgically joined to guide regenerating axons into the distal nerve stump. Even so, severe functional limitations persist after restorative surgery. Since most previous studies have used nerve transection, it is important to signal distinctions between different forms of nerve lesion. Regenerative and survival capacities could be differentially compromised in adult motoneurons following transection or avulsion of the peripheral nerve. However, crushing of a motor nerve causes an immediate and complete suppression of neuromuscular connectivity but, unlike transection, it preserves the endoneural tube, thus providing neurotrophic support and a physical guide for the growing proximal axonal endings (Moreno-López, 2010). A few weeks after nerve crushing, muscle re-innervation takes place without significant neuronal loss. Therefore, traumatic injury by crushing is a plausible model for the identification of molecules that regulate degenerative and regenerative processes after acquired peripheral neuropathies.

2.1 A model of acquired motor neuropathy: the crushing of the XIIth nerve

We have developed a model of acquired peripheral motor neuropathy induced by a traumatic insult that causes a well-characterized range of functional and synaptic impairments in the insulted motoneurons. This experimental model has been useful to test the role and effectiveness of diverse factors in degenerative/regenerative processes after nerve injury by means of functional and anatomical approaches. The hypoglossal system - hypoglossal motoneurons (HMNs), XIIth nerve and their target muscle (the tongue)- has been well characterized by our group in physiological and pathological conditions (González-Forero et al., 2004; Montero et al., 2008; 2010; Sunico et al., 2005; 2008; 2010; 2011). This motor system offers several advantages, since muscle and motoneuron activities can be accurately measured and its peripheral and central partners are easily accessible to carry out damage strategies, local microinjections and electrophysiological recordings.

Crushing the XIIth nerve immediately induces a complete suppression of neuromuscular connectivity, demonstrated by the complete absence in the tongue of the compound muscle action potential (CMAP) evoked by electrical stimulation of the injured nerve at the proximal portion (Fig. 1). CMAP was completely absent for 1, 3 or 7 days after crushing, even when supramaximal nerve stimulation was applied. These results indicate that our method of nerve crushing effectively disconnected most HMNs from their targets for at least 1 week. Evidence of muscle re-innervation was obtained at 15 days after crushing. Subsequently, there was a slow and progressive recovery of CMAP and at 30 days after crushing its amplitude was similar to the control condition (Fig. 1).

In the hypoglossal nucleus (HN), most motoneurons discharge bursts of action potentials synchronized with the inspiratory phase of breathing (Fig. 2). This characteristic activity persists even after animal decerebration and/or under anesthesia. The main alterations observed in the firing pattern of HMNs following XIIth nerve crushing were an overall reduction in firing rates and an almost complete loss of modulation by chemosensory afferents. The inspiratory activity of motoneurons was modulated by chemoreceptor-driven changes in response to alterations in end tidal CO_2 (ET_{CO2}). The activity bursts of HMNs increased when ET_{CO2} rose and decreased when ET_{CO2} declined. One week after XIIth nerve crushing the chemosensory-mediated responsiveness of HMNs to ET_{CO2} changes decreased (Fig. 2). Synaptic stripping of HMNs after nerve injury is at least partially responsible for reduced response of motoneurons to chemoreceptor-modulated inspiratory drive (Fig. 2).

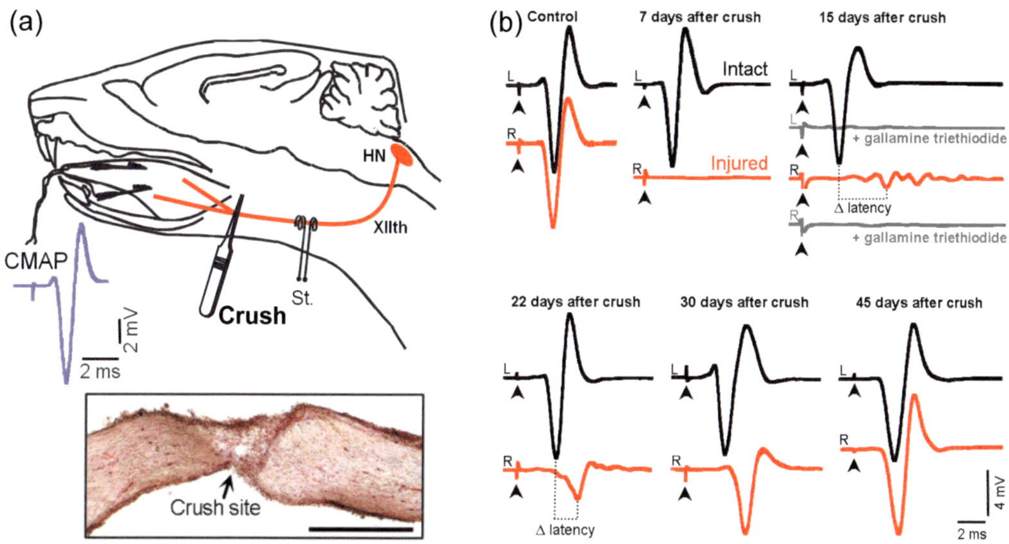

Fig. 1. Experimental design and time course of neuromuscular function recovery after XIIth nerve crushing. (a) To evaluate the time course of the neuromuscular function recovery, the compound muscle action potential (CMAP), evoked by electrical stimulation (St.) of the XIIth nerve, was recorded using electrodes implanted in the genioglossus muscle. Inset: Photomicrograph of a sagittal section at the level of the crushing site extracted 3 h after injury, stained by neutral red. Note that axons are fully transected but endoneural tube is preserved. Scale bar: 500 μm. (b) CMAPs evoked in the genioglossus muscle by single shock stimulation (arrowheads signal stimulus artifacts) of XIIth nerve in control and at 7, 15, 22, 30 and 45 days post-lesion. For comparison, CMAPs evoked by left (L, intact side) and right (R, crushed side) XIIth nerve stimulation are illustrated. Each trace represents an average of 10 individual traces. Dotted lines at 15 and 22 days represent how the Δ latency was calculated. Gray traces at 15 days represent the responses obtained in the same animal after injection of a neuromuscular blocker gallamine triethiodide in the genioglossus muscle. Note complete absence of CMAP on day 7 and the first signs of muscle re-innervation 15 days post-injury. Figure modified from Sunico et al., 2008 and Sunico & Moreno-López, 2010 (inset in (a)). © 2008 Elsevier Ltd and © 2010 Elsevier Ireland Ltd, respectively.

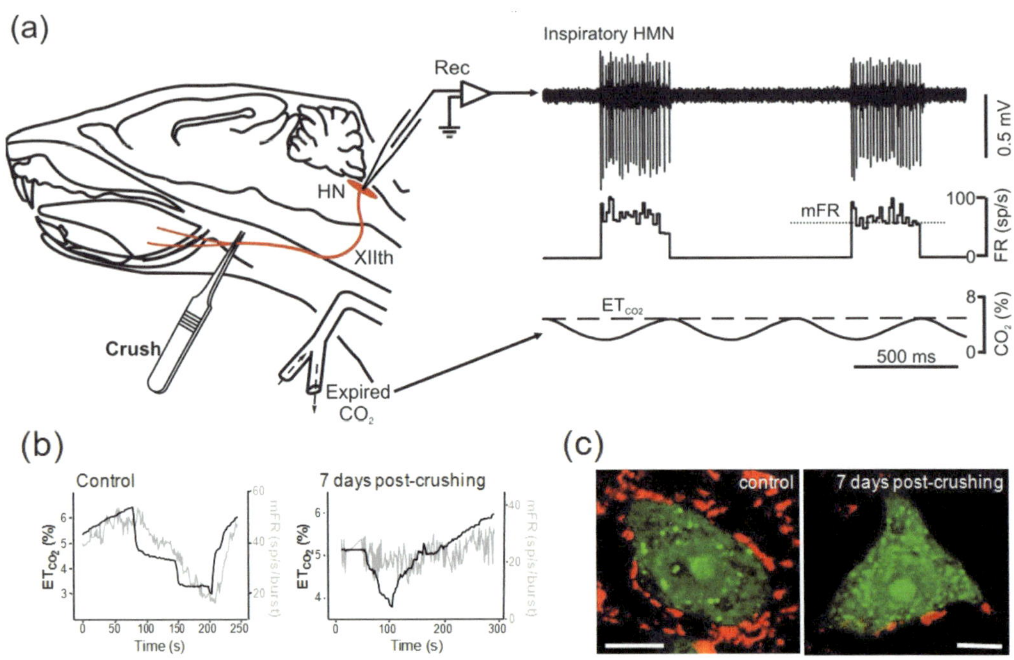

Fig. 2. XIIth nerve crushing induces a reduction of HMNs CO_2-modulated response and of their synaptic coverage. (a) Schematic diagram of the experimental preparation. Unitary discharge activity of HMNs and expired CO_2 were obtained in decerebrated, vagotomized rats, which had been injected with a neuromuscular blocking agent and lightly anesthetized. Right, characterization of firing properties of HMNs. From top to bottom, traces represent the extracellularly recorded spike discharge for a control inspiratory HMN, the instantaneous firing rate (FR, in spikes/s) and the partial pressure of CO_2 as a percentage of the expired air. Mean firing rate (mFR) per burst was measured and analyzed in relation to simultaneous ET_{CO2} measurements (dotted line in the middle trace). End-tidal CO_2 (ET_{CO2}) is indicated on the CO_2 record as a dashed line. (b) Illustrative examples of the time courses of the mean firing rate modulation (mFR, in spikes (sp)/s/burst; right y-axis; gray trace) relative to ET_{CO2} levels (left y-axis; black trace) for a control HMN and a motoneuron recorded 7 days after XIIth nerve crushing. (c) Confocal high-magnification photomicrographs of HMNs identified by the presence of a tongue-injected retrograde tracer (FluoroGold; green) in sections immunostained for the synaptic marker synaptophysin (red) obtained from control animals or 7 days after XIIth nerve crushing. Scale bars: 10 µm. Figure modified, with permission, from Gonzalez-Forero et al., 2004 (a); Sunico et al., 2005 (c) and Montero et al., 2010 (b). © 2004 The Physiological Society, © 2005 Society for Neuroscience and © 2010 The Physiological Society, respectively.

Up-regulation of NOS also happens as a consequence of different kinds of peripheral neuropathies. More specifically, after traumatic injury of a motor nerve, NOS expression is up-regulated at 3 different levels: in the damaged nerve, in the denervated muscle, and centrally at the injured motoneurons. In the distal stump of the affected nerve, all 3 major isoforms of NOS are up-regulated: iNOS is *de novo* expressed in dedifferentiated Schwann cells and in infiltrated macrophages, whereas nNOS is accumulated in the growing motor axons. However, eNOS, which is constitutively found in blood vessels, is overexpressed in *vasa nervorum* of the distal stump and around the injury site after the damage (Moreno-López, 2010). At the central level, nNOS, but not iNOS, is expressed *de novo* in the soma of motoneurons after traumatic motor nerve injury (Sunico et al., 2005). nNOS is then outwardly transported, accumulating in growing axons at the peripheral level (Moreno-López, 2010). However, eNOS induction has not been reported in injured motoneurons so far (Montero et al., 2010).

2.2 Using an AVV to accelerate and improve muscle re-innervation after acquired motor peripheral neuropathy

Evidences of NO as a harmful molecule for nerve regeneration show that systemic administration of N^{ω}-nitro-L-arginine methyl ester (L-NAME), a nonselective NOS inhibitor, improved motor nerve regeneration in mice after sciatic nerve transection (Zochodne & Levy, 2005). L-NAME also protected motoneurons from death and substantially increased the number that re-innervated the target muscle after facial nerve transection and repair, accompanied by improved motor function recovery (Wang et al., 2009). In the same direction, our studies showed that L-NAME treatment advanced the onset of neuromuscular reconnection after hypoglossal nerve crushing (Sunico et al., 2008). However, the pattern and time course of expression of each NOS isoform (Moreno-López, 2010) suggest that the NO from different origins could regulate diverse degenerative/regenerative processes after peripheral injury in a time-dependent manner. In nNOS or iNOS knockout mice, peripheral recovery was impaired after nerve injury due to delayed Wallerian degeneration, axon breakdown and Schwann cell reaction in the distal stump (Zochodne & Levy, 2005). Nevertheless, axon counts, myelination, and recovery of sensory and motor function in eNOS knockouts and wild-type mice were comparable after transection and reconstruction, although a delay of 2 days in revascularization was observed in eNOS knockout mice (Zochodne & Levy, 2005). The inherent risk of compensatory mechanisms for the disrupted enzyme during brain development is widespread in knockout animals. This may occur though a normally present redundant pathway and may be due to differences in expression of alternatively spliced isoforms of a particular NOS. For example, NOS catalytic activity levels in the brain of nNOS knockout mice are persistently low, which may mask the effect of nNOS deficiency (Moreno-López, 2010). Therefore, results obtained from knockouts, although useful, must be interpreted with caution.

Systemic application of relatively isoform-specific NOS inhibitors is another strategy that has been used to study the role of each isoform in degenerative/regenerative processes after nerve injury. nNOS or iNOS inhibition by the relatively specific inhibitors for nNOS 7-nitroindazole (7-NI), S-methyl-L-thiocitrulline (SMTC) and iNOS L-N6-(1-iminoethyl)-lysine hydrochloride (L-NIL), has contributed contradictory results. Whereas systemic administration of 7-NI, SMTC or L-NIL had beneficial effects on axonal regeneration after facial nerve transection and repair (Wang et al., 2009), positive effects were not obtained after XIIth nerve crushing by treatment with 7-NI or aminoguanidine (AG), another iNOS inhibitor (Sunico et al., 2008). Strikingly, administration of the relatively specific eNOS inhibitor L-N(5)-(l-iminoethyl)ornithine (L-NIO) accelerated the onset of muscle re-innervation after hypoglossal nerve crushing by promoting axonal regrowth (Sunico et al., 2008). Contradictions can be explained by differences in the lesion model and in the dose and relative specificity of NOS inhibitors (Moreno-López, 2010). In any case, these results pointed to eNOS as the major source of detrimental NO in axonal regeneration, at least in the first week after nerve injury.

In general, a strong consensus exists stating that NOS inhibition, at least during the first week after traumatic motor neuropathy, accelerates and improves motor function recovery. However, the administration route must be carefully taken into account. NO has important roles in the immunological, cardiovascular and nervous systems. Key physiological functions, such as learning, platelet aggregation, arterial blood pressure, and immune responses, could be disrupted by chronic and systemic NOS inhibition. NOS inhibition as a plausible treatment to improve functional recovery after nerve injury must bypass unwanted side effects of systemic administration of the inhibitors. The therapeutic strategy should entail specific inhibition of the proper NOS isoform that is detrimental to nerve regeneration and the selected NOS inhibitor should be locally administered (Moreno-López, 2010). Endothelial isoform has been described as having negative effects on functional recovery in the traumatic motor nerve injury model (Sunico et al., 2008), mainly inhibiting axonal regrowth. Due to the apparent involvement of eNOS in vasodilation of blood vessels and platelet aggregation, however, chronic systemic treatment with a specific eNOS inhibitor is not advised. Such a treatment can affect cardiovascular function, inducing hypertension and increasing the risk of thrombosis and atherosclerosis. Finally, systemic administration of NOS inhibitors is not advised because they cause motor deficits in mice and rats (Moreno-López, 2010). Feasible tools to improve motor function recovery after nerve injury without systemic side effects could involve local application of viral vectors. Promising results have been obtained by our group, which has reported that intraneural administration of an AVV expressing the dominant negative of eNOS (AVV-TeNOS) accelerated and improved motor function recovery after XIIth nerve crushing (Sunico et al., 2008).

To elucidate the role of eNOS, recombinant protein expression has been induced by viral transfection. There are different approaches to induce a full or partial "loss of function" using viral transgenesis. In this chapter we illustrate the use of a dominant negative protein, which interferes with the target protein or its function. To suppress eNOS activity, a recombinant AVV was used to express a truncated form of eNOS (TeNOS) under the control of the human cytomegalovirus (hCMV) promoter (Kantor et al., 1996). TeNOS, which lacks catalytic activity, acts as a dominant negative inhibitor of wild-type eNOS by heterodimerization with the native protein (Liu et al., 2011). As a viral control, a recombinant AVV was used to express the enhanced green fluorescent protein (eGFP) directed by the hCMV (AVV-eGFP). This gene therapy strategy successfully revealed the involvement of eNOS from the *nucleus tractus solitarii* in hypertension of spontaneously hypertensive rats (Kasparov et al., 2004; Waki et al., 2003; Waki et al., 2006; Paton et al., 2007). The expression of proteins under control of the hCMV promoter is characterized by a very rapid increase in expression, peaking 10 hr after transfection (Stokes et al., 2003).

Furthermore, when AVV-eGFP and AVV-TeNOS were injected in the nervous system, eGFP and TeNOS were expressed in glia and endothelial cells 7 days after transduction; expression diminished greatly at 14 days after vector injection (Waki et al., 2006). Therefore, a single intranerve injection of AVV-TeNOS could be expected to provide effective chronic inhibition of eNOS for at least 1 week in the transduced cells. It is noteworthy that this AVV did not retrogradely transduce motoneurons when injected into the nerve (Sunico et al., 2008; Moreno-López, 2010).

A single intranerve microinjection (3 μl) of AVV-TeNOS (2.2 x 10^{10} infective units/ml) on the day of the XIIth nerve crushing accelerated the recovery of neuromuscular transmission, resulting in a measurable CMAP 1 week after the damage (Fig. 3). Furthermore, the CMAP was fully recovered 22 days after the damage, which is 1 week earlier than in the untreated or eGFP transduced animals (Sunico et al., 2008). Stability of recovery was confirmed by the recording of a control-like CMAP from animals administered with AVV-TeNOS and studied at 62 days post-injury (Fig. 3). These results demonstrated that a single intraneural injection of the AVV-TeNOS efficiently accelerates the functional recovery of the neuromuscular junction after nerve injury (Sunico et al., 2008).

In addition, axonal regeneration was increased by AVV-TeNOS administration, compared with the AVV-eGFP treated group. Specifically, the number of retrogradely labeled motoneurons at 2 days after nerve crushing and intraneural injection of AVV-eGFP was significantly lower than that observed with AVV-TeNOS (Fig. 3). The number of retrogradely labeled HMNs at 7 days post-lesion in AVV-TeNOS-injected rats was similar to the control condition illustrating that AVV administration did not affect motoneuron viability (Sunico et al., 2008). Therefore, local eNOS inhibition with AVV-TeNOS speeds up neuromuscular functional recovery that is associated with accelerated axonal regeneration, among other possible mechanisms.

2.2.1 Cellular mechanisms that speed up axonal regrowth after nerve injury in AVV-TeNOS-treated animals

Schwann cells (SC) play a very important role in promoting axonal regeneration through the distal stump. After peripheral nerve axotomy, Wallerian degeneration involves axonal degradation as well as myelin breakdown and clearance in the distal stump of the injured nerve. For the subsequent axonal regeneration, SC dedifferentiation is required (Jessen & Mirsky, 2008). Thus, following nerve axotomy, SCs change from a myelin-producing state to a dedifferentiated, proliferating non-myelin-forming state (Stoll & Muller, 1999). In this dedifferentiated state, SCs are characterized by the formation of strands called bands of Bungner, which are the cellular substrate to guide growing axons, together with the up-regulation of several regeneration associated proteins, such as cell adhesion molecules, cytokines, neurotrophins, and growth factors that promote axonal regeneration (Araki et al., 2001; Stoll & Muller, 1999). More specifically, the growth-associated protein 43 kDa (GAP-43) is strongly up-regulated in regenerating axons and in dedifferentiated SCs (Curtis et al., 1992; Plantinga et al., 1993; Scherer et al., 1994). As soon as 1 day after transection or crushing of sciatic nerve, GAP-43 mRNA is significantly increased in the distal stump, remaining at high levels for at least 4 weeks (Plantinga et al., 1993). Thus, GAP-43 protein, which is involved in cell shape plasticity and motility (Curtis et al., 1992; Scherer et al., 1994), contributes to SC reorganization to form bands of Bungner in the degenerative/regenerative processes that take place after nerve injury.

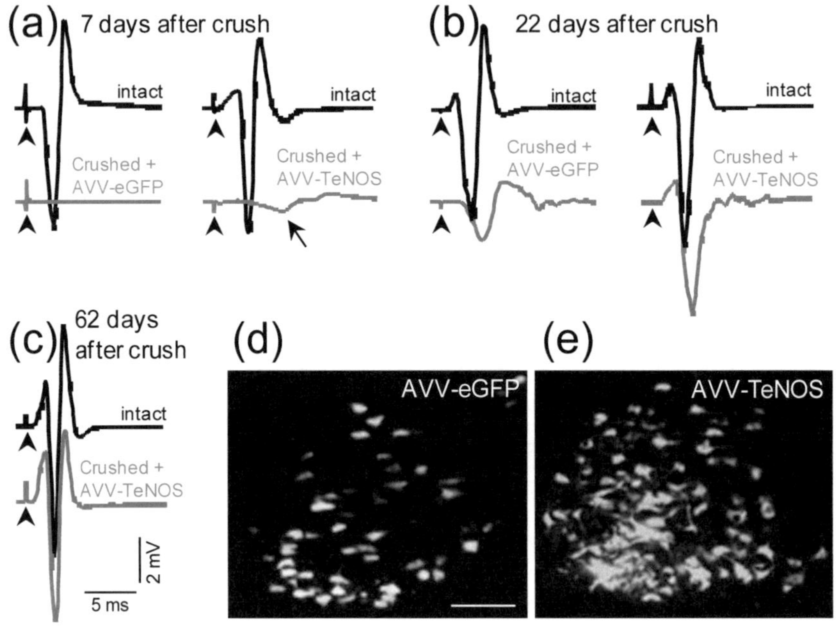

Fig. 3. Chronic intraneural inhibition of a dominant negative for eNOS using an AVV accelerates neuromuscular function recovery and axonal regeneration. (a)-(c) CMAPs evoked in the genioglossus muscle by single shock stimulation (arrowheads point to the stimulus artifact) of XIIth nerve at 7 (a), 22 (b), or 62 (c) days after intraneural injection of AVV-eGFP or AVV-TeNOS. For comparison, recordings obtained by stimulation of the left (intact) and right (crushed) XIIth nerve are illustrated. Each trace represents an average of 10 individual responses. (d), (e) Photomicrographs of coronal sections of the right HN showing FluoroGold-labeled motoneurons in animals injected with AVV-eGFP (d) or AVV-TeNOS (e) on the crushing day. FluoroGold was applied on day 2 post-crushing and the animals were perfused 7 days after retrograde marker application. Scale bar = 100 µm. Figure modified from Sunico et al., 2008. © 2008 Elsevier Ltd.

Given that AVV-TeNOS intraneural injection speeds up motor function recovery after XIIth nerve injury (Sunico et al., 2008), SCs were targeted to find out a feasible mechanism by which eNOS inhibition could enhance nerve regeneration, with the presumption that endothelial NO could be acting as a negative regulator of SC dedifferentiation after nerve crushing. To approach this issue, GAP-43 protein was analyzed in this study as a marker of regenerative processes, together with the density of SCs and bands of Bungner, in injured nerves after intraneural inhibition of eNOS. Indeed, our results indicate that endothelial NO confers a delaying action on SC dedifferentiation. As soon as 2 days following crushing of XIIth nerve together with AVV-TeNOS microinjection in the distal stump, GAP-43 immunoreactivity increases compared to control treatment with AVV-eGFP (Fig. 4). The reason for this, at least in part, could be an increase in GAP-43-positive cells, presumably SCs, after eNOS inhibition. Formation of bands of Bungner is also favored by TeNOS (Sunico & Moreno-López, 2010). Thereafter, all these data indicate that eNOS inhibition enhances the number of SCs and the subsequent formation of bands of Bungner after peripheral nerve injury (Fig. 4).

To summarize, negative regulators for myelination, which activates the SC dedifferentiation program, involve many extrinsic and intrinsic signals (Jessen & Mirsky, 2008). It is a well established fact that injury-related signals from neighboring SCs and neurons accelerate and influence SC dedifferentiation *in vivo* (Jessen & Mirsky, 2008). However, these recent studies also identify endothelial NO as a negative regulator of SC dedifferentiation, thus pointing to the vascular system as a source of signals that regulate some of the degenerative/regenerative processes that take place after peripheral nerve injuries (Sunico & Moreno-López, 2010). For this reason, the local endothelium is cautiously proposed in this chapter as a gene therapy target in the acute events that take place in peripheral neuropathies, and virally mediated eNOS antagonism is highlighted as a viable novel therapeutic strategy.

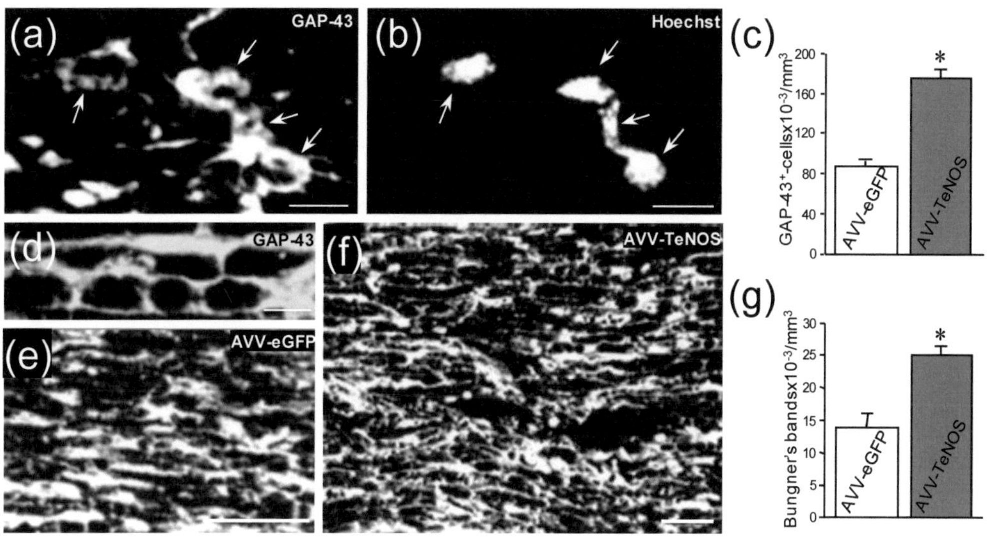

Fig. 4. TeNOS transgene increases the number of GAP-43 cells and bands of Bungner after XIIth nerve crushing. (a)-(c) GAP-43-immunoreactive (a) cells co-identified by Hoechst nuclear staining (b); the average number of GAP-43-positive cells (in thousands per cubic millimeter) at 4 and 5 mm distal to the injury site receiving the indicated adenoviruses is plotted (c). (d) Confocal high-magnification photomicrograph showing GAP-43-positive SCs forming two bands of Bunger disposed in parallel. (e)-(g) Confocal micrographs illustrating that after AVV-TeNOS injection the re-organization of SCs in bands of Bungner was more evident than in AVV-eGFP-treated injured nerves. The average number of bands of Bungner (in thousands per cubic millimeter) at 4 and 5 mm distal to the injury site receiving the indicated adenoviruses is plotted (g). Scale bars: (a), (b), (d), 10 µm; (e), (f), 50 µm. $^{*}P < 0.05$; non-parametric Mann-Whitney *U* test. Figure modified from Sunico & Moreno-López, 2010. © 2010 Elsevier Ireland Ltd.

2.3 Combinatory use of LVVs and AVVs to scrutinize the role of nNOS in central events occurring after traumatic nerve injury

Disconnection of motoneurons from their target myocytes interrupts mutual trophic relations, leading to deep alterations in the structural and physiological properties of both motoneurons and muscle fibers. Axotomy provokes changes in axonal, synaptic and intrinsic membrane properties, including enhanced somato-dendritic excitability, decreased axonal conduction speed, considerable loss of afferent synaptic contacts, and disorders in the firing properties and recruitment order of motor units (González-Forero et al., 2004; 2007). Synapse loss is the major feature underlying cognitive impairment in patients and/or animal models of AD, PD, MS, HD, and HIV-related dementia (Sunico et al., 2010; Moreno-López et al., 2011). Interestingly, synaptic alteration, rather than neuronal death, is the main factor responsible for the age-related downturn in neuronal function. Synapse loss also happens in several motor maladies, including ALS, progressive muscular atrophy, and traumatically-injured motor axons (Sunico et al., 2005; 2010). Interestingly, *de novo* expression of nNOS in motoneurons commonly occurs in response to the physical injury of a motor nerve and in the course of ALS. In both conditions, this event precedes synaptic withdrawal from motoneurons (Moreno-López et al., 2011). Changes in functional properties of injured cells also were prevented using various pharmacological agents targeting nNOS. NO-mediated disturbances involve changes in intrinsic membrane properties and anatomical synaptic deterioration that suggest a major pathological role of nNOS. However, nNOS is only one of the numerous proteins dysregulated after nerve damage. Therefore, the actual role for nNOS is less clear within the complex scenario created by multiple dysregulated proteins (Montero et al., 2010).

In an attempt to scrutinize whether nNOS up-regulation is sufficient to promote alterations after axonal injury on motoneurons, we have virally induced *de novo* expression of nNOS in non-axotomized HMNs together with complementary down-regulation of nNOS expression using virally mediated gene knock-down (Montero et al., 2010; Sunico et al., 2010). Replication-deficient recombinant AVVs (10^{10}-10^{11} infective units/ml), directing the expression of enhanced green or monomeric red fluorescent proteins (eGFP and mRFP, respectively) or nNOS, were injected into the tongue to retrogradely transduce HMNs (Fig. 5). AVVs expressed eGFP, mRFP, or nNOS downstream the hCMV promoter. The AVV-eGFP and AVV-mRFP vectors were used as controls to test virally induced side effects.

Neonatal HMNs were retrogradely transduced by injecting AVV-nNOS and/or AVV-eGFP into the genioglossus muscle. Ratiometric real-time NO imaging was used to record NO released around transduced HMNs in response to a glutamatergic stimulus (Fig. 5). For that purpose, the NO-sensitive fluorescent probe 1,2-diaminoanthraquinone sulphate (DAA) was perfused together with the reference dye Alexa 633. We found that the slope of DAA fluorescence increased around eGFP/nNOS-transduced motoneurons in response to glutamate, which was prevented by adding the NOS inhibitor L-NAME to the bath. This increase of NO created a gradient of concentration around the transduced HMNs, which in brain parenchyma showed a space constant of 12.3 μm. Thus, HMNs retrogradely transduced with AVV-nNOS express a functional enzyme that synthesizes NO in response to glutamatergic stimulation (Montero et al., 2010).

Retrograde cotransduction of adult HMNs, after injection in the tongue of AVV-eGFP/AVV-nNOS, induced a significant reduction in their synaptic coverage, as shown by immunohistochemistry and electron microscopy. Thus, nNOS transfection mimicked the effect of axonal injury on the synaptic coverage of HMNs. In this way, it seems clear that NO, synthesized by up-regulated nNOS in adult axotomized motoneurons, is not only necessary but also sufficient to trigger the molecular cascade leading to synapse withdrawal from HMN perikarya (Sunico et al., 2010; Moreno-López et al., 2011).

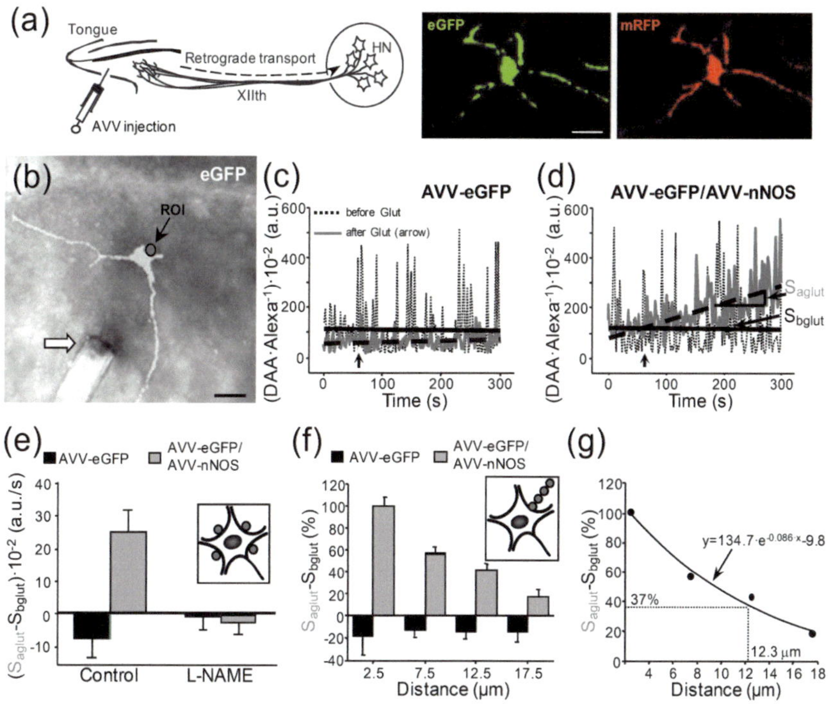

Fig. 5. AVV transfection of HMNs with functional nNOS. (a) Left, AVV injection into the tip of the tongue retrogradely transfected HMNs. Right, an illustrative example of a retrogradely cotransduced HMN after injection in the tip of the tongue of AVV-eGFP+AVV-mRFP. (b) Merged DIC and eGFP channels showing the tip of a pipette (arrow) ejecting dyes close to an eGFP-transfected HMN. The circle indicates the region of interest (ROI) used to construct the plot illustrated in (c). (c), (d) Time courses of the DAA/Alexa 633 ratio within a 5 µm diameter ROI placed just at the border of transfected HMNs by means of the indicated AVVs before and after addition to the perfusate of L-glutamate (500 µM; arrows). Slopes of the regression lines adjusted before (S_{bglut}) and after (S_{aglut}) glutamate addition are indicated in (d). The slope increase after Glut application in (d) result from a rise in DAA relative to Alexa fluorescence. This indicates that NO synthesized by transduced HMN interacts with the NO-sensitive dye DAA. (e) Averaged S_{aglut}–S_{bglut} was obtained from HMNs transfected with the specified AVVs and incubated with the indicated drugs. Drugs were added to the bath 5 min before glutamate. Inset, illustration signaling the location of ROIs analyzed per motoneuron. The average of S_{aglut}–S_{bglut} was taken as the representative HMN value. Prevention of the slope increase after Glut by pre-incubation with the NOS inhibitor L-NAME strongly suggests that the change in the slope is mediated by generation of NO. (f) NO gradient in brain tissue surrounding nNOS expressing HMNs. Average S_{aglut}–S_{bglut} was obtained from HMNs transfected with the indicated AVVs relative to the distance from the center of the ROI to the motoneuron border. Measures have been normalized relative to the value obtained in the ROI nearest to the motoneuron. Inset illustrates how ROIs were located for this type of measure. (g) Data presented in (f) were well fitted to the exponential decay equation used to calculate the theoretical space constant of the NO gradient created around AVV-nNOS transfected motoneurons. Scale bars: 50 µm. Figure modified, with permission, from Montero et al., 2010 (a) and Sunico et al., 2010 (b-g). © 2010 The Physiological Society and Society for Neuroscience, respectively.

For functional studies we injected AVV directly into the HN (Fig. 6). Five to 7 days after AVV administration, numerous neurons were identified as positively transfected at the injection site. Besides, a high number of astrocytes were also transfected, as confirmed by co-immunostaining against the astroglial cell marker glial fibrillary acidic protein (GFAP). Inspection of brainstem slices did not reveal eGFP-positive cell bodies in areas that project to the HN, such as the ventrolateral reticular formation (VLRF; Fig. 6). This argues against the possibility that our results could be affected by retrograde spread of AVV from the injection

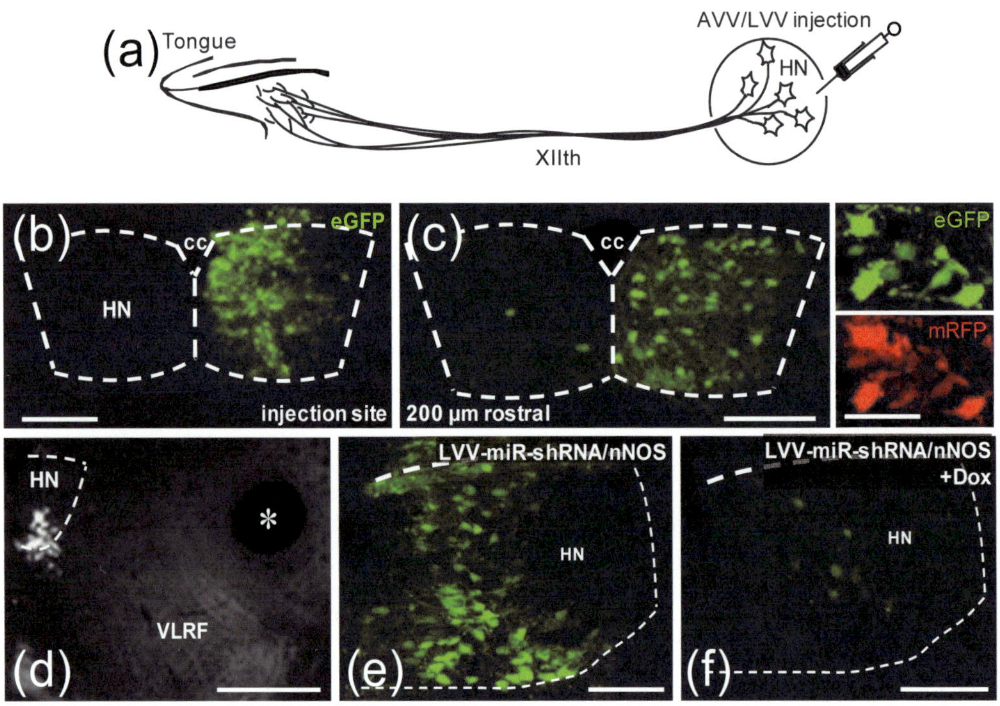

Fig. 6. Specificity of viral injections and transfections. (a) Schematic diagram of viral administration. AVV and LVV were administered into the HN. (b) Epifluorescence photomicrograph of a coronal section at the level of the HN obtained 6 days after intranuclear injection of AVV-eGFP. Note that injection was almost fully restricted to the HN; cc, central canal. (c) Photomicrograph of a coronal section obtained 7 days after viral administration at the indicated distance from the injection site showing a broad number of eGFP-expressing hypoglossal neurons. At this level a high frequency of co-transfection was observed after intranuclear injection of AVV-eGFP/AVV-mRFP (right panels). (d) Low magnification photomicrograph of a coronal section at the level of AVV-eGFP injection site, obtained 7 days after viral administration. Note the absence of infected neurons in neighboring regions, such as the ventrolateral reticular formation (VLRF), which project directly to the HN. Asterisk points to the mark that identifies the right side of the brainstem. (e), (f) Photomicrographs from coronal sections at the level of the injection place obtained 7 days after intranuclear injection of LVV-miR-shRNA/nNOS in untreated animals (e) and those receiving doxycycline (Dox) in the drinking water (f). Scale bars: (b), (e), (f) 250 µm; (c), (d) 500 µm; (c) right panels 100 µm. Figure modified from Montero et al., 2010. © 2010 The Physiological Society.

site. A large number of eGFP-positive neurons were identified, strictly within the HN, 200-300 μm rostrocaudal and ipsilateral to the injection site (Fig 6). Furthermore, astroglia was not transduced at these remote locations, as colocalization of eGFP and GFAP was absent there (Montero et al., 2010). Therefore, functional tests were performed in these areas away from the injection site to minimize any contaminating effects of nNOS transduction of astrocytes.

Unilateral AVV-nNOS microinjection in the HN of adult rats induced axotomy-like changes in HMNs such as alterations in axonal conduction properties and reduction in the responsiveness to synaptic drive (Montero et al., 2010). In AVV-eGFP-transfected animals, as in controls, the majority of HMNs display a characteristic respiratory pattern of bursts of action potentials that is synchronized with the inspiratory stage of breathing. In contrast, the mean firing rate in basal conditions (ET_{CO2}=4.8-5.2%) was considerably reduced after intranuclear microinjection of AVV-eGFP/AVV-nNOS (Fig. 7), likewise 1 week after hypoglossal nerve damage (Gonzalez-Forero et al., 2004). This reduction in the mean firing rate was prevented by chronic treatment with L-NAME or 7-NI, a relatively specific nNOS inhibitor. These results suggest that the reduction in the mean firing rate is evoked by NO synthesized by transduced nNOS in the HN.

To gain specificity in nNOS activity inhibition, we used a neuron-specific LVV to knock-down nNOS. This LVV system has been recently described (Liu et al., 2008; 2011). Briefly, for nNOS knock-down, we used a binary LVV system that requires co-operative action of 2 viral vectors. The first vector expresses tetracycline-sensitive transactivator Tet-off under control of an enhanced synapsin-1 promoter (Liu et al., 2008; 2011). The second LVV harbors an expression cassette for a miRNA30 (miR30)-based short hairpin (shRNA) interference system (Stegmeier et al., 2005) under control of a Tet-sensitive promoter. The system expresses a miRNA30-like hairpin targeting the gene of choice as a fusion with the eGFP, which facilitates targeting of the RNA duplex into the RNA-induced silencing pathway. Tet-off is able to bind tetracycline or similar molecules such as doxycycline (Dox); this renders it unable to bind to the Tet-sensitive promoter and blocks the expression of the hairpin (Fig. 6). This system is then referred to as LVV-miR-shRNA/nNOS.

nNOS-induced effects on mean firing rate were fully prevented by administration of LVV-miR-shRNA/nNOS before AVV-nNOS injection into the HN, indicating that nNOS expression in neurons, but not in glial or endothelial cells, affects mean firing rate (Fig 7).

In physiological conditions, the activity of HMNs increases when the ET_{CO2} rises, and decreases when the ET_{CO2} lowers. Axonal injury of HMNs induces a decrease in their response to chemoreceptor-modulated inspiratory drive (see Fig. 2; González-Forero et al., 2004) which was NO-mediated (Sunico et al., 2005). Strikingly, when HMNs are transduced with transgenic nNOS, their sensitivity to the chemoreceptor-modulated inspiratory drive is dramatically decreased, an alteration that was equivalent to the effects of crushing on motoneuron sensitivity to their afferent drive (Fig. 8). Chronic administration of L-NAME or 7-NI, as well as LVV-miR-shRNA/nNOS injection, protected against the changes in motoneuron sensitivity induced by *de novo* expression of nNOS. Altogether, these findings suggest that nNOS transgene-derived NO is sufficient to activate the molecular processes that lead to a decrease in motoneuron sensitivity to their afferent inputs.

NO-mediated synaptic withdrawal from motoneurons is an underlying factor that is at least partially responsible for functional changes induced by axonal injury of motoneurons

(Gonzalez-Forero et al., 2004; Sunico et al., 2005; 2010). We have recently reported that *de novo* synthesis of NO, induced by retrograde transduction of HMNs through muscle injection of AVV-nNOS, was sufficient to induce a withdrawal of synaptic boutons on HMNs (Sunico et al., 2010). This effect came together with a strong decline in the evoked excitatory postsynaptic potential on motoneurons *in vitro* (Sunico et al., 2010). Additionally, AVV-nNOS microinjection into the HN induced a reduction in the number of synaptic boutons apposed to HMNs, which could be prevented by preceding injection of LVV-miR-shRNA/nNOS (Fig. 8). Taken together, these observations indicate that main functional alterations induced in motoneurons by nNOS transgene expression or axotomy involve NO-directed synaptic re-arrangements.

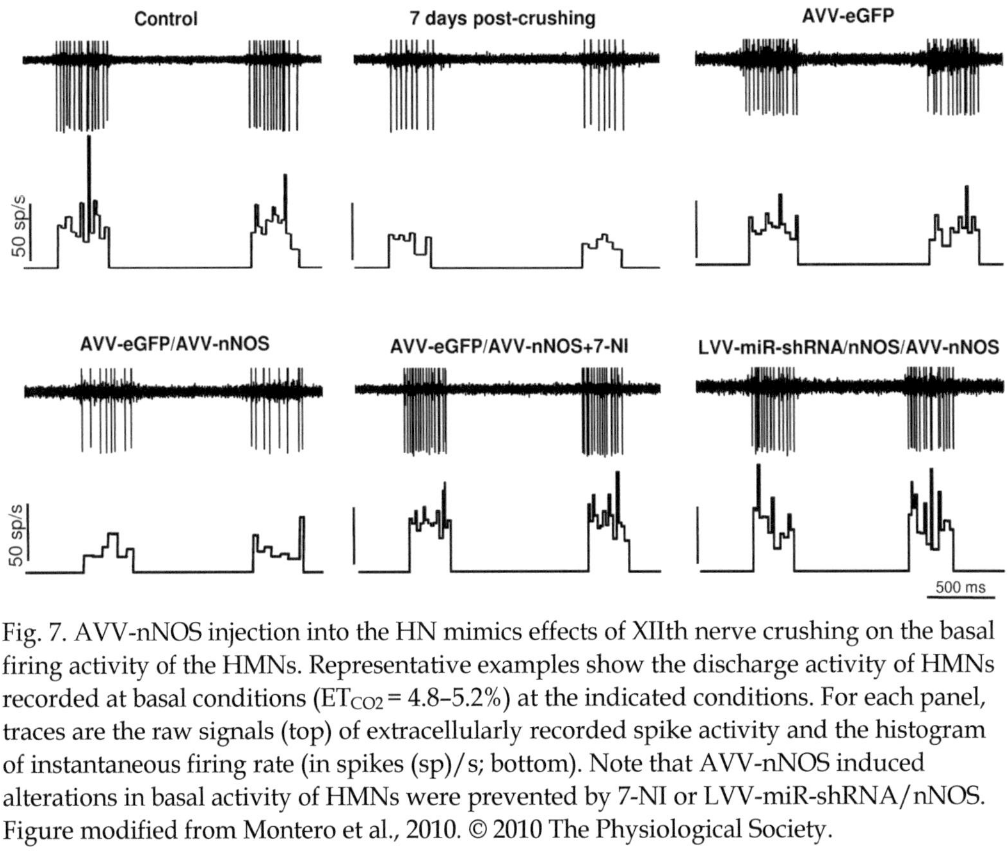

Fig. 7. AVV-nNOS injection into the HN mimics effects of XIIth nerve crushing on the basal firing activity of the HMNs. Representative examples show the discharge activity of HMNs recorded at basal conditions (ET_{CO2} = 4.8–5.2%) at the indicated conditions. For each panel, traces are the raw signals (top) of extracellularly recorded spike activity and the histogram of instantaneous firing rate (in spikes (sp)/s; bottom). Note that AVV-nNOS induced alterations in basal activity of HMNs were prevented by 7-NI or LVV-miR-shRNA/nNOS. Figure modified from Montero et al., 2010. © 2010 The Physiological Society.

In summary, we suggest that *de novo* expression of nNOS creates a repulsive gradient of NO around the motoneurons in an activity-dependent manner that can alter their inherent membrane properties as well as their synaptic coating. These results further point to nNOS as a pivotal target for the development of tools for the treatment of peripheral neuropathies and neurodegenerative disorders characteristically accompanied by central up-regulation of nNOS. Additionally, this opens a line of research for a strategy to elucidate the role of dysregulated proteins in the neuronal impairment taking place in the course of several neuropathological situations.

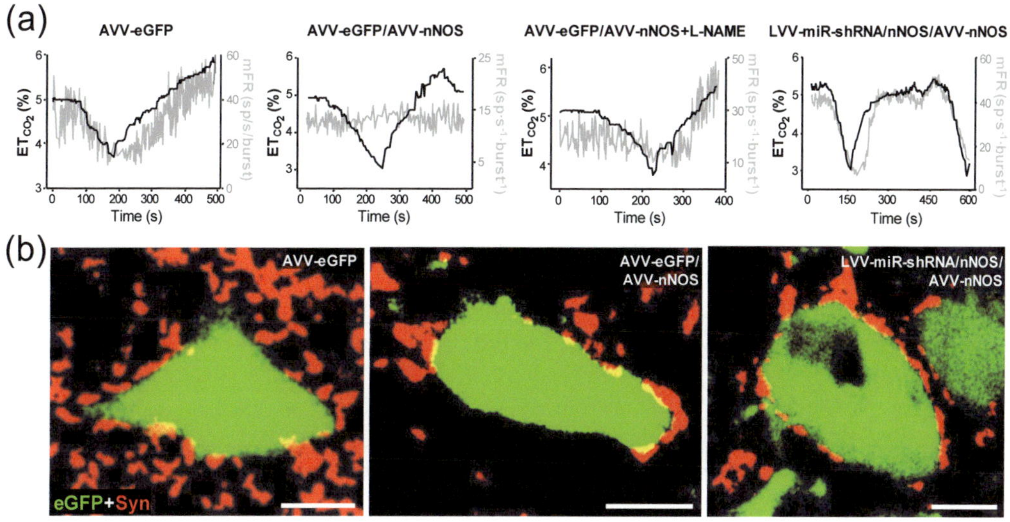

Fig. 8. AVV-nNOS injection into the HN mimics effects of XIIth nerve crushing on the chemoreceptor-modulated inspiratory activity of HMNs and on their synaptic coverage. (a) Illustrative examples of the time courses of the mean firing rate modulation (mFR, in spikes (sp)/s/burst; right y-axis) relative to ET_{CO2} levels (left y-axis) for HMNs recorded 7 days after the injection of the indicated viruses into the HN. Figure modified from Montero et al., 2010. © 2010 The Physiological Society.

3. Conclusions

Dysregulation of protein expression in specific cell populations of the central nervous system is a common hallmark in most neurodegenerative diseases. Ideally, this problem could be approached by somatic gene delivery targeted to specific cell types within a certain nucleus in order to increase or decrease the expression of a particular gene, with a precise control over the temporal expression of the transgenes. Transfection of cell lines with plasmids is a very efficient process, mainly thanks to the use of specific chemical reagents that increase the permeability of the cells. However, transfer of genes into a brain *in vivo* is still a challenging task. Nonetheless, gene delivery into brain cells using viral vectors has been successfully performed, even for long-term gene expression (Thomas et al., 2003; Papale et al., 2009). Likewise, viral vectors have been successfully used both *in vitro* and *in vivo* for the delivery of new genomic tools such as small interference RNAs (Snove and Rossi, 2006; Paddison, 2008).

As supported by our outcomes using an experimental model of peripheral neuropathy, the re-establishment of a functional gene through the insertion, removal, or modification of genes within cells and tissues is a very promising therapeutic alternative to chemicals for the treatment of human genetic disorders. Unfortunately, although in theory it could be considered as the holy grail, in practice each type of gene therapy still poses many challenges for use as a routine medical practice.

In germ line gene therapy, germ cells can be altered by the insertion of functional genes that integrate into their genomes, thus being inherited by later generations. However, numerous ethical, religious and technical reasons restrict this for application in human beings.

Conversely, in somatic gene therapy, the genes are introduced into somatic cells; therefore the effects will be restricted to the individual and will not be inherited by the offspring. However, we must be especially cautious with the vectors used for the gene delivery, particularly when viral vectors are used. Concerns about the risks of AVVs were raised during a gene therapy clinical trial in 1999, after an 18-year-old participant, Jesse Gelsinger, died because of a massive immune response triggered by the viral vector.

In our view, gene therapy represents a very promising tool that may ameliorate many human genetic diseases and neuropathological conditions accompanied by protein dysregulation at the expression and/or functional levels in the future. However, the nature of the diseases themselves and their genetic links must be more deeply understood before applying gene therapy. In the same way, the biological consequences of gene therapy need further evaluation, including its short-range and long-term side effects. Nonetheless, although gene therapy is still in its infancy, it has already been used *in vivo* with some success. The recent findings related to the treatment of acquired motor neuropathies described in this chapter highlight the therapeutic potential of this novel genetic tool.

4. Acknowledgement

Viral vectors were developed and real-time imaging experiments were performed in the Dr. Sergey Kasparov's laboratory (University of Bristol, UK). This work was supported by grants from the Ministerio de Ciencia e Innovación, (SAF2008-01415) and the Consejería de Innovación, Ciencia y Empresa from the Junta de Andalucía, (PAI2007-CTS-02606), both co-financed with FEDER funds and the Mútua Madrileña Foundation, Spain. We thank Elaine Lilly, Ph.D. (Writer's First Aid), for English language revision of the manuscript.

5. References

Curtis, R.; Stewart, H.J.; Hall, S.M.; Wilkin, G.P.; Mirsky, R. & Jessen, K.R. (1992). GAP-43 is expressed by nonmyelin-forming Schwann cells of the peripheral nervous system. *J Cell Biol* 116: 1455-64.

Gonzalez-Forero, D.; Portillo, F.; Sunico, C.R. & Moreno-López, B. (2004). Nerve injury reduces responses of hypoglossal motoneurones to baseline and chemoreceptormodulated inspiratory drive in the adult rat. *J Physiol* 557: 991-1011.

Gonzalez-Forero, D.; Portillo, F.; Gomez, L.; Montero, F.; Kasparov, S. & Moreno-López, B. (2007). Inhibition of resting potassium conductances by long-term activation of the NO/cGMP/protein kinase G pathway: A new mechanism regulating neuronal excitability. *J Neurosci* 27: 6302-6312.

Jessen, K.R. & Mirsky, R. (2008). Negative regulation of myelination: relevance for development, injury, and demyelinating disease. *Glia* 56: 1552-1565.

Kasparov, S.; Teschemacher, A.G.; Hwang, D.Y.; Kim, K.S.; Lonergan, T. & Paton, J.F. (2004). Viral vectors as tools for studies of central cardiovascular control. *Prog Biophys Mol Biol* 84: 251-277.

Liu, B.; Hewinson, J.; Xu, H.; Montero, F.; Sunico, C.R.; Portillo, F.; Paton, J.F.R.; Moreno-López, B. & Kasparov, S. (2011). *NOS antagonism using viral vectors as an experimental strategy: implications for in vivo studies of cardiovascular control and peripheral neuropathies.* In: *Nitric oxide, methods in molecular biology*, H.O. McCarthy, J.A. Coulter Eds, 197-223, Springer Science+Business Media, LLC 2011.

Liu, B.; Paton, J.F. & Kasparov, S. (2008). Viral vectors based on bidirectional cell specific mammalian promoters and transcriptional amplification strategy for use in vitro and in vivo. *BMC Biotechnol* 8: 49-57.

Montero, F.; Portillo, F.; González-Forero, D. & Moreno-López, B. (2008). The nitric oxide/cyclic guanosine monophosphate pathway modulates the inspiratory-related activity of hypoglossal motoneurons in the adult rat. *Eur J Neurosci* 28(1):107-116.

Montero, F.; Sunico, C.R.; Liu, B.; Paton, J.F.; Kasparov, S. & Moreno-López, B. (2010). Transgenic neuronal nitric oxide synthase expression induces axotomy-like changes in adult motoneurons. *J Physiol* 588: 3425-3443.

Moreno-López, B. (2010). Local isoform-specific NOS inhibition: a promising approach to promote motor function recovery after nerve injury. *J Neurosci Res* 88: 1846-1857.

Moreno-López, B.; Sunico, C.R. & González-Forero, D. (2011). NO orchestrates the loss of synaptic boutons from adult "sick" motoneurons: modeling a molecular mechanism. *Mol Neurobiol* 43(1): 41-66.

Paddison, P.J. (2008). RNA interference in mammalian cell systems. *Curr Top Microbiol Immunol* 320: 1-19.

Papale, A.; Cerovic, M. & Brambilla, R. (2009). Viral vector approaches to modify gene expression in the brain. *J Neurosci Methods* 15: 1-14.

Paton, J.F.; Waki, H.; Abdala, A.P.; Dickinson, J. & Kasparov, S. (2007). Vascular-brain signaling in hypertension: role of angiotensin II and nitric oxide. *Curr Hypertens Rep* 9: 242-247.

Plantinga, L.C.; Verhaagen, J.; Edwards, P.M.; Hol, E.M.; Bar, P.R. & Gispen, W.H. (1993). The expression of B-50/GAP-43 in Schwann cells is upregulated in degenerating peripheral nerve stumps following nerve injury. *Brain Res* 602: 69-76.

Scherer, S.S.; Xu, Y.T.; Roling, D.; Wrabetz, L.; Feltri, M.L. & Kamholz, J. (1994). Expression of growth-associated protein-43 kD in Schwann cells is regulated by axon-Schwann cell interactions and cAMP. *J Neurosci Res* 38: 575-589.

Snove, O. Jr. & Rossi, J.J. (2006). Expressing short hairpin RNAs in vivo. *Nat Methods* 3: 689-695.

Stegmeier, F.; Hu, G.; Rickles, R.J.; Hannon, G.J. & Elledge, S.J. (2005). A lentiviral microRNA-based system for single-copy polymerase II-regulated RNA interference in mammalian cells. *Proc Natl Acad Sci U S A* 102: 13212-7.

Stokes, C.E.; Murphy, D.; Paton, J.F. & Kasparov, S. (2003). Dynamics of a transgene expression in acute rat brain slices transfected with adenoviral vectors. *Exp Physiol* 88(4): 459-66.

Stoll, G. & Muller, H.W. (1999). Nerve injury, axonal degeneration and neural regeneration: basic insights. *Brain Pathol* 9: 313-325.

Sunico, C.R.; Domínguez, G.; García-Verdugo J.M.; Osta, R.; Montero F. & Moreno-López, B. (2011). Reduction in the motoneuron inhibitory/excitatory synaptic ratio in an early-symptomatic mouse model of amyotrophic lateral sclerosis. *Brain Pathol* 21: 1-15.

Sunico, C.R.; Gonzalez-Forero, D.; Domínguez, G.; García-Verdugo J.M. & Moreno-López, B. (2010). Nitric oxide induces pathological synapse loss by a protein kinase G-, Rho kinase-dependent mechanism preceded by myosin light chain phosphorylation. *J Neurosci* 30: 973-984.

Sunico, C.R. & Moreno-López, B. (2010). Evidence for endothelial nitric oxide as a negative regulator of Schwann cell dedifferentiation after peripheral nerve injury. *Neurosci Lett* 471: 119-124.

Sunico, C.R.; Portillo, F.; Gonzalez-Forero, D.; Kasparov, S. & Moreno-López, B. (2008). Evidence for a detrimental role of nitric oxide synthesized by endothelial nitric oxide synthase after peripheral nerve injury. *Neuroscience* 157: 40-51.

Sunico, C.R.; Portillo, F.; Gonzalez-Forero, D. & Moreno-López, B. (2005). Nitric oxide-directed synaptic remodeling in the adult mammal CNS. *J Neurosci* 25: 1448-1458.

Thomas, C.E.; Ehrhardt, A. & Kay, M.A. (2003). Progress and problems with the use of viral vectors for gene therapy. *Nat Rev Genet* 4: 346-358.

Waki, H.; Kasparov, S.; Wong, L.F.; Murphy, D.; Shimizu, T. & Paton, J.F. (2003). Chronic inhibition of endothelial nitric oxide synthase activity in nucleus tractus solitarii enhances baroreceptor reflex in conscious rats. *J Physiol* 546: 233-242.

Waki, H.; Murphy, D.; Yao, S.T.; Kasparov, S. & Paton, J.F. (2006). Endothelial NO synthase activity in nucleus tractus solitarii contributes to hypertension in spontaneously hypertensive rats. *Hypertension* 48: 644-650.

Wang, S.M.; Tsai, H.P.; Huang, J.J.; Huang, H.C.; Lin, J.L. & Liu, P.H. (2009). Inhibition of nitric oxide synthase promotes facial axonal regeneration following neurorrhaphy. *Exp Neurol* 216(2): 499-510.

Zochodne, D.W. & Levy, D. (2005). Nitric oxide in damage, disease and repair of the peripheral nervous system. *Cell Mol Biol (Noisy-le-grand)* 51(3): 255-67.

Part 4

Lentiviral Vector

13

Designing Lentiviral Gene Vectors

Oleg E. Tolmachov[1], Tanya Tolmachova[2] and Faisal A. Al-Allaf[3]
[1]*Cardiovascular Science, National Heart and Lung Institute, Faculty of Medicine, Imperial College London, London,*
[2]*Molecular Medicine, National Heart and Lung Institute, Faculty of Medicine, Imperial College London, London,*
[3]*Department of Medical Genetics, Faculty of Medicine, Umm Al-Qura University, Makkah,*
[1,2]*UK*
[3]*Saudi Arabia*

1. Introduction

Gene therapy relies on the delivery of therapeutic genes into patients' cells. The micro-devices used to reach the cells and to transfer the gene payload are called gene vectors. Viral packaging machinery is often utilized to generate the particles transporting the cargo genes. Lentiviruses, a subgroup of retroviruses, are highly suitable for remodeling into gene transfer vectors because they offer the stability of transgene expression, the ability to reach the nuclei of the therapeutically important non-dividing cells and are known to have a low immunogenic profile. Well studied members of the lentiviruses include human immunodeficiency viruses 1 and 2 (HIV-1 and HIV-2), feline immunodeficiency virus (FIV) and equine infectious anemia virus (EIAV).

It is important not to confuse "gene delivery vectors" and "gene cloning vectors". While the former are microparticles delivering genes, the latter are replicating vehicles for the amplification of nucleic acid sequences. "Gene delivery vectors" and "gene cloning vectors" coincide when the naked DNA of replicating bacterial plasmids or replication competent viruses is used for gene delivery into cells. Viral gene delivery vectors are normally non-replicating and should correctly be referred to as "viral vectors", not "viruses". Particles of viral vectors can be referred to as "virions" or "transducing particles", because viral gene transfer is traditionally described as "transduction". Replication deficient viral gene vector particles are similar to "defective interfering particles", that is, faulty non-self-viable virions arising during natural viral infections and competing with non-defective virions, which were described in virology literature many years ago.

Native lentiviral envelope proteins, which determine the cell range of viral infectivity (tropism) and mediate the fusion of viral and cellular membranes, are always composed from two non-covalently attached subunits, one of which (e.g. gp41 glycoprotein in HIV-1) is membrane-embedded and the other is an external subunit (e.g. gp120 glycoprotein in HIV-1). This arrangement makes lentiviruses notoriously unstable because of their tendency to shed the external subunit of the envelope protein. As the virion's stability is a pre-requisite for the effective purification and concentration of viral vector preparations, in lentiviral gene vectors native lentiviral envelope proteins are routinely replaced with stable heterologous viral envelope glycoproteins, most commonly G-protein of Vesicular Stomatitis Virus (VSV) or, alternatively, G protein of Rabies Virus. Both VSV and Rabies Virus belong to the family of rhabdoviruses. VSV-G protein has a broad tropism towards lipid membranes while rabies G has a distinct tropism to neural cells. The interchangeable use of envelope proteins by viruses belonging to different groups is very common and is called "pseudotyping". Lentiviral vectors can be pseudotyped with many other proteins, including artificially designed proteins, in order to improve infectivity for a particular cell type or, alternatively, to restrict the viral tropism. The rules of efficient pseudotyping are not yet completely clear, but one of the obvious requirements is the ability of the "cytoplasmic tails" of the membrane-embedded putative envelope proteins to fit into the available space between the viral capsid and the lipid envelope of the virion. Sometimes lentiviral vectors are pseudotyped by a cocktail of various viral, cellular or artificial membrane proteins. The structure of the lentiviral gene vector virion is presented in Figure 1.

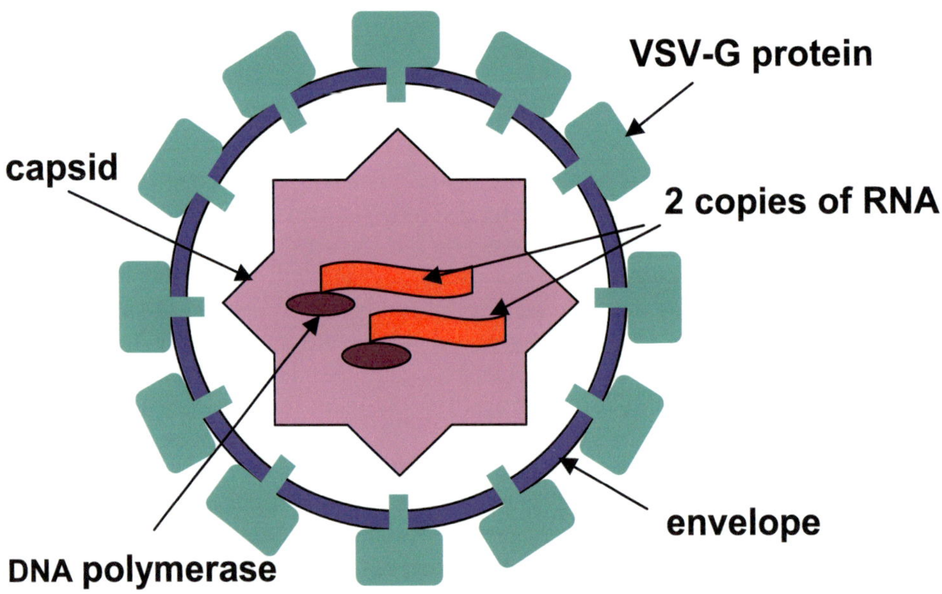

Fig. 1. A typical lentiviral vector particle

Lentiviral vectors are a promising tool for both *in vivo* and *ex vivo* gene therapy (Srinivasakumar 2001; Maier, von Kalle et al. 2010). These vectors can be used for therapeutic strategies relying on both transgene expression and gene correction (Al-Allaf, Coutelle et al. 2010). In addition, lentiviral gene vectors are extensively used in basic biomedical research to deliver genes for the expression of proteins and RNAs, e.g. shRNAs for gene knockdown. Lentiviral gene vectors are also being investigated as vaccines for immunization.

In some situations the use of classical lentiviral vectors can be compounded by the following problems: 1) insertional mutagenesis with a potential for malignant transformation; 2) relative difficulty of obtaining high titre concentrated viral vector preparations and the related problem of transduction inhibitors in the viral preparations; 3) toxicity of the commonly used VSV-G envelope protein at high multiplicity of infection; 4) limited insert capacity because of the RNA size packaging constraints specified by the lentiviral Gag complex.

Some of the above problems can be overcome. For example, contamination of lentiviral vector preparations with some inhibitors of infection can be avoided by the viral preparation concentration and purification by chromatography methods, which can be sufficiently gentle in comparison to ultracentrifugation based methods, which often result in a substantial fraction of the viral vector particles becoming inactivated. The reduction of viral vector losses during concentration is important, in particular because defective virions can compete with the functional virions and inhibit transduction (Geraerts, Willems et al. 2006). Perhaps the most dramatic improvement of the lentiviral vectors was the introduction of non-integrating lentiviral vectors, which do not cause genomic mutations arising via the random genomic integration of the classical lentiviral vectors (Section 5 of this review).

Lentiviral vectors can be assembled through transient co-transfection of the lentiviral vector backbone plasmid with helper plasmids expressing viral packaging functions or by stably transfected packaging cell lines. The first production method is currently a preferred choice because of its greater flexibility. A small undesirable possibility of reconstitution of the replication competent virus in the cells used for the lentiviral vector packaging can compromise safety. So, the chances of formation of a complete viral genome are customarily reduced by splitting genes for helper packaging functions between separate plasmids. For example, a common three-plasmid transient co-transfection packaging system employs a helper plasmid with genes for the structural Gag polyprotein, the catalytic GagPol polyprotein and the accessory HIV-1 Rev and Tat proteins (e.g. psPAX2) plus a helper plasmid for an envelope protein (e.g. VSV-G plasmid pMD2G). In a four-plasmid packaging system the genes for the Gag and GagPol functions on the one hand and the Rev function on the other hand are split between two different helper plasmids (with the Tat function missing altogether). Universally used cell lines for the packaging of lentiviral vectors in transient co-transfection are HEK293 cell line and its derivatives. HEK293 cells were produced by selecting an individual immortalised clone among a mixed population of human embryonic kidney cells transformed with DNA fragments of adenovirus type 5. HEK293 cells can be efficiently transfected by the calcium phosphate method, protocols involving cationic lipids (e.g. Fugene 6 and Fugene HD) or electroporation. Contamination of plasmid DNA with co-purifying bacterial lypopolysaccharides should be avoided, as these endotoxins can substantially reduce the efficiency of transfection. HEK293T cells, which were derived from HEK293 cells and stably express large Simian Virus 40 (SV40) large T-antigen, are purported to generate retroviral and lentiviral vector preparations with particularly high titres. Thus, at present HEK293T and closely related HEK293FT cells are predominantly used for lentiviral vector production via transient co-transfection of the backbone vector plasmid and the helper plasmids. The abundance of lentiviral vector genomic RNA and levels of expression of VSV-G protein, Gag and GagPol polyproteins plus the accessory protein Rev in the packaging cells are of paramount importance for the resultant lentiviral vector titre. The ratio of a lentiviral backbone vector plasmid DNA and non-vector helper packaging plasmids is used to regulate the relative amount of genomic RNA and packaging proteins. In part, the optimal balance depends on the known toxicity of the excess VSV-G protein to mammalian cells. Clontech-Takara and ThermoFisherScientific-OpenBiosystems offer mixtures of plasmids with tetracycline-inducible expression of the *trans*-acting packaging functions. As an alternative to plasmids, adenoviral vectors (Kuate, Stefanou et al. 2004) or baculoviral vectors (Lesch, Laitinen et al. 2011) can be used to deliver

DNA cassettes for the transient expression of lentiviral packaging proteins and the lentiviral vector backbone modules. Clearly, this method can broaden the range of cell lines suitable for lentiviral packaging, as receptors for adenoviruses are commonly expressed by different types of cells.

The process of cell transduction by a viral vector follows the infection pathway of the cognate virus. There are several parameters characterizing the transduction of cells with a viral vector. Firstly, efficiency of transduction, defined as percentage of transduced cells out of all cells treated with a viral vector preparation, is a common and readily-obtained read-out quantity in transduction experiments. The second commonly used parameter is end-point titre, which is the number of "transduction units" per volume of the viral vector preparation with the number of transduced cells (corresponding to the "transduction units") estimated when one of the highest dilutions of the viral preparation is used to infect the cells. The third important parameter describing transduction by a viral vector is the multiplicity of infection, that is, the average number of functional transducing particles infecting one cell. The infection of a cell by a lentiviral vector normally results in the establishment of one or several copies of the corresponding provirus. The efficiency of the transduction of the cell population by a retroviral vector, which is a function of the multiplicity of infection, correlates with a number of proviruses in the genome of the infected cell (Kustikova, Wahlers et al. 2003). Thus, the obtained transgene copy number reflects the multiplicity of infection. Expression of retroviral envelope proteins is known to block superinfection (i.e. extra-infection by the same virus) of the infected cells through the depletion of the cognate cellular receptor molecules during their intracellular transport. This mechanism, though, does not apply to VSV-G protein pseudotyped lentiviral vectors, which neither have protein cellular receptors, nor code for an envelope protein under typical circumstances. Therefore, it is possible to increase the number of the lentiviral vector proviruses and, hence, transgene copy number by repeated rounds of superinfection.

As an alternative to gene delivery with packaged lentiviral vectors, the cargo genes within lentiviral vector DNA sequences can be transferred *in situ* "on the back" of other viral gene vectors, such as adenoviral or herpes virus based vectors. These, "dual-viral systems", e.g. adenovirus-retrovirus hybrid vectors, can deliver attenuated lentiviral vectors competent for replication and packaging in order to achieve "a booster effect" due to lentiviral vector spread *in situ* (Dalba, Bellier et al. 2007). In addition, such delivery systems allow for the exploitation of the cellular tropism of some well-established non-lentiviral vectors, particularly vectors based on non-enveloped viruses which lack membrane-imbedded anti-receptors suitable for pseudotyping (Soifer, Higo et al. 2002).

The stable maintenance of lentiviral vectors makes them a highly suitable tool for various cell-fate mapping studies and also as sensors of cell differentiation. Tracing cells with a specific differentiation status is important in biomedical research, e.g. in stem cell studies (Gallo, Grimaldi et al. 2008). The packaging size constraints make it a challenge to avoid cross-talk between various elements within lentiviral vectors and, therefore, require the thoughtful design of lentiviral vectors with tissue specific transgene expression (Hager, Frame et al. 2008).

2. Elements of lentiviral vector backbone plasmids

The lentiviral vector genome has the size of about 10 kb and can be conveniently amplified by cloning its complete or partial DNA copy in the bacterial plasmid cloning vectors. Such lentiviral vector backbone plasmids are similar to other vector plasmids for mammalian gene expression, which were recently reviewed (Tolmachov 2009). The immediate purpose of the lentiviral vector backbone plasmid is to serve as a template for the transcription generating viral vector genomic RNA, which can be packaged into the lentiviral vector particles. The bacterial portion of the vector plasmid is not transcribed and, therefore, is not included in the genomic RNA of the viral vector. Thus, a typical lentiviral vector backbone plasmid consists of a bacterial plasmid portion, lentiviral elements required for viral vector RNA packaging and intracellular transport, a marker gene and/or a cargo gene and elements for their regulation, optional chromatin-control elements and sites for convenient plasmid DNA re-engineering (Figure 2).

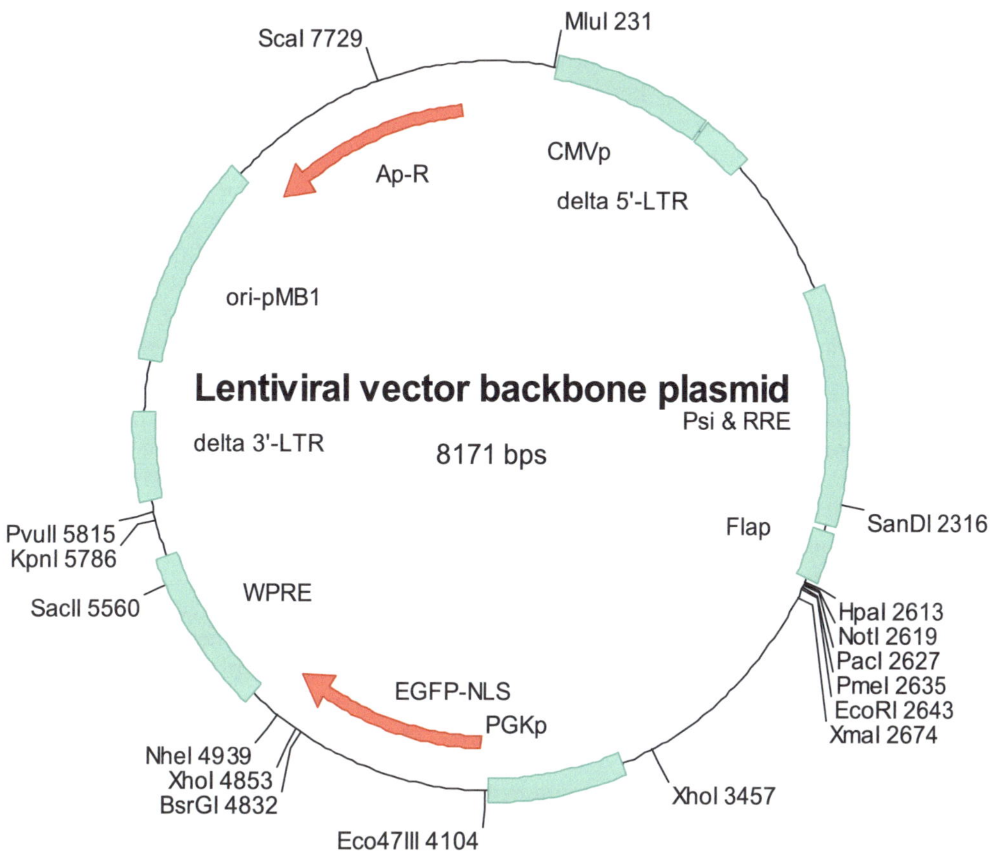

CMVp – the immediate early CMV promoter; delta 5′-LTR and delta 3′-LTR – the long terminal repeats with some deletions; Psi & RRE – the packaging sequence ψ and the Rev Response Element (RRE); PGKp – the mouse phosphoglycerol kinase promoter; EGFP-NLS – the gene for nuclear targeted enhanced GFP protein; ori-pMB1 – the multicopy origin of replication originating from the wild type plasmid pMB1; Ap-R – the ampicillin resistance marker, the gene for β-lactamase.

Fig. 2. A typical lentiviral vector backbone plasmid

Evolution has shaped both bacterial plasmid and viral genomes as mosaic assemblies, which can be disassembled into individual functional units that can then be assembled back into new chimeras. Thus, the genomes of lentiviral vectors consist of a number of genetic elements, of which lentiviral elements *per se* are only a fraction (often less than 30% of the vector genome). Lentiviral sequences essential for lentiviral gene vectors are Long Terminal Repeats (LTRs, which can be complete or partially deleted) for proviral integration and the packaging ψ sequence within the genome region proximal to the 5'-LTR. A viral life cycle involving tight nucleic acid packaging into protein shells (capsids) requires compactness from the viral genetic elements. Thus, terse genetic elements from various unrelated viruses are particularly suitable for employment within lentiviral vector constructs. Various cargo genes can be delivered with lentiviral vectors. Because of the lentiviral packaging size constraints, the shorter, cDNA-based, versions of the genes are normally preferable. As the space within the lentiviral capsid is limited, one would only include an intron within a lentiviral vector born cargo gene if it provides an important regulatory function for the gene's expression.

Other regulatory genetic elements within lentiviral vectors include viral or cellular promoters and enhancers, splicing control elements if an intron is included, RNA stabilizing components like Woodchuck hepatitis virus Post-transcriptional Regulatory Element (WPRE) and, with a pinch of salt, polyadenylation signals (see discussion in Section 2.4).

Thus, the lentiviral vector backbone plasmid normally includes a bacterial plasmid segment, *cis*-elements of the lentiviral packaging machinery and an elective strong promoter to drive the synthesis of lentiviral vector's genomic RNA, cargo genes (e.g. marker genes, therapeutic genes) and genetic elements for their control. Optionally, lentiviral vector backbone plasmids can also contain sites for efficient transport of vector RNA from nucleus, for episomal maintenance of proviruses, site-specific genomic integration and also sites alleviating plasmid manipulation, e.g. polylinkers with restriction enzyme recognition sites.

2.1 Bacterial plasmid segment

Lentiviral vector backbone plasmids are propagated in bacteria and hence need to contain a bacterial origin of replication to drive the DNA amplification. Plasmid origins of replication are traditionally classified into a "stringent control of the plasmid copy number" group and a "relaxed control of the plasmid copy number" group. High number of plasmid copies per cell, which is typical for the "relaxed control" group, insures the high yield of the plasmid DNA. However a high plasmid copy number can place substantial stress onto the host cells, thereby decreasing their growth rate and, thus, resulting in occasional accumulation of cells with the shortened, "deletion", plasmid mutants or cells lacking the plasmid altogether. In contrast, replicons from a "stringent control" group have a lower number of plasmid copies per cell and hence comparatively small plasmid DNA yields, however plasmids driven by these replicons only rarely place a selective disadvantage onto their host cells. In addition, stable maintenance of the stringent control replicons is insured by their "partition" functions, which are responsible for the faithful distribution of plasmids between daughter cells after cell divisions. Classic relaxed control replicons are derived from plasmids ColE1 and pMB1, while typical stringent control replicons originate from plasmids RSF1010, pSC101, F-factor, and bacteriophage P1. A particularly convenient replication system, which is used in the lentiviral vector backbone plasmids, is borrowed from the plasmid R6K. This plasmid has several origins of replication, all dependent on the Π-protein encoded by the plasmid's *pir* gene. Thus, a lentiviral backbone plasmid with R6Kγ replicon can replicate only in the bacterial strains expressing the Π-protein. The copy number of ori-R6Kγ-driven plasmids can be increased substantially if the plasmid is transferred to an array of strains expressing various "copy-up" mutant versions of the Π-protein, thus giving the flexibility to choose the optimal copy number for a particular lentiviral backbone plasmid.

To select bacterial tranformants during plasmid modifications and to prevent plasmid loss using selective pressure for plasmid-containing cells, the bacterial plasmid segment should include a suitable selection marker. The standard solution is to employ an antibiotic selection gene such as the ampicillin resistance gene for β-lactamase or the chloramphenicol resistance gene for chloramphenicol acetyl transferase. Large scale preparations of plasmid DNA with antibiotic resistance genes might lead to the undesirable escape of these genes into environment. Thus, genetic systems, which rely on a short RNA-expressing gene as a plasmid selection marker, can be contrived (Luke, Carnes et al. 2009).

Regrettably, it is relatively common for lentiviral vector backbone plasmids to suffer from structural and maintenance instability in bacteria. There are several common factors contributing to this instability. Lentiviral vector backbone plasmids are necessarily greater than 9 kb in size; if their replication is driven by a replication origin with "relaxed control" of the plasmid copy number, spontaneously arising deletion mutants have a propensity to replicate faster and, as a result, tend to establish dominance in the mixed plasmid population. Plasmid deletions can occur through homologous or illegitimate recombination between inverted repeats of the lentiviral LTRs. A mosaic of eukaryotic sequences within the lentiviral vector backbone plasmid might contain cryptic bacterial promoters, which could be able to drive the expression of toxic RNAs and polypeptides creating a negative selection pressure on the population of bacterial cells harbouring the desired plasmids. It should be noted that the ampicillin resistance gene coding for β-lactamase, which is often used in the commercially available lentiviral backbone plasmids as a selection marker, is poorly suited for long-term bacterial selection in liquid cultures. This is because wild type β-lactamase is secreted in *Escherichia coli* and can destroy ampicillin before the bacterial culture is fully grown. Thus, if a particular lentiviral backbone plasmid would have a maintenance problem, the overgrowth of plasmidless cells in liquid culture would not be stopped by ampicillin. In such a situation, the use of alternative non-ampicillin-based selection marker is recommended. Alternatively, as much bacterial cultivation as possible should be performed on a solid agar medium containing ampicillin, where the spread of ampicillin-destroying β-lactamase is slower. For example, a seeding stock for a liquid plasmid maxi-preparation culture can be grown from an individual colony on agar plates with ampicillin instead of a liquid overnight culture. Non-secreted, cytosolic, mutant versions of β-lactamase were described and can be used for efficient selection of bacteria harbouring maintenance-compromised lentiviral vector backbone plasmids.

2.2 *Cis*-acting elements of the lentiviral molecular machinery

The standard purpose of lentiviral vector backbone plasmids is to provide a template for the synthesis of lentiviral vector genomic RNA, which can be successfully packaged into lentiviral vector virions, reverse transcribed and integrated within the cellular genome. The Ψ-sequence close to the 5′-LTR is strictly required for the packaging of RNA by the Gag polyprotein. A substantial portion of the sequences within the LTRs of the lentiviral genome is required for chromosomal integration. However, some sequences within the LTRs can be removed without reduction in the integration efficiency. Wild-type retroviral and lentiviral genomes contain a promoter within their 5′-LTR to drive expression of genomic RNA. The promoter sequences can be deleted from the 5′-LTR DNA segment in the lentiviral vector backbone plasmids and a strong constitutive promoter capable of directing synthesis of the vector genomic RNA, e.g.

immediate early CMV promoter, can be placed externally to the bracket of the lentiviral sequences within the plasmids. As the accessory lentiviral protein Tat is required for the activation of the promoter within the wild type 5′-LTR of HIV-1, the use of an external promoter for genomic RNA synthesis allows exclusion of the Tat gene from the packaging system with the consequent reduction in the probability for the re-constitution of the replication competent virus and the corresponding improvement in safety (Dull, Zufferey et al. 1998). A substantial fraction of the currently used lentiviral vectors are "self-inactivating" (SIN) due to a deletion within their 3′-LTR. Indeed, as the DNA-copy of the 5′-LTR of the vector provirus is always synthesized by reverse transcription from the template of the 3′-LTR, proviruses of the SIN vectors lack sequences required for the re-constitution of the lentiviral promoter within the 5′-LTR segment of the vector provirus and the synthesis of the lentiviral vector genomic RNA from the provirus template. Thus, the SIN-vectors cannot be re-distributed from the target cells, which is beneficial for their safety profile.
Lentiviruses possess molecular machinery to enter into the nuclei of postmitotic, non-dividing cells with an intact nuclear envelope. Lentiviral nuclear-penetration apparatus is in part dependent on the triple-stranded structure created during reverse transcription of the lentiviral genomic RNA, "the central DNA flap" (Riviere, Darlix et al. 2010). Central Polypurine Tract (cPPT) and Central Termination Sequence (CTS) are required for the formation of "the flap". Therefore, DNA sequences for cPPT and CTS need to be present in the plasmid template of the nuclear penetrating lentiviral vectors.
Rev protein of HIV-1 is known to increase lentiviral vector titres by promoting the export of genomic RNA from the nucleus. This export depends on the Rev Response Element (RRE) sequence within genomic RNA. Therefore, the RRE sequence is a desirable building block for inclusion into the lentiviral vector backbone plasmids.

2.3 Marker genes for mammalian cells

The concentration of lentiviral vector particles can be assessed by their ability to transduce cells and by physical measurements estimating the number of virions in a volume. A substantial number of virions in lentiviral preparations can be infection defective, so transduction data are vital for the evaluation of the titre of functional lentiviral vector particles. Convenient markers for the assessment of efficiency of transduction and for the fate mapping of transduced cells include genes for fluorescent proteins, drug resistance proteins, luciferase and cell surface antigens. More practical markers are easily detected in live cells, while others require fixation of the live material. Enzyme coding genes, such as the *lacZ* gene for bacterial β-galactosidase, can be used as transduction markers, but lost some of their initial popularity because of the need to fix and, thus, to kill the transduced cells before colour reaction with enzymatic substrates. In addition, the *lacZ* gene is large (3075 bp), and occupies a substantial portion of the permissible payload size within lentiviral vectors. Similarly, detection of intracellular proteins by immunostaining requires cells to be killed by permeabilization of their membranes and fixation. Thoughtful choice of the viral vector marker is important for the straightforward collection of data and their faithful interpretation. Most marker proteins are small and do not illicit a substantial immune reaction *in vivo*. It is important to plan a convenient intracellular localization of the marker proteins as this can affect their activity and can minimize background signal. Genetic determinants used to direct proteins to a specific subcellular compartment include nuclear localization signals (NLS), chromosome binding moieties (e.g. histon H2B) and domains for plasma membrane association, endoplasmic reticulum retention, targeting to mitochondria, peroxisomes, Golgi-apparatus, actin filaments and microtubules. Fused signal sequences or protein domains must not interfere with the marker protein multimer formation if the quaternal protein structure is required for its activity.

Drug resistance (normally antibiotic resistance) genes are especially suitable for tasks requiring the establishment of stably transduced cell clones originating from individual transduced cells. The choice of a particular drug resistance gene can be affected by its size. The gene for blasticidin resistance, *bsr*, is 423 bp long and is particularly compact. In contrast, the gene for hygromycin resistance is 1038 bp long, and, therefore, is a less attractive choice if the available space within the lentiviral vector is limited. Different drugs cause cell death with dissimilar rates and their minimal inhibitory concentrations vary for different types of cells. The number of surviving transduced cell clones is typically higher at lower drug concentrations. Other frequently used antibiotic resistance markers include genes for resistance to zeocin, puromycin and neomycin analogue G418. Drug sensitivity genes, such as HSV thymidine kinase (TK), can also be delivered by lentiviral vectors. These genes are highly instrumental for cell suicide systems in cancer gene therapy, but are difficult to use as transduction markers.

Fluorescent proteins are remarkably convenient as gene transfer markers because they can be detected both in live and fixed cells. The largest family of fluorescent proteins originates from the green fluorescent protein (GFP) of jellyfish *Aequoria victoria.* Systematic protein engineering efforts produced mutant derivatives of GFP with increased brightness and widely different excitation and emission spectra (e.g. blue, cyan and yellow fluorescent proteins). Similarly, dsRed protein of coral *Discosoma sp.* was used to create a family of proteins including the orange fluorescent protein mOrange and the far-red fluorescent protein E2-Crimson. A number of specialized versions of fluorescent proteins were obtained, e.g. reduced half-life GFP for the collection of dynamic gene expression data. Fluorescently activated cell sorting (FACS) is the method of choice both for analytical analysis of the transduced fluorescent cells and for their preparative isolation. Fluorescence-based microscopy is another convenient and informative method; however, 3-D imaging of fluorescent material is complicated by the extinction of both excitation and emission light in the thick slices. Still, the image data collected from thin slices can be assembled into 3-D images using computational algorithms. Computational algorithms can be also applied for "image de-convolution" in order to achieve some improvement of image quality using fluorescence data obtained directly on the thick specimens.

The titre of a lentiviral vector depend to a large degree on the type of the marker used for analysis. Indeed, the titre determined by detecting the fluorescent transduction markers is usually higher than the titre obtained by counting drug resistant cell clones.

Genes for luminescence proteins can be transferred by lentiviral vectors and used as cell tracers (Reumers, Deroose et al. 2008). Luciferases from North American firefly *Photinus pyralis* and sea pansy *Renilla reniformis* are commonly used. The two luciferases use different substrates for light production, this can be exploited to create internal control for luminescence in "dual luciferase reporter assays" used, e.g., for promoter strength testing or shRNA/siRNA analysis. The "baseline" luciferase marker (normally *Renilla* luciferase) can be delivered for expression on a separate vector or on the same vector. A version of firefly luciferase with enhanced expression in mammalian cells (luc2) was developed by Promega by codon optimization (as discussed in Section 2.4) and elimination of predicted transcription factor binding sites within the reporter gene sequence. On the basis of luc2,

Promega developed luciferases with a higher rate of degradation such as luc2P (containing PEST protein degradation signal ("degron") on the C-terminus or luc2CP (containing CL1 and PEST protein degrons on the C-terminus). PEST is a 40 amino acid sequence present in the C-terminal region of mouse ornithine decarboxylase. CL1 is a 16 amino acid degron from yeast. This signal was also optimized for expression in mammalian cells. Versions of luciferase with the degradation signals improve responsiveness to factors enhancing or inhibiting luciferase expression. Other specialized versions of luciferases are available. For example, secreted firefly luciferase is convenient to measure the luciferase activity of live cells in tissue culture. *Renilla* luciferase-neo^R fusion protein was generated and can be used for both cell clone selection and as an internal luminescence control. *In vivo* "whole animal" detection of luminescence is a common approach with no excitation light being required and with the efficient amplification of emitted photons. However, low spatial resolution limits due to light dispersion in the animal restrict the expediency of this approach.
Surface antigen markers, e.g. extracellular domain of CD4, truncated low-affinity nerve growth factor (LNGFR) or truncated mouse MHC class I molecule H-2K^k can be used as cell markers for antibody-mediated conjugation with paramagnetic particles, which can be used for both magnetic cell sorting and magnetic resonance imaging (So, Hotee et al. 2005). The intracellular domains of these proteins are removed to avoid signal transduction and the extracellular domains are supplied with GPI-lipidation signal for plasma-membrane anchoring (as in Miltenyi Biotec MAC Select™ system). Background signal during whole-animal imaging can be avoided by using species-specific monoclonal antibodies for the cell surface marker proteins in a heterologous host organism.

2.4 Genetic elements for controlling the expression of marker genes and cargo genes in lentiviral vectors

In general, *cis*-acting elements strictly required for gene expression in eukaryotes are a minimal promoter and a transcription terminator. Genes coding for proteins (cistrons) also necessarily contain: 1) the translation start codon ATG with the surrounding Kozak consensus sequence controlling translation initiation; 2) the protein coding sequence; 3) the stop codon. Protein-encoding genes are transcribed by eukaryotic Polymerase II from Polymerase II specific promoters. The sequence of the Polymerase II promoters is variable; however, "TATA-box" with the consensus sequence 5'-TATAAAA-3' is normally found 20-25 bp upstream of the transcription start site. In addition, minimal Polymerase II promoters often contain "CAT-box" with the consensus sequence 5'-GGCCAATCT-3' at the position -70 relative to the transcription start site. The Kozak consensus sequence is important for expression of protein-coding transgenes born on lentiviral vectors. The DNA template for one of the strong versions of the Kozak sequence can be written down as 5'-gccaccATGgcg-3'.
The Polymerase II transcripts, e.g. mRNAs, are nearly always modified by the addition of 7-methylguanosine (the "cap") to their 5'-ends and the addition of the homopolymeric tail of adenosine nucleotides to their 3'-ends. Polyadenylation of eukaryotic mRNAs is important for their protection from exonucleolytic attack and for their export out of nucleus. It also serves as a means of transcription termination. For mRNA to be polyadenylated, it should contain a specific signal sequence downstream of its polypeptide coding sequence. In general, a DNA sequence for the functional "polyadenylation signal" (pA signal), which is suitable for insertion into lentiviral vector backbone plasmids, is several hundred nucleotides long and is borrowed from a mammalian gene or a viral genome. Commonly

used pA signal sites are taken from the rabbit β-globin gene, human growth hormone gene and human herpes virus (HSV) thymidine kinase (TK) gene. The sequence 5′-AAUAAA-3′ located 10-30 nucleotides upstream of the cleavage site is highly conserved but is not strictly required for the polyadenylation of mammalian mRNAs. A very important feature of the lentiviral vector backbone is the pA signal in its 3′-LTR. This signal functions as a terminator for wild type lentiviral RNAs including complete lentiviral genomic RNA. As the 3′-LTR sequence itself is strictly required for chromosomal integration in lentiviruses, any foreign pA signals which can cause premature termination of the genomic RNA are bound to reduce the amount of transductionally active genomic RNA, and, therefore, to diminish drastically the titre of the functional lentiviral vector particles (Hager, Frame et al. 2008). Thus, foreign pA signals within lentiviral vectors should be either avoided altogether, or weakened, or positioned to terminate the transcription of the anti-genomic DNA strand only. With this challenge in view, it should be noted that while most pA signal sites act unidirectionally, a pA signal borrowed from SV40 viral genome is known to terminate RNA and to promote polyadenylation irrespective of transcription direction. A brief look at the transcription map of SV40 can explain this fluke. Indeed, two opposing transcription waves of SV40 meet and terminate at its polyadenylation signal site, which is, therefore, an overlap of two opposing polyadenylation signals.

Natural Polymerase II promoters are nearly always supplemented with one or several "enhancers", that is, genetic elements, which up-regulate the activity of the promoter through binding to specific nuclear proteins, so-called "transcription factors". Size limitations of the lentiviral payload and insufficiently precise enhancer localization data restrict the use of enhancers in the lentiviral vectors. However, small enhancer elements can still be used where, for example, tissue-specific or inducible transgene expression is desired.

A typical eukaryotic protein-coding gene is a patchwork of coding exons and non-coding introns, so that the translation-grade mRNA is produced by the splicing of the primary transcript. The result of the splicing is the establishment of the phosphodiester bond between the AG dinucleotide at the 3′-end of the preceding exon and the G nucleotide at the 5′-end of the subsequent exon within the transcript (Hiller and Platzer 2008). The interlacing sequences, the introns, are flanked with a "splice-donor" consensus sequence 5′-GTRAGT-3′ at their 5′-ends and a "splice-acceptor" sequence 5-YAG-3′ at their 3′-ends (where R is A or G, Y is C or T). In addition, introns contain a "branch point" 5′-YTRAY-3′ and a polypyrimidine tract, which are functionally important for successful splicing. As the payload space within the lentiviral vectors is limited, the standard practice is to include the genes in their complementary DNA (cDNA) form, that is, as spliced versions without introns. The introns, however, are not entirely inert genetically and occasionally take part in the regulation of gene expression. In such situations, the inclusion of small regulatory introns within lentiviral vectors can be considered (Le Hir, Nott et al. 2003).

Coding sequences delivered by lentiviral vectors are often derived from non-mammalian organisms where the translation machinery is adapted to a non-mammalian profile of codon frequencies. Unusual codons, also called "hungry codons", can cause undesirable pauses during translation and reduce the efficiency of gene expression. Therefore, the optimization of codon frequencies for the genes, which are born on the lentiviral vectors, is often advantageous. If the frequencies in a coding sequence are adapted to the human codon usage profile, the sequence is said to be "humanized" (Zeeberg 2002; Burgess-Brown, Sharma et al. 2008).

The stability of genomic RNA of lentiviral vectors is crucial for attaining high lentiviral vector titres and stability of the lentiviral vector encoded mRNAs is important for efficient transgene expression. It was discovered that an element from Woodchuck Hepatitis Virus (WHV) genome can operate at a post-transcriptional level to improve transgene expression. The sequence, called WHV Post-transcriptional Regulatory Element (WPRE) is thought to act by expediting the export of RNA from the nucleus with the concomitant reduction of the intra-nuclear RNA degradation. WPRE and a similar element from Human Hepatitis Virus (HBV) are extensively used in lentiviral vectors, where they are normally positioned immediately upstream from the 3′-LTR, primarily because of their vector titre enhancing properties. WPRE, as defined originally, was known to cause tumours in rodents, therefore, a safer version of WPRE with deleted sequences for the WHV X protein and its promoter was generated (Schambach, Bohne et al. 2006).

Cistrons are not the only cargo genes delivered by the lentiviral vectors. Other payload genes include the genes for RNAi-exploiting "micro" RNAs (miRNAs) or their artificial analogues, "short hairpin" RNAs (shRNAs). These genes are transcribed by RNA Polymerases III or I from the corresponding promoters. The benefits of the lentiviral vectors, such as the relative stability of transgene expression and the ability to transduce postmitotic cells, considerably broaden the versatility of gene knock-down experiments with shRNAs (Rubinson, Dillon et al. 2003). A range of suitable lentiviral vectors, exploiting the high activity of hybrid miRNA-30-shRNA design, are offered by ThermoFisherScientific-OpenBiosystems (Silva, Li et al. 2005).

In summary, *cis*-acting elements regulating gene expression act in concert and in a cell-type-specific manner. The inherent mosaicism of lentiviral genetic organization allows interchangeable use of an extensive array of genetic elements for the generation of new lentiviral vectors. However, some combinations of genetic determinants are less functional than others, so the optimization of the lentiviral vector set-up is usually required.

2.5 Genetic elements for epigenetic maintenance of transgene expression

It is a relatively common occurrence for transgene expression to die out both in terms of the reduction of the fraction of expressing cells and the decrease of the efficiency of expression. Integrated lentiviral proviruses are faithfully maintained in mammalian cells, so the reasons for the shutdown of transgene expression are mostly epigenetic. Malfunction of the transgene expression control elements is often blamed, indeed, the phenomenon is sometimes referred to as "promoter shut down". Certainly, different promoters have various capabilities to maintain long-term transgene expression. In particular, some promoters tend to turn off in cell populations where they are not normally active. The shutdown of transgene expression is particularly common in cell populations undergoing differentiation (Bagchi, Kumar et al. 2006). Natural chromosomal integration of lentiviruses tends to occur in transcriptionally active areas of the genome where heterochromatin and DNA methylation are unlikely to interfere with transgene expression. However, as the cells differentiate, the pattern of heterochromatization and DNA methylation changes and some of the proviruses find themselves in the transcriptionally silent areas of the genome.

There are many levels at which the longevity of transgene expression can be addressed through the lentiviral vector design, including: 1) control of the provirus amenity to methylation (e.g. purposeful exclusion of the methylation-prone CpG islands); 2) chromatin re-modeling control via *cis*-acting proviral elements; 3) choice of non-immunogenic transgene products to prevent cell elimination via immune reaction *in vivo*; 4) choice of a suitable tissue-specific promoter-enhancer combination; 5) achieving the high copy number of proviruses; 6) control of the provirus integration sites via the preferences of the viral integrase or via harnessing the site-specific integration systems.

In principle, the protection of proviruses from heterochromatin can be achieved with genomic insulators or other similar anti-heterochromatin elements. However, experiments with known insulators show that their effects on transgene expression from lentiviral proviruses are multi-vectorial depending on the cell context (Grandchamp, Henriot et al. 2011). Ideally, targeting proviruses to a continuously active locus (e.g. human homologue of the mouse Rosa 26 locus) can resolve the transgene expression shutdown problem. An alternative solution is to escape chromatin-remodeling events by creating episomally maintained lentiviral proviruses (Section 5).

2.6 Elements alleviating manipulation of lentiviral vector backbone plasmids

The fairly large size of the lentiviral vector backbone plasmids means they contain a limited number of unique sites for restriction nucleases. Thus, it is often desirable to introduce artificial clusters of suitable unique restriction sites (polylinkers) to simplify the modification of these plasmids. Alternatively, selection schemes involving site-specific recombination can be used for repetitive modifications, e.g. for marker exchange or promoter exchange. In this scenario, the introduction of suitable site-specific recombination sites into the lentiviral vector backbone plasmid is required.

As discussed in Section 2.1, lentiviral vector backbone plasmids are occasionally structurally unstable and/or poorly maintained. These plasmids are particularly vulnerable during initial establishment in bacteria. Instability of nascent recombinant plasmids can result in a practical unfeasibility of seemingly straightforward DNA cloning strategies. For example, the generation of new lentiviral vector backbone plasmids through inefficient ligation of two DNA fragments with blunt ends is normally very challenging. In such situations we recommend splitting the DNA cloning procedure into separate cloning steps, each one relying on either effective positive selection of new recombinant plasmids or on efficient ligation. For example, the insertion of additional DNA sequences into lentiviral vector backbone plasmids can take advantage of the "pop-in-pop-out" cloning strategy. In this approach, a plasmid containing the desired insert and marked with antibiotic resistance marker 1 is first fused with the lentiviral vector backbone plasmid marked with antibiotic resistance marker 2 using positive selection of the co-integrate plasmid with two antibiotics. The desired new lentiviral vector backbone plasmid is then obtained by removing the unwanted plasmid sequences from the resultant bi-replicon plasmid using restriction digestion and efficient intra-molecular ligation reaction. Clearly, this strategy for insertions into a lentiviral vector backbone plasmid requires the thoughtful placement of restriction sites conveniently accommodating both the "pop-in" step and the "pop-out" step.

3. Engineering lentiviral vectors for the concomitant expression of several transgenes

The genome sizes of non-defective wild type HIV-1 isolates are close to 9.5 kb. The lentiviral packaging size constraints are dictated by the geometry of the viral capsid and are thought to be fairly permissive of the smaller than wild type genome versions, but remarkably intolerant of the larger than wild type variants. As lentiviral sequences required for genomic RNA packaging and chromosomal integration constitute about 2 kb, the available gene payload space within HIV-1 based lentiviral vectors should not be much more than 7.5 kb. Thus, the insert size capacity of the lentiviral vectors is completely appropriate for the vast majority of the monogenic applications but can present a challenge in situations where the delivery of several genes by a single vector is required. Therefore, various possible methods of gene cargo reduction have been explored.

The expression of two or more cistrons from a single promoter can be achieved by the employment of internal ribosome entry site (IRES) elements, which are normally borrowed from viral genomes (Fux, Langer et al. 2004). The IRES sequences (about 0.5 kb) are inserted between the coding frames to facilitate translation of the downstream coding frames from the same transcript. IRES efficiency is not absolute and it is a common occurrence for the subsequent gene in the expression cassette to be expressed at a lower level than the preceding gene. As the length of the intercistronic inserts is an important factor in the IRES efficiency, the expression of the downstream genes can be improved by increasing or decreasing the sizes of the IRES inserts (Attal, Theron et al. 1999).

Another common method used to compress the gene expression cassettes is to produce gene products as polyproteins, that is, large polypeptides, which are split into individual proteins by proteases recognizing the appropriate amino acid sequence cleavage motifs between the protein modules. In fact, lentiviruses use the same principle themselves as the Gag polyprotein is proteolytically processed inside the viral particles to form nucleocapsid, capsid, matrix proteins and the GagPol polyprotein is processed to form additionally viral protease, integrase and reverse transcriptase. The usual proteolytic signal, 2A, which is used in recombinant lentiviral gene vectors, is, however, borrowed not from lentiviruses but from the Foot-and-Mouth Disease Virus belonging to the family of picornaviruses. Multiple copies of the 2A sequence can be successfully used to indicate the desired break-up of the polyproteins. The method has its limitations as protein misfolding might occur, which would require some extra chaperone support.

Quite often there is no need to separate several proteins as they can perform several functions remaining as a single polypeptide chain. In general, multifunctional fusion proteins are produced by the fusion of the coding sequences in the same translation frame. Some spacer peptides might be used to intercalate between the fused polypeptides to improve folding and to facilitate the functional activity of the individual protein domains. There are two common methods to achieve protein fusion: 1) the stop codon of the upstream coding unit is deleted and the start codon of the downstream coding unit is retained to obtain alternative translation starts; 2) both the stop codon of the upstream coding unit and the start codon of the downstream coding unit are deleted. It is important to remember that many proteins are naturally proteolytically processed and this processing can be upset by protein fusion or can interfere with the desired fusion. For example, many proteins are secreted into the lumen of the endoplasmic reticulum (ER) with the concomitant cleavage of the leader peptide by the signal peptidase. If incorporated within the downstream portion of the fusion protein, the signal peptide cleavage sequence can cause undesired fission of the fusion protein. Thus, potential problems associated with building of novel fusion proteins include protein misfolding, incorrect intracellular localization and unexpected sensitivity to a protease attack. In addition, *in vivo* use of fusion proteins might be impeded by unwanted immunogenicity of the newly-created epitopes.

Mimicking wild type lentiviruses, splicing signals can be exploited to generate multiple mRNAs for different proteins from a single primary transcript (Zhu, Chung et al. 2001). However, internal splicing signals reduce the amount of the full size genomic RNA of the lentiviral vectors and, therefore, are bound to be detrimental for the vectors' titres.

On some occasions several cargo genes within one lentiviral vector can be arranged to be driven by their individual promoters. This option is discussed in the following Section 4.

4. Multiple transcription modules in lentiviral vectors

The most straightforward way to arrange two transcription cassettes within the lentiviral vector is to assemble them in a tandem with the orientation coinciding with the transcription direction for the primary genomic RNA (that is, from 5'-LTR to 3'-LTR). Extreme caution is recommended in the employment of foreign pA signals in both cassettes, as they can interfere with the production of functional genomic RNA of the lentiviral vector. The production of functional genomic RNA and transcription from the two gene expression cassettes can all rely on the pA signal within 3'-LTR and a postranscriptional enhancer, such as WPRE, positioned immediately upstream from the 3'-LTR. Such tandem arrangement of two gene expression units is prone to overriding any regulatory features of the downstream promoter by the topmost upstream promoter. Thus, a regulated promoter (e.g. a tissue specific promoter) should be positioned in the upstream gene expression unit while a constitutive and ubiquitous promoter should be positioned downstream (Gallo, Grimaldi et al. 2008; Kita-Matsuo, Barcova et al. 2009). As the lentiviral promoter in the 5'-LTR can override any regulatory features of the downstream promoters, versions of the lentiviral vectors with a deleted 5'-LTR promoter are preferable for tandem assemblies of expression cassettes, which include a regulated promoter. There are multiple situations, both in gene therapy and in general biomedical research, where an induced transgene expression is required. In particular, heat (Vilaboa and Voellmy 2006), light (Schoenenberger, Gerosa et al. 2009; Deisseroth 2011) and gas-born acetaldehyde (Weber, Rimann et al. 2004) were used for induction of gene expression in mammalian cells (Goverdhana, Puntel et al. 2005).

An alternative solution for the arrangement of two expression cassettes within a lentiviral vector genome is an assembly with the divergent orientation of the transcription. The advantage of the divergent orientation of the promoters is that it excludes any cross-talk between two gene expression units. Therefore, two highly regulated promoters can be employed in the same vector. An expression cassette positioned along the transcription of the genomic RNA can still use pA signal in 3'-LTR while a counter-genomic-transcription unit requires its own pA signal. Care should be taken to use an exclusively unidirectional pA signal and not to use a DNA fragment with two opposing pA signals, which can cause the disruption of the functional genomic RNA production.

Lentiviral vectors with tissue-specific promoters can be used for the long-term expression of transgenes in gene therapy and also as sensors of cell differentiation, an important task in stem-cell-based therapy. There are two principal types of genetic sensors: a "responsive" type with a real-time reaction to the cell's state and a "fate-mapping" type, which, once activated, can permanently retain the sensor state during any epigenetic changes happening while cells differentiate or react to outside stimuli. As promoters and enhancers are pivotal elements of the gene expression control, the ability of lentiviral vectors to accommodate several transcription cassettes is an important consideration in the gene vector choice.

A flexible way to regulate gene expression is via cistron inversion relative to a promoter (Atasoy, Aponte et al. 2008; Sohal, Zhang et al. 2009). Thus, a site-specific recombinase, such as Cre-recombinase, can react with the cognate recombination sites within lentiviral vector provirus to activate or to block gene expression. Similarly, controlled excision or inversion of a transcription terminator can be used as a regulatory contrivance. The expression of some genes, e.g. cell suicide genes in cancer gene therapy, requires extra tight control, which can be achieved via a parallel or cascade arrangement of two control elements such as an inducible promoter and a cistron-inversion system (Sektas, Hasan et al. 2001). Lentiviral vectors seem to be particularly suited for the assembly of complex gene expression control systems destined for delivery to postmitotic cell populations as their packaging size constraints are less prohibitive than the packaging size constraints of competing Adeno-Associated Virus (AAV) based gene vectors.

5. Generating non-integrating lentiviral vectors

One of the current trends in vectorology is for viral vectors to acquire some of the advantageous features of non-viral vectors and for non-viral vectors to borrow attractive bits of the viral machinery. A clear example of that trend is the rapid coming to the fore of non-integrating lentiviral vectors, which are transducing particles still bearing a substantial resemblance to lentiviruses and yet deficient in typical for retroviruses random chromosomal integration of their proviruses (Nightingale, Hollis et al. 2006; Philippe, Sarkis et al. 2006; Yanez-Munoz, Balaggan et al. 2006; Apolonia, Waddington et al. 2007; Philpott and Thrasher 2007; Bayer, Kantor et al. 2008; Sarkis, Philippe et al. 2008; Rahim, Wong et al. 2009). Importantly, non-integrating lentiviral vectors retain the nuclear-penetrating ability, the flexibility of virion envelope engineering and capacity to package nucleic acids of the therapeutically relevant size that are otherwise characteristic of the lentiviral gene vectors (Wanisch and Yanez-Munoz 2009). The benefits of the non-integrative vectors for gene therapy arise from the absence of malignancy provoking insertional mutagenesis, which can occur because of the disruption of the tumour supressor genes or activation of expression of the oncogenes after proviral integration.

Non-integrating lentiviral vectors are prepared with modified lentiviral packaging systems, which employ a modified GagPol polyprotein containing mutations specifically inactivating the lentiviral integrase function. If a regular lentiviral vector backbone plasmid is used in the packaging procedure, the resultant vector virions can deliver transgenes to the nucleoplasm, where the transgenes can stay and be expressed until they are diluted out in cell divisions. Therefore, such vectors are suitable either for transient transduction of dividing cells or for relatively stable transduction of non-dividing cells, where the lentiviral vector genomes can persist. To achieve better maintenance of the transgenes, non-integrating lentiviral vectors have to be supplemented with either site-specific integration machinery (Lombardo, Genovese et al. 2007; Moldt, Staunstrup et al. 2008) or episomal maintenance apparatus (Wong, Argyros et al. 2009; Argyros, Wong et al. 2011).

Provirus integration can be made harmless by its targeting to a benign locus within the target cell genome (Moldt, Staunstrup et al. 2008). The lentiviral integrase itself can be engineered into a site-directed recombination enzyme by its fusion with site-specific "tethering" domains (Ferris, Wu et al. 2010). Robust and error-free site-specific integration into mammalian cells lacking pre-engineered integration sites is, however, difficult to achieve. Thus, compact episomal replicons from SV40, polyoma, papilloma viruses or

EBNA1-Rep1 DNA segment of Epstein-Barr virus (EBV) can be used to support maintenance of non-integrating lentiviral vectors in the nucleoplasm of dividing cells. Viral replicons are often completely adequate for research use of gene vectors, however they are rarely acceptable for therapeutic applications. Indeed, expression of the large SV40 T-antigen and, hence, malignant transformation of the recipient host cells is required for SV40-origin-based replication. EBNA1 expression does not result in a typical malignant transformation but can still tilt the cells towards the undesired immortalisation (Humme, Reisbach et al. 2003). Alternative benign episomal replicons are being sought; encouragingly, the scaffold/matrix attachment region (S/MAR) from the human β-interferon gene was reported to support episomal replication (Wong, Argyros et al. 2011).

6. How to enhance the transduction of cells with lentiviral vectors

The titre of lentiviral vector particles in the cell culture supernatant hardly ever exceeds $1x10^8$ TU/ml and, depending on a particular lentiviral vector backbone, is often much lower. Therefore, the use of concentrated lentiviral vector preparations is a popular, even though relatively involved, approach to achieve high efficiency of transduction with small volumes of the applied viral vector suspension. In addition to increased titres, concentrated lentiviral vector preparations benefit from concomitant purification of viral vector particles from transduction inhibitors, which are commonly present in the cell culture supernatants. Ultracentrifugation is a traditional method to concentrate lentiviral vector virions, however it is often accompanied by the loss of a substantial fraction of the active lentiviral vector particles. The particles are, in part, inactivated because of the contact between the vector pellet and air. To make the pellet more compact, ultracentrifugation is performed in swing-out bucket rotors and conical-bottom tubes supplemented with appropriate adaptors. Centrifugal force can also cause deterioration of sedimenting vector particles, so a bottom layer of dense sucrose solution is recommended as a "cushion" for better survival of the vector virions. The cushion is also important because a considerable portion of the lentiviral vector preparation can be lost due to incomplete wash-off of the viral vector pellet from the tube or its poor re-suspension. VSV-G pseudotyped lentiviral vectors have relatively short half-life of 8-9 hrs at 37 °C and are better stored at -80 °C.

Similarly to other virions, lentiviral vector particles can be precipitated using "molecular crowding" agents such as polyethylene glycol (PEG), which can soak up water molecules and create micro-pockets with an extra-high virion concentration. Thus, precipitation of virions can be achieved by a proprietary reagent "Lenti-X™ concentrator" supplied by Clontech-Takara. Precipitated lentiviral vector particles can be pelleted by low-speed centrifugation and re-suspended in a smaller volume. However, some non-lentiviral material from cell culture supernatants tends to co-precipitate with virions complicating the re-suspension step. Therefore, additional viral vector purification is required, which is often performed by ion exchange chromatography. Lentiviral vector particles are eluted from the ion exchange column in a high salt solution, which can be toxic to cells. Therefore, the medium for lentiviral vector particles should be exchanged to the desired one using dialysis, gel filtration or ultrafiltration. Ultrafiltration also provides a means for additional concentration of the viral vector.

A completely different strategy for the lentiviral vector concentration is to bind the vector particles to a coated plastic surface, which can then be used as a substrate for the cells to be infected. A recombinant derivative of human fibronectin called RetroNectin™, which was originally used for surface immobilisation of amphotropic retroviral vectors, can be used to trammel VSV-G pseudotyped lentiviral vectors on a plastic surface (Clontech-Takara). Lentiviral vector virions can also be concentrated, including directly at the recipient cell surfaces, after conjugation to paramagnetic particles and attraction by magnet.

Receptors for VSV-G protein are ubiquitous, but still poorly defined. Various types of cells are transduced by VSV-G-pseudotyped lentiviral vectors with different efficiency. A higher efficiency of transduction can often be achieved by a better match of the recipient cells' type and the type of the envelope protein used to pseudotype lentiviral vector particles. Lentiviral transduction is normally dramatically enhanced by polycations, such as hexadimethrine bromide (Polybrene), presumably because they modify the electrostatic interaction between the cells and the vector particles. The polycations' transduction enhancer activity is highly cell specific. Alternative polycations, such as positively charged lipid dioctadecylamidoglycylspermine (DOGS), can be more effective than Polybrene for specific cell populations (Tolmachov, Ma et al. 2006). Transduction efficiency can be further increased by a very unusual and poorly understood method called "spinfection". The recipient cells are overlaid by a viral vector suspension and centrifuged at low speed for 45 min or more. In most circumstances, such a centrifugation step results in a distinct increase in the transduction efficiency, perhaps because of the changes in the trajectories of vector-laden endosomal vesicles due to the centrifugal force.

Lentiviral vectors are able to transduce non-dividing cells. However, higher efficiencies of transduction are achieved with dividing cells, indicating that the nuclear envelope still constitutes a difficult barrier to negotiate for the entering lentiviral vector particles. Therefore, growth factors that stimulate cell division can be applied to increase the efficiency of the lentiviral transduction.

In addition to the measurement of the transduction activity, a lentiviral vector titre can be estimated using physical methods such as electron microscopy or enzyme-linked immunosorbent assay (ELISA) for capsid protein (such as "p24-antigen" of HIV-1). The titre of viral vector particles can be inferred from the concentration of genomic RNA determined by quantitative (real time) PCR. As the proportion of defective viral vector particles can vary depending on the procedures used to isolate and to concentrate the vector, such projections should rely on individually built calibration plots relating the physical titre and the transduction-based titre for a specific set of the viral vector production protocols.

7. Conclusion

Lentiviral gene vectors are generated by the packaging of the RNA transcribed in mammalian cells from vector backbone plasmids propagated in bacteria. Such plasmids contain bacterial and eukaryotic sets of elements. The bacterial set is comprised of a plasmid origin of replication, a bacterial selection marker, an optional partition region for stable maintenance in bacteria and plasmid DNA manipulation prop-ups like multiple cloning sites and site-specific recombination sites. The eukaryotic set consists of the lentiviral *cis*-acting determinants for nuclear export of vector genomes, their packaging, entry into the target nuclei and chromosomal integration, plus a cargo gene or multiple cargo genes with their regulatory elements, an optional marker gene and the elements required for stable maintenance of transgenes in human cells. The bacterial set of elements is lost after vector genome RNA is produced and packaged into lentiviral transducing particles. Different cargo genes can be delivered with lentiviral vectors including genes for proteins, shRNA and miRNA. Currently lentiviral vectors are packaged in mammalian cells only (Lesch, Laitinen et al. 2011). The development of straightforward lentiviral vector production systems in easily cultured insect cells and yeast would be desirable (Tolmachov 2006).

8. References

Al-Allaf, F. A., C. Coutelle, et al. (2010). "LDLR-Gene therapy for familial hypercholesterolaemia: problems, progress, and perspectives." Int Arch Med 3: 36.

Apolonia, L., S. N. Waddington, et al. (2007). "Stable gene transfer to muscle using non-integrating lentiviral vectors." Mol Ther 15(11): 1947-54.

Argyros, O., S. P. Wong, et al. (2011). "Development of S/MAR minicircles for enhanced and persistent transgene expression in the mouse liver." J Mol Med 89(5): 515-29.

Atasoy, D., Y. Aponte, et al. (2008). "A FLEX switch targets Channelrhodopsin-2 to multiple cell types for imaging and long-range circuit mapping." J Neurosci 28(28): 7025-30.

Attal, J., M. C. Theron, et al. (1999). "Effect of intercistronic length on internal ribosome entry site (IRES) efficiency in bicistronic mRNA." Gene Expr 8(5-6): 299-309.

Bagchi, B., M. Kumar, et al. (2006). "CMV promotor activity during ES cell differentiation: potential insight into embryonic stem cell differentiation." Cell Biol Int 30(6): 505-13.

Bayer, M., B. Kantor, et al. (2008). "A large U3 deletion causes increased in vivo expression from a nonintegrating lentiviral vector." Mol Ther 16(12): 1968-76.

Burgess-Brown, N. A., S. Sharma, et al. (2008). "Codon optimization can improve expression of human genes in Escherichia coli: A multi-gene study." Protein Expr Purif 59(1): 94-102.

Dalba, C., B. Bellier, et al. (2007). "Replication-competent vectors and empty virus-like particles: new retroviral vector designs for cancer gene therapy or vaccines." Mol Ther 15(3): 457-66.

Deisseroth, K. (2011). "Optogenetics." Nat Methods 8(1): 26-9.

Dull, T., R. Zufferey, et al. (1998). "A third-generation lentivirus vector with a conditional packaging system." J Virol 72(11): 8463-71.

Ferris, A. L., X. Wu, et al. (2010). "Lens epithelium-derived growth factor fusion proteins redirect HIV-1 DNA integration." Proc Natl Acad Sci U S A 107(7): 3135-40.

Fux, C., D. Langer, et al. (2004). "New-generation multicistronic expression platform: pTRIDENT vectors containing size-optimized IRES elements enable homing endonuclease-based cistron swapping into lentiviral expression vectors." Biotechnol Bioeng 86(2): 174-87.

Gallo, P., S. Grimaldi, et al. (2008). "A lentiviral vector with a short troponin-I promoter for tracking cardiomyocyte differentiation of human embryonic stem cells." Gene Ther 15(3): 161-70.

Geraerts, M., S. Willems, et al. (2006). "Comparison of lentiviral vector titration methods." BMC Biotechnol 6: 34.

Goverdhana, S., M. Puntel, et al. (2005). "Regulatable gene expression systems for gene therapy applications: progress and future challenges." Mol Ther 12(2): 189-211.

Grandchamp, N., D. Henriot, et al. (2011). "Influence of insulators on transgene expression from integrating and non-integrating lentiviral vectors." Genet Vaccines Ther 9(1): 1.

Hager, S., F. M. Frame, et al. (2008). "An internal polyadenylation signal substantially increases expression levels of lentivirus-delivered transgenes but has the potential to reduce viral titer in a promoter-dependent manner." Hum Gene Ther 19(8): 840-50.

Hiller, M. and M. Platzer (2008). "Widespread and subtle: alternative splicing at short-distance tandem sites." Trends Genet 24(5): 246-55.

Humme, S., G. Reisbach, et al. (2003). "The EBV nuclear antigen 1 (EBNA1) enhances B cell immortalization several thousandfold." Proc Natl Acad Sci U S A 100(19): 10989-94.

Kita-Matsuo, H., M. Barcova, et al. (2009). "Lentiviral vectors and protocols for creation of stable hESC lines for fluorescent tracking and drug resistance selection of cardiomyocytes." PLoS One 4(4): e5046.

Kuate, S., D. Stefanou, et al. (2004). "Production of lentiviral vectors by transient expression of minimal packaging genes from recombinant adenoviruses." J Gene Med 6(11): 1197-205.

Kustikova, O. S., A. Wahlers, et al. (2003). "Dose finding with retroviral vectors: correlation of retroviral vector copy numbers in single cells with gene transfer efficiency in a cell population." Blood 102(12): 3934-7.

Le Hir, H., A. Nott, et al. (2003). "How introns influence and enhance eukaryotic gene expression." Trends Biochem Sci 28(4): 215-20.

Lesch, H. P., A. Laitinen, et al. (2011). "Production and purification of lentiviral vectors generated in 293T suspension cells with baculoviral vectors." Gene Ther, in press.

Lombardo, A., P. Genovese, et al. (2007). "Gene editing in human stem cells using zinc finger nucleases and integrase-defective lentiviral vector delivery." Nat Biotechnol 25(11): 1298-306.

Luke, J., A. E. Carnes, et al. (2009). "Improved antibiotic-free DNA vaccine vectors utilizing a novel RNA based plasmid selection system." Vaccine 27(46): 6454-9.

Maier, P., C. von Kalle, et al. (2010). "Retroviral vectors for gene therapy." Future Microbiol 5: 1507-23.

Moldt, B., N. H. Staunstrup, et al. (2008). "Genomic insertion of lentiviral DNA circles directed by the yeast Flp recombinase." BMC Biotechnol 8: 60.

Nightingale, S. J., R. P. Hollis, et al. (2006). "Transient gene expression by nonintegrating lentiviral vectors." Mol Ther 13(6): 1121-32.

Philippe, S., C. Sarkis, et al. (2006). "Lentiviral vectors with a defective integrase allow efficient and sustained transgene expression in vitro and in vivo." Proc Natl Acad Sci U S A 103(47): 17684-9.

Philpott, N. J. and A. J. Thrasher (2007). "Use of nonintegrating lentiviral vectors for gene therapy." Hum Gene Ther 18(6): 483-9.

Rahim, A. A., A. M. Wong, et al. (2009). "Efficient gene delivery to the adult and fetal CNS using pseudotyped non-integrating lentiviral vectors." Gene Ther 16(4): 509-20.

Reumers, V., C. M. Deroose, et al. (2008). "Noninvasive and quantitative monitoring of adult neuronal stem cell migration in mouse brain using bioluminescence imaging." Stem Cells 26(9): 2382-90.
Riviere, L., J. L. Darlix, et al. (2010). "Analysis of the viral elements required in the nuclear import of HIV-1 DNA." J Virol 84(2): 729-39.
Rubinson, D. A., C. P. Dillon, et al. (2003). "A lentivirus-based system to functionally silence genes in primary mammalian cells, stem cells and transgenic mice by RNA interference." Nat Genet 33(3): 401-6.
Sarkis, C., S. Philippe, et al. (2008). "Non-integrating lentiviral vectors." Curr Gene Ther 8(6): 430-7.
Schambach, A., J. Bohne, et al. (2006). "Woodchuck hepatitis virus post-transcriptional regulatory element deleted from X protein and promoter sequences enhances retroviral vector titer and expression." Gene Ther 13(7): 641-5.
Schoenenberger, P., D. Gerosa, et al. (2009). "Temporal control of immediate early gene induction by light." PLoS One 4(12): e8185.
Sektas, M., N. Hasan, et al. (2001). "Expression plasmid with a very tight two-step control: Int/att-mediated gene inversion with respect to the stationary promoter." Gene 267(2): 213-20.
Silva, J. M., M. Z. Li, et al. (2005). "Second-generation shRNA libraries covering the mouse and human genomes." Nat Genet 37(11): 1281-8.
So, P. W., S. Hotee, et al. (2005). "Generic method for imaging transgene expression." Magn Reson Med 54(1): 218-21.
Sohal, V. S., F. Zhang, et al. (2009). "Parvalbumin neurons and gamma rhythms enhance cortical circuit performance." Nature 459(7247): 698-702.
Soifer, H., C. Higo, et al. (2002). "A novel, helper-dependent, adenovirus-retrovirus hybrid vector: stable transduction by a two-stage mechanism." Mol Ther 5(5 Pt 1): 599-608.
Srinivasakumar, N. (2001). "HIV-1 vector systems." Somat Cell Mol Genet 26(1-6): 51-81.
Tolmachov, O. (2006). "A heterologous system for assembly of retroviral gene vectors: intracellular budding in yeast?" Med Hypotheses 67(4): 807-9.
Tolmachov, O. (2009). "Designing plasmid vectors." Methods Mol Biol 542: 117-29.
Tolmachov, O., Y. L. Ma, et al. (2006). "Overexpression of connexin 43 using a retroviral vector improves electrical coupling of skeletal myoblasts with cardiac myocytes in vitro." BMC Cardiovasc Disord 6: 25.
Vilaboa, N. and R. Voellmy (2006). "Regulatable gene expression systems for gene therapy." Curr Gene Ther 6(4): 421-38.
Wanisch, K. and R. J. Yanez-Munoz (2009). "Integration-deficient lentiviral vectors: a slow coming of age." Mol Ther 17(8): 1316-32.
Weber, W., M. Rimann, et al. (2004). "Gas-inducible transgene expression in mammalian cells and mice." Nat Biotechnol 22(11): 1440-4.
Wong, S. P., O. Argyros, et al. (2009). "Strategies for the episomal modification of cells." Curr Opin Mol Ther 11(4): 433-41.
Wong, S. P., O. Argyros, et al. (2011). "Non-viral S/MAR vectors replicate episomally in vivo when provided with a selective advantage." Gene Ther 18(1): 82-7.

Yanez-Munoz, R. J., K. S. Balaggan, et al. (2006). "Effective gene therapy with nonintegrating lentiviral vectors." Nat Med 12(3): 348-53.

Zeeberg, B. (2002). "Shannon information theoretic computation of synonymous codon usage biases in coding regions of human and mouse genomes." Genome Res 12(6): 944-55.

Zhu, X., I. Chung, et al. (2001). "Coexpression of normal and mutated CD40 ligand with deletion of a putative RNA lariat branchpoint sequence in X-linked hyper-IgM syndrome." Clin Immunol 99(3): 334-9.

14

Gene Regulatable Lentiviral Vector System

Yasutsugu Suzuki[1,2] and Youichi Suzuki[1]
[1]*Yong Loo Lin School of Medicine, National University of Singapore*
[2]*Graduate School of Biostudies, Kyoto University*
[1]*Singapore*
[2]*Japan*

1. Introduction

The basic principle of current gene therapy is to deliver genetic material to a population of cells in the body, thereby preventing a disease or improving the clinical status of a patient. One of key factors for successful gene therapy is the development of effective delivery. To date, a plethora of gene delivery systems, termed "vectors", have been developed, and these fall into two broad categories: nonviral and viral vectors. Basically, the nonviral vector systems involve delivery of naked DNA or RNA into target cells with the aid of physical or chemical mediators such as cationic lipids. In terms of their simplicity, producibility, and immunogenicity, nonviral vector systems hold advantages over viral vector systems. However, in terms of the efficiency of gene delivery and expression, the viral vector systems are considered as more ideal (Goverdhana et al., 2005; Verma & Weitzman, 2005).

Although a variety of gene-transfer vectors based on RNA and DNA viruses have been adapted to deliver foreign genes to target cells *in vitro* and *in vivo*, most viral vectors are derived from adenoviruses and retroviruses. Adenoviruses are DNA viruses that are characterized by a nonenveloped icosahedral virion containing a double-stranded linear DNA genome of 30-36 kb (Berk, 2007). The virus enters the target cell by endocytosis via interactions between the fiber protein on the virion and the adenoviral receptor on the cell surface followed by the subsequent binding of a second virion protein, penton, to a cellular integrin protein. Inside the cell, uncoating of virions takes place in the cytoplasm where the viral DNA genome remains associated with a core-derived protein that promotes efficient nuclear entry of the viral genome. Within the nucleus, viral DNA exists as an episome, consequently replication of the viral genome takes place in the nucleus (Leopold et al., 1998). Adenovirus genes are mainly divided into two classes, early and late, based on the time of expressions during the replication. Many of the recombinant adenovirus vectors used in gene transfer have been generated by the deletion and/or mutation of the early genes which are mostly involved in the activation of other viral genes, replication of the viral DNA genome, modulation of host immune responses, and inhibition of host cell apoptosis (Armentano et al., 1995; Armentano et al., 1999; Bett et al., 1994; Brough et al., 1997; Danthinne& Imperiale, 2000; Fallaux et al., 1996; Flint & Shenk, 1997; Gao et al., 1996; Graham et al., 1977; Imler et al., 1996; Wang et al., 1995; Yeh et al., 1996). More recently, the helper-dependent adenoviral vectors, so-called "gutted" vectors, have been created by removing most of the viral genes from adenoviral genome (Kochanek et al., 1996; Lowenstein et al., 2002; Ng et al., 2001; Parks et al., 1996; Umana et al., 2001). Although the gutted vectors need to employ a helper virus that provides all the viral proteins necessary for vector production (Kochanek et al., 1996; Lowenstein et al., 2002; Ng et al., 2001; Parks et al., 1996; Umana et al., 2001), defect of all the viral-coding sequences theoretically allows the cloning of large DNA fragments up to 36 kb (Goverdhana et al., 2005). Although their tropism for the airway epithelial cells meant that adenovirus-based vectors were originally developed for the treatment of genetic lung diseases such as cystic fibrosis (Flotte et al., 2007), one of the major advantages of adenoviral vectors is that they are able to infect a wide variety of cells in a cell-cycle independent manner (Bergelson et al., 1997; Cullen, 2001; Tomko et al., 1997; Whittaker et al., 2000). However, one limitation is the persistence of transgene expression; adenoviral vector-mediated gene expression is short-term, ranging from two weeks to a few months. Thus, this vector is more appropriate for use in treatment of diseases that require high and transient gene expression (Robbins & Ghivizzani, 1998).

In contrast with adenoviral vectors, retroviruses have a substantial advantage as vectors for the sustained expression of a transgene in target cells (Verma & Weitzman, 2005). Retroviruses are enveloped RNA viruses belonging to the *Retroviridae* family. The retroviral particle contains two copies of linear, positive sense, single-stranded RNA of 7-13 kb in length. All members of the *Retroviridae* family harbors at the minimum three essential genes: *gag* for structural proteins, *pol* for enzymes, and *env* for envelope. In the retroviral genome, the *gag* gene is positioned upstream of the *pol* gene, and the Pol polyprotein is generated as a fusion protein with the Gag polyprotein (Gag-Pol). As we shall see in the next section, the viral RNA genome is converted into a double-stranded DNA copy by reverse transcriptase (RT), a processing product of Pol, soon after the entry into the target cell (reverse transcription). Subsequently, the viral DNA is transported to the nucleus and covalently joined with cellular chromatin. This joining step is called integration and it is catalyzed by integrase (IN), another processing product of Pol. The integration step as well as the reverse transcription is hallmark of retroviral infection. Once integrated, the viral DNA serves as a template for the transcription of viral genes, enabling sustained gene expression in infected cells. The integrated viral DNA also contains *cis*-acting sequences termed the long terminal repeat (LTR) at its termini, which consist of 3′ unique elements (U3), repeat elements (R), and 5′ unique elements (U5). The 5′ LTR sequence functions as the promoter sequence for gene expression, in which viral RNA transcription is initiated at the U3-R, and the transcripts are polyadenylated at the R-U5 boundary of the 3′ LTR. The development of retrovirus as a gene transfer vector was first achieved with oncoretroviruses in the 1980s (Mann et al., 1983; Miller & Rosman, 1989; Shimotohno & Temin, 1981; Tabin et al., 1982; Watanabe & Temin, 1983; Wei et al., 1981); nowadays Moloney murine leukemia virus (MoMLV), one of the well characterized oncoretroviruses, is commonly used for therapeutic applications (Anderson et al., 1990; Blaese et al., 1993; Guild et al., 1988; Levine& Friedmann, 1991; Miller, 1992a, b). However, the important limitation of the MoMLV-derived vector is its cell cycle dependency: this virus lacks the ability to infect non-dividing cells (Harel et al., 1981; Hatziioannou & Goff, 2001; Lewis & Emerman, 1994; Miller et al., 1990; Roe et al., 1993). Unlike the MoMLV, lentiviruses, a separate genus of the *Retroviridae* family including human immunodeficiency virus type-1 (HIV-1), can infect both dividing and non-dividing cells (Bukrinsky et al., 1992; Hatziioannou & Goff, 2001; Lewis et al., 1992; Lewis &

Emerman, 1994). The ability to infect non-dividing cells is not restricted to *in vitro* cell culture as lentivirus-derived vectors are capable of transducing certain quiescent or terminally differentiated cells such as macrophages and microglia (Miyake et al., 1998; Naldini et al., 1996; Weinberg et al., 1991). This property makes the lentivirus an attractive choice for gene transfer vector (Suzuki & Craigie, 2007).

It is well known that HIV-1 is the causative agent for acquired immunodeficiency syndrome (AIDS). Currently, the standard AIDS treatment, termed highly active antiretroviral therapy (HAART), is to use cocktail of antiretroviral drugs that targets different HIV-1 enzymes including reverse transcriptase and protease. However, although it successfully causes suppression of HIV-1 RNA detected in plasma for a prolonged period of time and dramatic decrease of patient mortality (Palella et al., 1998; Volberding & Deeks, 2010), this pharmacological therapy is facing problems such as drug resistance and side effects in administrated individuals (Meadows & Gervay-Hague, 2006; Richman, 2001). Hence, viral vector-based gene therapy should offer a new approach to supplement the need for current drug regimens for the treatment of HIV/AIDS (Poluri et al., 2003; Strayer et al., 2005). Genetic modification of HIV-susceptible cells or hematopoietic stem cells (HSCs) by expressing anti-HIV transgenes should be one of the goals of the HIV gene therapy (Kitchen et al., 2011). In this regard, the lentiviral vector has the potential advantage for transduction because of its ability to infect quiescent cells including HSC (Miyoshi et al., 1999). However, incorporation of anti-HIV genes into an HIV-based lentiviral vector can create problems for production of the vector itself; expression of the anti-HIV trans gene in the producer cells can interfere with vector production (Banerjea et al., 2003; Li et al., 2003; Mautino & Morgan, 2002c). One way to avoid this difficulty is to introduce a gene regulatable system in which the target transgene is kept silent during vector production and expression is subsequently induced on following infection of the vector in target cells.

Several regulatable gene expression systems have been developed and applied to viral vectors including lentiviral vectors (Goverdhana et al., 2005; Weber & Fussenegger, 2004). In this chapter, we focus on recent development of the gene-regulatable lentiviral vectors and discuss the suitability of the vectors for anti-HIV therapy.

2. Biology of HIV-1 replication

2.1 Genomic organization and gene expression

Lentiviruses, as represented by HIV-1, are also called complex retroviruses, which are characterized by a set of additional regulatory and accessory genes encoded in the viral genome (Cullen, 1991; Frankel & Young, 1998). In the case of HIV-1, the DNA genome converted from the RNA genome is about 9.7 kb and contains nine ORFs; in addition to the *gag*, *pol*, and *env* genes that are typical of all retroviruses, there are two regulatory (*tat* and *rev*) and four accessory (*vif*, *vpr*, *vpu*, and *nef*) genes (Fig. 1). These protein-coding regions are flanked by 5′ and 3′ LTR that are required for reverse transcription, integration, and gene expression steps.

The complexity of HIV-1 is also characterized by its specific pattern of viral gene regulation (Kingsman & Kingsman, 1996). The HIV-1 LTR harbors several *cis*-acting sequences required for the initiation of viral RNA expression. The U3 region of the LTR is composed of a series of control elements that recruit a variety of transcription factors (Brady & Kashanchi, 2005), and consequently, transcription of viral RNA initiates at the U3-R junction. However, the transcription activity of the U3 is basically low, and *trans*-acting proteins are required to enhance the viral RNA synthesis from the 5′ LTR. Viral regulatory protein, Tat is one of these transactivators (Brady & Kashanchi, 2005). Tat interacts not with DNA, but with an RNA bulge of a stem-loop structure formed at the 5′ end of nascent transcripts, which is known as the transactivation response region (TAR) (Berkhout et al., 1989; Feng & Holland, 1988). Binding of Tat to the TAR then recruits an active transcription elongation complex consisting of cyclin T1 (CycT1), CDK9, and some other factors (Brady & Kashanchi, 2005). Subsequently, CDK9 leads the hyperphosphorylation of the C-terminal domain of RNA polymerase II, in turn resulting in a dramatic stimulation of transcriptional processivity (Brady & Kashanchi, 2005).

More than 30 species of RNA are transcribed from the integrated HIV-1 DNA; these fall into three size classes of mRNA based on the pattern of splicing: unspliced, partially spliced, and multiply spliced RNAs. (Kingsman & Kingsman, 1996; Purcell & Martin, 1993; Schwartz et al., 1990). The unspliced transcript is full-length RNA (about 9 kb) that is packaged as the viral genome into new viral particles but it also functions as mRNA to produce Gag and Gag-Pol polyproteins. The partially spliced transcripts (about 4 kb) encode Vif, Vpr, Vpu, and Env proteins. At early times after infection, however, the multiply spliced RNAs are predominant, and their encoded proteins, Tat, Rev, and Nef are highly produced (Kim et al., 1989).

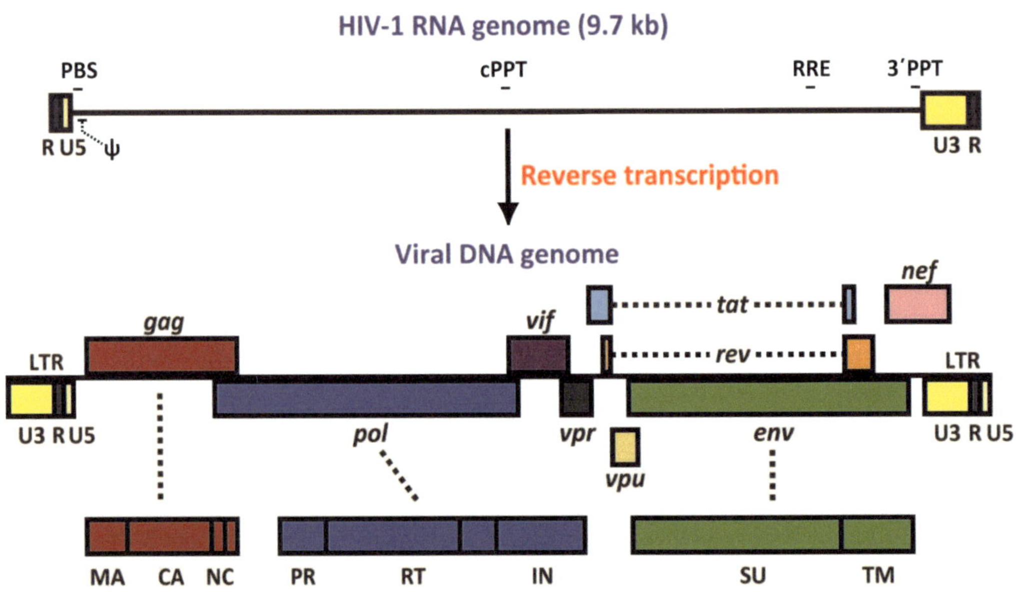

Fig. 1. Organization of the HIV-1 genome.

2.2 Replication cycle

HIV-1 infection begins with the binding of the viral envelope (Env) glycoprotein gp120 (surface envelope protein: SU) to the CD4 receptor molecule on the surface of host cells. Consequently, the main target cells for HIV-1 infection are the $CD4^{+}$ subset of helper T cells and monocyte/macrophage lineages (Dalgleish et al., 1984; Landau et al., 1988; Stevenson, 2003). The gp120-CD4 interaction triggers a conformational change in the gp120 that facilitates subsequent binding to a secondary cellular receptor (coreceptor). While most HIV-1 strains use either the α-chemokine receptor CXCR4 or the β-chemokine receptor CCR5 as the coreceptor, other chemokine receptors or related proteins have been reported to serve as coreceptors for HIV-1 infection (Berger et al., 1999). This coreceptor usage is the basis for the differential cell-type tropism of HIV-1 strains. Formation of the gp120-CD4-coreceptor complex then induces refolding of the gp41 subunit of the Env (transmembrane envelope protein: TM), which allows the membrane fusion process between the virus and target cell (Melikyan, 2008).

After penetrating the cell membrane, the viral nucleoprotein core, which contains genomic RNA, is released into the cytoplasm, followed by the uncoating of the viral core that is required for the formation of the reverse transcription complex (RTC) (Arhel, 2010; Bukrinskaya et al., 1998; Fassati & Goff, 2001). Reverse transcription, one of the defining steps of retrovirus infection, takes place in the RTC and it is initiated from the 3′ end of the $tRNA^{Lys3}$ that is annealed to the primer binding site (PBS) near the 5′ end of the viral RNA genome. During the reverse transcription reaction, RT firstly synthesizes the minus-strand DNA along with the concomitant degradation of the RNA template by its RNase H activity (Basu et al., 2008). Subsequent synthesis of plus-strand DNA involves priming from two polyprine tracts (PPT), short RNA segments resistant to RNase H digestion, at the 3′ terminus (3′ PPT) and the center (central PPT: cPPT) of the HIV-1 genome. Once the 3′ end of the plus-strand DNA reaches the 5′ end of the cPPT, DNA synthesis proceeds by displacing the existing DNA fragments and stops at a central termination sequence (CTS) in the minus-strand DNA, resulting in a 99 bp triple-strand DNA structure in the center of the HIV-1 DNA (Arhel, 2010; Charneau et al., 1992; Charneau et al., 1994).

The newly synthesized full-length viral DNA remains associated with viral and cellular proteins in a large nucleoprotein complex called the preintegration complex (PIC) (Engelman, 2003). The HIV-1 PIC has been shown to contain RT, IN, matrix (MA), nucleocapsid (NC), and Vpr proteins (Lewinski & Bushman, 2005; Suzuki & Craigie, 2007). In addition to viral proteins, several cellular proteins have been reported as components of the HIV PIC (Suzuki & Craigie, 2007). As mentioned above, unlike many oncoretroviruses, HIV-1 is able to infect non-dividing cells. Thus, the HIV-1 PIC is believed to carry karyophilic signals that direct transport across an intact nuclear membrane in non-dividing cells. Although the molecular mechanisms underlying the active transport of HIV-1 PIC into the nucleus is still poorly understood, several viral and cellular factors have been shown to be implicated in the nuclear import of the HIV-1 PIC (Fassati, 2006; Suzuki & Craigie, 2007; Yamashita & Emerman, 2006). Cell cycle-independent infection of HIV-1 is particularly important in the pathogenesis of the virus and the development of HIV-1-based lentiviral vectors (Blankson et al., 2002; Kaul et al., 2001; Somia & Verma, 2000).

Following nuclear transport of the PIC, integration of viral DNA into the host chromatin takes place. IN is a key component of the PIC that catalyzes the integration. This reaction proceeds via three coordinated steps: 3′ end processing of the viral DNA, joining to the target DNA, and repairing of the gaps between viral DNA and target DNA. IN is responsible for the 3′ end processing and DNA joining steps, but the gap repair step is likely to be carried out by yet-to-be-identified cellular enzymes (Engelman, 2003) (Fig. 2).

The integrated DNA, called the provirus, is acted upon by cellular transcription factors to express viral genes. Early populations of the transcripts are the multiply spliced class of mRNA that encodes Tat, Rev, and Nef proteins (Kingsman & Kingsman, 1996). Tat enhances production of viral mRNAs by more than two log via interaction with TAR and a cellular elongation complex (Brady & Kashanchi, 2005). There is then an increase in the partially spiced and unspliced mRNAs along with a concomitant decrease in the multiply spliced mRNAs, which is caused by the accumulation of Rev protein. Rev is also required for the nuclear export of partially spliced and unspliced mRNAs. These classes of viral RNAs contain a highly structured *cis*-acting element termed Rev response element (RRE) that is located in the *env* coding region. Rev bears a leucine-rich nuclear export signal (NES) and, via association with the RRE, mediates nuclear-to-cytoplasmic transport of the partially spliced and unspliced RNAs, resulting in production of Gag, Gag-Pol, Env, and accessory proteins (Pollard & Malim, 1998).

Following the synthesis of the full-length viral RNA genome and the viral proteins, these components are assembled together to produce new viruses. In HIV-1, the assembly process takes place at the plasma membrane (Ono, 2010). Gag protein plays a central role in the formation of virions; this protein is synthesized as a 55 kDa precursor protein for matrix (MA), capsid (CA)), and nucleocapsid (NC) proteins. The Gag precursor proteins are rapidly targeted to the plasma membrane where they multimerize. Although the multimerization of the Gag is sufficient to give rise to virus like particles, incorporation of Gag-Pol proteins is integral to the formation of infectious virions (Wu et al., 1997). Gag-Pol is a 160 kDa multidomain protein consisting of RT, IN, and protease (PR), and it too relocates to the plasma membrane, where Gag and Gag-Pol are assembled into virus particles. In the HIV-1 genome, Gag and Pol are encoded by overlapping ORF; Gag-Pol is generated by a ribosomal frameshifting during translation of the *gag* gene. This translation mechanism limits intracellular synthesis of Gag-Pol at 10- to 20-fold-lower than Gag (Haraguchi et al., 2010). Env glycoprotein, which is synthesized in the rough endoplasmic reticulum (ER), reaches the cell surface and is incorporated into virus particles. The MA domain of Gag has been suggested to be important for the recruitment of Env into virions (Ono, 2010). Encapsidation of the viral genomic RNA is directed by an interaction between the NC domain of Gag and the packaging signal (or ψ-site located in the 5′ region of the *gag* initiation codon. The ψ sequence also acts as a dimerization signal for the viral RNA genome. Eventually, the virus particle is pinched off the host cell membrane (budding). Recent evidence has revealed that a number of cellular proteins in the vacuolar protein sorting (VPS) pathway are involved in the HIV-1 budding process. After release from the plasma membrane, virus particles undergo a maturation step, in which Gag and Gag-Pol precursor proteins are cleaved by the viral PR to yield the functional mature proteins of infectious HIV-1 (Vogt, 1996) (Fig. 2).

Accessory proteins (i.e. Vif, Vpr, Vpu, and Nef) are dispensable for viral replication in many *in vitro* cell culture systems, but these proteins are likely to be required for efficient replication and pathogenicity of HIV-1 *in vivo* (Malim & Emerman, 2008).

3. Development of HIV-1-derived lentiviral vectors

Although retrovirus vectors derived from oncoretroviruses were introduced first, in recent years, attention of the viral vector research has been focused on lentiviruses such as HIV-1 and equine infectious anemia virus (EIAV) due to their ability to infect non-dividing cells. In particular, HIV-1 should be one of the most practical gene transfer vectors for gene therapy applications because this is the best studied retrovirus. However, HIV-1 is a human pathogen that causes destruction the of $CD4^+$ helper T lymphocytes and the subsequent loss of immune competence (Forsman & Weiss, 2008). Therefore, considerable efforts have been devoted to develop efficient HIV-1-derived lentiviral vectors with improved biosafety features.

So far, three different generations of HIV-1-based lentiviral vectors have been established, which is based on the level of safety improvements in viral vector production (Fig. 3).

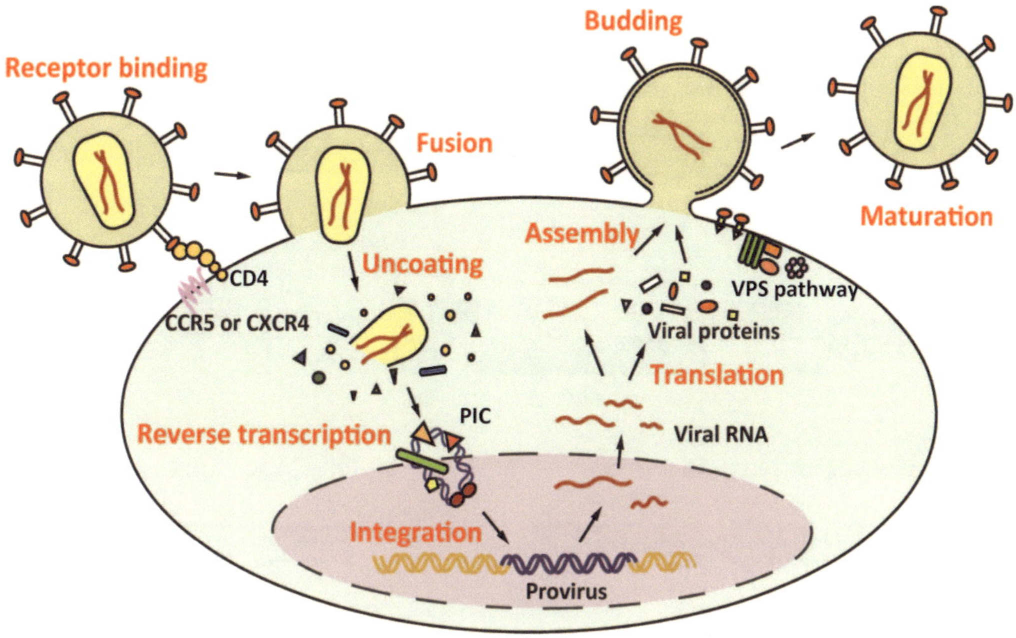

Fig. 2. Schematic representation of HIV-1 replication. HIV-1 enters target cells by first binding to the CD4 receptor and a coreceptor (CCR5 or CXCR4), this allows fusion between the cellular and viral membranes. After entry, the viral nucleoprotein core containing the genomic RNA is released into cytoplasm. Reverse transcription takes place in a nucleoprotein complex termed the RTC. The synthesis of full-length viral DNA produces an integration-competent nucleoprotein complex called the PIC and this nucleoprotein complex mediates integration of viral DNA into chromatin. Integrated viral DNA, called the provirus, serves as a transcription template for the synthesis of viral mRNA and genomic RNA. Following the synthesis of viral proteins, the viral components are assembled together to produce new virions, the virus particles then undergo a maturation step to generate infectious HIV-1.

3.1 First-generation lentiviral vectors

One of the key safety concerns in the use of HIV-derived vectors is the generation of replication competent lentiviruses (RCL). Earlier development of lentiviral vectors was achieved by transient transfection of human embryonic kidney (HEK293T) cells with three separate plasmid DNAs encoding i) the lentiviral vector genome which was composed of the wild-type 5′ and 3′ LTR, a part of the *gag* gene corresponding to the ψ sequence, a part of the *env* gene containing the RRE, an internal promoter, and the desired gene (transfer vector plasmid), ii) the HIV-1 genome containing all viral genes with the exception of the *env* gene (packaging plasmid), and iii) the vesicular stomatitis virus G protein (VSV-G) that improves the stability and broadens the cellular tropism of lentiviral vectors (Burns et al., 1993; Naldini et al., 1996). However, in this vector production system, there is a potential risk for the generation of RCL; a recombination event would occur during subsequent reverse transcription in transduced cells between two RNAs that are derived from the transfer vector plasmid and the packaging plasmid and incidentally copackaged within the same virion (Fig. 3A).

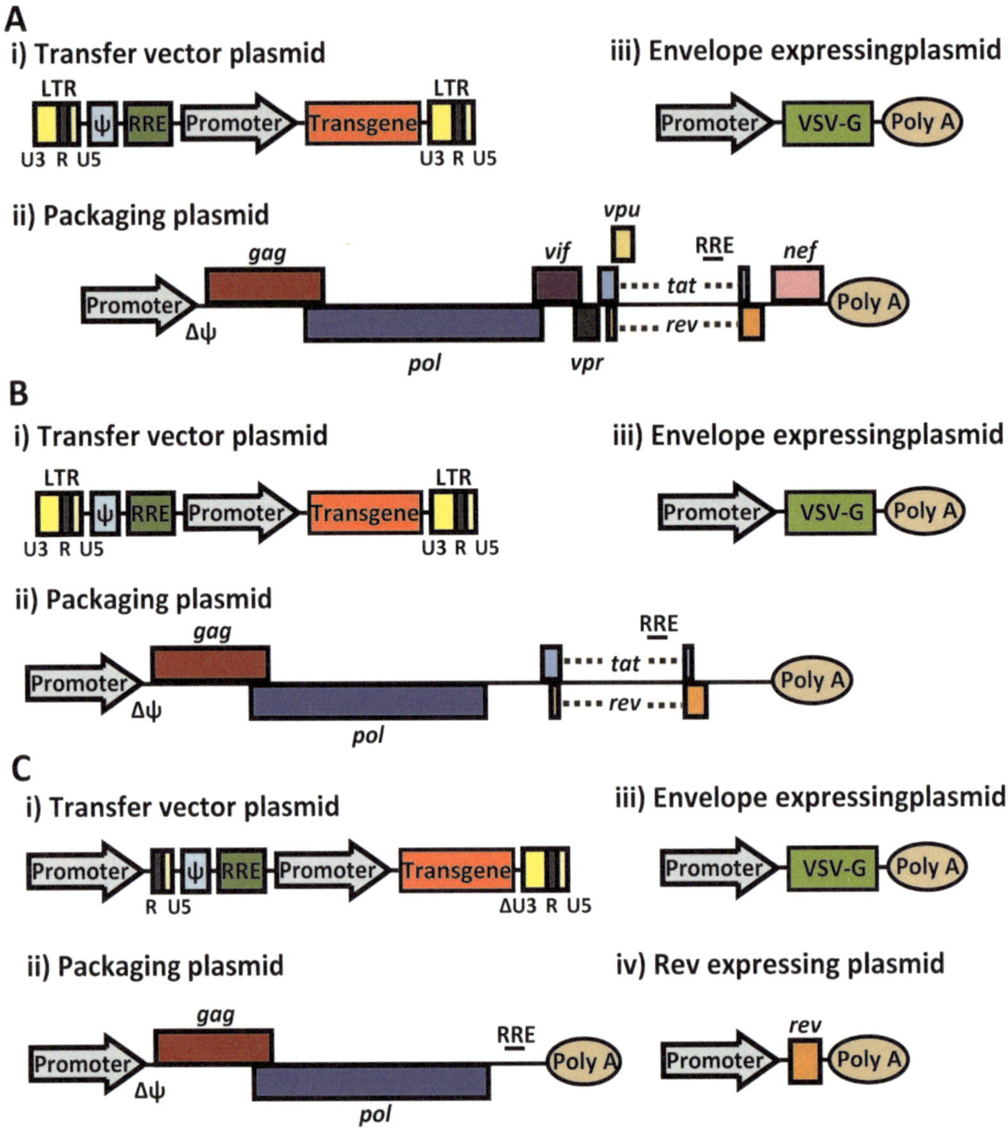

Fig. 3. Schematic representation of HIV-1-derived lentiviral vector packaging constructs. The first-generation lentiviral vectors (A) are produced by three separate plasmid DNAs encoding the vector genome, all HIV-1 genes except for *env* gene, and Env protein (VSV-G). To reduce the potential risk of the generation of replication competent viruses, all accessory genes (*vif*, *vpr*, *vpu*, and *nef*) are removed from (or mutated in) the packaging plasmids in second-generation lentiviral vectors (B). In third-generation lentiviral vectors, the enhancer/promoter unit is deleted from the U3 region of the 3′ LTR (ΔU3) in transfer vector plasmids (SIN vector). Additionally the U3 region of the 5′ LTR is replaced with the CMV promoter, enabling Tat-independent production of the lentiviral vectors (C). LTR, long terminal repeat; ψ, packaging signal; RRE, Rev response element.

3.2 Second-generation lentiviral vectors

The second-generation lentiviral vectors basically employ a similar three-plasmid system as the first generation vectors. Yet, in order to overcome the safety issue attributable to the first-generation vectors, the second-generation lentiviral vectors were generated without production of all accessory proteins (Vif, Vpr, Vpu, and Nef) via mutation or deletion of these genes from the packaging plasmid (Gasmi et al., 1999; Kim et al., 1998; Zufferey et al., 1997) (Fig. 3B).

3.3 Third-generation lentiviral vectors

The second-generation vectors, however, still carry the transcriptionally active LTR elements that could induce the homologous recombination between the vector genome and wild-type HIV-1. This would be particularly problematic if the lentiviral vectors are used for gene therapy of HIV/AIDS. Thus, further improvements were made in the third-generation lentiviral vectors. To minimize the transcriptional activity of the LTR in transduced cells, the enhancer/promoter unit was deleted from the U3 region of the 3′ LTR in transfer vector plasmids. During reverse transcription in the transduced cells, this deletion is transferred to the 5′ LTR of the lentiviral DNA, thereby reducing promoter activity of the integrated provirus (self-inactivating [SIN] vector) (Miyoshi et al., 1998; Zufferey et al., 1998). Additionally, the U3′region of the 5′ LTR in the transfer vector plasmid was replaced with the cytomegalovirus (CMV) promoter, which enabled Tat-independent transcription of the lentiviral vector genome in producer cells (Dull et al., 1998; Miyoshi et al., 1998). In these SIN vectors, there is no compete HIV-1 U3 sequence. Moreover, expression of Rev protein is directed by a separate plasmid, but not by the packaging plasmid encoding *gag* and *pol* genes (Wagner et al., 2000) (Fig. 3C). Currently, third-generation SIN lentiviral vector system offers the best safety profile in terms of generation of RCL because this vector requires only three HIV-1 genes (*gag*, *pol*, and *rev*) for production, however safety improvement in the design of HIV-1-derived lentiviral vectors is still one of the challenging areas in gene therapy study

4. Incorporation of regulatable gene expression systems in HIV-1-derived lentiviral vectors

Lentiviral vectors hold great promise for a gene therapy approach to inherited and acquired diseases. In these particular clinical settings, it would be more beneficial to reversibly control transgene expression in a dose and time dependent manner as illustrated in the field of angiogenesis and Parkinson's disease (Ma et al., 2002; Yancopoulos et al., 2000). To meet the standards required for clinical applications, a number of regulatable gene expression systems have been developed, and some of them are indeed incorporated into viral vectors including HIV-1-derived lentiviral vectors (reviewed in Goverdhana et al., 2005).

Although early development of the regulatable gene expression systems was based on naturally occurring inducible cellular promoters that respond to exogenous signals, these types of systems had limitations due to the pleiotropic effects of the inducer, high levels of "leaky" background expression and poor performance in inducibility. Therefore, recent efforts have been mostly focused on the development of chimeric gene regulatable systems derived from prokaryotic, eukaryotic, and viral elements, which are designed to enhance specificity and activity of transgene expression (Fussenegger, 2001).

4.1 Tetracycline-regulated system

The most widely used inducible system in lentiviral vectors is the tetracycline (Tet)-regulated system. This system was originally based on binding of the Tet-controlled repressor (tetR), a 23.6 kDa protein of *Escherichia coli* (*E. coli*), to the operator sequence of *E. coli* Tet resistance gene (Baron & Bujard, 2000), but further developed to be operated in mammalian cells by the generation of a chimeric protein in which tetR is fused with herpes simplex virus (HSV) VP16 protein, a eukaryotic transactivator (Tet-controlled transactivator: tTA) (Gossen & Bujard, 1992). In the absence of Tet or its derivatives such as doxycycline (Dox), the tTA binds the Tet-response element (TRE) that is composed of seven tandem copies of Tet operator (tetO) sequences and placed upstream of the CMV minimal promoter (Baron & Bujard, 2000). This type of original Tet-regulated system, called Tet-off system, has been incorporated into HIV-1-derived lentiviral vectors (Gascon et al., 2008; Haack et al., 2004; Kafri et al., 2000; Vigna et al., 2002) (Fig. 4A). In the first study that employed the Tet-off system in the context of a lentiviral vector, transgene induction by the withdrawal of Dox resulted in a more than 500-fold increase in the expression level of a GFP reporter gene (Kafri et al., 2000). Of note, the Dox-dependent regulation of GFP expression was also confirmed in the brain cells of rats that had been transduced by the lentiviral vector and then administered Dox through drinking water, indicating applicability of the gene regulatable lentiviral vectors *in vivo* (Kafri et al., 2000). However, even in the presence of Dox, high levels of basal GFP expression was observed, which would be attributed to the transcriptional interference arising from the neighboring CMV promoter or the wild-type HIV-1 LTR.

In addition to the background activity in the repressed state, the major limitation of the Tet-off system is the requirement of continuous administration of Tet or Dox to suppress transgene expression. To overcome this limitation, another type of Tet-controlled gene expression system was established by introduction of several permutations in the tTA protein of the Tet-off system. The mutant tTA binds the tetO sequences only in the presence of Tet/Dox: it exhibits opposite function (Gossen et al., 1995). Because this modified version of regulatable system, the so-called Tet-on system, shows rapid kinetics of gene upregulation compared to Tet-off system, several HIV-1-derived lentiviral vectors have been constructed using the Tet-on system as well (Johansen et al., 2002; Koponen et al., 2003; Pluta et al., 2005; Reiser et al., 2000; Vogel et al., 2004) (Fig. 4B).

One more approach to permit tight control of transgenes in the context of a lentiviral vector is demonstrated in the Tet-regulated system that employs a chimeric tetR fused with the Krüppel-associated box (KRAB) domain, a transcriptional regulator found in many DNA binding zinc-finger proteins (Szulc et al., 2006; Wiznerowicz & Trono, 2003). Binding of the KRAB domain-containing repressor protein to DNA recruits various heterochromatin-inducing factors, thereby suppressing activity of cellular RNA polymerases (RNAPs) II and III. This transcriptional silencing can be exerted no farther than 2-3 kb away from the repressor binding site. In the new design of Tet-regulated lentiviral vector system, the tetO site was inserted upstream of the RNAP III promoter-driven small hairpin RNA (shRNA) expression cassette which was located in the U3 region of lentiviral vector genome, and the activity of tetO-linked shRNA expression unit was tightly suppressed in the presence of KRAB-fused tTA and in the absence of Dox. The KRAB-fused tTA/Dox-dependent inhibition of transcriptional activity was also observed in the internal RNAP II promoter for a reporter transgene within the same vector genome. However, when the transduced cells were treated with Dox, shRNA was produced to achieve RNA interference, which was correlated with the expression of the reporter transgene (Szulc et al., 2006; Wiznerowicz & Trono, 2003).

One drawback of the Tet-regulated system is that there is a requirement to deliver two distinct expression units into a target cell: one is for transactivator (e.g. tTA) expression and the other is for transgene expression. In a binary lentiviral vector approach in which tTA and transgene expression cassettes are cloned into separate vectors, a population cells that is singly transduced with either tTA or transgene would be produced, resulting in low inducibility as a whole. This can be a bottleneck, particularly in relevant applications of the Tet-regulated lentiviral vector systems in clinical use. Single vector systems that contain the entire regulatable component in a unique vector is one of the solutions to guarantee simultaneous expression of the two expression units in the target gene, and these have indeed been established (Gascon et al., 2008; Kafri et al., 2000; Szulc et al., 2006; Vogel et al., 2004).

4.2 Mifepristone-inducible system

This gene regulatable system (also called GeneSwitch system) is based on a mutated human progesterone receptor that responds to the synthetic progestin antagonist but fails to bind natural progestins or other steroids (Burcin et al., 1999; Wang et al., 1994). Similar to Tet-regulated system, this system requires two components: the regulator (transactivator) protein and the inducible promoter sequence that drives transgene expression. The regulator is a hybrid protein consisting of a GAL4 DNA-binding domain from *Saccharomyces cerevisiae*, a ligand-binding domain of mutant progesterone receptor, and an activation domain of the p65 subunit of human NF-κB (Burcin et al., 1999). The inducible transgene expression unit contains six copies of the GAL4 upstream activating sequences (UAS) and the TATA box sequence in its promoter (Abruzzese et al., 1999). The progestin antagonist commonly used as an inducer for the GeneSwitch system is mifepristone (MFP, RU486). The regulator protein initially exists as an inactive monomeric form. However, in the presence of MFP, it binds to the MFP and undergoes a conformational change, causing the regulator protein to become an active homodimer. The active form of the regulator is able to bind to GAL4 UAS and induce transgene expression (Nordstrom, 2003) (Fig. 4C).

Sirin and Park have incorporated the MFP-inducible gene expression system into HIV-1-derived lentiviral vectors (Sirin & Park, 2003). In their design, two different SIN lentiviral vectors were constructed, in which either the regulator protein expression unit or the inducible transgene expression unit was cloned. When human cell lines (HeLa and Huh7 cells) were infected with both lentiviral vectors, up to a 275-fold increase in the number of reporter fluorescent protein-positive cells was observed at 48 hours following MFP treatment. Similar effective induction was also detected in cells transduced by a lentiviral vector expressing the human α_1-antitrypsin (hAAT) with an extremely low level of basal hAAT expression (Sirin & Park, 2003).

Although an *in vitro* study using adenovirus vector expressing the chloramphenicol acetyl transferase (CAT) as a reporter transgene gene demonstrates that induction level of the GeneSwitch system is lower than that of the Tet-regulated (Tet-on) system (Molin et al., 1998), the GeneSwitch system holds some advantages in its application to human gene therapy. The majority of components of the regulator protein are derived from human proteins, which has less impact on cell viability and immunogenicity. In addition, MFP has been approved by the Food and Drug Administration (FDA) for use in humans (Ulmann et al., 1995), and the concentration of MFP need for transgene induction is significantly lower than the concentration for its anti-progesterone effect (Nordstrom, 2003).

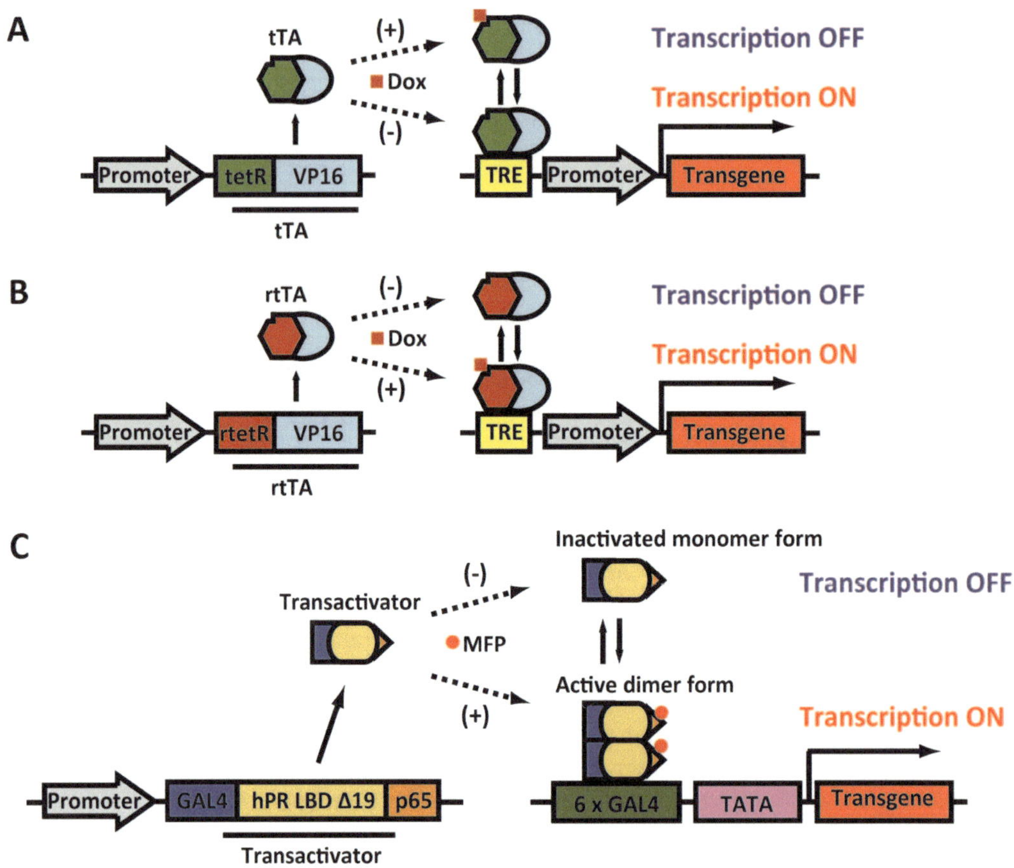

Fig. 4. Diagrams of two regulatable gene expression systems. The Tetracycline-regulated system is the most widely used inducible system in lentiviral vectors. In a Tet-off system (A), the Tet-controlled transactivator (tTA), a chimeric protein of *E. Coli* Tet-controlled repressor (tetR) and HSV VP16, binds the Tet-response element (TRE) upstream of the CMV promoter in the absence of Tet or Dox. On the other hand, in the Tet-on system (B), several mutations are introduced into the tTA (rtTA) so that this transactivator binds the TRE in the presence of Dox. The Mifepristone-inducible system (GeneSwitch) has been also incorporated into HIV-1-derived lentiviral vectors. In this system, the transactivator is a chimeric protein that comprises the GAL4 DNA-binding domain from *Saccharomyces cerevisiae* fused to the ligand-binding domain of a mutant progesterone receptor (hPR LBD Δ19) and the activation domain of the p65 subunit of human NF-*k*B. In the presence of mifepristone (MFP), the chimeric transactivator binds to the six copies of GAL4 upstream of the activating sequences and induce transgene expression (C). TATA, TATA box sequence.

4.3 Ecdysone-regulated system

The *Drosophila melanogaster* ecdysone receptor (EcR)-based gene regulatable system has been adapted to lentiviral vectors (Galimi et al., 2005). EcR is a member of the nuclear receptor superfamily that mediates a cascade of morphological changes in *Drosophila,* triggered by the steroid hormone ecdysone. Ecdysone regulates gene expressions by interacting with the functional EcR, which in turn induces binding of the EcR to DNA regulatory elements

EcREs) near target genes (No et al., 1996). The ecdysone-regulated gene expression system incorporated into lentiviral vectors employed two elements: i) the dimeric regulator protein of the EcR fused with HSV VP16 activation domain (VgEcR) and the retinoid X receptor (RXR), and ii) the hybrid promoter between the glucocorticoid response element and that of type II nuclear receptors (E/GRE) (Galimi et al., 2005). Upon exposure to ecdysone or synthetic analogues such as ponasterone A, the VgECR/RXR heterodimer binds to the E/GRE, resulting in induction of transgene expression (Saez et al., 2000). One advantage of the ecdysone-regulated gene expression system is the pharmacological profile of the inducer that allows for fast distribution and clearance after administration *in vivo* (Saez et al., 2000). Additionally, the inducible promoter is not responsive to natural nuclear receptors (No et al., 1996).

In the single vector approach, the inducible GFP expression cassette containing E/GRE as well as a CNV promoter-driven bicistronic unit for VgEcR and RXR expressions were cloned into an HIV-1-derived SIN lentiviral vector. However, this ecdysone-regulated system was also applicable to the binary vector system, in which the VgEcR/RXR expression unit was in one lentiviral vector and the inducible transgene expression unit was in the second vector. The latter approach would be of value in deliver of longer transgene. These lentiviral vectors have been shown to successfully deliver the ponA-inducible GFP expression units *in vitro* and *ex vivo* (Galimi et al., 2005).

4.4 Other regulatable systems

Besides the Tet- MFP-, and ecdysone-regulated systems, different types of inducible lentiviral vectors have been generated based on the other chimeric regulatable systems, which include streptogramin-adjustable expression system derived from *Streptomyces coelicolor* (Mitta et al., 2004) and gaseous acetaldehyde-inducible expression system derived from *Aspergillus nidulans* (Hartenbach & Fussenegger, 2005). Although some endogenous cellular elements that respond to exogenous signals or stress have been adapted to HIV-1- and EIAV-derived lentiviral vectors (Beutelspacher et al., 2005; Hurttila et al., 2008; Parker et al., 2009), the pleiotropic effects exerted by the inducing agent would be a drawback in a human therapeutic context (Fussenegger, 2001).

5. Application of a gene regulatable lentiviral vector for HIV-1 inhibition

Lentiviral vector-mediated gene therapy has the potential to improve the clinical state of a patient with HIV-1. This goal would be accomplished by *ex vivo* transduction of anti-HIV genes into $CD4^+$ virus target cells such as helper T cells and macrophages or $CD34^+$ progenitor cells (HSCs), making them resistant to HIV-1 infection (intracellular immunization approach) (Baltimore, 1988; Kitchen et al., 2011). So far, various studies have reported the delivery of anti-HIV genes by HIV-1-based lentiviral vectors *in vitro* and *in vivo*, and the anti-HIV genes can be categorized as either RNA- or protein-based (Mukhtar et al., 2000) (Banerjea et al., 2003; Dropulic et al., 1996; Klimatcheva et al., 2001; Li et al., 2003; Mautino et al., 2001; Mautino & Morgan, 2002a, b, c). Among the RNA-based anti-HIV genes include a ribozyme that cleaves the U5 region of HIV-1 RNA by its enzymatic activity (Dropulic et al., 1996), an antisense RNA that hybridizes the transcripts of HIV-1 *env* gene to inhibit translation of Env (Mautino & Morgan, 2002a, c), and small interfering RNA (siRNA) that induces sequence-specific degradation of HIV-1 RNA (Banerjea et al., 2003). In the protein-based approach, the transdominant negative mutant of Rev (TdRev) is best described as an anti-HIV gene used in the setting of lentiviral vectors (Klimatcheva et al., 2001; Mautino et al., 2001; Mautino & Morgan, 2002c; Mukhtar et al., 2000). The TdReV named RevM10 is a derivative of HIV-1 Rev in which two amino acid mutations are introduced in the C-terminus activation domain, and hampers nuclear export of HIV-1 mRNAs via the formation of inactive multimers with WT Rev (Hope et al., 1992; Malim et al., 1989). It should be noted that RevM10 has been already tested in phase I clinical trials to treat HIV infection via transduction of the gene into $CD34^+$ cells with MoMLV-derived retroviral vectors (Kang et al., 2002; Kitchen et al., 2011; Podsakoff et al., 2005).

Although a promising approach for HIV gene therapy, constitutive expression of anti-HIV genes in the context of HIV-1-derived lentiviral vectors could encounter a problem of self-inhibition of the vector particle production, resulting in significant decrease of viral infectious titer (Mautino & Morgan, 2002b). This problem of self-inhibition can be solved by several means. If the anti-HIV gene targets specific sequences in the HIV-1 RNA, one strategy to avoid the self-inhibition would be to engineer nucleotide sequences of lentiviral vector genome and packaging genes in order that anti-HIV gene will exclusively recognize wild-type virus in transduced cells. As for TdRev, the inhibition of vector production could be overcome by replacement of the HIV-1 Rev-dependent nuclear export element (e.g. RRE) with the one derived from another lentiviruses, conferring Rev-independent property on the lentiviral vectors (Mautino et al., 2001; Taylor et al., 2008). But, if the anti-HIV genes are designed to target HIV-1 at more fundamental process such as virion formation and budding processes, an ideal strategy would be the incorporation of regulatable transgene expression system into lentiviral vectors, in which expression of the anti-HIV gene is "OFF" during vector production and turned "ON" in the target cells.

In order to assess the availability of gene regulatable systems in inhibition of HIV-1, we have generated HIV-1-derived lentiviral vectors harboring the MFP-inducible transgene expression unit (Shinoda et al., 2009). In the study, two SIN lentiviral vectors were designed to incorporate the MFP-inducible unit in either the forward or the reverse orientation with respect to the direction of transfer vector genome (designated as forward and reverse vectors, respectively), since it has been reported that promoter activity of the internal gene expression unit could be affected by its orientation and/or the presence of adjacent LTR (Chen et al., 1992; Reiser et al., 2000; Sirin & Park, 2003). When firefly luciferase gene, which does not interfere with HIV-1 production, was inserted into the MFP-inducible lentiviral vectors, substantial levels of infectious vectors could be yielded from the forward and reverse vector systems by co-transfection with packaging plasmid DNAs in HEK293T cells. However, the infectious titer obtained by the forward vector was more than 10-fold higher than reverse vector, and even in the absence of transactivator and inducer, significant level of the leaky expression of luciferase was observed in the forward vector plasmid transfected-cells, but not in the reverse vector-transfected cells (Shinoda et al., 2009). It can be speculated that the higher background activity in the forward vector was due to the enhancement of gene expression by orientation-dependent *cis*-acting element such as the woodchuck post-regulatory element (WPRE) and/or the weak promoter activity of the 5′ LTR. Importantly, this tight suppression of inducible unit in the reverse vector was reflected in its ability to produce infectious vectors when a transdominant negative mutant of human VPS4B protein in the VPS pathway, which inhibits budding process of HIV-1, was used as a transgene. Transfection of the reverse vector plasmid containing VPS4B dominant-negative mutant yielded infectious lentiviral vector, transfection of the forward vector could not generate infectious vectors, demonstrating the self-inhibition by the leaky expression of

VPS4B dominant-negative mutant from the forward vector plasmid in vector producing cells (Shinoda et al., 2009). As expected, subsequent transduction of the transactivator-expressing cells with the infectious reverse vector bearing the VPS4B mutant resulted in significant inhibition of wild-type HIV-1 production only in the presence of MFP (Shinoda et al., 2009). Thus, this previous study demonstrates that the gene regulatable lentiviral vector system has the capability to transduce anti-HIV gene and subsequently block HIV-1 budding without the problem of self-inhibition during vector production.

6. Conclusion and future direction

Lentiviral vectors derived from HIV-1 are attractive gene delivery vehicles in terms of stable and long-term transgene expression in dividing and non-dividing cells. Although strong promoters used to achieve high levels of transgene expression are put into general use in the lentiviral vectors, incorporation of regulatable gene expression system confers transcriptional flexibility to the vector, which expands the potential of the lentiviral vectors for a wide array of gene transfer applications, particularly when undesired side effect would be expected by the constitutive expression of transgene. Nevertheless, many obstacles must be overcome for the clinical application of gene regulatable lentiviral vectors in gene therapy. One of the obstacles is that all the components of a regulatory system should be incorporated into a single vector, limiting the cloning capacity for transgene. Another issue is that there is no gene regulatory system approved by the FDA for clinical use. However, if their safety and efficacy are validated, development of gene regulatable lentiviral vector systems will be a next promising step toward achieving successful gene therapy for otherwise incurable diseases.

7. Acknowledgment

We are grateful Wei Xin Chin for proofreading and comments on the manuscript.

8. References

Abruzzese, R.V.; Godin, D.; Burcin, M.; Mehta, V.; French, M.; Li, Y.; O'Malley, B.W.; Nordstrom, J.L. (1999). Ligand-dependent regulation of plasmid-based transgene expression in vivo. *Hum. Gene Ther.*, Vol. 10, No. 9, pp. 1499-1507

Anderson, W.F.; Blaese, R.M.; Culver, K. (1990). The ADA human gene therapy clinical protocol: Points to Consider response with clinical protocol, July 6, 1990. *Hum. Gene Ther.*, Vol. 1, No. 3, pp. 331-362

Arhel, N. (2010). Revisiting HIV-1 uncoating. *Retrovirology*, Vol. 7, pp. 96

Armentano, D.; Sookdeo, C.C.; Hehir, K.M.; Gregory, R.J.; St George, J.A.; Prince, G.A.; Wadsworth, S.C.; Smith, A.E. (1995). Characterization of an adenovirus gene transfer vector containing an E4 deletion. *Hum. Gene Ther.*, Vol. 6, No. 10, pp. 1343-1353

Armentano, D.; Smith, M.P.; Sookdeo, C.C.; Zabner, J.; Perricone, M.A.; St George, J.A.; Wadsworth, S.C.; Gregory, R.J. (1999). E4ORF3 requirement for achieving long-term transgene expression from the cytomegalovirus promoter in adenovirus vectors. *J. Virol.*, Vol. 73, No. 8, pp. 7031-7034

Baltimore, D. (1988). Gene therapy. Intracellular immunization. *Nature,* Vol. 335, No. 6189, pp. 395-396

Banerjea, A.; Li, M.J.; Bauer, G.; Remling, L.; Lee, N.S.; Rossi, J.; Akkina, R. (2003). Inhibition of HIV-1 by lentiviral vector-transduced siRNAs in T lymphocytes differentiated in SCID-hu mice and CD34+ progenitor cell-derived macrophages. *Mol. Ther.,* Vol. 8, No. 1, pp. 62-71

Baron, U.; Bujard, H. (2000). Tet repressor-based system for regulated gene expression in eukaryotic cells: principles and advances. *Methods Enzymol.,* Vol. 327, pp. 401-421

Basu, V.P.; Song, M.; Gao, L.; Rigby, S.T.; Hanson, M.N.; Bambara, R.A. (2008). Strand transfer events during HIV-1 reverse transcription. *Virus Res.,* Vol. 134, No. 1-2, pp. 19-38

Bergelson, J.M.; Cunningham, J.A.; Droguett, G.; Kurt-Jones, E.A.; Krithivas, A.; Hong, J.S.; Horwitz, M.S.; Crowell, R.L.; Finberg, R.W. (1997). Isolation of a common receptor for Coxsackie B viruses and adenoviruses 2 and 5. *Science,* Vol. 275, No. 5304, pp. 1320-1323

Berger, E.A.; Murphy, P.M.; Farber, J.M. (1999). Chemokine receptors as HIV-1 coreceptors: roles in viral entry, tropism, and disease. *Annu. Rev. Immunol.,* Vol. 17, pp. 657-700

Berk, A.J. (2007). *Adenoviridae*: The Viruses and Their Replication, In *Fields Virology,* Knipe, D.M.; Howley, P.M., Vol. 2, pp. 2355, Lippincott Williams & Wilkins, Philadelphia

Berkhout, B.; Silverman, R.H.; Jeang, K.T. (1989). Tat trans-activates the human immunodeficiency virus through a nascent RNA target. *Cell,* Vol. 59, No. 2, pp. 273-282

Bett, A.J.; Haddara, W.; Prevec, L.; Graham, F.L. (1994). An efficient and flexible system for construction of adenovirus vectors with insertions or deletions in early regions 1 and 3. *Proc. Natl. Acad. Sci. USA,* Vol. 91, No. 19, pp. 8802-8806

Beutelspacher, S.C.; Ardjomand, N.; Tan, P.H.; Patton, G.S.; Larkin, D.F.; George, A.J.; McClure, M.O. (2005). Comparison of HIV-1 and EIAV-based lentiviral vectors in corneal transduction. *Exp. Eye Res.,* Vol. 80, No. 6, pp. 787-794

Blaese, R.M.; Culver, K.W.; Chang, L.; Anderson, W.F.; Mullen, C.; Nienhuis, A.; Carter, C.; Dunbar, C.; Leitman, S.; Berger, M.; et al. (1993). Treatment of severe combined immunodeficiency disease (SCID) due to adenosine deaminase deficiency with $CD34^+$ selected autologous peripheral blood cells transduced with a human ADA gene. Amendment to clinical research project, Project 90-C-195, January 10, 1992. *Hum. Gene Ther.,* Vol. 4, No. 4, pp. 521-527

Blankson, J.N.; Persaud, D.; Siliciano, R.F. (2002). The challenge of viral reservoirs in HIV-1 infection. *Annu. Rev. Med.,* Vol. 53, No. pp. 557-593

Brady, J.; Kashanchi, F. (2005). Tat gets the "green" light on transcription initiation. *Retrovirology* Vol. 2, pp. 69

Brough, D.E.; Hsu, C.; Kulesa, V.A.; Lee, G.M.; Cantolupo, L.J.; Lizonova, A.; Kovesdi, I. (1997). Activation of transgene expression by early region 4 is responsible for a high level of persistent transgene expression from adenovirus vectors in vivo. *J. Virol.* Vol. 71, No. 12, pp. 9206-9213

Bukrinskaya, A.; Brichacek, B.; Mann, A.; Stevenson, M. (1998). Establishment of a functional human immunodeficiency virus type 1 (HIV-1) reverse transcription complex involves the cytoskeleton. *J. Exp. Med.,* Vol. 188, No. 11, pp. 2113-2125

Bukrinsky, M.I.; Sharova, N.; Dempsey, M.P.; Stanwick, T.L.; Bukrinskaya, A.G.; Haggerty, S.; Stevenson, M. (1992). Active nuclear import of human immunodeficiency virus type 1 preintegration complexes. *Proc. Natl. Acad. Sci. USA,* Vol. 89, No. 14, pp. 6580-6584

Burcin, M.M.; Schiedner, G.; Kochanek, S.; Tsai, S.Y.; O'Malley, B.W. (1999). Adenovirus-mediated regulable target gene expression in vivo. *Proc. Natl. Acad. Sci. USA,* Vol. 96, No. 2, pp. 355-360

Burns, J.C.; Friedmann, T.; Driever, W.; Burrascano, M.; Yee, J.K. (1993). Vesicular stomatitis virus G glycoprotein pseudotyped retroviral vectors: concentration to very high titer and efficient gene transfer into mammalian and nonmammalian cells. *Proc. Natl. Acad. Sci. USA,* Vol. 90, No. 17, pp. 8033-8037

Charneau, P.; Alizon, M.; Clavel, F. (1992). A second origin of DNA plus-strand synthesis is required for optimal human immunodeficiency virus replication. *J. Virol.,* Vol. 66, No. 5, pp. 2814-2820

Charneau, P.; Mirambeau, G.; Roux, P.; Paulous, S.; Buc, H.; Clavel, F. (1994). HIV-1 reverse transcription. A termination step at the center of the genome. *J. Mol. Biol.,* Vol. 241, No. 5, pp. 651-662

Chen, B.F.; Hsieh, C.L.; Chen, D.S.; Hwang, L.H. (1992). Improved gene expression by a U3-based retroviral vector. *Biochem. Biophys. Res. Commun.,* Vol. 184, No. 1, pp. 330-337

Cullen, B.R. (1991). Human immunodeficiency virus as a prototypic complex retrovirus. *J. Virol.,* Vol. 65, No. 3, pp. 1053-1056

Cullen, B.R. (2001). Journey to the center of the cell. *Cell,* Vol. 105, No. 6, pp. 697-700

Dalgleish, A.G.; Beverley, P.C.; Clapham, P.R.; Crawford, D.H.; Greaves, M.F.; Weiss, R.A. (1984). The CD4 (T4) antigen is an essential component of the receptor for the AIDS retrovirus. *Nature,* Vol. 312, No. 5996, pp. 763-767

Danthinne, X.; Imperiale, M.J. (2000). Production of first generation adenovirus vectors: a review. *Gene Ther.,* Vol. 7, No. 20, pp. 1707-1714

Dropulic, B.; Hermankova, M.; Pitha, P.M. (1996). A conditionally replicating HIV-1 vector interferes with wild-type HIV-1 replication and spread. *Proc. Natl. Acad. Sci. USA,* Vol. 93, No. 20, pp. 11103-11108

Dull, T.; Zufferey, R.; Kelly, M.; Mandel, R.J.; Nguyen, M.; Trono, D.; Naldini, L. (1998). A third-generation lentivirus vector with a conditional packaging system. *J. Virol.,* Vol. 72, No. 11, pp. 8463-8471

Engelman, A. (2003). The roles of cellular factors in retroviral integration. *Curr. Top. Microbiol. Immunol.,* Vol. 281, pp. 209-238

Fallaux, F.J.; Kranenburg, O.; Cramer, S.J.; Houweling, A.; Van Ormondt, H.; Hoeben, R.C.; Van Der Eb, A.J. (1996). Characterization of 911: a new helper cell line for the titration and propagation of early region 1-deleted adenoviral vectors. *Hum. Gene Ther.,* Vol. 7, No. 2, pp. 215-222

Fassati, A. (2006). HIV infection of non-dividing cells: a divisive problem. *Retrovirology,* Vol. 3, pp. 74

Fassati, A.; Goff, S.P. (2001). Characterization of intracellular reverse transcription complexes of human immunodeficiency virus type 1. *J. Virol.,* Vol. 75, No. 8, pp. 3626-3635

Feng, S.; Holland, E.C. (1988), HIV-1 tat trans-activation requires the loop sequence within tar. *Nature,* Vol. 334, No. 6178, pp. 165-167

Flint, J.; Shenk, T. (1997). Viral transactivating proteins. *Annu. Rev. Genet.*, Vol. 31, pp. 177-212

Flotte, T.R.; Ng, P.; Dylla, D.E.; McCray, P.B., Jr.; Wang, G.; Kolls, J.K.; Hu, J. (2007). Viral vector-mediated and cell-based therapies for treatment of cystic fibrosis. *Mol. Ther.*, Vol. 15, No. 2, pp. 229-241

Forsman, A.; Weiss, R.A. (2008). Why is HIV a pathogen? *Trends Microbiol.*, Vol. 16, No. 12, pp. 555-560

Frankel, A.D.; Young, J.A. (1998). HIV-1: fifteen proteins and an RNA. *Annu. Rev. Biochem.*, Vol. 67, pp. 1-25

Fussenegger, M. (2001). The impact of mammalian gene regulation concepts on functional genomic research, metabolic engineering, and advanced gene therapies. *Biotechnol., Prog.* Vol. 17, No. 1, pp. 1-51

Galimi, F.; Summers, R.G.; van Praag, H.; Verma, I.M.; Gage, F.H. (2005). A role for bone marrow-derived cells in the vasculature of noninjured CNS. *Blood,* Vol. 105, No. 6, pp. 2400-2402

Gao, G.P.; Yang, Y.; Wilson, J.M. (1996). Biology of adenovirus vectors with E1 and E4 deletions for liver-directed gene therapy. *J. Virol.* Vol. 70, No. 12, pp. 8934-8943

Gascon, S.; Paez-Gomez, J.A.; Diaz-Guerra, M.; Scheiffele, P.; Scholl, F.G. (2008). Dual-promoter lentiviral vectors for constitutive and regulated gene expression in neurons. *J. Neurosci. Methods,* Vol. 168, No. 1, pp. 104-112

Gasmi, M.; Glynn, J.; Jin, M.J.; Jolly, D.J.; Yee, J.K.; Chen, S.T. (1999). Requirements for efficient production and transduction of human immunodeficiency virus type 1-based vectors. *J. Virol.*, Vol. 73, No. 3, pp. 1828-1834

Gossen, M.; Bujard, H. (1992). Tight control of gene expression in mammalian cells by tetracycline-responsive promoters. *Proc. Natl. Acad. Sci. USA,* Vol. 89, No. 12, pp. 5547-5551

Gossen, M.; Freundlieb, S.; Bender, G.; Muller, G.; Hillen, W.; Bujard, H. (1995). Transcriptional activation by tetracyclines in mammalian cells. *Science,* Vol. 268, No. 5218, pp. 1766-1769

Goverdhana, S.; Puntel, M.; Xiong, W.; Zirger, J.M.; Barcia, C.; Curtin, J.F.; Soffer, E.B.; Mondkar, S.; King, G.D.; Hu, J.; Sciascia, S.A.; Candolfi, M.; Greengold, D.S.; Lowenstein, P.R.; Castro, M.G. (2005). Regulatable gene expression systems for gene therapy applications: progress and future challenges. *Mol. Ther.,* Vol. 12, No. 2, pp. 189-211

Graham, F.L.; Smiley, J.; Russell, W.C.; Nairn, R. (1977). Characteristics of a human cell line transformed by DNA from human adenovirus type 5. *J. Gen. Virol.,* Vol. 36, No. 1, pp. 59-74

Guild, B.C.; Finer, M.H.; Housman, D.E.; Mulligan, R.C. (1988). Development of retrovirus vectors useful for expressing genes in cultured murine embryonal cells and hematopoietic cells in vivo. *J. Virol.,* Vol. 62, No. 10, pp. 3795-3801

Haack, K.; Cockrell, A.S.; Ma, H.; Israeli, D.; Ho, S.N.; McCown, T.J.; Kafri, T. (2004). Transactivator and structurally optimized inducible lentiviral vectors. *Mol. Ther.,* Vol. 10, No. 3, pp. 585-596

Haraguchi, H.; Sudo, S.; Noda, T.; Momose, F.; Kawaoka, Y.; Morikawa, Y. (2010). Intracellular localization of human immunodeficiency virus type 1 Gag and GagPol products and virus particle release: relationship with the Gag-to-GagPol ratio. *Microbiol. Immunol.*, Vol. 54, No. 12, pp. 734-746

Harel, J.; Rassart, E.; Jolicoeur, P. (1981). Cell cycle dependence of synthesis of unintegrated viral DNA in mouse cells newly infected with murine leukemia virus. *Virology*, Vol. 110, No. 1, pp. 202-207

Hartenbach, S.; Fussenegger, M. (2005). Autoregulated, bidirectional and multicistronic gas-inducible mammalian as well as lentiviral expression vectors. *J. Biotechnol.*, Vol. 120, No. 1, pp. 83-98

Hatziioannou, T.; Goff, S.P. (2001). Infection of nondividing cells by Rous sarcoma virus. *J. Virol.*, Vol. 75, No. 19, pp. 9526-9531

Hope, T.J.; Klein, N.P.; Elder, M.E.; Parslow, T.G. (1992). trans-dominant inhibition of human immunodeficiency virus type 1 Rev occurs through formation of inactive protein complexes. *J. Virol.*, Vol. 66, No. 4, pp. 1849-1855

Hurttila, H.; Koponen, J.K.; Kansanen, E.; Jyrkkanen, H.K.; Kivela, A.; Kylatie, R.; Yla-Herttuala, S.; Levonen, A.L. (2008). Oxidative stress-inducible lentiviral vectors for gene therapy. *Gene Ther.*, Vol. 15, No. 18, pp. 1271-1279

Imler, J.L.; Chartier, C.; Dreyer, D.; Dieterle, A.; Sainte-Marie, M.; Faure, T.; Pavirani, A.; Mehtali, M. (1996). Novel complementation cell lines derived from human lung carcinoma A549 cells support the growth of E1-deleted adenovirus vectors. *Gene Ther.*, Vol. 3, No. 1, pp. 75-84

Johansen, J.; Rosenblad, C.; Andsberg, K.; Moller, A.; Lundberg, C.; Bjorlund, A.; Johansen, T.E. (2002). Evaluation of Tet-on system to avoid transgene down-regulation in ex vivo gene transfer to the CNS. *Gene Ther.*, Vol. 9, No. 19, pp. 1291-1301

Kafri, T.; van Praag, H.; Gage, F.H.; Verma, I.M. (2000). Lentiviral vectors: regulated gene expression. *Mol. Ther.*, Vol. 1, No. 6, pp. 516-521

Kang, E.M.; De Witte, M.; Malech, H.; Morgan, R.A.; Carter, C.; Leitman, S.F.; Childs, R.; Barrett, A.J.; Little, R.; Tisdale, J.F. (2002). Gene therapy-based treatment for HIV-positive patients with malignancies. *J. Hematother. Stem Cell Res.*, Vol. 11, No. 5, pp. 809-816

Kaul, M.; Garden, G.A.; Lipton, S.A. (2001). Pathways to neuronal injury and apoptosis in HIV-associated dementia. *Nature*, Vol. 410, No. 6831, pp. 988-994

Kim, S.Y.; Byrn, R.; Groopman, J.; Baltimore, D. (1989). Temporal aspects of DNA and RNA synthesis during human immunodeficiency virus infection: evidence for differential gene expression. *J. Virol.*, Vol. 63, No. 9, pp. 3708-3713

Kim, V.N.; Mitrophanous, K.; Kingsman, S.M.; Kingsman, A.J. (1998). Minimal requirement for a lentivirus vector based on human immunodeficiency virus type 1. *J. Virol.*, Vol. 72, No. 1, pp. 811-816

Kingsman, S.M.; Kingsman, A.J. (1996). The regulation of human immunodeficiency virus type-1 gene expression. *Eur. J. Biochem.*, Vol. 240, No. 3, pp. 491-507

Kitchen, S.G.; Shimizu, S.; An, D.S. (2011). Stem cell-based anti-HIV gene therapy. *Virology*, Vol. 411, No. 2, pp. 260-272

Klimatcheva, E.; Planelles, V.; Day, S.L.; Fulreader, F.; Renda, M.J.; Rosenblatt, J. (2001). Defective lentiviral vectors are efficiently trafficked by HIV-1 and inhibit its replication. *Mol. Ther.*, Vol. 3, No. 6, pp. 928-939

Kochanek, S.; Clemens, P.R.; Mitani, K.; Chen, H.H.; Chan, S.; Caskey, C.T. (1996). A new adenoviral vector: Replacement of all viral coding sequences with 28 kb of DNA independently expressing both full-length dystrophin and beta-galactosidase. *Proc. Natl. Acad. Sci. USA,* Vol. 93, No. 12, pp. 5731-5736

Koponen, J.K.; Kankkonen, H.; Kannasto, J.; Wirth, T.; Hillen, W.; Bujard, H.; Yla-Herttuala, S. (2003). Doxycycline-regulated lentiviral vector system with a novel reverse transactivator rtTA2S-M2 shows a tight control of gene expression in vitro and in vivo. *Gene Ther.,* Vol. 10, No. 6, pp. 459-466

Landau, N.R.; Warton, M.; Littman, D.R. (1988). The envelope glycoprotein of the human immunodeficiency virus binds to the immunoglobulin-like domain of CD4. *Nature,* Vol. 334, No. 6178, pp. 159-162

Leopold, P.L.; Ferris, B.; Grinberg, I.; Worgall, S.; Hackett, N.R.; Crystal, R.G. (1998). Fluorescent virions: dynamic tracking of the pathway of adenoviral gene transfer vectors in living cells. *Hum. Gene Ther.,* Vol. 9, No. 3, pp. 367-378

Levine, F.; Friedmann, T. (1991). Gene therapy techniques. *Curr. Opin. Biotechnol.,* Vol. 2, No. 6, pp. 840-844

Lewinski, M.K.; Bushman, F.D. (2005). Retroviral DNA integration--mechanism and consequences. *Adv. Genet.,* Vol. 55, pp. 147-181

Lewis, P.; Hensel, M.; Emerman, M. (1992). Human immunodeficiency virus infection of cells arrested in the cell cycle. *EMBO J.,* Vol. 11, No. 8, pp. 3053-3058

Lewis, P.; Emerman, M. (1994). Passage through mitosis is required for oncoretroviruses but not for the human immunodeficiency virus. *J. Virol.,* Vol. 68, No. 1, pp. 510-516

Li, M.J.; Bauer, G.; Michienzi, A.; Yee, J.K.; Lee, N.S.; Kim, J.; Li, S.; Castanotto, D.; Zaia, J.; Rossi, J.J. (2003). Inhibition of HIV-1 infection by lentiviral vectors expressing Pol III-promoted anti-HIV RNAs. *Mol. Ther.,* Vol. 8, No. 2, pp. 196-206

Lowenstein, P.R.; Thomas, C.E.; Umana, P.; Gerdes, C.A.; Verakis, T.; Boyer, O.; Tondeur, S.; Klatzmann, D.; Castro, M.G. (2002). High-capacity, helper-dependent, "gutless" adenoviral vectors for gene transfer into brain. *Methods Enzymol.,* Vol. 346, pp. 292-311

Ma, Y.; Feigin, A.; Dhawan, V.; Fukuda, M.; Shi, Q.; Greene, P.; Breeze, R.; Fahn, S.; Freed, C.; Eidelberg, D. (2002). Dyskinesia after fetal cell transplantation for parkinsonism: a PET study. *Ann. Neurol.,* Vol. 52, No. 5, pp. 628-634

Malim, M.H.; Bohnlein, S.; Hauber, J.; Cullen, B.R. (1989). Functional dissection of the HIV-1 Rev trans-activator--derivation of a trans-dominant repressor of Rev function. *Cell,* Vol. 58, No. 1, pp. 205-214

Malim, M.H.; Emerman, M. (2008). HIV-1 accessory proteins--ensuring viral survival in a hostile environment. *Cell Host Microbe.,* Vol. 3, No. 6, pp. 388-398

Mann, R.; Mulligan, R.C.; Baltimore, D. (1983). Construction of a retrovirus packaging mutant and its use to produce helper-free defective retrovirus. *Cell,* Vol. 33, No. 1, pp. 153-159

Mautino, M.R.; Keiser, N.; Morgan, R.A. (2001). Inhibition of human immunodeficiency virus type 1 (HIV-1) replication by HIV-1-based lentivirus vectors expressing transdominant Rev. *J. Virol.,* Vol. 75, No. 8, pp. 3590-3599

Mautino, M.R.; Morgan, R.A. (2002a). Enhanced inhibition of human immunodeficiency virus type 1 replication by novel lentiviral vectors expressing human immunodeficiency virus type 1 envelope antisense RNA. *Hum. Gene Ther.,* Vol. 13, No. 9, pp. 1027-1037

Mautino, M.R.; Morgan, R.A. (2002b). Gene therapy of HIV-1 infection using lentiviral vectors expressing anti-HIV-1 genes. *AIDS Patient Care STDS*, Vol. 16, No. 1, pp. 11-26

Mautino, M.R.; Morgan, R.A. (2002c). Inhibition of HIV-1 replication by novel lentiviral vectors expressing transdominant Rev and HIV-1 env antisense. *Gene Ther.*, Vol. 9, No. 7, pp. 421-431

Meadows, D.C.; Gervay-Hague, J. (2006). Current developments in HIV chemotherapy. *ChemMedChem*, Vol. 1, No. 1, pp. 16-29

Melikyan, G.B. (2008). Common principles and intermediates of viral protein-mediated fusion: the HIV-1 paradigm. *Retrovirology*, Vol. 5, pp. 111

Miller, A.D.; Rosman, G.J. (1989). Improved retroviral vectors for gene transfer and expression. *Biotechniques* Vol. 7, No. 9, pp. 980-990

Miller, A.D. (1992a). Human gene therapy comes of age. *Nature*, Vol. 357, No. 6378, pp. 455-460

Miller, A.D. (1992b). Retroviral vectors. *Curr. Top. Microbiol. Immunol.*, Vol. 158, pp. 1-24

Miller, D.G.; Adam, M.A.; Miller, A.D. (1990). Gene transfer by retrovirus vectors occurs only in cells that are actively replicating at the time of infection. *Mol. Cell. Biol.*, Vol. 10, No. 8, pp. 4239-4242

Mitta, B.; Weber, C.C.; Rimann, M.; Fussenegger, M. (2004). Design and in vivo characterization of self-inactivating human and non-human lentiviral expression vectors engineered for streptogramin-adjustable transgene expression. *Nucleic Acids Res.*, Vol. 32, No. 12, pp. e106

Miyake, K.; Suzuki, N.; Matsuoka, H.; Tohyama, T.; Shimada, T. (1998). Stable integration of human immunodeficiency virus-based retroviral vectors into the chromosomes of nondividing cells. *Hum. Gene Ther.*, Vol. 9, No. 4, pp. 467-475

Miyoshi, H.; Blomer, U.; Takahashi, M.; Gage, F.H.; Verma, I.M. (1998). Development of a self-inactivating lentivirus vector. *J. Virol.*, Vol. 72, No. 10, pp. 8150-8157

Miyoshi, H.; Smith, K.A.; Mosier, D.E.; Verma, I.M.; Torbett, B.E. (1999). Transduction of human $CD34^+$ cells that mediate long-term engraftment of NOD/SCID mice by HIV vectors. *Science*, Vol. 283, No. 5402, pp. 682-686

Molin, M.; Shoshan, M.C.; Ohman-Forslund, K.; Linder, S.; Akusjarvi, G. (1998). Two novel adenovirus vector systems permitting regulated protein expression in gene transfer experiments. *J. Virol.*, Vol. 72, No. 10, pp. 8358-8361

Mukhtar, M.; Duke, H.; BouHamdan, M.; Pomerantz, R.J. (2000). Anti-human immunodeficiency virus type 1 gene therapy in human central nervous system-based cells: an initial approach against a potential viral reservoir. *Hum. Gene Ther.*, Vol. 11, No. 2, pp. 347-359

Naldini, L.; Blomer, U.; Gallay, P.; Ory, D.; Mulligan, R.; Gage, F.H.; Verma, I.M.; Trono, D. (1996). In vivo gene delivery and stable transduction of nondividing cells by a lentiviral vector. *Science*, Vol. 272, No. 5259, pp. 263-267

Ng, P.; Beauchamp, C.; Evelegh, C.; Parks, R.; Graham, F.L. (2001). Development of a FLP/frt system for generating helper-dependent adenoviral vectors. *Mol. Ther.*, Vol. 3, No. 5, pp. 809-815

No, D.; Yao, T.P.; Evans, R.M. (1996). Ecdysone-inducible gene expression in mammalian cells and transgenic mice. *Proc. Natl. Acad. Sci. USA*, Vol. 93, No. 8, pp. 3346-3351

Nordstrom, J.L. (2003). The antiprogestin-dependent GeneSwitch system for regulated gene therapy. *Steroids,* Vol. 68, No. 10-13, pp. 1085-1094

Ono, A. (2010), Relationships between plasma membrane microdomains and HIV-1 assembly. *Biol. Cell* Vol. 102, No. 6, pp. 335-350

Palella, F.J., Jr.; Delaney, K.M.; Moorman, A.C.; Loveless, M.O.; Fuhrer, J.; Satten, G.A.; Aschman, D.J.; Holmberg, S.D. (1998). Declining morbidity and mortality among patients with advanced human immunodeficiency virus infection. HIV Outpatient Study Investigators. *N. Engl. J. Med.,* Vol. 338, No. 13, pp. 853-860

Parker, D.G.; Brereton, H.M.; Klebe, S.; Coster, D.J.; Williams, K.A. (2009). A steroid-inducible promoter for the cornea. *Br. J. Ophthalmol.,* Vol. 93, No. 9, pp. 1255-1259

Parks, R.J.; Chen, L.; Anton, M.; Sankar, U.; Rudnicki, M.A.; Graham, F.L. (1996). A helper-dependent adenovirus vector system: removal of helper virus by Cre-mediated excision of the viral packaging signal. *Proc. Natl. Acad. Sci. USA,* Vol. 93, No. 24, pp. 13565-13570

Pluta, K.; Luce, M.J.; Bao, L.; Agha-Mohammadi, S.; Reiser, J. (2005). Tight control of transgene expression by lentivirus vectors containing second-generation tetracycline-responsive promoters. *J. Gene Med.,* Vol. 7, No. 6, pp. 803-817

Podsakoff, G.M.; Engel, B.C.; Carbonaro, D.A.; Choi, C.; Smogorzewska, E.M.; Bauer, G.; Selander, D.; Csik, S.; Wilson, K.; Betts, M.R.; Koup, R.A.; Nabel, G.J.; Bishop, K.; King, S.; Schmidt, M.; von Kalle, C.; Church, J.A.; Kohn, D.B. (2005). Selective survival of peripheral blood lymphocytes in children with HIV-1 following delivery of an anti-HIV gene to bone marrow CD34(+) cells. *Mol. Ther.,* Vol. 12, No. 1, pp. 77-86

Pollard, V.W.; Malim, M.H. (1998). The HIV-1 Rev protein. *Annu. Rev. Microbiol.,* Vol. 52, pp. 491-532

Poluri, A.; van Maanen, M.; Sutton, R.E. (2003). Genetic therapy for HIV/AIDS. *Expert Opin. Biol. Ther.,* Vol. 3, No. 6, pp. 951-963

Purcell, D.F.; Martin, M.A. (1993). Alternative splicing of human immunodeficiency virus type 1 mRNA modulates viral protein expression, replication, and infectivity. *J. Virol.,* Vol. 67, No. 11, pp. 6365-6378

Reiser, J.; Lai, Z.; Zhang, X.Y.; Brady, R.O. (2000). Development of multigene and regulated lentivirus vectors. *J. Virol.,* Vol. 74, No. 22, pp. 10589-10599

Richman, D.D. (2001). HIV chemotherapy. *Nature,* Vol. 410, No. 6831, pp. 995-1001

Robbins, P.D.; Ghivizzani, S.C. (1998). Viral vectors for gene therapy. *Pharmacol. Ther.,* Vol. 80, No. 1, pp. 35-47

Roe, T.; Reynolds, T.C.; Yu, G.; Brown, P.O. (1993). Integration of murine leukemia virus DNA depends on mitosis. *EMBO J.,* Vol. 12, No. 5, pp. 2099-2108

Saez, E.; Nelson, M.C.; Eshelman, B.; Banayo, E.; Koder, A.; Cho, G.J.; Evans, R.M. (2000). Identification of ligands and coligands for the ecdysone-regulated gene switch. *Proc. Natl. Acad. Sci. USA,* Vol. 97, No. 26, pp. 14512-14517

Schwartz, S.; Felber, B.K.; Benko, D.M.; Fenyo, E.M.; Pavlakis, G.N. (1990). Cloning and functional analysis of multiply spliced mRNA species of human immunodeficiency virus type 1. *J. Virol.,* Vol. 64, No. 6, pp. 2519-2529

Shimotohno, K.; Temin, H.M. (1981). Formation of infectious progeny virus after insertion of herpes simplex thymidine kinase gene into DNA of an avian retrovirus. *Cell,* Vol. 26, No. 1, pp. 67-77

Shinoda, Y.; Hieda, K.; Koyanagi, Y.; Suzuki, Y. (2009). Efficient transduction of cytotoxic and anti-HIV-1 genes by a gene-regulatable lentiviral vector. *Virus Genes* Vol. 39, No. 2. pp. 165-175

Sirin, O.; Park, F. (2003). Regulating gene expression using self-inactivating lentiviral vectors containing the mifepristone-inducible system. *Gene,* Vol. 323, pp. 67-77

Somia, N.; Verma, I.M. (2000). Gene therapy: trials and tribulations. *Nat. Rev. Genet.,* Vol. 1, No. 2, pp. 91-99

Stevenson, M. (2003). HIV-1 pathogenesis. *Nat. Med.,* Vol. 9, No. 7, pp. 853-860

Strayer, D.S.; Akkina, R.; Bunnell, B.A.; Dropulic, B.; Planelles, V.; Pomerantz, R.J.; Rossi, J.J.; Zaia, J.A. (2005). Current status of gene therapy strategies to treat HIV/AIDS. *Mol. Ther.,* Vol. 11, No. 6, pp. 823-842

Suzuki, Y.; Craigie, R. (2007). The road to chromatin - nuclear entry of retroviruses. *Nat. Rev. Microbiol.,* Vol. 5, No. 3, pp. 187-196

Szulc, J.; Wiznerowicz, M.; Sauvain, M.O.; Trono, D.; Aebischer, P. (2006). A versatile tool for conditional gene expression and knockdown. *Nat. Methods,* Vol. 3, No. 2, pp. 109-116

Tabin, C.J.; Hoffmann, J.W.; Goff, S.P.; Weinberg, R.A. (1982). Adaptation of a retrovirus as a eucaryotic vector transmitting the herpes simplex virus thymidine kinase gene. *Mol. Cell. Biol.,* Vol. 2, No. 4, pp. 426-436

Taylor, J.A.; Vojtech, L.; Bahner, I.; Kohn, D.B.; Laer, D.V.; Russell, D.W.; Richard, R.E. (2008). Foamy virus vectors expressing anti-HIV transgenes efficiently block HIV-1 replication. *Mol. Ther.,* Vol. 16, No. 1, pp. 46-51

Tomko, R.P.; Xu, R.; Philipson, L. (1997). HCAR and MCAR: the human and mouse cellular receptors for subgroup C adenoviruses and group B coxsackieviruses. *Proc. Natl. Acad. Sci. USA,* Vol. 94, No. 7, pp. 3352-3356

Ulmann, A.; Peyron, R.; Silvestre, L. (1995). Clinical uses of mifepristone (MFP). *Ann. N. Y. Acad. Sci.,* Vol. 761, pp. 248-260

Umana, P.; Gerdes, C.A.; Stone, D.; Davis, J.R.; Ward, D.; Castro, M.G.; Lowenstein, P.R. (2001). Efficient FLPe recombinase enables scalable production of helper-dependent adenoviral vectors with negligible helper-virus contamination. *Nat. Biotechnol.,* Vol. 19, No. 6, pp. 582-585

Verma, I.M.; Weitzman, M.D. (2005). Gene therapy: twenty-first century medicine. *Annu. Rev. Biochem.,* Vol. 74, pp. 711-738

Vigna, E.; Cavalieri, S.; Ailles, L.; Geuna, M.; Loew, R.; Bujard, H.; Naldini, L. (2002), Robust and efficient regulation of transgene expression in vivo by improved tetracycline-dependent lentiviral vectors. *Mol. Ther.,* Vol. 5, No. 3, pp. 252-261

Vogel, R.; Amar, L.; Thi, A.D.; Saillour, P.; Mallet, J. (2004). A single lentivirus vector mediates doxycycline-regulated expression of transgenes in the brain. *Hum. Gene Ther.,* Vol. 15, No. 2, pp. 157-165

Vogt, V.M. (1996). Proteolytic processing and particle maturation. *Curr. Top. Microbiol. Immunol.,* Vol. 214, pp. 95-131

Volberding, P.A.; Deeks, S.G. (2010). Antiretroviral therapy and management of HIV infection. *Lancet,* Vol. 376, No. 9734, pp. 49-62

Wagner, R.; Graf, M.; Bieler, K.; Wolf, H.; Grunwald, T.; Foley, P.; Uberla, K. (2000). Rev-independent expression of synthetic gag-pol genes of human immunodeficiency virus type 1 and simian immunodeficiency virus: implications for the safety of lentiviral vectors. *Hum. Gene Ther.*, Vol. 11, No. 17, pp. 2403-2413

Wang, Q.; Jia, X.C.; Finer, M.H. (1995). A packaging cell line for propagation of recombinant adenovirus vectors containing two lethal gene-region deletions. *Gene Ther.*, Vol. 2, No. 10, pp. 775-783

Wang, Y.; O'Malley, B.W., Jr.; Tsai, S.Y.; O'Malley, B.W. (1994). A regulatory system for use in gene transfer. *Proc. Natl. Acad. Sci. USA*, Vol. 91, No. 17, pp. 8180-8184

Watanabe, S.; Temin, H.M. (1983). Construction of a helper cell line for avian reticuloendotheliosis virus cloning vectors. *Mol. Cell. Biol.*, Vol. 3, No. 12, pp. 2241-2249

Weber, W.; Fussenegger, M. (2004), Approaches for trigger-inducible viral transgene regulation in gene-based tissue engineering. *Curr. Opin. Biotechnol.* Vol. 15, No. 5, pp. 383-391

Wei, C.M.; Gibson, M.; Spear, P.G.; Scolnick, E.M. (1981). Construction and isolation of a transmissible retrovirus containing the src gene of Harvey murine sarcoma virus and the thymidine kinase gene of herpes simplex virus type 1. *J. Virol.*, Vol. 39, No. 3, pp. 935-944

Weinberg, J.B.; Matthews, T.J.; Cullen, B.R.; Malim, M.H. (1991). Productive human immunodeficiency virus type 1 (HIV-1) infection of nonproliferating human monocytes. *J. Exp. Med.*, Vol. 174, No. 6, pp. 1477-1482

Whittaker, G.R.; Kann, M.; Helenius, A. (2000). Viral entry into the nucleus. *Annu. Rev. Cell Dev. Biol.* Vol. 16, pp. 627-651

Wiznerowicz, M.; Trono, D. (2003). Conditional suppression of cellular genes: lentivirus vector-mediated drug-inducible RNA interference. *J. Virol.*, Vol. 77, No. 16, pp. 8957-8961

Wu, X.; Liu, H.; Xiao, H.; Conway, J.A.; Hunter, E.; Kappes, J.C. (1997). Functional RT and IN incorporated into HIV-1 particles independently of the Gag/Pol precursor protein. *EMBO J.*, Vol. 16, No. 16, pp. 5113-5122

Yamashita, M.; Emerman, M. (2006). Retroviral infection of non-dividing cells: old and new perspectives. *Virology*, Vol. 344, No. 1, pp. 88-93

Yancopoulos, G.D.; Davis, S.; Gale, N.W.; Rudge, J.S.; Wiegand, S.J.; Holash, J. (2000). Vascular-specific growth factors and blood vessel formation. *Nature*, Vol. 407, No. 6801, pp. 242-248

Yeh, P.; Dedieu, J.F.; Orsini, C.; Vigne, E.; Denefle, P.; Perricaudet, M. (1996). Efficient dual transcomplementation of adenovirus E1 and E4 regions from a 293-derived cell line expressing a minimal E4 functional unit. *J. Virol.*, Vol. 70, No. 1, pp. 559-565

Zufferey, R.; Dull, T.; Mandel, R.J.; Bukovsky, A.; Quiroz, D.; Naldini, L.; Trono, D. (1998). Self-inactivating lentivirus vector for safe and efficient in vivo gene delivery. *J. Virol.*, Vol. 72, No. 12, pp. 9873-9880

Zufferey, R.; Nagy, D.; Mandel, R.J.; Naldini, L.; Trono, D. (1997). Multiply attenuated lentiviral vector achieves efficient gene delivery in vivo. *Nat. Biotechnol.*, Vol. 15, No. 9, pp. 871-875

15

Dendritic Cells and Lentiviral Vectors: Mapping the Way to Successful Immunotherapy

Cleo Goyvaerts[1], Grazyna Kochan[2], David Escors[3] and Karine Breckpot[1]
[1]*Laboratory of Molecular and Cellular Therapy,*
Department of Physiology-Immunology, Vrije Universiteit Brussel, Jette,
[2]*Oxford Structural Genomics Consortium, University of Oxford, Oxford,*
[3]*Division of Infection and Immunity, University College London, London,*
[1]*Belgium*
[2,3]*United Kingdom*

1. Introduction

Professional antigen presenting cells, in particular dendritic cells (DCs) are central players in the immune response (Steinman & Banchereau 2007). Their function is dual; on the one hand DCs evoke strong immune responses against antigens that are considered hazardous, on the other hand DCs induce tolerance against self-antigens. To that end, DCs need to present antigen-derived peptides in the context of MHC class I or class II molecules to $CD8^+$ and $CD4^+$ T cells, respectively. It is the context in which these peptides are presented that determines the outcome of the immune response, immune activation *versus* tolerance. Consequently, DCs have become targets for immunotherapy against not only cancer and infectious disease, but also autoimmune diseases and transplantation rejection (Palucka *et al.*).

Key to successful DC-based immunotherapy is the delivery of the antigen of interest, be it cancer, viral or auto-antigens, to DCs, as well as the delivery of molecules that dictate the immune stimulatory capacity of the DCs. Therefore, it is not surprising that much effort has been put in the development of vectors for genetic modification of DCs (Breckpot *et al.* 2004c). Of these lentiviral vectors (LVs), often derived from human immunodeficiency virus type 1 (HIV-1) are amongst the most efficient gene delivery vehicles, for both *in vitro* and *in vivo* modification of DCs (Escors & Breckpot ; Breckpot *et al.* 2007a). In addition, these LVs were demonstrated to activate the innate immune system through interaction with amongst others Toll-like receptors (TLRs), a characteristic that makes LVs even better suited for immunotherapeutic approaches against cancer and infectious diseases (Breckpot *et al.* ; Brown *et al.* 2006a). As immune activation of DCs is critical for the induction of antigen-specific immunity, several strategies have been developed to further strengthen the immune response by introduction of immune modulating molecules or by modulation of well-known activation pathways such as the nuclear factor-kappaB (NF-κB), mitogen activated protein kinase (MAPK) p38 and MAPK c-Jun N-terminal kinases (JNK) pathways (Breckpot & Escors 2009a). Although LVs inherently activate DCs, they have also been evaluated for their ability to switch of the stimulatory capacity of DCs, thus to generate tolerogenic DCs. The strategies exploited therefore are similar to the strategies employed to activate DCs and include introduction of single inhibitory molecules and modulation of pathways that

regulate the tolerogenic potential of DCs, such as the MAPK extracellular signal-regulated kinase (ERK) pathway (Arce *et al.* ; Gould & Favorov 2003).
In the remainder of this chapter, we will give a comprehensive overview on how DCs have evolved to the cell type of choice for manipulation of the immune system, why LVs are successful for the genetic modification of DCs and which developments have led to the use of LVs to generate stimulatory or tolerogenic DCs. We will further touch upon the concerns that are raised in terms of translating the use of LVs to the clinic, *i.e.* the biosafety of LVs, summarizing strategies to avoid off-target transduction, and linked herewith insertional mutagenesis. Finally, we will conclude this chapter with our view on the future perspectives for the use of LVs to manipulate DCs, hence the immune system.

2. Dendritic cells

Dendritic cells (DCs) as we know them today were described during the mid 1970s by Ralph Steinman and co-workers as a rare subset of accessory cells, which are characterized by stellate cytoplasmatic protrusions. It was this tree-like morphology that led to their name (Dendron is Greek for tree) (Steinman & Cohn 1973). DCs are a heterogeneous population for which individual DC subtypes have been described. These DC subtypes differ in tissue distribution, surface marker expression and their capacity to stimulate T cells (Palucka *et al.*). Moreover, DCs have a remarkable functional plasticity. On the one hand DCs can induce immune responses against invading pathogens (non-self). On the other hand DCs can induce T cell anergy/depletion, and regulatory T cells (Treg) to avoid unwanted immune reactions against auto-antigens (self) (Fig. 1). This Janus-like functional behaviour is correlated with complex decision-making processes, triggered by the presence or absence of so called danger signals, hence resulting in the expression of stimulatory and/or inhibitory molecules, respectively (Coquerelle & Moser). Although, we are still deciphering the DC system in its complexity, DCs have entered the clinic as a cellular therapeutic.

2.1 Dendritic cell subsets

Originally it was thought that DCs were of myeloid origin. Studies demonstrating *in vitro* generation of DCs from monocytes (Sallusto & Lanzavecchia 1994), and *in vivo* studies demonstrating the differentiation of phagocytic monocytes to DCs (Randolph *et al.* 1999) supported this idea. Later on, the existence of lymphoid DCs was evidenced (Wu *et al.* 1996; Wu *et al.* 1998). These $CD11c^+$ MHC class II^+ myeloid and lymphoid DC subtypes were afterwards termed $CD8^-$ DCs or $CD8^+$ DCs, respectively. Together they are called conventional DCs (cDCs). Importantly, it was demonstrated in several *in vivo* studies that both $CD8^-$ and $CD8^+$ DC subsets could be generated from either lymphoid (Martin *et al.* 2000; Traver *et al.* 2000), or myeloid progenitors (Traver *et al.* 2000), mounting the question whether these subsets are really distinct or represent different developmental states. cDCs can be found within lymph nodes, spleen, and thymus, but not in bone marrow (Steinman & Cohn 1973). They are believed to cross-present antigens to T cells (den Haan & Bevan 2002), as such stimulate a T helper type 2 (T_H2, humoral) and type 1 (T_H1, cellular) immune response (Maldonado-Lopez *et al.* 1999). In humans, DCs expressing BDCA-1 (CD1c) and BDCA-3 (CD141) are considered the counterparts of mouse cDCs. However, these human DC subsets are often termed myeloid instead of conventional. Human myeloid DCs are characterized by their ability to produce high amounts of interleukin (IL)-12 in response to several stimuli (van Duin *et al.* 2006), thus to induce cellular immunity.

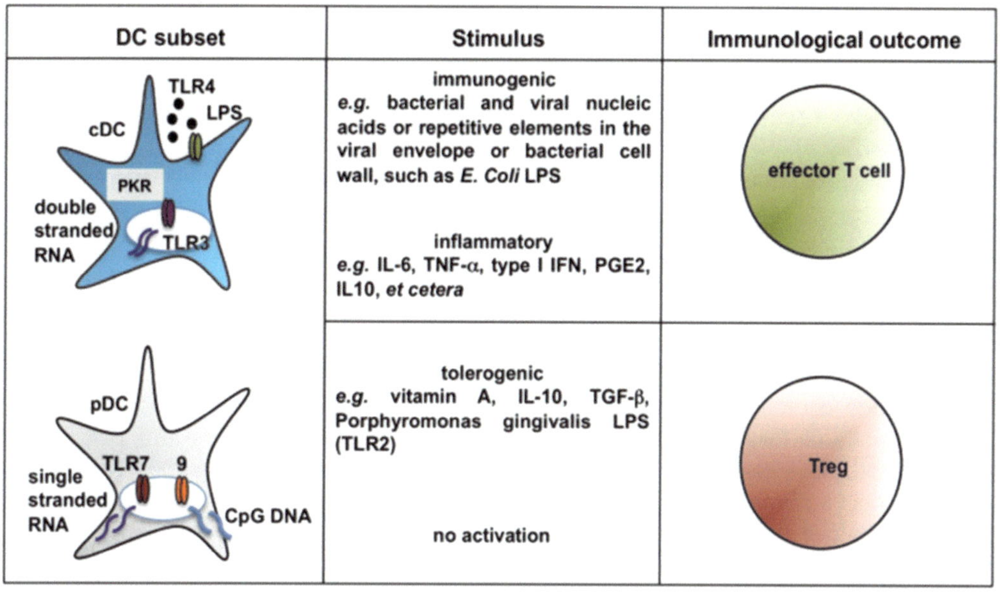

Fig. 1. **Schematic representation of DC subsets and their functional plasticity.** Generally DC subsets are divided into cDCs (blue) and pDCs (grey). These DC subsets differ in tissue distribution, expression of PRRs, hence their ability to sense pathogens and subsequently stimulate appropriate T cell responses. Dependent on the stimuli these DCs encounter they will become tolerogenic or immunogenic, hence induce tolerance (Treg, red) or immunity (effector T cells, green), respectively.

Another DC subset, the plasmacytoid DCs (pDCs) were described a decade ago (Siegal *et al.* 1999). Whereas mouse pDCs express CD11c, human pDCs express low to undetectable levels of CD11c. Instead, human pDCs are characterized by the expression of CD4, CD45RA, as well as the expression of high levels of CD123 (IL-3 receptor) and the c-type lectin receptor BDCA2. Recently, it was described that pDCs can be further divided into subclasses based on the expression of CD2 (Matsui *et al.* 2009). pDCs reside in the same tissues as cDCs, and can moreover be found in bone marrow (Nakano *et al.* 2001), where they are believed to be a precursor for cDCs (Soumelis & Liu 2006; Segura *et al.* 2009). Nonetheless, pDCs, isolated from mice and humans, are functionally distinct from cDCs. In their resting state, pDCs play an important role in the induction of tolerance (Martin *et al.* 2002). However, pDCs are best known for the ability to produce high amounts of type I interferon (IFN) in response to viral infection (O'Keeffe *et al.* 2002; Fitzgerald-Bocarsly *et al.* 2008). In fact, pDCs control the progress of a virus infection at various levels: (i) through non-specific blockade of viral replication by type I IFN, (ii) by promoting the maturation of pDCs as well as other DC subsets (Fonteneau *et al.* 2004), and (iii) through the specific stimulation of adaptive anti-viral $CD8^+$ T cell responses (Di Pucchio *et al.* 2008).

The last DC subset to be discussed, the epidermal Langerhans' cells (LCs), was in fact described in 1868 by Paul Langerhans (Merad & Manz 2009), almost a century before the description of cDCs (Steinman & Cohn 1973). LCs are characterized by the expression of Langerin and Birbeck granules. Furthermore, they are characterized by their long life span (weeks) when compared to other DC types (3-10 days) (Kamath *et al.* 2002). Upon activation LCs migrate through the dermis into regional lymph nodes to present antigens to T cells

(Romani *et al.* 2003). Because of this migration they are categorized as migratory DCs, a category, which also comprises other non-lymphoid tissue residing DCs, amongst which dermal DCs. LCs and dermal DCs are often grouped as skin DCs. It is generally accepted that these have a potent T cell stimulatory capacity (Romani *et al.* 2003; Larregina & Falo 2005; He *et al.* 2006). Nevertheless, as for pDCs and cDCs, a possible tolerogenic capacity has been reported for skin DCs (Grabbe *et al.* 1995; Kaplan *et al.* 2005).

2.2 Dendritic cells and the regulation of immune responses

In addition to subsets with functional specialization, DCs are endowed with a remarkable functional plasticity. The hypothesis is that distinct DC activation stages play a role in the induction of tolerance *versus* immunity. This is correlated with the two-signal model of T cell stimulation, in which it is proposed that a productive T cell response requires recognition of MHC/peptide complexes by the T cell receptor (TCR) (signal 1) along with signalling through co-stimulatory molecules (signal 2). Indeed, steady-state cDCs and pDCs, have been described to induce T cell tolerance (Jonuleit *et al.* 2001; Mahnke *et al.* 2002; Martin *et al.* 2002), whereas both activated DC types have been shown to induce immunity (Salio *et al.* 2003; Cerundolo *et al.* 2004; Salio *et al.* 2004).

Immature DCs efficiently take up pathogens, apoptotic cells and particulate antigens from the environment by phagocytosis, macropinocytosis, or endocytosis; process these but are considered inefficient in presenting these to T cells (Wilson *et al.* 2004). Hence, immature DCs are believed to induce tolerance (Steinbrink *et al.* 1997; Lutz & Schuler 2002). Indeed, in steady-state conditions DCs remain immature and tissue-resident, express small amounts of MHC and co-stimulatory molecules hence induce T cell anergy instead of T cell activation upon DC-T cell interaction (Hawiger *et al.* 2001). Furthermore, injection of immature DCs in humans induces tolerance (Dhodapkar *et al.* 2001; Jonuleit *et al.* 2001; Dhodapkar & Steinman 2002). In contrast, activated DCs are considered to be immunogenic. Maturation of DCs can be induced by a variety of signals, such as microorganisms (Rescigno *et al.* 2000; Beyer *et al.* 2001), cytokines (Jonuleit *et al.* 1997), interaction with $CD4^+$ T_H cells (Caux *et al.* 1994; Mackey *et al.* 1998a; Mackey *et al.* 1998b) and chemicals like haptens (Aiba *et al.* 1997; Aiba & Tagami 1998; Aiba & Tagami 1999). DC maturation is associated with several coordinated events, including: (i) loss of endocytic and phagocytic receptors; (ii) changes in morphology; (iii) up-regulation of MHC and co-stimulatory molecules, such as CD40, CD80 and CD86, adhesion molecules and chemokine receptors, such as CCR7 (Tuyaerts *et al.* 2007a). The latter is one of the first changes and enables DCs to migrate from the periphery to the T cell areas of draining lymphoid organs (Forster *et al.* 2008). Here DCs present antigenic peptides in the context of MHC molecules to T cells. The phenotypic changes, high expression of antigen presenting, co-stimulatory and adhesion molecules, make mature DCs potent inducers of T cell immunity. However, the view that immature DCs induce tolerance and mature DCs induce immunity is simplified. It has been demonstrated that mature DCs can contribute to T cell tolerance through the induction of Treg (Verhasselt *et al.* 2004). It was suggested that the maturation trigger dictates the T cell polarizing or tolerating immune functions of the DCs. Some stimuli have been demonstrated to promote induction of T_H1 responses, hence cellular immunity, whereas others hamper full DC maturation and cytokine production, hence promote tolerance.

2.3 Stimulatory dendritic cells

The immune system is constantly faced with choices. When confronted with a microbe, it must first decide whether to respond or not. If it chooses to respond, then it must decide what kind of response to launch. A hallmark of the mammalian immune system is its ability to launch qualitatively distinct types of responses against different pathogens (Pulendran *et al.* 2008). Immune responses against T cell-dependent antigens can be divided in (i) $CD4^+$ T_H1 responses, which are characterized by high secretion of IFN-γ, and induced against intracellular microbes, (ii) $CD4^+$ T_H2 responses, which are characterized by the secretion of cytokines, such as IL-5 and IL-13, and induced against extracellular pathogens, (iii) $CD4^+$ T_H17 responses, characterized by the secretion of IL-17, and induced against fungi (Bettelli *et al.* 2007; Reiner 2007), and finally (iv) Treg responses, with suppressive activity, and which are essential to maintain tolerance to host antigens (Wing & Sakaguchi). Treg can also be induced by some microbial stimuli (Belkaid 2007), and are abundantly present in the blood, lymphoid organs and tumours of cancer patients (Vence *et al.* 2007; Ahmadzadeh *et al.* 2008), as such Treg enable evasion from the immune system.

For the treatment of cancer and infectious diseases, a $CD4^+$ T_H1 response is required to induce a strong $CD8^+$ cytotoxic T cell (CTL) response (Breckpot & Escors 2009a). These CTLs will then kill the target cells. To activate T cells, at least two signals are required (i) antigen recognition and (ii) co-stimulation. In the presence of tolerogenic mechanisms, as it is the case in cancer, an additional third signal is required. This is obtained by triggering of innate sensing pathways (Breckpot & Escors 2009a). As co-stimulatory molecules are not expressed by immature DCs, it goes without saying that DC activation (maturation) is a key event that determines the T cell stimulatory potential of DCs.

Differentiation of immature to mature DCs requires pathogen recognition. Groups of pathogens express similar structures such as bacterial and viral nucleic acids or repetitive elements in the bacterial cell wall or within the viral envelope, enabling the recognition of a wide variety of pathogens. These structures are called pathogen-associated molecular patterns (PAMPs) and are recognized on DCs by pathogen recognition receptors (PRRs). The best-studied PRRs are the TLRs, although other PRRs, such as Nod-like receptors, RIG-I-like receptors, as well as some members of the C-type lectin family, are described. Distinct pathogens express different PAMPs and this combination works as a fingerprint that triggers a specific set of PRRs (Akira *et al.* 2006; Barton & Kagan 2009; Geijtenbeek & Gringhuis 2009). As such complex signalling networks are activated. These cooperate, integrate and finally converge into a few pathways, of which the NF-κB and the MAPK pathways are examples (Rescigno *et al.* 1998; Sato *et al.* 1999; Re & Strominger 2001; Caparros *et al.* 2006; Kawai & Akira 2008). These are described in detail elsewhere (Breckpot & Escors 2009c).

The concept of co-stimulation was first introduced by Kevin Lafferty and co-workers (Lafferty *et al.* 1979). In the last decades, a large number of co-stimulatory molecules have been identified, which can be divided in members of the (i) B7 and (ii) tumour necrosis factor (TNF) type family. B7.1 (CD80) and B7.2 (CD86) are textbook examples of the B7 family. These transmit strong co-stimulatory signals to T cells through interactions with CD28 on T cells (Greenwald *et al.* 2005). Recently, this group was expanded with a number of new members including ICOS ligand, PD-L1 (B7-H1), PD-L2 (B7-DC), B7-H3 and B7-H4. All these molecules are expressed on DCs. The corresponding CD28 members that are inducible expressed on T cells are ICOS, PD-1 and BTLA. It is important to mention that not all B7 family members are co-stimulatory. In fact, many of these new members have been linked to induction of tolerance hence they are discussed in the next section. The TNF type family of co-stimulatory molecules, includes CD70, OX40L, GITRL and 4-1BBL, which are expressed on DCs and their corresponding receptors CD27, OX40 (CD134), GITR and 4-1BB (CD137), expressed on T cells (Watts 2005). Some co-stimulatory molecules exemplified by

CD83, which is expressed on mature DCs, but also on T cells, can't be classified in either group. So far, no receptor has been identified for this molecule (Hirano *et al.* 2006; Aerts-Toegaert *et al.* 2007; Prechtel *et al.* 2007).
Initial activation of naive T cells generally occurs through interactions with CD28, after which they differentiate into effector T cells, and up-regulate other co-stimulatory molecules. Depending on the stimulus, expression of co-stimulatory ligands on DCs will vary. Their relative expression will ultimately determine the quality of the T cell stimulation hence the T cell function. It has to be mentioned that the importance of co-stimulatory molecules is not limited to the stimulation of effector T cells, but can moreover involve modulation of Treg, as described for GITRL and OX40L. It has been shown that triggering of GITR results in alleviation of Treg suppression of effector T cells. Although Treg constitutively express GITR, the effect of GITR-GITRL interactions is not mediated through functional impairment of Treg, but rather protection of effector T cells against Treg (Stephens *et al.* 2004). However, whether these observations in mice can be translated to a human setting remains unclear (Tuyaerts *et al.* 2007b). Direct inhibitory effects on Treg suppression have been shown for OX40L (Valzasina *et al.* 2005), which upon binding with OX40 on Treg mediates down-regulation of Foxp3 and the Tregs' suppressive capacity (Vu *et al.* 2007). For other co-stimulatory molecules (CD70 and 4-1BBL), of which its receptors are also expressed on Treg, no unequivocal effect on Treg function has been described.

2.4 Tolerogenic dendritic cells

In physiological conditions, the organism is in direct contact with millions of innocuous antigens of different origins. Many of them are bacterial antigens, such as those present within the gut. Others vary from pollen, yeast, dust mites and chemicals of all sorts. Until recently, it was thought that the immune system was constantly and restlessly fighting potentially dangerous organisms and antigens. This view has certainly become obsolete, and it is not inaccurate to consider the immune system in a kind of steady-state in which tolerance is the default outcome and has to be maintained at all costs, except when a real threat arises. Therefore, several tolerogenic mechanisms are constantly in place.
One of the first mechanisms to be described is central tolerance, in which auto-reactive T cells are eliminated in the thymus by clonal deletion (Griesemer *et al.* 2010). Although this mechanism is essential to eliminate most auto-reactive T cells, it can't explain the aetiology of autoimmune disorders in which self-antigens are clearly recognised. Even though clonal deletion is efficient, it does not eliminate all auto-reactive T cells. Interestingly, many auto-reactive T cells that survive clonal deletion further differentiate into natural $Foxp3^+$ $CD4^+$ Treg (Sakaguchi *et al.* 2008; Griesemer *et al.* 2010). These are strong and intrinsic immunosuppressive, and are part of the central tolerance. Research on Treg has recently exploded, although ample experimental evidence of their existence was provided during the 1970s (Rich & Pierce 1973; Ha *et al.* 1974; Taussig 1974). However, early studies were abandoned partly by the inexistence of specific cell markers associated with suppressive T cells. Nevertheless, Sakaguchi and colleagues demonstrated that high expression of CD25 and Foxp3 was characteristic for natural Treg (Hori *et al.* 2003; Sakaguchi 2003), which re-awakened research into this fundamental T cell type. Importantly, many of the early studies drew similar conclusions to more recent studies on Treg (Basten *et al.* 1974; Kirchner *et al.* 1974; Polak & Turk 1974). Even so, clonal deletion and natural Treg activity can't explain tolerance towards many other auto- and foreign antigens, which are not present in the thymus. Theoretically strong immune responses should constantly arise towards a wide

variety of antigens. However, this is not the case, and the organism still remains tolerant towards most antigens. Differentiation of inducible Treg specific for peripheral antigens can partially fill this experimental and conceptual gap. Inducible Treg derive from naïve $CD4^+$ T cells and can be broadly classified into Tr1 ($CD4^+$ $CD25^+$ IL-10^+ or TGF-β^+) and T_H3 ($CD4^+$ $CD25^+$ $Foxp3^+$) cells (Mahnke *et al.* 2003; O'Garra *et al.* 2004; Peng *et al.* 2004; Arce *et al.* 2011). For differentiation of inducible Treg to occur, antigens have to be captured, processed and presented in a tolerogenic context. DCs, which induce Treg differentiation and inhibition of effector T cell expansion, are termed tolerogenic DCs.

There is no compelling evidence demonstrating that tolerogenic DCs are a truly specialised cell type that is exclusively devoted to suppress immune responses. In fact, tolerogenic DCs encompass a wide range of DCs which acquire immune suppressive activities in particular circumstances. Firstly, it is well known that steady state DCs can capture antigens in peripheral tissues and migrate to secondary lymphoid organs. Antigen presentation by immature DCs leads to T cell inactivation (anergy), apoptosis and Treg differentiation (Dhodapkar *et al.* 2001; Hawiger *et al.* 2001; Bonifaz *et al.* 2002; Kretschmer *et al.* 2005). Secondly, DCs located in certain anatomical parts such as the mucosa and gut, are intrinsically tolerogenic. Interestingly, retinoic-acid (vitamin A) metabolising enzymes are critical in their suppressive functions. Mucosal DCs in contact with many microbial-derived antigens are potently immunosuppressive, particularly after TLR2 signal transduction (Dillon *et al.* 2006; Ilarregui *et al.* 2009; Manicassamy *et al.* 2009). Treatment of DCs with lectin ligands such as galectin 1 or potent immunosuppressive cytokines also renders them tolerogenic (Corinti *et al.* 2001; Ghiringhelli *et al.* 2005; Dillon *et al.* 2006; Rutella *et al.* 2006; Ilarregui *et al.* 2009; Arce *et al.* 2011). Importantly, certain types of specialised myeloid-derived cells with very potent intrinsic immunosuppressive capacities have been found in recent years. These cells are known as myeloid-derived suppressor cells and inhibit T cell proliferation through a variety of mechanisms (Li *et al.* 2009; Srivastava *et al.* 2010). In addition, certain types of monocytes are immunosuppressive cells, and are involved in establishing tolerance after organ transplantation (Garcia *et al.* 2010). According to the expression of surface molecules, tolerogenic DCs are generally considered to be immature. This is characterised by low levels of MHC and co-stimulatory molecules (Rutella *et al.* 2006; Escors *et al.* 2008; Breckpot & Escors 2009b; Arce *et al.* 2010). It is believed that because of their immature phenotype antigen presentation is inefficient, and expansion of effector T cells is hampered. However, phenotypical mature DCs can also be potently tolerogenic. These mature tolerogenic DCs exert their suppressive activities through secretion of high levels of immunosuppressive cytokines (Rutella *et al.* 2006).

The mechanisms by which tolerogenic DCs exert their activity are certainly varied in nature, and it is likely that several of these take place simultaneously. As mentioned, tolerogenic immature DCs are thought to lead to inefficient antigen presentation to naive T cells. Therefore, expansion of effector T cells is, if not prevented, at least severely reduced. However, there is evidence that these DCs do present antigens, although the interaction between immature DCs and T cells is transient and leads to T cell anergy, apoptosis or Treg differentiation (Rothoeft *et al.* 2006). An important characteristic that seems to be common in all tolerogenic DCs is the secretion of potent immunosuppressive cytokines during antigen presentation (Ghiringhelli *et al.* 2005; Dillon *et al.* 2006; Escors *et al.* 2008; Ilarregui *et al.* 2009; Arce *et al.* 2010; Saraiva & O'Garra 2010). In fact, at least in the presence of TGF-β, strong TCR stimulation during antigen presentation greatly enhances $Foxp3^+$ Treg differentiation. Tolerogenic DCs can also secrete high amounts of IL-10, a potent immunosuppressive cytokine, resulting in differentiation of mainly Tr1 cells (Kuhn *et al.* 1993; Saraiva & O'Garra 2010). In addition IL-10 autocrine and paracrine activities keep DCs in an immature stage (Takayama *et al.* 1998; Corinti *et al.* 2001). DCs can also up-regulate surface expression of molecules with T cell inhibitory activities. This is the case for some members of the B7 family. One of the most extensively studied immunosuppressive members is PD-L1, the ligand of the T cell inhibitory receptor PD-1. Binding of PD-L1 to PD-1 on T cells, especially in the case of chronic antigen exposure, renders T cells inactive (exhausted) (Sakuishi *et al.* 2010). This is a critical mechanism by which many tumour cells exert their immunosuppressive activities towards effector $CD8^+$ T cells. PD-L1 is expressed ubiquitously, but it is likely that its expression on DCs and other professional antigen presenting cells has a more specific role. Importantly, binding of PD-L1 expressed on DCs to CD80 on T cells has been shown to be required for TGF-β dependent antigen-specific Treg differentiation (Wang *et al.* 2008). A second PD-1 ligand was described that is specifically expressed on DCs and macrophages, termed PD-L2. However, it is unclear whether PD-L2 is truly immunosuppressive (Radhakrishnan *et al.* 2009). Recently, other B7 family members have also been shown to exert immunosuppressive activities (Sica *et al.* 2003). Finally, another interesting mechanism is up-regulation of amino acid-metabolising enzymes. Intriguingly, many of these are triggered by TGF-β (Belladonna *et al.* 2009). It has been known for some time that increased arginase activity in DCs suppresses immune responses (Munder 2009; Norian *et al.* 2009). Indoleamine 2,3-dioxygenase up-regulation, a tryptophan-metabolising enzyme, suppresses immune responses (Fallarino *et al.* 2002; Mellor & Munn 2004). Interestingly, Tregs can induce DCs to up-regulate several of these metabolic enzymes, resulting in infectious tolerance that amplifies the suppressive capacities of regulatory DCs and T cells (Cobbold *et al.* 2009).

3. Lentiviral vectors

Viruses are excellent candidates for the development of efficient gene delivery systems. As intracellular obligate parasites, they are specialized in the delivery of their genome to cells. Therefore it is no surprise that viruses have always been of interest for gene therapeutic applications. Nowadays a large number of viruses have been evaluated, *e.g.* adenovirus, adeno-associated virus, herpes virus, poxvirus, retrovirus, lentivirus, *et cetera* (Escors & Breckpot 2010). The first human gene therapy trial was performed in the 1970s and applied an arginase encoding Shope papilloma virus to treat hyperargininemia (Friedmann & Roblin 1972). By 1985, gene transfer with viral vectors to mammalian cells was performed routinely and the use of the γ-retroviral Murine leukaemia virus for gene delivery was introduced (Mann *et al.* 1983). This seemed promising as these viruses integrate their cargo into the host genome. It was Brenner *et al* (Brenner *et al.* 1993) who demonstrated the proof-of-principle of γ-retroviral gene transfer in hematopoietic stem cells (HSCs). The first clinical trial using γ-retroviral vectors (RVs) was carried out by Anderson and colleagues to correct severe combined immunodeficiency (SCID) in 1991 (Anderson *et al.* 1990). The majority of clinical gene therapy trials today use γ-RVs, despite their relative low stability, the low titers and their inability to transduce quiescent cells. More importantly, worrisome incidents of RV induced insertional mutagenesis were reported (Pincha *et al.* 2010). Lentiviruses, which as γ-retroviruses are members of the *Retroviridae*, were suggested to be an attractive alternative, since they are capable of transducing both dividing and non-dividing cells (Bukrinsky *et al.* 1993; Lewis & Emerman 1994). Moreover, their integration into the host genome is, in contrast to γ-retroviruses, associated with lower genotoxicity (Montini *et al.* 2006).

At the end of the 1990s, the use of recombinant LVs was boosted, especially for transduction of non-dividing cells (Akkina *et al.* 1996; Naldini *et al.* 1996a; Naldini *et al.* 1996b; Reiser *et al.* 1996). Another 10 years later the first clinical trial using LV modified cells for the treatment of HIV infection was completed (Lu *et al.* 2004).

3.1 Development of recombinant lentiviral vectors

Lentiviruses are characterized by a diploid 7-12 kb single stranded RNA genome with positive polarity that is reverse transcribed to double stranded DNA upon host cell entry (Coffin 1997). Diploidy permits genetic recombination, which accounts partially for their success as procreators of the acquired immunodeficiency syndrome, a disease that develops by slowly affecting the immune systems' function (lenti meaning slow). Lentiviruses include primate and non-primate retroviruses, *e.g.* HIV and simian immunodeficiency virus, and caprine arthritis-encephalitis virus, equine infectious anaemia virus, Maedi-visna virus, feline immunodeficiency virus and bovine immunodeficiency virus, respectively (Breckpot *et al.* 2008; Escors & Breckpot 2010). The spherical virion measures about 80-120 nm in diameter, has a mass of 2.5 x 10^5 kDA and a density of 1.16 g/ml in sucrose density gradient. Its envelope consists of a plasma membrane derived phospholipid bilayer loaded with surface (SU) and transmembranary (TM) glycoproteins and is supported on the inside by the non-glycosylated structural matrix (MA) proteins (Fig. 2). Within the envelope the nucleocapsid, comprised of capsid (CA) proteins, surrounds the viral genome, which is packaged together with nucleocapsid (NC) proteins and a few copies of the enzymes reverse transcriptase (RT), integrase (IN) and protease (PR).

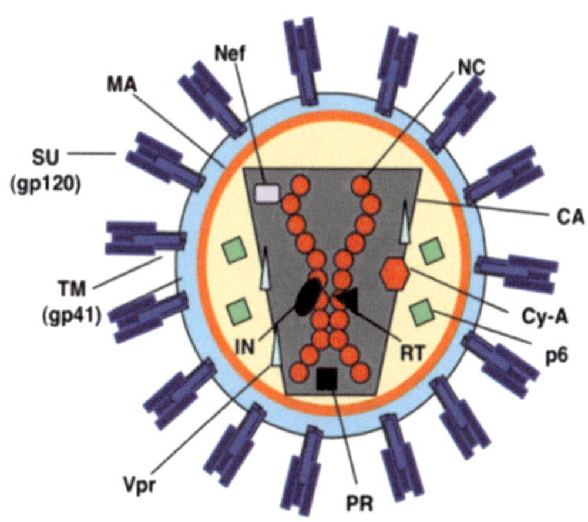

Fig. 2. **Schematic representation of a retroviral particle.** The viral envelope consists of a lipid bilayer loaded with viral proteins. These are composed of TM and SU components, linked *via* a disulphide bridge and encoded by de *env genes*. Internal non-glycosylated proteins are coded by the *gag* region of the viral genome and comprise MA, CA and NC proteins. The products of the *pol* - coding region are the RT and IN, while the PR is coded by the *pro* gene that resides between the *gag* and the *pol* gene.

The replication cycle of lentiviruses starts with the attachment of the viral envelope proteins to specific receptors on the host cell surface (Flint S.J. 2009). This interaction defines the tropism and results in conformational changes of SU and TM, which allows the hydrophobic fusion peptide of TM to insert in the cellular membrane, as such allowing the release of the nucleocapsid complex in the cytoplasm (Schaffer *et al.* 2008). The reverse transcription process sets off by primer binding of a viral tRNA and produces successively the negative and positive linear DNA strands till the DNA molecule called provirus is formed. Important are its *cis*-acting ends called long terminal repeats (LTRs) that are shown juxtaposed in preparation for integration (Fig. 3). As a unique characteristic of lentiviruses, viral DNA and IN gain access to the nucleus by formation of a pre-integration complex. Therefore, the lentiviral genome contains not only a 3′ polypurine tract (PPT), as other retroviruses, but also a central PPT (Fig. 3) (Charneau & Clavel 1991). The latter sequence together with a central termination sequence (CTS) controls the formation of a stable 99-nucleotide long plus strand overlap in the linear DNA molecule in *cis,* which enables active pro-viral nuclear import (Follenzi *et al.* 2000; Zennou *et al.* 2000). The subsequent integrative recombination is catalyzed by the IN, which uses the outer *att* sequences on the LTRs to grab the pro-viral DNA and results in random insertion of the viral DNA in the host genome. Transcription of the integrated provirus is mediated by cellular RNA polymerase II and results in different subsets of RNA molecules namely: mRNA molecules and new viral single stranded RNA genomes. The most important viral genes encoding mRNA molecules are: (i) the *env* (*envelope*) gene which encodes SU and TM; (ii) the *gag* (*group specific antigen*) gene which encodes the internal structural proteins MA, CA and NC; (iii) the *pol* (*polymerase*) gene which codes for the enzymes IN and RT including a DNA polymerase as well as its associated RNase H activity and finally (iv) the *pro* (*protease*) gene which encodes PR. Based on genomic organization retroviruses can be divided in simple and complex viruses. The simple viral genomes only encode the three genes, *gag, pol,* and *env*, common to all retroviruses, such as α-, β-, and γ-retroviruses. In contrast, complex viruses have a genome that encodes several accessory genes that affect viral gene expression and/or pathogenesis. Lentiviruses encode not only two extra regulatory genes *tat* and *rev* but also several accessory genes such as *vpr, vpu, vif* and *nef.* After transcription of the unspliced full-length viral RNA and translation of the mRNA encoding viral proteins, everything is transported to the cytoplasm where virion maturation occurs. The *cis*-acting packaging signal, ψ (psi), is required to ensure viral genome packaging and subsequent budding of the particle from the cell to give rise to infectious virions.

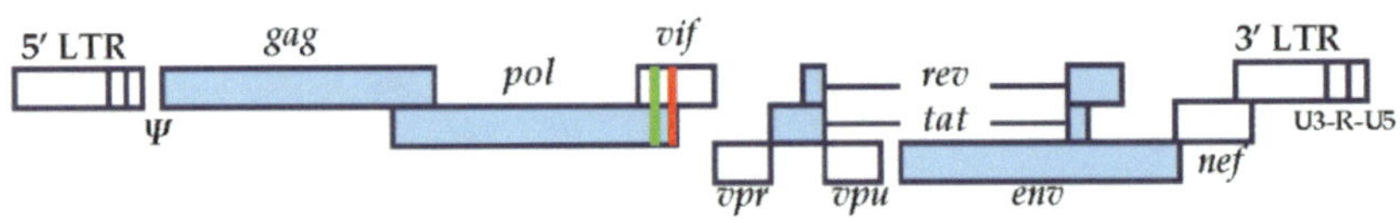

Fig. 3. **Schematic representation of the pro-viral HIV-1 genome.** All genes of the provirus (*gag, pol, pro, vif, vpr, vpu, rev, tat, env* and *nef*) are flanked on either side by identical 'long terminal repeats' (LTRs) that consist of a U3, R and U5 fragment. The pro-viral transcriptional control elements like the actual promoter and enhancer sequences can be found in the U3 regions. Ψ represents the encapsidation signal. Unlike most retroviruses, HIV and other LVs have two copies of the PPT, one at the border of the 3′LTR (3′ polypurine tract) and the other located within the *pol-coding* region (central polypurine tract [red line] together with a central termination sequence [green line]).

Given the fact that lentiviruses are pathogenic, it is crucial to develop a recombinant LV that is replication deficient, safe and efficient in transduction of target cells. Therefore, LVs have been vigorously modified, which has contributed to their widespread use as a gene delivery shuttle. A safety concern is the possible generation of replication-competent LVs (RCLs) as a consequence of genetic recombination (Wu *et al.* 2000). Therefore, LVs are produced by transient transfection of producer cells (HEK 293T) with at least three plasmids. This allows separation of *cis*- and *trans*-acting sequences. Generally the following plasmids are used: (i) a packaging, (ii) a transfer, and (iii) an envelope plasmid. All plasmids have been scrutinized to enhance their performance in terms of safety and efficacy (Breckpot *et al.* 2007a).

The packaging plasmid provides all viral structural and enzymatic sequences, encoded by *gag* and *pol,* to make an infective virion in *trans.* Based on the packaging plasmid recombinant LVs can be divided into different generations. The first generation is represented by a plasmid encoding the entire *gag* and *pol* sequence in *trans* to enable packaging of the transfer construct together with the viral regulatory genes *tat* and *rev* and the virulence genes *vif, vpr, vpu* and *nef.* The second generation plasmid is multiply attenuated by removal of the four virulence genes without any negative effect on transduction efficacy as these genes seemed dispensable for the efficient generation of HIV-derived LVs (Zufferey *et al.* 1997). In the third generation, the *rev* gene is expressed from a separate plasmid (Dull *et al.* 1998). Furthermore also the *tat* sequence could be removed by insertion of a strong constitutional promoter in the 5′ LTR of the transfer vector. More recently the importance of the development of non-integrating LVs (NILVs) has been brought to the attention because of the oncogene transactivation incidents in some clinical trials with γ-RVs. Although the LV integration profile seems more favourable than that of γ-RVs (Montini *et al.* 2009), several groups tested the transduction efficacy of NILVs by mutating the catalytic triad within the IN gene of the packaging plasmid (Wanisch & Yanez-Munoz 2009). Improved safety without major reduction in efficacy was demonstrated (Negri *et al.* 2007; Karwacz *et al.* 2009; Wanisch & Yanez-Munoz 2009). Downsides are the lower titers, higher doses needed and the fact that there still is a chance for integration of about 0.1 to 2.3% (Apolonia *et al.* 2007). An alternative to IN deficiency is site-specific integration into a safe harbour sequence of the target cell. Several strategies have been described, *e.g.* Cre-loxP carrying LVs, use of the zinc finger nuclease or meganuclease technology, *et cetera* (Matrai *et al.* 2010; Michel *et al.* 2010; Silva *et al.* 2011). Furthermore, the discovery that the LEDGF/p75 protein controls the site of integration of HIV-derived LVs presents new possibilities to control mutagenesis (Ciuffi 2008; Silvers *et al.* 2010).

The transfer plasmid is the only plasmid derived from the viral genome where all viral coding regions are replaced by the expression cassette. An important improvement for safety was the development of so called self-inactivating (SIN) vectors (Zufferey *et al.* 1998). These rely on the introduction of a deletion in the U3 region of the 3′ LTR. This deletion will be transferred to the 5′ LTR of the pro-viral DNA during reverse transcription, which abolishes production of full-length vector RNA in transduced cells. This has several advantages: (i) it minimizes the risk for emerging RCLs, (ii) it reduces the chance that cellular coding sequences located adjacent to the integrated pro-viral sequence will be aberrantly expressed due to the promoter activity in the 3′ LTR and (iii) it prevents transcriptional interference between the LTRs and an internal promoter. As the expression of genes delivered by LVs is often inefficient, several strategies were developed to ameliorate this. Firstly, the promoter within the expression cassette can be varied. Instead of using strong constitutive promoters, such as the promoter of cytomegalovirus or spleen focus forming virus, one can choose a cell-specific promoter as these are less sensitive to promoter inactivation and less likely to activate the host-cell defence machinery (Liu *et al.*

2004). Secondly, the incorporation of the cPPT and CTS into the transfer plasmid not only improved LV yields, but also provided enhanced transgene expression by mediating active nuclear import of the provirus (Follenzi *et al.* 2000; Sirven *et al.* 2000). Addition of posttranscriptional regulatory elements such as the Woodchuck hepatitis virus regulatory element (WPRE) has also been explored (Zufferey *et al.* 1999). Although some groups demonstrated improved gene expression by modification of polyadenylation, RNA export and/or translation, others reported only a negligible benefit (Breckpot *et al.* 2003). Another issue is epigenetic silencing and heterochromatin formation nearby the inserted provirus, which hampers its transcription. This silencing process can be avoided by the insertion of insulators or with vectors containing an enhancer-less ubiquitously acting chromatin-opening element (Zhang *et al.* 2007; Nielsen *et al.* 2009). To improve safety, the incorporation of a suicide-gene has been proposed to eliminate cells that are transformed as a consequence of LV integration (Tseng *et al.* 2009). Finally the discovery of RNA interference opens novel possibilities for LVs in terms of stable gene silencing (Gu *et al.* ; Arrighi *et al.* 2004), as well as for LV de-targeting strategies (Brown *et al.* 2006b).
Last but not least also the envelope plasmid is variable. Since wild-type HIV-1 glycoproteins have a restricted tropism and do not allow production of high titer LV preparations, heterologous glycoproteins are used for LV production. This process is termed pseudotyping and most commonly the envelope of the vesicular stomatitis virus (VSV.G) is used. This rhabdovirus envelope glycoprotein interacts with an ubiquitous receptor and subsequently confers a broad host-cell range and high vector particle stability (Burns *et al.* 1993; Marsac *et al.* 2002; Schaffer *et al.* 2008).

3.2 Lentiviral vectors for the *in vitro* modification of dendritic cells

Efficient transduction of human DCs with transgenic vectors has been challenging for several reasons. Human DCs are usually generated from peripheral blood-derived quiescent $CD14^+$ progenitors or from mitotically hypoactive primitive $CD34^+$-derived progenitor cells. Therefore, the capacity of LVs to transduce quiescent and non-dividing cells turned out to be an important asset for DC transduction. The first successful transduction of human monocyte-derived DCs with LVs was described by Unutmaz *et al* (Unutmaz *et al.* 1999) in 1999. Since then, several research groups have reported successful transduction of human monocyte-derived (Gruber *et al.* 2000; Schroers *et al.* 2000; Dyall *et al.* 2001; Firat *et al.* 2002; Breckpot *et al.* 2003; Lizee *et al.* 2004), human $CD34^+$-derived DCs (Salmon *et al.* 2000; Oki *et al.* 2001; Sumimoto *et al.* 2002) and mouse bone marrow-derived DCs (Metharom *et al.* 2001; Breckpot *et al.* 2003) with varying efficiencies. Transgene expression was found to be stable in monocyte-derived DCs (Gruber *et al.* 2000; Breckpot *et al.* 2003) and $CD34^+$-derived DCs (Oki *et al.* 2001). However, for mouse DCs, the kinetics are somewhat more complicated, due to a process which is called pseudotransduction (Dullaers *et al.* 2004), and which results in a wrong estimation of the transduction efficiency when analyzed early after transduction. Nevertheless, DCs can be modified at high efficiency (Breckpot *et al.* 2003). Importantly, there is quite some variability in transduction efficiency among different reports. This most likely reflects the diversity in DC sources, techniques and vectors used for transduction (Breckpot *et al.* 2004a).

3.3 Lentiviral vectors for the *in vivo* modification of dendritic cells

As broad-tropism LVs efficiently transduced mouse and human DCs *in vitro*, it was next questioned whether these LVs can be used to transduce DCs *in vivo*, as such circumvent the labour-intensive, time- and money-consuming procedure of generating DCs *ex vivo*. Dullaers *et al* (Dullaers *et al.* 2006) used a PCR-based method to demonstrate the presence of the LV delivered transgene in the draining lymph node at days 2 and 10, but not day 25 post administration of LVs in the footpad. These data were confirmed in flow cytometry, demonstrating that the PCR signal correlated with a small percentage (less than 1%) of transduced CD11c$^+$ cells (unpublished data Dullaers *et al*). Using the same injection route, Esslinger *et al* (Esslinger *et al.* 2003) showed transduction of CD11c$^+$ cells in the lymph node by immunohistochemical analysis, whereas He *et al* (He & Falo 2006) were able to demonstrate by flow cytometry that transduced DCs present in the lymph node after footpad injection of GFP encoding LVs originated from locally transduced migratory skin DC. More recently, a new imaging technique, *in vivo* bioluminescence imaging, was used to visualize cells transduced *in situ* with Firefly luciferase encoding LVs upon footpad injection (Breckpot *et al.*). Intravenous administration of LVs also leads to transduction of DCs in the spleen (VandenDriessche *et al.* 2002; Palmowski *et al.* 2004; Arce *et al.* 2009). These studies indicate that LVs, independent of the route of administration transduce DCs *in situ* and have instigated the exploration of LVs as an off-the-shelf vaccine.

4. Exploitation of lentivirally transduced dendritic cells in anti-cancer immunotherapy

Active anti-tumour immunotherapy is based on the delivery of tumour antigens (Boon & van der Bruggen 1996) in a way that induces therapeutic immunity. As several tumour-induced tolerogenic mechanisms are in place it is not sufficient to stimulate effector T cells, it is moreover critical to circumvent suppressive immune cells, such as Treg. Such anti-tumour immunity can only be induced by professional antigen presenting cells, in particular DCs, and requires presentation of the tumour antigen-derived peptides to both CD4$^+$ and CD8$^+$ T cells in the context of strong co-stimulation. As mentioned previously LVs have been tested as vehicles, for *ex vivo* and *in vivo* antigen delivery to DCs. In the following section we will discus the induction of potent T cell mediated immune responses that can control tumour growth by *ex vivo*, as well as *in situ* LV transduced DCs. Finally, we will discuss some strategies that have been explored to enhance the performance of LV-based vaccines.

4.1 Evaluation of *ex vivo* lentiviral vector transduced dendritic cells as a cellular anti-tumour vaccine

Since the beginning of the millennium, several reports on the use of tumour antigen encoding LVs for the *ex vivo* modification of DCs have been published. As it is of paramount importance that tumour antigen-derived peptides are efficiently processed and presented on the DC surface in order to efficiently prime and activate tumour antigen-specific T cells, it was first evaluated whether LV transduced DCs activate established T cell lines. Note, strategies in which the tumour antigen encoding genetic sequence is fused to the sequence encoding class II targeting signals, such as the first 80 amino acids of the invariant chain (Ii80), were employed to obtain not only presentation of antigenic peptides in MHC class I, but furthermore in MHC class II in order to activate CD8$^+$ and CD4$^+$ T cells, respectively (Bonehill *et al.* 2005). As mentioned before, the activation of IFN-γ producing CD4$^+$ T_H1 cells supports priming and maintenance of CTLs, moreover in anti-tumour immunotherapy, it has been shown that these CD4$^+$ T_H1 cells mediate tumour rejection

(Bonehill *et al.* 2003). Both human and mouse LV transduced DCs were able to activate established CD8+ and CD4+ T cell lines specific for epitopes derived from various relevant tumour antigens, such as MAGE-3 (Breckpot *et al.* 2003), Melan-A (Firat *et al.* 2002; Sumimoto *et al.* 2002) and tyrosinase (Lizee *et al.* 2004) in the human system and for the surrogate antigen ovalbumin (OVA) (Breckpot *et al.* 2003; He *et al.* 2005), as well as for TRP-2 (Metharom *et al.* 2001) in the murine system.

Moreover, several groups reported on the *in vitro* priming of naive T cells against tumour antigens using LV transduced human DCs. Firat *et al* (Firat *et al.* 2002) stimulated CD8+ T cells in bulk with monocyte-derived DCs that were transduced with LVs encoding a melanoma poly-epitope and demonstrated expansion of tetramer+ CD8+ T cells, which could specifically lyse gp100 and Melan-A peptide-pulsed targets. We showed priming of both CD8+ and CD4+ T cells against the poorly immunogenic melanoma antigen MAGE-A3 after *in vitro* stimulation with DCs transduced with LVs encoding the fusion protein Ii80MAGEA3 (Breckpot *et al.* 2003). The primed CD8+ T cells were further cloned and characterized enabling the identification of a novel HLA-Cw7 restricted MAGE-A3 peptide (Breckpot *et al.* 2004b). A number of groups evaluated the potential of mouse DCs transduced with LVs as a cellular anti-tumour vaccine *in vivo*. Herein, the induced immune response was characterized and tested for protection against tumour growth. We showed that immunization with DCs transduced with OVA encoding LVs induced a strong CTL response, resulting in specific lyses of OVA-expressing tumour cells after *in vitro* restimulation (Breckpot *et al.* 2003) or *in vivo* upon delivery of autologous OVA peptide-pulsed spleen cells (Dullaers *et al.* 2006). He *et al* (He *et al.* 2005) confirmed these data. It was moreover demonstrated that these CTL responses were protective against a subsequent challenge with a lethal dose of OVA-expressing B16 melanoma cells and slowed down the outgrowth of pre-existing tumours (He *et al.* 2005; Dullaers *et al.* 2006). Later on, it was shown with endogenous tumour antigens that the results obtained with the strong immunogenic OVA were not an overestimation of the potential of LV transduced DCs as a cellular therapeutic. Tumour antigens such as TRP-2 (Metharom *et al.* 2001) and erbB2 (mouse analogue of human Her-2/neu) (Mossoba *et al.* 2008) were used to demonstrate induction of strong CTL responses and decreased tumour growth. Importantly, Wang *et al.* (Wang *et al.* 2006) extended these data in a mouse hepatoma model, immunized with LV transduced DCs expressing three hepatoma-associated antigens, which are self-antigens that are highly expressed in tumour cells, demonstrating CD4+ and CD8+ T cell responses against all three hepatoma antigens, as well as regression of established tumours. Delivery of multiple tumour antigens might overcome the problem of tumour escape due to antigen loss (Dullaers *et al.* 2006). Finally, it has to be noted that several groups compared DCs transduced with LVs to DCs pulsed with (tumour) antigen-derived peptides (He *et al.* 2005; Metharom *et al.* 2005) or electroporated with mRNA (Dullaers *et al.* 2004), two strategies that were approved in the clinic, demonstrating that LV modified DCs elicited stronger and longer-lasting anti-tumour T cell responses.

These studies suggest that *ex vivo* LV transduced DCs are effective in therapeutic treatment of cancer. However, this strategy has important drawbacks common to all DC-based vaccination approaches. Because the vaccine is patient-specific it requires specialized personnel and facilities for vaccine production. Consequently, there is a high cost and considerable time required for vaccine production and quality control. It is for that reason that direct administration of LVs *in vivo* has gained substantial interest.

4.2 Evaluation of lentiviral vectors as an off-the-shelf anti-tumour vaccine

For LVs to be an effective vaccine they have to transduce DCs *in situ*, a pre-requisite that is fulfilled. Furthermore, the *in vivo* transduced DCs need to process the transgene, have to be activated so they migrate to lymphoid organs, where they subsequently present transgene-derived epitopes in the context of MHC molecules and strong co-stimulation to T cells. Hence, the degree of tumour antigen-specific CTL induction can be considered as a reliable measure for the value of direct administration of tumour antigen encoding LVs in tumour immunology. Antigen-specific CTLs could be generated upon direct administration of LVs using HLA-Cw3 as a model antigen (Esslinger *et al.* 2003). Similar results were obtained in HLA-A transgenic mice using a LV encoding a minigene containing the dominant human Melan-A HLA-A*0201 epitope (Chapatte *et al.* 2006) or human telomerase reverse transcriptase (hTERT) (Adotevi *et al.* ; Rusakiewicz *et al.*). Using OVA as an antigen, it was confirmed that direct administration of LVs resulted in a higher number of IFN-γ producing $CD8^+$ T cells, which had a higher lytic capacity as compared to those primed with *ex vivo* transduced DCs (Dullaers *et al.* 2006). Memory CTL responses were also significantly stronger upon LV administration. Other studies with tumour antigens such as NY-ESO (Palmowski *et al.* 2004), TRP-2 (Kim *et al.* 2005), TRP-1 (Liu *et al.* 2009) and CEA (Loisel-Meyer *et al.* 2009), have also shown potent immune responses upon vaccination with LVs. Comparison of *in vivo* administration of LVs to the peptide or DNA vaccination strategy was performed in a HLA-A transgenic mice, by Chapatte *et al* (Chapatte *et al.* 2006) and Rusakiewicz *et al* (Rusakiewicz *et al.*), demonstrating that stronger tumour-specific immune responses were elicited when immunization was performed with LVs.

Reference	Dose	Route	Antigen
Esslinger et al	2×10^7 EFU	sc (footpad, tail base)	Cw3, mini Melan-A
Palmowski et al	1×10^6 PFU	iv (tail vein)	NY-ESO
Kim et al	1.6×10^6 PFU	sc (footpad)	TRP-2
Rowe et al	1×10^7 IU	iv (tail vein)	OVA
Dullaers et al	2×10^7 TU	sc (footpad)	OVA
He et al	1×10^6 TU	sc (footpad)	OVA
Chapatte et al	2×10^7 EFU	sc (tail base)	Melan-A
Liu et al	2.5×10^7 TU	sc (footpad)	TRP-1
Loisel-Meyer	0.15×10^6 TU	sc (footpad)	CEA
Rusakiewicz et al	1×10^7 TU	sc (footpad)	hTERT

Table 1. **Summary of the studies evaluating LVs as an off-the-shelf vaccine.**

Although $CD4^+$ T cell responses were shown to be necessary for the priming and maintenance of CTLs when DCs are used for vaccination, not much data is available on the role of $CD4^+$ T cell help in the induction of CTLs upon immunization with LVs. Esslinger *et al* (Esslinger *et al.* 2003) showed that CD4 depletion reduces the primary CTL response upon direct administration of LVs. Similarly, we (Dullaers *et al.* 2006) showed that although there was a larger requirement for $CD4^+$ T cell help during the primary response in case of immunization with *ex vivo* transduced DCs compared to direct administration of LVs; $CD4^+$ T cell depletion strongly reduced the capacity to mount a recall CTL response in both cases. Interestingly, Marzo *et al* (Marzo *et al.* 2004) showed that in the case of a VSV infection, a functional $CD8^+$ T cell memory response can be generated in the absence of $CD4^+$ T cells, this in contrast to an infection with *Listeria monocytogenes*. These authors suggest that the difference might be due to the fact that VSV can directly infect DC whereas *L. monocytogenes* antigens need to be cross-presented. Since, the currently applied LVs are pseudotyped with VSV envelopes, it needs to be further examined to what extent the CTL response is $CD4^+$ T cell-dependent.

The generation of specific T cell responses is a convenient read-out for the success of a vaccination strategy however; there are many examples of discrepancies between immune responses and anti-tumour responses (Rosenberg *et al.* 2005). Therefore, it is critical to evaluate the effect of LV vaccination on tumour growth. Rowe *et al* (Rowe *et al.* 2006) showed significantly improved protection of mice vaccinated with LVs encoding OVA against a subsequent tumour challenge. Similarly, Dullaers *et al* (Dullaers *et al.* 2006) showed that direct administration of LVs offers increased protection to a subsequent tumour challenge compared to DC vaccination and a significantly improved survival of tumour bearing mice. Other studies using TRP-2 (Kim *et al.* 2005), TRP-1 (Liu *et al.* 2009) or CEA (Loisel-Meyer *et al.* 2009) as tumour antigen, demonstrated improved survival of tumour bearing mice receiving LVs encoding these tumour antigens. Liu *et al* (Liu *et al.* 2009) showed that this type of immunization could result in complete regression of small subcutaneous tumours, which correlated with enhanced numbers of functional $CD8^+$ T cells in the tumour environment. Therefore, these studies highlight the potential of LVs encoding tumour antigens as an anti-cancer therapeutic.

These studies demonstrate that administration of LVs doesn't provoke immunological tolerance, but rather elicits powerful CTL responses against transgene-encoded proteins. This suggests a certain degree of immunogenicity of LVs or components within LV preparations, leading to activation of innate viral-sensing pathways and as a consequence induction of strong adaptive immunity. Therefore, it is not surprising that several studies addressed the immunogenicity of LVs. LVs are generally derived from HIV-1, for which activation of pDCs through TLR7 triggering has been demonstrated (Fonteneau *et al.* 2004; Beignon *et al.* 2005). It was demonstrated *in vivo* that activation of pDCs by recombinant LVs is mediated by several mechanisms. Brown *et al.* (Brown *et al.* 2006a) reported a TLR7-dependent type I IFN response, whereas a role for TLR9 was demonstrated by Pichlmair *et al* (Pichlmair *et al.* 2007), who demonstrated that VSV.G pseudotyped LV preparations contain tubulovesicular structures of cellular origin, which carry nucleic acids. These structures triggered TLR9 in pDCs, whereas LVs pseudotyped with a γ-retroviral envelope didn't (Lopes *et al.* 2008), suggesting that this particular mechanism is not necessary for potent immune stimulation. More recently, Rossetti *et al* (Rossetti *et al.*) demonstrated that also human blood-derived pDCs are activated in a TLR7/9-dependent way by LVs *in vitro*. These observations were not surprising as the pDC subset is the DCs subset that is best equipped to sense viral infections. However, recombinant LVs also target cDCs. Therefore, this DC subset should not be neglected when the LV immunogenicity is discussed. Gruber *et al* (Gruber *et al.* 2000) reported that transduction of cDCs at low MOI didn't result in DC activation, whereas Tan *et al.* (Tan *et al.* 2005) described that transduction of cDCs at high MOI results in up-regulation of adhesion, stimulatory and antigen presenting molecules. Furthermore, these DCs displayed enhanced allo-stimulatory capacities and an altered cytokine secretion pattern. To clarify these results, we (Breckpot *et al.* 2007b) transduced DCs with LVs at varying MOI, confirming that transduction of DCs with LVs at low MOI results in considerable transgene delivery, without activation, whereas transduction at high

MOI indeed leads to DC maturation. A role for protein kinase R, a cytosolic receptor that interacts with double stranded RNA during LV replication, and several TLRs was suggested (Breckpot *et al.* 2007b). In our recent *in vivo* study, we demonstrated that cDCs are activated upon LV infection. More importantly, we showed that this activation was dependent on retroviral reverse transcription and critically dependent on the signal adaptor molecules MyD88 and TRIF, hence TLR signalling. Experiments with TLR knock out DCs demonstrated that both TLR3 and TLR7 are involved in the DC activation (Breckpot *et al.*).
It is important to stress that induction of therapeutic anti-tumour immunity is critically dependent on an inflammatory environment in order to overcome tolerance, and active inhibitory mechanisms exerted by suppressive immune cells, such as Treg, as well as tumour cells. Such an inflammatory environment can be achieved by strong activation of the innate arm of the immune system, in particular through the engagement of TLRs. This was highlighted by Yang *et al* (Yang *et al.* 2004) and by Lang *et al* (Lang *et al.* 2005), who demonstrated that tolerance of antigen-specific CTLs could be broken by persistent TLR ligation. In that respect, we demonstrated that DCs activated by LVs *via* TLR3 and TLR7, efficiently expanded antigen-specific CTLs, whereas DCs lacking either TLR lacked this CTL inducing capacity (Breckpot *et al.*). Furthermore, it has been described that signalling through certain combinations of TLRs on DCs not only provided a synergy with respect to the production of stimulatory cytokines such as IL-12, which is essential in the differentiation of $CD4^+$ T cells to a T_H1 phenotype (Gautier *et al.* 2005; Napolitani *et al.* 2005), but also offered protection from suppressive Treg that actively quench the anti-tumour immune response (Warger *et al.* 2006). As a consequence, much research efforts have been put in designing approaches that enhance the intrinsic immunogenicity of LV-based vaccines. Some of these will be discussed in the next section.

4.3 Engineering lentiviral vectors to enhance the immune stimulatory capacity of dendritic cells

To enhance the immunogenic potential of LVs, and concomitantly prevent the actions of tolerogenic mechanisms over transduced DCs, LVs can be engineered to not only deliver the tumour antigen but also deliver molecules that enhance DC activation. Based on our growing knowledge on the importance of TLRs for DC activation and which activation pathways are triggered by these TLRs, several TLR-based strategies have been developed to enhance the immune stimulatory capacity of DCs upon LV transduction.
Over the years LPS, which binds to TLR4 has been extensively used to activate DCs *in vitro* (Ardeshna *et al.* 2000; Arrighi *et al.* 2001; da Silva Correia *et al.* 2001). LPS-mediated activation remarkably enhances stimulation of DC-mediated immune responses *in vitro*, and overcomes suppression by Treg, a critical factor in anti-tumour immunology (Pasare & Medzhitov 2003). However, its clinical use is limited by its cytotoxicity. Therefore, the feasibility of using RVs encoding a constitutive active TLR4 (caTLR4) for DC maturation has been evaluated (Xu *et al.* 2007). This was achieved by linking the cytoplasmic domain of TLR4 to the extracellular single-chain immunoglobulin anti-erbB2. However, no activation of an immortalized DC line, JAWSII was observed, although a similar strategy, *i.e.* electroporation with mRNA encoding caTLR4, was recently shown to activate human DCs, resulting in priming of Melan-A CTL responses (Bonehill *et al.* 2008). Using a similar cloning strategy Xu *et al* (Xu *et al.* 2007) generated RVs encoding MyD88 or IRAK-1, two major adaptor molecules in TLR triggered activation pathways. Again they used the JAWSII DC line to evaluate the chimeric proteins, demonstrating that only the IRAK-1 chimera

mediated IL-12 and TNF-α secretion, and enhanced OVA-specific $CD4^+$ T cell responses. Akazawa *et al* (Akazawa *et al.* 2007) expressed MyD88 and TRIF, another major TLR signal transduction molecule in mouse DCs using LVs. MyD88-modified DCs produced IL-6 and IL-12, but didn't up-regulate phenotypic markers, whereas TRIF expression stimulated IFN-β production and increased levels of CD86. Both MyD88 and TRIF increased the allo-stimulatory capacity of the modified DCs, and tumour outgrowth was delayed after immunization with these DCs.

Introduction of MyD88 or IRAK-1 in DCs activates the NF-κB pathway. NF-κB is a well-studied transcription factor that targets genes associated with DC maturation. Sustained NF-κB activation in DCs using LVs has been achieved by expressing Kaposi's sarcoma associated human herpes virus vFLIP (Rowe *et al.* 2009). In this case, DC maturation was enhanced by up-regulation of MHC, adhesion (ICAM-1) and co-stimulatory molecules (CD80, CD86, CD40), and increased secretion of TNF-α and IL-12. vFLIP-modified DCs significantly increased antigen-specific CTL responses resulting in enhanced anti-tumour immunity (Karwacz *et al.* 2009; Rowe *et al.* 2009). Another effective approach leading to sustained NF-κB activation consists of down-regulating the negative feedback molecule, A20 of which the expression is under the immediate control of NF-κB. A20 deactivates several adaptor molecules of the TNFR, IL-1/TLR signalling pathways by ubiquitinating/de-ubiquitinating activity (Vereecke *et al.* 2009). Therefore, A20 down-regulation could result in prolonged NF-κB activation, resulting in DCs with enhanced stimulatory capacity. LV delivered A20-targeted shRNA (Song *et al.* 2008) and direct introduction of siRNA (Breckpot *et al.* 2009) were applied to down-regulate A20 in mouse and human DCs, respectively. These approaches showed that A20 controls DC maturation, cytokine production and immunostimulatory potency. Human DCs with down-regulated A20 expression had an increased NF-κB activity and showed enhanced and sustained IL-10 and IL-12 secretion. These DCs were more potent in stimulating Melan-A CTL responses (Breckpot *et al.* 2009). Mouse DCs with down-regulated A20 expression showed enhanced expression of co-stimulatory molecules and pro-inflammatory cytokines. Moreover, these DCs hyper-activated tumour-specific CTL and T_H cells, which were refractory to Treg suppression (Song *et al.* 2008).

Besides LVs that target the NF-κB pathway, LVs have been engineered to increase the DC's immunogenicity by introducing specific genes that modulate intracellular MAPK pathways. p38 was activated by expressing MKK6 mutants containing glutamate and aspartate residues in their activation loop, mimicking phosphorylated serine or threonine residues (Raingeaud *et al.* 1996). A fusion protein between MKK7 and JNK1 was expressed to achieve constitutive JNK1 phosphorylation (Escors *et al.* 2008). Expression of constitutive activators prevents inactivation by phosphatase-dependent negative feedback mechanisms, which may counteract tolerogenic mechanisms in anti-tumour immunity. In the absence of TLR stimulation, p38 activation resulted in a DC maturation phenotype different from full maturation as achieved by LPS treatment (Escors *et al.* 2008). Particularly, there was specific up-regulation of co-stimulatory molecules and absence of significant secretion of pro-inflammatory cytokines (Escors *et al.* 2008). Interestingly, co-expression of OVA with the p38 activator in DCs significantly increased antigen-specific $CD4^+$ and $CD8^+$ T cell responses leading to increased anti-tumour immunity (Escors *et al.* 2008; Karwacz *et al.* 2009). Additionally, MAPK p38 constitutive activation also increased $CD8^+$ T cell responses to human tumour antigens NY-ESO in a humanized HLA-A2 mouse model and Melan-A in a human DC-T cell culture (Escors *et al.* 2008). Specific activation of JNK1 in DCs showed only a moderate up-regulation of co-stimulatory molecules and no significant secretion of pro-inflammatory cytokines, confirming previous studies, which suggested that JNK marginally controls DC maturation (Nakahara *et al.* 2004; Escors *et al.* 2008). On the other hand, increased antigen-specific CD8$^+$ T cell expansion was achieved in mice after subcutaneous vaccination with LV expressing MKK7-JNK1, suggesting that JNK1 may play a subtle but important role in DCs *in vivo* (Escors *et al.* 2008).

5. Exploitation of lentivirally transduced dendritic cells for the induction of tolerance

There are many ways in which DCs have been utilised for the treatment of autoimmune disorders. This chapter will focus on genetic modification using LVs, rather than providing an extensive review of all DC-based methods. Because the achievement of immune suppression is more challenging than inducing activation, there are a limited number of reports on the use of LVs as immunosuppressive (tolerogenic) therapeutic agents.

An obvious approach to genetically modify DCs for the treatment of autoimmune disorders is to express potent immunosuppressive cytokines. In fact, there are a few reports of DC modification using mainly RVs expressing immunosuppressive cytokines for the treatment of inflammatory diseases (Lee *et al.* 1998; Takayama *et al.* 1998; Morita *et al.* 2001). The equivalent approach has been undertaken by transduction of DCs using LVs expressing IL-10 in an OVA-dependent model of experimental asthma (Henry *et al.* 2008). *In vivo* intratracheal injection of OVA-pulsed DCs modified with LVs expressing IL-10 effectively inhibited airway inflammation and asthma-associated symptoms. Interestingly, it was demonstrated that host IL-10 expression was absolutely required for the IL-10 DCs to inhibit asthma (Henry *et al.* 2008). Therefore, IL-10 expression from DCs was playing an indirect role in inhibiting disease. Interestingly, a significant increase in Foxp3$^+$ Treg expressing IL-10 were expanded, and their adoptive transfer prevented OVA-sensitized mice from eosinophilia after OVA challenge (Henry *et al.* 2008).

An attractive option for programming tolerogenic DCs is to modulate signalling pathways involved in differentiation of immunosuppressive DCs. This approach regulates expression of gene clusters, which act in a concerted action in physiological functional tolerogenic DCs. There is quite a wide range of experimental evidence linking MAPK ERK activation to immune suppression and tolerance (Agrawal *et al.* 2006; Caparros *et al.* 2006; Dillon *et al.* 2006; Escors *et al.* 2008). Constitutive activation of the ERK pathway can be readily achieved by expression of constitutively active MEK1 mutants, the upstream ERK kinase (Pages *et al.* 1994; Raingeaud *et al.* 1996; Escors *et al.* 2008; Anastasaki *et al.* 2009). Particularly, DCs modified with a LV expressing a MEK1 mutant with a deletion in the coding region of the nuclear export signal, together with two activating mutations resulted in DCs with a marked immature phenotype (Escors *et al.* 2008). ERK-activated mouse and human DCs showed a pronounced CD40 down-regulation and secretion of significant amounts of TGF-β (Escors *et al.* 2008; Arce *et al.* 2010). These DCs were strongly immunosuppressive, leading to differentiation of antigen-specific Foxp3$^+$ Treg *in vivo* and *in vitro* (Arce *et al.* 2010). These differentiated Treg strongly proliferated after a second antigen encounter in inflammatory conditions. A LV vaccine based on an ERK activator was successfully applied for the treatment of inflammatory arthritis in a mouse model (Arce *et al.* 2010). This therapeutic approach could be applied even when the specific arthritogenic antigen was not specifically targeted. Application in human therapy could follow a similar approach in which simultaneous ERK activation and expression of an endogenous antigen could be used to inhibit arthritis even though the arthritogenic antigens are not well characterized and may vary between patients.

Interestingly, constitutive activation of the type I IFN signalling pathway was also immunosuppressive in DCs. Expression of a constitutively active IRF3 mutant (IRF3 2D) in mouse DCs induced expression of high levels of IL-10 (Escors *et al.* 2008). Interestingly, vaccination with a LV co-expressing IRF3 2D with an OVA-containing transgene resulted in systemic expansion of OVA-specific Foxp3^{+} Treg (Escors *et al.* 2008). In physiological conditions, phosphorylated IRF3 dimerizes and translocates to the nucleus where it transactivates type I IFN promoters, leading to IFN-β production, a potent antiviral cytokine (Fitzgerald *et al.* 2003). Interestingly, it has been known for some time that components of the type I interferon pathway are in fact immunosuppressive (Chang *et al.* 2007). This is also the basis of the use of type I IFNs for the treatment of multiple sclerosis (Comabella *et al.* 2002; Billiau 2006). Very interestingly, production of both IFN-β and IL-10 share a common pathway when activated by TLR signalling (Hacker *et al.* 2006; Chang *et al.* 2007). It has been proposed that phosphorylated IRF3 may link IFN-β production with IL-10 secretion through a MyD88-dependent pathway (Escors *et al.* 2008). Taking advantage of this, activators of the type I IFN pathway could be expressed in DCs for the treatment of autoimmune disorders such as multiple sclerosis.

An alternative to constitutive activation of immunosuppressive pathways is to specifically inhibit pro-inflammatory signalling pathways. Possibly, one of the major pro-inflammatory pathways in DCs is NF-κB (Breckpot & Escors 2009b). Consequently, silencing of components from the NF-κB pathway could theoretically prevent DC maturation and induce immune suppression and tolerance. For instance, this has been successfully applied by silencing Rel-B in DCs by delivery of a specific shRNA using LVs (Zhang *et al.* 2009). Rel-B silencing was sufficient to confer DCs resistance to TLR-derived maturation signals and to inhibit experimental autoimmune myasthenia gravis in a mouse model (Zhang *et al.* 2009). Interestingly, just by inhibiting NF-κB, DCs acquired tolerogenic activities characterised by inhibition of T cell proliferation and differentiation of Foxp3^{+} Treg.

Another interesting approach is the exploitation of naturally occurring negative feedback mechanisms of pro-inflammatory pathways. This has been achieved by over-expressing suppressor of cytokine signalling 3 (SOCS-3) in DCs using LVs (Li *et al.* 2006). SOCS comprise a family of cytoplasmic proteins induced by cytokine-mediated signal transduction. They form part of a negative feedback mechanism that limits cytokine-induced signalling. Expression of SOCS3 in mouse DCs results in immature DCs with down-regulated MHC molecules and reduced CD86 (Li *et al.* 2006). These modified DCs exhibit an impaired signalling by IL-12 and IL-23, and reduced expression of these cytokines. More importantly, enhanced secretion of IL-10 was observed, which polarised T cell responses towards a T_H2 type. Interestingly, SOCS3-expressing DCs could efficiently inhibit the development of EAE, an experimental model for human multiple sclerosis (Li *et al.* 2006).

Recently, a LV-based shRNA delivery system was successfully applied for the treatment of experimental collagen-induced arthritis without specific targeting of the arthritogenic antigen (collagen) (Lai Kwan Lam *et al.* 2008). Direct administration of a LV encoding a siRNA specific for B cell activating factor (BAFF) to the inflamed joint was sufficient to inhibit arthritis. BAFF is a member of the TNF family which is mainly involved in regulating B cell maturation and functions (Batten *et al.* 2000; Yang *et al.* 2010). Interestingly, elevated BAFF levels have been found in the serum of patients suffering from several autoimmune disorders including rheumatoid arthritis. Very interestingly, it was demonstrated that LVs preferentially transduced DCs in the inflamed joint, and that BAFF silencing in these DCs interfered with DC maturation. Local BAFF silencing inhibited pro-inflammatory T cell development and inhibited production of pro-inflammatory cytokines such as IL-17, IL-23 and IL-6 (Lai Kwan Lam *et al.* 2008). Importantly, these authors clearly demonstrated that (i) LVs can be directly administered to the site of inflammation, (ii) they preferentially transduce local DCs and (iii) it is not strictly necessary to target the arthritogenic antigen.

In addition to manipulation of signalling pathways, there are small peptides with broad activities including immune suppression. Direct intraperitoneal immunisation with a LV encoding vasointestinal peptide (VIP) reduced the severity of collagen-induced arthritis in a mouse model (Delgado *et al.* 2008). Interestingly, vaccination with this LV significantly inhibited the secretion of a wide array of pro-inflammatory cytokines both systemically and in the joint. This tolerogenic LV-vaccination expanded Foxp3$^+$ Treg (Delgado *et al.* 2008). However, VIP has a variety of physiological functions apart from its immunosuppressive properties. Therefore, in this case, it would be desirable to modify DCs *ex vivo* with a VIP-expressing LV followed by *in vivo* transfer (Toscano *et al.* 2010). In fact, VIP expression in DCs was sufficient to keep them in an immature stage, leading to secretion of high levels of IL-10 (Toscano *et al.* 2010). *In vivo* administration of VIP-expressing DCs had beneficial therapeutic effects in EAE mice and in the cecal ligation and puncture model, both models relevant for multiple sclerosis and sepsis in humans (Toscano *et al.* 2010).

6. Limitations of lentiviral vectors for direct *in vivo* application

Although the HIV-based vector system is by far the best developed among the various LVs, a variety of quality, safety, efficacy, regulatory and ethical concerns slacken the frequent employment of HIV-based vectors in a clinical setting. In view of DC modulation, the scope of this review will be limited to the biological risks and immunogenic consequences of LV-based vaccination. Safety seems the most pressing issue as LVs are derived from an integrating pathogenic agent, lethal in humans. As mentioned, one of the main adverse events to consider is the potential generation of RCLs. However, to date no RCLs have been reported for LV packaging systems. This can be partially explained by the separation of *cis-* and *trans*-acting sequences during LV production, but also by the fact that SIN LVs are less likely to produce RCLs (Pauwels *et al.* 2009). A major setback for viral gene therapy clinical trials was caused by the development of leukaemia in five patients of two separate γ-RV gene therapy trials for X-linked SCID as a consequence of insertional activation of the LMO2 gene (proto-oncogene) by the LTR enhancer. As genomic integration is common to all retroviruses, the associated risk of insertional mutagenesis and/or transactivation of adjacent sequences must be taken into account for LVs as well (Howe *et al.* 2008). However, as these observations were made with γ-RV it would be to hasty to extrapolate this risk to the multiply attenuated recombinant LV system used today. An *in vitro* mapping study comparing RV and LV integration in transduced human HSCs revealed that RV but not LV hot spots were highly enriched in proto-oncogenes, cancer-associated and growth-controlling genes, suggesting that LVs have a lower propensity for integrating in potentially dangerous regions within the human genome (Cattoglio *et al.* 2007). Furthermore, an *in vivo* genotoxicity assay using a tumour-prone murine model, also showed differences in the oncogenic potential of RVs and LVs. Herein, it was shown that LTRs co-determine the vector's genotoxic potential, supporting the choice of SIN LVs (Montini *et al.* 2009). Recently, immune-deficient mice received LV transduced HSCs, and were followed for 2-6 months. No LV-associated adverse events were observed, and none of the mice had detectable levels of HIV p24 antigen in their sera (Bauer *et al.* 2008). More recently also the concept of clonal dominance came forward for LVs in a phase I/II clinical trial using HSCs transduced by a SIN LV with chromatin insulators (Bank *et al.* 2005). This clonal dominance seems to be due to growth and/or survival advantage conferred by gene-activating or -suppressing effects of the integrated LV. Importantly, such induced clonal dominance didn't lead to malignant transformation (Fehse & Roeder 2008). Additional potential adverse events are seroconversion of the subject to components of the HIV-1 vector, mobilization and subsequent spread of mobilized vector particles to previously untransduced cells and tissues, and transmission of exogenous DNA to cells of the germ line (Romano *et al.* 2003).

In view of LV based vaccination, the induced innate and adaptive immune reactions against the LV particle, transduced cells and/or its transgene product, act as a double-edged sword. This immunogenicity may aggravate a robust immune reaction, which is possibly advantageous in the context of *e.g.* anti-tumour immunotherapy. However, unwanted immune responses may curtail the induction of tolerance, which is desired for the treatment of *e.g.* transplantation rejection or autoimmune diseases. As broad tropism LVs are capable of transducing DCs but also other cell types, this can have important consequences in view of the immunological outcome. On the one hand transgene expression by non-DCs could lead to uptake of cellular remains from these cells by DCs followed by antigen presentation in the context of MHC class II and *via* cross-presentation in the context of MHC class I. In this way not only a CTL response is triggered, but also T_H cells, which are important to induce a proper CTL response (Matrai *et al.* 2010). On the other hand DCs also play an important role in the induction and maintenance of peripheral tolerance against self-antigens (Steinman 2007). In this context, persistent expression of the transgene by a non-DC, as a consequence of LV integration in a terminally differentiated long-living cell, could also lead to induction of peripheral tolerance (Follenzi *et al.* 2004). Thus, upon broad tropism LV vaccination, the antigen-specific immune response could be initiated by transduced DCs (direct priming), and theoretically by non-lymphoid cells (cross-priming). However, the latter might also counteract the envisaged immune response, which makes it hard to predict the immunological outcome. Therefore, targeting of LVs to DCs, the cell type of choice to induce immunity or tolerance has been explored. Two different approaches have been successfully attempted (i) transcriptional targeting in which DC-specific promoters are exploited and (ii) transductional targeting in which DC-specific LV entry is achieved. Transcriptional targeting has been extensively discussed by Frecha *et al* (Frecha *et al.* 2008).

We believe that transductional targeting of LVs to DCs is a very interesting strategy to tackle safety and efficacy concerns all at once, since: (i) DCs have a relative short half-life, which decreases the chance for malignant transformation after insertional mutagenesis, since this is a multi-step process (Fehse & Roeder 2008), (ii) there is no risk for transmission of exogenous DNA to the germ line, (iii) non-DC transduction is prevented which can overcome unwanted interference with the desired immune response, (iv) DC subset-specific targeting paves the way to fundamental research on the exact role of each DC subset in the development of diseases, as well as their therapeutic importance.

As the LV tropism is determined by the envelope glycoprotein, pseudotyping allows the generation of LVs with a specific transduction pattern. To date, there is no natural DC-

specific envelope glycoprotein identified. In first instance, it was attempted to modify existing envelope proteins by means of genetic engineering to obtain DC-specific binding without disrupting membrane fusion. An example of this application is the construction of a LV where the VSV.G envelope is replaced by a chimeric version of a scFv, coupled to a (i) N-terminal end of the VSV.G protein (Dreja & Piechaczyk 2006), (ii) the amphotrophic MLV protein (Gennari *et al.* 2009), (iii) the sindbis virus envelope protein (Morizono *et al.* 2009; Zhang *et al.* 2010) or (iv) the H-protein of the measle virus envelope, which is than combined with its F-protein (Ageichik *et al.*). However, these manipulations result in viral particles with low stability and limited binding- and fusion capacities. Alternatively, the sindbis glycoprotein can be mutated in its heparin sulphate receptor (HSR) binding part whereby it exclusively binds to DC-SIGN, a DC-specific glycoprotein (Yang *et al.* 2008). Importantly, with this strategy DC-specific transduction could be demonstrated *in vivo*. It was moreover demonstrated that a strong T cell response could be generated that induced tumour regression. An alternative method to target LVs to specific cell types was proposed by Chandrashekran *et al* (Chandrashekran *et al.* 2004). Since RVs and LVs obtain their envelope after budding from the cell membrane of the producer cell line, every glycoprotein that is expressed on this membrane, will be incorporated in the viral envelope. Through this mechanism a membrane bound form of stem cell factor (mbSCF) was incorporated in the membrane of a RV producing cell line, which produced ecotropic RVs. This envelope doesn't allow transduction of human cells. However, binding of the mbSCF onto its receptor, c-kit, resulted in the transduction of human c-kit$^+$ cells by the mbSCF-containing and ecotropic envelope pseudotyped RVs. This strategy was later on expanded by Yang *et al* to LVs (Yang *et al.* 2006). They incorporated a fusogenic protein (derived from influenza A or sindbis virus), as well as an antibody against CD20 in the plasmamembrane of the LV producing cell line. Subsequently LVs were produced, which transduced B cells both *in vitro* and *in vivo*. Importantly, Zhang *et al* (Zhang et al.) engineered a truncated version of VSV.G (VSV.GS), which resulted in a binding-defective, but fusogenic envelope, which still confers vector stability hence allows production of high titer LVs. It was shown that LVs that incorporate the VSV.GS together with mbSCF in their viral surface efficiently transduced c-kit$^+$ cells. This strategy could be translated to DCs, where DC-specific molecules, such as BDCA-2 or DEC-205 are targeted (Dzionek *et al.* 2001; Bonifaz *et al.* 2004; Yang *et al.* 2008).
As molecular cloning of classic antibodies or fragments thereof is challenging, alternatives have been explored. One of these is the use of antibodies from members of the family of *Camilidae* (*i.e.* dromedaries, camels, llamas), which produce a unique class of antibodies composed of two identical heavy chains as opposed to the conventional (four-chain) antibody repertoire (Hamers-Casterman *et al.* 1993). The antigen-binding part of the molecule is composed of only one single variable region (termed VHH, or Nanobody, Nb). These antigen-specific antibody fragments offer many advantages: (i) they are highly soluble, (ii) they can refold after denaturation whilst retaining their binding capacity, (iii) cloning and selection of antigen-specific Nbs obviate the need for construction and screening of large libraries, (iv) as Nbs can be fused to other proteins, it should be possible to present them on the cell membrane of a producer cell line, thus generating LVs that incorporated a DC-specific Nb in their envelope during budding as described above .

7. Conclusion and future perspectives

To date, numerous studies have demonstrated that LVs are excellent candidates for the treatment of immunological pathologies such as cancer and infectious diseases. This can be explained by their capacity to transduce DCs *in vivo*, which is followed by efficient expression, processing and presentation of the introduced transgenes *via* MHC class I and class II molecules, thereby (re) activating an effector and T_H1 response, respectively. Although LVs comprise an intrinsic immunogenic potential, crucial for effective activation of transduced DCs, they have been exploited as a means to induce antigen-specific tolerance for the treatment of diseases with an autoimmune aetiology and transplantation rejection as well. Although this seems contradictory, this duality endows the LV with the potential to become the vaccine tool of choice with an infinite number of application possibilities. Although we are convinced of the LVs' potential as an immunotherapeutic, we give a concise overview of the extra improvements we believe are necessary to moderate the translation of the LVs from bench to bedside.

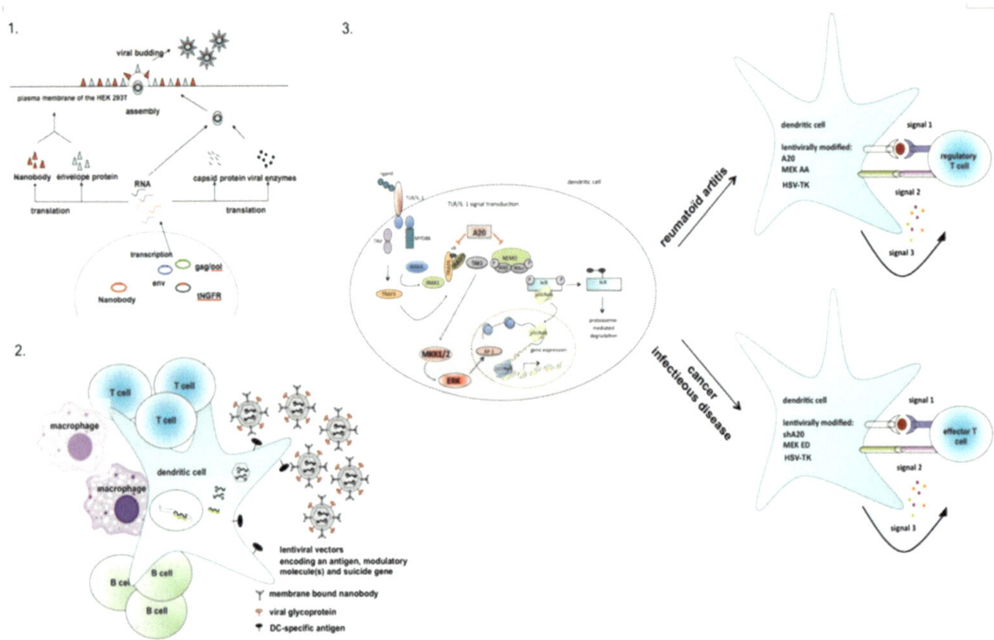

Fig. 4. **Schematic representation of what we believe is the ultimate strategy to successfully exploit the advantageous of LVs and DCs for immunotherapeutic purposes.** Herein, LVs encoding antigen and immune modulating molecules are pseudotyped with a binding-defective but fusogenic envelope glycoprotein, as well as a DC-specific Nb (1). The latter will dictate binding of the LVs to DCs, after which the envelope mediates fusion (2). Subsequently, the DCs are rendered immunogenic or tolerogenic, depending on the envisaged therapy, and the DCs present antigen-derived peptides in the context of MHC class I and class II molecules, hence induce effector T cells or Treg (3).

A first improvement will be the overall use of third generation LVs to curtail the risk of RCLs. Secondly, the use of NILVs is believed to be an inevitable strategy to diminish the LVs' potential to induce insertional mutagenesis. A third improvement to increase both safety and efficacy lies within transductional targeting of the LV to DCs *in vivo*. Therefore we propose to exploit the Nb display technology to target LVs to DCs in combination with

LV-based modulation of two signal transduction pathways within the DCs (Fig. 4). The Nb display technology is based on the natural budding mechanism of LVs as they are released from the LV producing cell. This mechanism allows the incorporation of a binding-defective but fusogenic glycoprotein together with a DC-specific Nb in the plasmamembrane of the LV producer cells and subsequently in the viral envelope. The DC-specific Nb will bind to its antigen on the DC surface whereupon the fusogenic envelope induces transduction. In this way LVs shuttle their cargo into the DC. Subsequently DCs can be conditioned to become either stimulatory or tolerogenic for the introduced transgene(s). For this purpose we can modulate adaptor molecules, such as the MAPK ERK, which switches on a tolerogenic pathway (Arce *et al.*) or A20, which inhibits the stimulatory NF-κB pathway (Song *et al.* 2008). Down-regulation of both will elevate the DC' immunogenic potential, whereas their up-regulation could ameliorate its tolerogenic potential. We strongly believe that this strategy can pave the way toward a safe and multifunctional LV toolbox.

8. Acknowledgements

The Oxford Structural Genomics Consortium is a registered UK charity (1097737) that receives funds from the Canadian Institutes of Health Research, The Canadian Foundation for Innovation, Genome Canada through the Ontario Genomics Insitute, GlaxoSmithKline, Karolinska Institutet, the Knut and Alice Wallenberg Foundations, the Ontario Innovation Trust, the Ontario Ministry for Research and Innovation, Merck & Co., Inc., the Novartis Research Foundation, the Swedish Foundation for Strategic Research and the Wellcome Trust. David Escors, Cleo Goyvaerts and Karine Breckpot are funded by an Arthritis Research UK career development fellowship (18433), the research committee of the 'Vrije Universiteit Brussel' (OZR) and the Research foundation Flanders (FWO-V), respectively. The research performed at the Laboratory of Molecular and Cellular Therapy is funded by FWO-V, the Agency of Innovation by Science and Technology (IWT), the Interuniversity Attraction Poles Program, the 'Stichting tegen Kanker' and the Belgian State - Belgian Science Policy.

9. References

Adotevi O, Mollier K, Neuveut C, Dosset M, Ravel P, Fridman WH, Tartour E, Charneau P, Wain-Hobson S, Langlade-Demoyen P Targeting human telomerase reverse transcriptase with recombinant lentivector is highly effective to stimulate antitumor CD8 T-cell immunity in vivo. *Blood.* 115, 3025-3032.

Aerts-Toegaert C, Heirman C, Tuyaerts S, Corthals J, Aerts JL, Bonehill A, Thielemans K, Breckpot K (2007). CD83 expression on dendritic cells and T cells: correlation with effective immune responses. *Eur J Immunol.* 37, 686-695.

Ageichik A, Buchholz C, Collins MK Lentiviral vectors targeted to MHC II are effective in immunization. *Hum Gene Ther.*

Agrawal A, Dillon S, Denning TL, Pulendran B (2006). ERK1-/- mice exhibit Th1 cell polarization and increased susceptibility to experimental autoimmune encephalomyelitis. *J Immunol.* 176, 5788-5796.

Ahmadzadeh M, Felipe-Silva A, Heemskerk B, Powell DJ, Jr., Wunderlich JR, Merino MJ, Rosenberg SA (2008). FOXP3 expression accurately defines the population of intratumoral regulatory T cells that selectively accumulate in metastatic melanoma lesions. *Blood.* 112, 4953-4960.

Aiba S, Tagami H (1998). Dendritic cell activation induced by various stimuli, e.g. exposure to microorganisms, their products, cytokines, and simple chemicals as well as adhesion to extracellular matrix. *J Dermatol Sci.* 20, 1-13.

Aiba S, Tagami H (1999). Dendritic cells play a crucial role in innate immunity to simple chemicals. *J Investig Dermatol Symp Proc.* 4, 158-163.

Aiba S, Terunuma A, Manome H, Tagami H (1997). Dendritic cells differently respond to haptens and irritants by their production of cytokines and expression of co-stimulatory molecules. *Eur J Immunol.* 27, 3031-3038.

Akazawa T, Shingai M, Sasai M, Ebihara T, Inoue N, Matsumoto M, Seya T (2007). Tumor immunotherapy using bone marrow-derived dendritic cells overexpressing Toll-like receptor adaptors. *FEBS Lett.* 581, 3334-3340.

Akira S, Uematsu S, Takeuchi O (2006). Pathogen recognition and innate immunity. *Cell.* 124, 783-801.

Akkina RK, Walton RM, Chen ML, Li QX, Planelles V, Chen IS (1996). High-efficiency gene transfer into CD34+ cells with a human immunodeficiency virus type 1-based retroviral vector pseudotyped with vesicular stomatitis virus envelope glycoprotein G. *J Virol.* 70, 2581-2585.

Anastasaki C, Estep AL, Marais R, Rauen KA, Patton EE (2009). Kinase-activating and kinase-impaired cardio-facio-cutaneous syndrome alleles have activity during zebrafish development and are sensitive to small molecule inhibitors. *Human molecular genetics.* 18, 2543-2554.

Anderson WF, Blaese RM, Culver K (1990). The ADA human gene therapy clinical protocol: Points to Consider response with clinical protocol, July 6, 1990. *Hum Gene Ther.* 1, 331-362.

Apolonia L, Waddington SN, Fernandes C, Ward NJ, Bouma G, Blundell MP, Thrasher AJ, Collins MK, Philpott NJ (2007). Stable gene transfer to muscle using non-integrating lentiviral vectors. *Mol Ther.* 15, 1947-1954.

Arce F, Breckpot K, Stephenson H, Karwacz K, Ehrenstein MR, Collins M, Escors D Selective ERK activation differentiates mouse and human tolerogenic dendritic cells, expands antigen-specific regulatory T cells, and suppresses experimental inflammatory arthritis. *Arthritis Rheum.* 63, 84-95.

Arce F, Breckpot K, Stephenson H, Karwacz K, Ehrenstein MR, Collins M, Escors D (2010). Selective ERK activation suppresses inflammatory arthritis via tolerogenic dendritic cells and antigen-specific regulatory T cells. *Arthritis and rheumatism.* DOI 10.1002/art.30099.

Arce F, Breckpot K, Stephenson H, Karwacz K, Ehrenstein MR, Collins M, Escors D (2011). Selective ERK activation differentiates mouse and human tolerogenic dendritic cells, expands antigen-specific regulatory T cells, and suppresses experimental inflammatory arthritis. *Arthritis and rheumatism.* 63, 84-95.

Arce F, Rowe HM, Chain B, Lopes L, Collins MK (2009). Lentiviral vectors transduce proliferating dendritic cell precursors leading to persistent antigen presentation and immunization. *Mol Ther.* 17, 1643-1650.

Ardeshna KM, Pizzey AR, Devereux S, Khwaja A (2000). The PI3 kinase, p38 SAP kinase, and NF-kappaB signal transduction pathways are involved in the survival and maturation of lipopolysaccharide-stimulated human monocyte-derived dendritic cells. *Blood.* 96, 1039-1046.

Arrighi JF, Pion M, Wiznerowicz M, Geijtenbeek TB, Garcia E, Abraham S, Leuba F, Dutoit V, Ducrey-Rundquist O, van Kooyk Y, Trono D, Piguet V (2004). Lentivirus-mediated RNA interference of DC-SIGN expression inhibits human immunodeficiency virus transmission from dendritic cells to T cells. *J Virol.* 78, 10848-10855.

Arrighi JF, Rebsamen M, Rousset F, Kindler V, Hauser C (2001). A critical role for p38 mitogen-activated protein kinase in the maturation of human blood-derived dendritic cells induced by lipopolysaccharide, TNF-alpha, and contact sensitizers. *J Immunol.* 166, 3837-3845.

Bank A, Dorazio R, Leboulch P (2005). A phase I/II clinical trial of beta-globin gene therapy for beta-thalassemia. *Ann N Y Acad Sci.* 1054, 308-316.

Barton GM, Kagan JC (2009). A cell biological view of Toll-like receptor function: regulation through compartmentalization. *Nat Rev Immunol.* 9, 535-542.

Basten A, Miller JF, Sprent J, Cheers C (1974). Cell-to-cell interaction in the immune response. X. T-cell-dependent suppression in tolerant mice. *J Exp Med.* 140, 199-217.

Batten M, Groom J, Cachero TG, Qian F, Schneider P, Tschopp J, Browning JL, Mackay F (2000). BAFF mediates survival of peripheral immature B lymphocytes. *J Exp Med.* 192, 1453-1466.

Bauer G, Dao MA, Case SS, Meyerrose T, Wirthlin L, Zhou P, Wang X, Herrbrich P, Arevalo J, Csik S, Skelton DC, Walker J, Pepper K, Kohn DB, Nolta JA (2008). In vivo biosafety model to assess the risk of adverse events from retroviral and lentiviral vectors. *Mol Ther.* 16, 1308-1315.

Beignon AS, McKenna K, Skoberne M, Manches O, DaSilva I, Kavanagh DG, Larsson M, Gorelick RJ, Lifson JD, Bhardwaj N (2005). Endocytosis of HIV-1 activates plasmacytoid dendritic cells via Toll-like receptor-viral RNA interactions. *J Clin Invest.* 115, 3265-3275.

Belkaid Y (2007). Regulatory T cells and infection: a dangerous necessity. *Nat Rev Immunol.* 7, 875-888.

Belladonna ML, Orabona C, Grohmann U, Puccetti P (2009). TGF-beta and kynurenines as the key to infectious tolerance. *Trends in molecular medicine.* 15, 41-49.

Bettelli E, Korn T, Kuchroo VK (2007). Th17: the third member of the effector T cell trilogy. *Curr Opin Immunol.* 19, 652-657.

Beyer T, Herrmann M, Reiser C, Bertling W, Hess J (2001). Bacterial carriers and virus-like-particles as antigen delivery devices: role of dendritic cells in antigen presentation. *Curr Drug Targets Infect Disord.* 1, 287-302.

Billiau A (2006). Anti-inflammatory properties of Type I interferons. *Antiviral research.* 71, 108-116.

Bonehill A, Heirman C, Thielemans K (2005). Genetic approaches for the induction of a CD4+ T cell response in cancer immunotherapy. *J Gene Med.* 7, 686-695.

Bonehill A, Heirman C, Tuyaerts S, Michiels A, Zhang Y, van der Bruggen P, Thielemans K (2003). Efficient presentation of known HLA class II-restricted MAGE-A3 epitopes by dendritic cells electroporated with messenger RNA encoding an invariant chain with genetic exchange of class II-associated invariant chain peptide. *Cancer Res.* 63, 5587-5594.

Bonehill A, Tuyaerts S, Van Nuffel AM, Heirman C, Bos TJ, Fostier K, Neyns B, Thielemans K (2008). Enhancing the T-cell stimulatory capacity of human dendritic cells by co-electroporation with CD40L, CD70 and constitutively active TLR4 encoding mRNA. *Mol Ther.* 16, 1170-1180.

Bonifaz L, Bonnyay D, Mahnke K, Rivera M, Nussenzweig MC, Steinman RM (2002). Efficient targeting of protein antigen to the dendritic cell receptor DEC-205 in the steady state leads to antigen presentation on major histocompatibility complex class I products and peripheral CD8+ T cell tolerance. *J Exp Med.* 196, 1627-1638.

Bonifaz LC, Bonnyay DP, Charalambous A, Darguste DI, Fujii S, Soares H, Brimnes MK, Moltedo B, Moran TM, Steinman RM (2004). In vivo targeting of antigens to maturing dendritic cells via the DEC-205 receptor improves T cell vaccination. *J Exp Med.* 199, 815-824.

Boon T, van der Bruggen P (1996). Human tumor antigens recognized by T lymphocytes. *J Exp Med.* 183, 725-729.

Breckpot K, Aerts JL, Thielemans K (2007a). Lentiviral vectors for cancer immunotherapy: transforming infectious particles into therapeutics. *Gene Ther.* 14, 847-862.

Breckpot K, Aerts-Toegaert C, Heirman C, Peeters U, Beyaert R, Aerts JL, Thielemans K (2009). Attenuated expression of A20 markedly increases the efficacy of double-stranded RNA-activated dendritic cells as an anti-cancer vaccine. *J Immunol.* 182, 860-870.

Breckpot K, Corthals J, Heirman C, Bonehill A, Michiels A, Tuyaerts S, De Greef C, Thielemans K (2004a). Activation of monocytes via the CD14 receptor leads to the enhanced lentiviral transduction of immature dendritic cells. *Hum Gene Ther.* 15, 562-573.

Breckpot K, Dullaers M, Bonehill A, van Meirvenne S, Heirman C, de Greef C, van der Bruggen P, Thielemans K (2003). Lentivirally transduced dendritic cells as a tool for cancer immunotherapy. *J Gene Med.* 5, 654-667.

Breckpot K, Emeagi P, Dullaers M, Michiels A, Heirman C, Thielemans K (2007b). Activation of immature monocyte-derived dendritic cells after transduction with high doses of lentiviral vectors. *Hum Gene Ther.* 18, 536-546.

Breckpot K, Emeagi PU, Thielemans K (2008). Lentiviral vectors for anti-tumor immunotherapy. *Curr Gene Ther.* 8, 438-448.

Breckpot K, Escors D (2009a). Dendritic cells for active anti-cancer immunotherapy: targeting activation pathways through genetic modification. *Endocr Metab Immune Disord Drug Targets.* 9, 328-343.

Breckpot K, Escors D (2009b). Dendritic Cells for Active Anti-cancer Immunotherapy: Targeting Activation Pathways Through Genetic Modification. *Endocrine, metabolic & immune disorders drug targets.* 9, 328-343.

Breckpot K, Escors D (2009c). Dendritic cells for active anti-cancer immunotherapy: targeting activation pathways through genetic modification. *Current Drug Targets.*

Breckpot K, Escors D, Arce F, Lopes L, Karwacz K, Van Lint S, Keyaerts M, Collins M HIV-1 lentiviral vector immunogenicity is mediated by Toll-like receptor 3 (TLR3) and TLR7. *J Virol.* 84, 5627-5636.

Breckpot K, Heirman C, De Greef C, van der Bruggen P, Thielemans K (2004b). Identification of new antigenic peptide presented by HLA-Cw7 and encoded by several MAGE genes using dendritic cells transduced with lentiviruses. *J Immunol.* 172, 2232-2237.

Breckpot K, Heirman C, Neyns B, Thielemans K (2004c). Exploiting dendritic cells for cancer immunotherapy: genetic modification of dendritic cells. *J Gene Med.* 6, 1175-1188.

Brenner MK, Rill DR, Holladay MS, Heslop HE, Moen RC, Buschle M, Krance RA, Santana VM, Anderson WF, Ihle JN (1993). Gene marking to determine whether autologous marrow infusion restores long-term haemopoiesis in cancer patients. *Lancet.* 342, 1134-1137.

Brown BD, Sitia G, Annoni A, Hauben E, Sergi Sergi L, Zingale A, Roncarolo MG, Guidotti LG, Naldini L (2006a). In vivo administration of lentiviral vectors triggers a type I interferon response that restricts hepatocyte gene transfer and promotes vector clearance. *Blood.*

Brown BD, Venneri MA, Zingale A, Sergi Sergi L, Naldini L (2006b). Endogenous microRNA regulation suppresses transgene expression in hematopoietic lineages and enables stable gene transfer. *Nat Med.* 12, 585-591.

Bukrinsky MI, Haggerty S, Dempsey MP, Sharova N, Adzhubel A, Spitz L, Lewis P, Goldfarb D, Emerman M, Stevenson M (1993). A nuclear localization signal within HIV-1 matrix protein that governs infection of non-dividing cells. *Nature.* 365, 666-669.

Burns JC, Friedmann T, Driever W, Burrascano M, Yee JK (1993). Vesicular stomatitis virus G glycoprotein pseudotyped retroviral vectors: concentration to very high titer and efficient gene transfer into mammalian and nonmammalian cells. *Proc Natl Acad Sci U S A.* 90, 8033-8037.

Caparros E, Munoz P, Sierra-Filardi E, Serrano-Gomez D, Puig-Kroger A, Rodriguez-Fernandez JL, Mellado M, Sancho J, Zubiaur M, Corbi AL (2006). DC-SIGN ligation on dendritic cells results in ERK and PI3K activation and modulates cytokine production. *Blood.* 107, 3950-3958.

Cattoglio C, Facchini G, Sartori D, Antonelli A, Miccio A, Cassani B, Schmidt M, von Kalle C, Howe S, Thrasher AJ, Aiuti A, Ferrari G, Recchia A, Mavilio F (2007). Hot spots of retroviral integration in human CD34+ hematopoietic cells. *Blood.* 110, 1770-1778.

Caux C, Massacrier C, Vanbervliet B, Dubois B, Van Kooten C, Durand I, Banchereau J (1994). Activation of human dendritic cells through CD40 cross-linking. *J Exp Med.* 180, 1263-1272.

Cerundolo V, Hermans IF, Salio M (2004). Dendritic cells: a journey from laboratory to clinic. *Nat Immunol.* 5, 7-10.

Chandrashekran A, Gordon MY, Casimir C (2004). Targeted retroviral transduction of c-kit+ hematopoietic cells using novel ligand display technology. *Blood.* 104, 2697-2703.

Chang EY, Guo B, Doyle SE, Cheng G (2007). Cutting edge: involvement of the type I IFN production and signaling pathway in lipopolysaccharide-induced IL-10 production. *J Immunol.* 178, 6705-6709.

Chapatte L, Colombetti S, Cerottini JC, Levy F (2006). Efficient induction of tumor antigen-specific CD8+ memory T cells by recombinant lentivectors. *Cancer Res.* 66, 1155-1160.

Charneau P, Clavel F (1991). A single-stranded gap in human immunodeficiency virus unintegrated linear DNA defined by a central copy of the polypurine tract. *J Virol.* 65, 2415-2421.

Ciuffi A (2008). Mechanisms governing lentivirus integration site selection. *Curr Gene Ther.* 8, 419-429.

Cobbold SP, Adams E, Farquhar CA, Nolan KF, Howie D, Lui KO, Fairchild PJ, Mellor AL, Ron D, Waldmann H (2009). Infectious tolerance via the consumption of essential amino acids and mTOR signaling. *Proc Natl Acad Sci U S A.* 106, 12055-12060.

Coffin JH, SH.; Varmus, HE. (1997). *Retroviruses.* Woodbury, NY: Cold Spring Harbor Laboratory Press.

Comabella M, Imitola J, Weiner HL, Khoury SJ (2002). Interferon-beta treatment alters peripheral blood monocytes chemokine production in MS patients. *Journal of neuroimmunology.* 126, 205-212.

Coquerelle C, Moser M DC subsets in positive and negative regulation of immunity. *Immunol Rev.* 234, 317-334.

Corinti S, Albanesi C, la Sala A, Pastore S, Girolomoni G (2001). Regulatory activity of autocrine IL-10 on dendritic cell functions. *J Immunol.* 166, 4312-4318.

da Silva Correia J, Soldau K, Christen U, Tobias PS, Ulevitch RJ (2001). Lipopolysaccharide is in close proximity to each of the proteins in its membrane receptor complex. transfer from CD14 to TLR4 and MD-2. *J Biol Chem.* 276, 21129-21135.

Delgado M, Toscano MG, Benabdellah K, Cobo M, O'Valle F, Gonzalez-Rey E, Martin F (2008). In vivo delivery of lentiviral vectors expressing vasoactive intestinal peptide complementary DNA as gene therapy for collagen-induced arthritis. *Arthritis and rheumatism.* 58, 1026-1037.

den Haan JM, Bevan MJ (2002). Constitutive versus activation-dependent cross-presentation of immune complexes by CD8(+) and CD8(-) dendritic cells in vivo. *J Exp Med.* 196, 817-827.

Dhodapkar MV, Steinman RM (2002). Antigen-bearing immature dendritic cells induce peptide-specific CD8(+) regulatory T cells in vivo in humans. *Blood.* 100, 174-177.

Dhodapkar MV, Steinman RM, Krasovsky J, Munz C, Bhardwaj N (2001). Antigen-specific inhibition of effector T cell function in humans after injection of immature dendritic cells. *J Exp Med.* 193, 233-238.

Di Pucchio T, Chatterjee B, Smed-Sorensen A, Clayton S, Palazzo A, Montes M, Xue Y, Mellman I, Banchereau J, Connolly JE (2008). Direct proteasome-independent cross-presentation of viral antigen by plasmacytoid dendritic cells on major histocompatibility complex class I. *Nat Immunol.* 9, 551-557.

Dillon S, Agrawal S, Banerjee K, Letterio J, Denning TL, Oswald-Richter K, Kasprowicz DJ, Kellar K, Pare J, van Dyke T, Ziegler S, Unutmaz D, Pulendran B (2006). Yeast zymosan, a stimulus for TLR2 and dectin-1, induces regulatory antigen-presenting cells and immunological tolerance. *J Clin Invest.* 116, 916-928.

Dreja H, Piechaczyk M (2006). The effects of N-terminal insertion into VSV-G of an scFv peptide. *Virol J.* 3, 69.

Dull T, Zufferey R, Kelly M, Mandel RJ, Nguyen M, Trono D, Naldini L (1998). A third-generation lentivirus vector with a conditional packaging system. *J Virol.* 72, 8463-8471.

Dullaers M, Breckpot K, Van Meirvenne S, Bonehill A, Tuyaerts S, Michiels A, Straetman L, Heirman C, De Greef C, Van Der Bruggen P, Thielemans K (2004). Side-by-side comparison of lentivirally transduced and mRNA-electroporated dendritic cells: implications for cancer immunotherapy protocols. *Mol Ther.* 10, 768-779.

Dullaers M, Van Meirvenne S, Heirman C, Straetman L, Bonehill A, Aerts JL, Thielemans K, Breckpot K (2006). Induction of effective therapeutic antitumor immunity by direct in vivo administration of lentiviral vectors. *Gene Ther.* 13, 630-640.

Dyall J, Latouche JB, Schnell S, Sadelain M (2001). Lentivirus-transduced human monocyte-derived dendritic cells efficiently stimulate antigen-specific cytotoxic T lymphocytes. *Blood.* 97, 114-121.

Dzionek A, Sohma Y, Nagafune J, Cella M, Colonna M, Facchetti F, Gunther G, Johnston I, Lanzavecchia A, Nagasaka T, Okada T, Vermi W, Winkels G, Yamamoto T, Zysk M, Yamaguchi Y, Schmitz J (2001). BDCA-2, a novel plasmacytoid dendritic cell-specific type II C-type lectin, mediates antigen capture and is a potent inhibitor of interferon alpha/beta induction. *J Exp Med.* 194, 1823-1834.

Escors D, Breckpot K Lentiviral vectors in gene therapy: their current status and future potential. *Arch Immunol Ther Exp (Warsz).* 58, 107-119.

Escors D, Breckpot K (2010). Lentiviral vectors in gene therapy: their current status and future potential. *Arch Immunol Ther Exp (Warsz).* 58, 107-119.

Escors D, Lopes L, Lin R, Hiscott J, Akira S, Davis RJ, Collins MK (2008). Targeting dendritic cell signalling to regulate the response to immunisation. *Blood.* 111, 3050-3061.

Esslinger C, Chapatte L, Finke D, Miconnet I, Guillaume P, Levy F, MacDonald HR (2003). In vivo administration of a lentiviral vaccine targets DCs and induces efficient CD8(+) T cell responses. *J Clin Invest.* 111, 1673-1681.

Fallarino F, Vacca C, Orabona C, Belladonna ML, Bianchi R, Marshall B, Keskin DB, Mellor AL, Fioretti MC, Grohmann U, Puccetti P (2002). Functional expression of indoleamine 2,3-dioxygenase by murine CD8 alpha(+) dendritic cells. *Int Immunol.* 14, 65-68.

Fehse B, Roeder I (2008). Insertional mutagenesis and clonal dominance: biological and statistical considerations. *Gene Ther.* 15, 143-153.

Firat H, Zennou V, Garcia-Pons F, Ginhoux F, Cochet M, Danos O, Lemonnier FA, Langlade-Demoyen P, Charneau P (2002). Use of a lentiviral flap vector for induction of CTL immunity against melanoma. Perspectives for immunotherapy. *J Gene Med.* 4, 38-45.

Fitzgerald KA, McWhirter SM, Faia KL, Rowe DC, Latz E, Golenbock DT, Coyle AJ, Liao SM, Maniatis T (2003). IKKepsilon and TBK1 are essential components of the IRF3 signaling pathway. *Nat Immunol.* 4, 491-496.

Fitzgerald-Bocarsly P, Dai J, Singh S (2008). Plasmacytoid dendritic cells and type I IFN: 50 years of convergent history. *Cytokine Growth Factor Rev.* 19, 3-19.

Flint S.J. ELW, . Racaniello V.R, Skalka A.M. (2009). *Principles of virology.* Washington, DC: ASM Press.

Follenzi A, Ailles LE, Bakovic S, Geuna M, Naldini L (2000). Gene transfer by lentiviral vectors is limited by nuclear translocation and rescued by HIV-1 pol sequences. *Nat Genet.* 25, 217-222.

Follenzi A, Battaglia M, Lombardo A, Annoni A, Roncarolo MG, Naldini L (2004). Targeting lentiviral vector expression to hepatocytes limits transgene-specific immune response and establishes long-term expression of human antihemophilic factor IX in mice. *Blood.* 103, 3700-3709.

Fonteneau JF, Larsson M, Beignon AS, McKenna K, Dasilva I, Amara A, Liu YJ, Lifson JD, Littman DR, Bhardwaj N (2004). Human immunodeficiency virus type 1 activates plasmacytoid dendritic cells and concomitantly induces the bystander maturation of myeloid dendritic cells. *J Virol.* 78, 5223-5232.

Forster R, Davalos-Misslitz AC, Rot A (2008). CCR7 and its ligands: balancing immunity and tolerance. *Nat Rev Immunol.* 8, 362-371.

Frecha C, Szecsi J, Cosset FL, Verhoeyen E (2008). Strategies for targeting lentiviral vectors. *Curr Gene Ther.* 8, 449-460.

Friedmann T, Roblin R (1972). Gene therapy for human genetic disease? *Science.* 175, 949-955.

Garcia MR, Ledgerwood L, Yang Y, Xu J, Lal G, Burrell B, Ma G, Hashimoto D, Li Y, Boros P, Grisotto M, van Rooijen N, Matesanz R, Tacke F, Ginhoux F, Ding Y, Chen SH, Randolph G, Merad M, Bromberg JS, Ochando JC (2010). Monocytic suppressive cells mediate cardiovascular transplantation tolerance in mice. *J Clin Invest.* 120, 2486-2496.

Gautier G, Humbert M, Deauvieau F, Scuiller M, Hiscott J, Bates EE, Trinchieri G, Caux C, Garrone P (2005). A type I interferon autocrine-paracrine loop is involved in Toll-like receptor-induced interleukin-12p70 secretion by dendritic cells. *J Exp Med.* 201, 1435-1446.

Geijtenbeek TB, Gringhuis SI (2009). Signalling through C-type lectin receptors: shaping immune responses. *Nat Rev Immunol.* 9, 465-479.

Gennari F, Lopes L, Verhoeyen E, Marasco W, Collins MK (2009). Single-chain antibodies that target lentiviral vectors to MHC class II on antigen-presenting cells. *Hum Gene Ther.* 20, 554-562.

Ghiringhelli F, Puig PE, Roux S, Parcellier A, Schmitt E, Solary E, Kroemer G, Martin F, Chauffert B, Zitvogel L (2005). Tumor cells convert immature myeloid dendritic cells into TGF-beta-secreting cells inducing CD4+CD25+ regulatory T cell proliferation. *J Exp Med.* 202, 919-929.

Gould DJ, Favorov P (2003). Vectors for the treatment of autoimmune disease. *Gene Ther.* 10, 912-927.

Grabbe S, Steinbrink K, Steinert M, Luger TA, Schwarz T (1995). Removal of the majority of epidermal Langerhans cells by topical or systemic steroid application enhances the effector phase of murine contact hypersensitivity. *J Immunol.* 155, 4207-4217.

Greenwald RJ, Freeman GJ, Sharpe AH (2005). The B7 family revisited. *Annu Rev Immunol.* 23, 515-548.

Griesemer AD, Sorenson EC, Hardy MA (2010). The role of the thymus in tolerance. *Transplantation.* 90, 465-474.

Gruber A, Kan-Mitchell J, Kuhen KL, Mukai T, Wong-Staal F (2000). Dendritic cells transduced by multiply deleted HIV-1 vectors exhibit normal phenotypes and functions and elicit an HIV-specific cytotoxic T-lymphocyte response in vitro. *Blood.* 96, 1327-1333.

Gu W, Payne E, Sun S, Burgess M, McMillan NA Inhibition of cervical cancer cell growth in vitro and in vivo with dual shRNAs. *Cancer Gene Ther.*

Ha TY, Waksman BH, Treffers HP (1974). The thymic suppressor cell. I. Separation of subpopulations with suppressor activity. *J Exp Med.* 139, 13-23.

Hacker H, Redecke V, Blagoev B, Kratchmarova I, Hsu LC, Wang GG, Kamps MP, Raz E, Wagner H, Hacker G, Mann M, Karin M (2006). Specificity in Toll-like receptor signalling through distinct effector functions of TRAF3 and TRAF6. *Nature.* 439, 204-207.

Hamers-Casterman C, Atarhouch T, Muyldermans S, Robinson G, Hamers C, Songa EB, Bendahman N, Hamers R (1993). Naturally occurring antibodies devoid of light chains. *Nature.* 363, 446-448.

Hawiger D, Inaba K, Dorsett Y, Guo M, Mahnke K, Rivera M, Ravetch JV, Steinman RM, Nussenzweig MC (2001). Dendritic cells induce peripheral T cell unresponsiveness under steady state conditions in vivo. *J Exp Med.* 194, 769-779.

He Y, Falo LD (2006). Induction of T cell immunity by cutaneous genetic immunization with recombinant lentivector. *Immunologic research.* 36, 101-117.

He Y, Zhang J, Donahue C, Falo LD, Jr. (2006). Skin-derived dendritic cells induce potent CD8(+) T cell immunity in recombinant lentivector-mediated genetic immunization. *Immunity.* 24, 643-656.

He Y, Zhang J, Mi Z, Robbins P, Falo LD, Jr. (2005). Immunization with lentiviral vector-transduced dendritic cells induces strong and long-lasting T cell responses and therapeutic immunity. *J Immunol.* 174, 3808-3817.

Henry E, Desmet CJ, Garze V, Fievez L, Bedoret D, Heirman C, Faisca P, Jaspar FJ, Gosset P, Jacquet AP, Desmecht D, Thielemans K, Lekeux P, Moser M, Bureau F (2008). Dendritic cells genetically engineered to express IL-10 induce long-lasting antigen-specific tolerance in experimental asthma. *J Immunol.* 181, 7230-7242.

Hirano N, Butler MO, Xia Z, Ansen S, von Bergwelt-Baildon MS, Neuberg D, Freeman GJ, Nadler LM (2006). Engagement of CD83 ligand induces prolonged expansion of CD8+ T cells and preferential enrichment for antigen specificity. *Blood.* 107, 1528-1536.

Hori S, Nomura T, Sakaguchi S (2003). Control of regulatory T cell development by the transcription factor Foxp3. *Science*. 299, 1057-1061.

Howe SJ, Mansour MR, Schwarzwaelder K, Bartholomae C, Hubank M, Kempski H, Brugman MH, Pike-Overzet K, Chatters SJ, de Ridder D, Gilmour KC, Adams S, Thornhill SI, Parsley KL, Staal FJ, Gale RE, Linch DC, Bayford J, Brown L, Quaye M, Kinnon C, Ancliff P, Webb DK, Schmidt M, von Kalle C, Gaspar HB, Thrasher AJ (2008). Insertional mutagenesis combined with acquired somatic mutations causes leukemogenesis following gene therapy of SCID-X1 patients. *J Clin Invest*. 118, 3143-3150.

Ilarregui JM, Croci DO, Bianco GA, Toscano MA, Salatino M, Vermeulen ME, Geffner JR, Rabinovich GA (2009). Tolerogenic signals delivered by dendritic cells to T cells through a galectin-1-driven immunoregulatory circuit involving interleukin 27 and interleukin 10. *Nat Immunol*. 10, 981-991.

Jonuleit H, Kuhn U, Muller G, Steinbrink K, Paragnik L, Schmitt E, Knop J, Enk AH (1997). Pro-inflammatory cytokines and prostaglandins induce maturation of potent immunostimulatory dendritic cells under fetal calf serum-free conditions. *Eur J Immunol*. 27, 3135-3142.

Jonuleit H, Schmitt E, Steinbrink K, Enk AH (2001). Dendritic cells as a tool to induce anergic and regulatory T cells. *Trends Immunol*. 22, 394-400.

Kamath AT, Henri S, Battye F, Tough DF, Shortman K (2002). Developmental kinetics and lifespan of dendritic cells in mouse lymphoid organs. *Blood*. 100, 1734-1741.

Kaplan DH, Jenison MC, Saeland S, Shlomchik WD, Shlomchik MJ (2005). Epidermal langerhans cell-deficient mice develop enhanced contact hypersensitivity. *Immunity*. 23, 611-620.

Karwacz K, Mukherjee S, Apolonia L, Blundell MP, Bouma G, Escors D, Collins MK, Thrasher AJ (2009). Nonintegrating lentivector vaccines stimulate prolonged T-cell and antibody responses and are effective in tumor therapy. *J Virol*. 83, 3094-3103.

Kawai T, Akira S (2008). Toll-like receptor and RIG-I-like receptor signaling. *Ann N Y Acad Sci*. 1143, 1-20.

Kim JH, Majumder N, Lin H, Watkins S, Falo LD, Jr., You Z (2005). Induction of therapeutic antitumor immunity by in vivo administration of a lentiviral vaccine. *Hum Gene Ther*. 16, 1255-1266.

Kirchner H, Chused TM, Herberman RB, Holden HT, Lavrin DH (1974). Evidence of suppressor cell activity in spleens of mice bearing primary tumors induced by Moloney sarcoma virus. *J Exp Med*. 139, 1473-1487.

Kretschmer K, Apostolou I, Hawiger D, Khazaie K, Nussenzweig MC, von Boehmer H (2005). Inducing and expanding regulatory T cell populations by foreign antigen. *Nat Immunol*. 6, 1219-1227.

Kuhn R, Lohler J, Rennick D, Rajewsky K, Muller W (1993). Interleukin-10-deficient mice develop chronic enterocolitis. *Cell*. 75, 263-274.

Lafferty KJ, Warren HS, Woolnough JA (1979). A mediator acting as a costimulator for the development of cytotoxic responses in vitro. *Adv Exp Med Biol*. 114, 497-501.

Lai Kwan Lam Q, King Hung Ko O, Zheng BJ, Lu L (2008). Local BAFF gene silencing suppresses Th17-cell generation and ameliorates autoimmune arthritis. *Proc Natl Acad Sci U S A*. 105, 14993-14998.

Lang KS, Recher M, Junt T, Navarini AA, Harris NL, Freigang S, Odermatt B, Conrad C, Ittner LM, Bauer S, Luther SA, Uematsu S, Akira S, Hengartner H, Zinkernagel RM (2005). Toll-like receptor engagement converts T-cell autoreactivity into overt autoimmune disease. *Nat Med*. 11, 138-145.

Larregina AT, Falo LD, Jr. (2005). Changing paradigms in cutaneous immunology: adapting with dendritic cells. *J Invest Dermatol*. 124, 1-12.

Lee WC, Zhong C, Qian S, Wan Y, Gauldie J, Mi Z, Robbins PD, Thomson AW, Lu L (1998). Phenotype, function, and in vivo migration and survival of allogeneic dendritic cell progenitors genetically engineered to express TGF-beta. *Transplantation*. 66, 1810-1817.

Lewis PF, Emerman M (1994). Passage through mitosis is required for oncoretroviruses but not for the human immunodeficiency virus. *J Virol*. 68, 510-516.

Li H, Han Y, Guo Q, Zhang M, Cao X (2009). Cancer-expanded myeloid-derived suppressor cells induce anergy of NK cells through membrane-bound TGF-beta 1. *J Immunol*. 182, 240-249.

Li Y, Chu N, Rostami A, Zhang GX (2006). Dendritic cells transduced with SOCS-3 exhibit a tolerogenic/DC2 phenotype that directs type 2 Th cell differentiation in vitro and in vivo. *J Immunol*. 177, 1679-1688.

Liu BH, Wang X, Ma YX, Wang S (2004). CMV enhancer/human PDGF-beta promoter for neuron-specific transgene expression. *Gene Ther*. 11, 52-60.

Liu Y, Peng Y, Mi M, Guevara-Patino J, Munn DH, Fu N, He Y (2009). Lentivector immunization stimulates potent CD8 T cell responses against melanoma self-antigen tyrosinase-related protein 1 and generates antitumor immunity in mice. *J Immunol*. 182, 5960-5969.

Lizee G, Gonzales MI, Topalian SL (2004). Lentivirus vector-mediated expression of tumor-associated epitopes by human antigen presenting cells. *Hum Gene Ther*. 15, 393-404.

Loisel-Meyer S, Felizardo T, Mariotti J, Mossoba ME, Foley JE, Kammerer R, Mizue N, Keefe R, McCart JA, Zimmermann W, Dropulic B, Fowler DH, Medin JA (2009). Potent induction of B- and T-cell immunity against human carcinoembryonic antigen-expressing tumors in human carcinoembryonic antigen transgenic mice mediated by direct lentivector injection. *Molecular cancer therapeutics*. 8, 692-702.

Lopes L, Dewannieux M, Gileadi U, Bailey R, Ikeda Y, Whittaker C, Collin MP, Cerundolo V, Tomihari M, Ariizumi K, Collins MK (2008). Immunization with a lentivector that targets tumor antigen expression to dendritic cells induces potent CD8+ and CD4+ T-cell responses. *J Virol*. 82, 86-95.

Lu X, Yu Q, Binder GK, Chen Z, Slepushkina T, Rossi J, Dropulic B (2004). Antisense-mediated inhibition of human immunodeficiency virus (HIV) replication by use of an HIV type 1-based vector results in severely attenuated mutants incapable of developing resistance. *J Virol*. 78, 7079-7088.

Lutz MB, Schuler G (2002). Immature, semi-mature and fully mature dendritic cells: which signals induce tolerance or immunity? *Trends Immunol*. 23, 445-449.

Mackey MF, Barth RJ, Jr., Noelle RJ (1998a). The role of CD40/CD154 interactions in the priming, differentiation, and effector function of helper and cytotoxic T cells. *J Leukoc Biol.* 63, 418-428.

Mackey MF, Gunn JR, Maliszewsky C, Kikutani H, Noelle RJ, Barth RJ, Jr. (1998b). Dendritic cells require maturation via CD40 to generate protective antitumor immunity. *J Immunol.* 161, 2094-2098.

Mahnke K, Qian Y, Knop J, Enk AH (2003). Induction of CD4+/CD25+ regulatory T cells by targeting of antigens to immature dendritic cells. *Blood.* 101, 4862-4869.

Mahnke K, Schmitt E, Bonifaz L, Enk AH, Jonuleit H (2002). Immature, but not inactive: the tolerogenic function of immature dendritic cells. *Immunol Cell Biol.* 80, 477-483.

Maldonado-Lopez R, De Smedt T, Michel P, Godfroid J, Pajak B, Heirman C, Thielemans K, Leo O, Urbain J, Moser M (1999). CD8alpha+ and CD8alpha- subclasses of dendritic cells direct the development of distinct T helper cells in vivo. *J Exp Med.* 189, 587-592.

Manicassamy S, Ravindran R, Deng J, Oluoch H, Denning TL, Kasturi SP, Rosenthal KM, Evavold BD, Pulendran B (2009). Toll-like receptor 2-dependent induction of vitamin A-metabolizing enzymes in dendritic cells promotes T regulatory responses and inhibits autoimmunity. *Nat Med.* 15, 401-409.

Mann R, Mulligan RC, Baltimore D (1983). Construction of a retrovirus packaging mutant and its use to produce helper-free defective retrovirus. *Cell.* 33, 153-159.

Marsac D, Loirat D, Petit C, Schwartz O, Michel ML (2002). Enhanced presentation of major histocompatibility complex class I-restricted human immunodeficiency virus type 1 (HIV-1) Gag-specific epitopes after DNA immunization with vectors coding for vesicular stomatitis virus glycoprotein-pseudotyped HIV-1 Gag particles. *J Virol.* 76, 7544-7553.

Martin P, Del Hoyo GM, Anjuere F, Arias CF, Vargas HH, Fernandez LA, Parrillas V, Ardavin C (2002). Characterization of a new subpopulation of mouse CD8alpha+ B220+ dendritic cells endowed with type 1 interferon production capacity and tolerogenic potential. *Blood.* 100, 383-390.

Martin P, del Hoyo GM, Anjuere F, Ruiz SR, Arias CF, Marin AR, Ardavin C (2000). Concept of lymphoid versus myeloid dendritic cell lineages revisited: both CD8alpha(-) and CD8alpha(+) dendritic cells are generated from CD4(low) lymphoid-committed precursors. *Blood.* 96, 2511-2519.

Marzo AL, Vezys V, Klonowski KD, Lee SJ, Muralimohan G, Moore M, Tough DF, Lefrancois L (2004). Fully functional memory CD8 T cells in the absence of CD4 T cells. *J Immunol.* 173, 969-975.

Matrai J, Chuah MK, VandenDriessche T (2010). Recent advances in lentiviral vector development and applications. *Mol Ther.* 18, 477-490.

Matsui T, Connolly JE, Michnevitz M, Chaussabel D, Yu CI, Glaser C, Tindle S, Pypaert M, Freitas H, Piqueras B, Banchereau J, Palucka AK (2009). CD2 distinguishes two subsets of human plasmacytoid dendritic cells with distinct phenotype and functions. *J Immunol.* 182, 6815-6823.

Mellor AL, Munn DH (2004). IDO expression by dendritic cells: tolerance and tryptophan catabolism. *Nature reviews.* 4, 762-774.

Merad M, Manz MG (2009). Dendritic cell homeostasis. *Blood*. 113, 3418-3427.

Metharom P, Ellem KA, Schmidt C, Wei MQ (2001). Lentiviral vector-mediated tyrosinase-related protein 2 gene transfer to dendritic cells for the therapy of melanoma. *Hum Gene Ther*. 12, 2203-2213.

Metharom P, Ellem KA, Wei MQ (2005). Gene transfer to dendritic cells induced a protective immunity against melanoma. *Cell Mol Immunol*. 2, 281-288.

Michel G, Yu Y, Chang T, Yee JK (2010). Site-specific gene insertion mediated by a Cre-loxP-carrying lentiviral vector. *Mol Ther*. 18, 1814-1821.

Montini E, Cesana D, Schmidt M, Sanvito F, Bartholomae CC, Ranzani M, Benedicenti F, Sergi LS, Ambrosi A, Ponzoni M, Doglioni C, Di Serio C, von Kalle C, Naldini L (2009). The genotoxic potential of retroviral vectors is strongly modulated by vector design and integration site selection in a mouse model of HSC gene therapy. *J Clin Invest*. 119, 964-975.

Montini E, Cesana D, Schmidt M, Sanvito F, Ponzoni M, Bartholomae C, Sergi Sergi L, Benedicenti F, Ambrosi A, Di Serio C, Doglioni C, von Kalle C, Naldini L (2006). Hematopoietic stem cell gene transfer in a tumor-prone mouse model uncovers low genotoxicity of lentiviral vector integration. *Nat Biotechnol*. 24, 687-696.

Morita Y, Yang J, Gupta R, Shimizu K, Shelden EA, Endres J, Mule JJ, McDonagh KT, Fox DA (2001). Dendritic cells genetically engineered to express IL-4 inhibit murine collagen-induced arthritis. *J Clin Invest*. 107, 1275-1284.

Morizono K, Pariente N, Xie Y, Chen IS (2009). Redirecting lentiviral vectors by insertion of integrin-tageting peptides into envelope proteins. *J Gene Med*. 11, 549-558.

Mossoba ME, Walia JS, Rasaiah VI, Buxhoeveden N, Head R, Ying C, Foley JE, Bramson JL, Fowler DH, Medin JA (2008). Tumor protection following vaccination with low doses of lentivirally transduced DCs expressing the self-antigen erbB2. *Mol Ther*. 16, 607-617.

Munder M (2009). Arginase: an emerging key player in the mammalian immune system. *British journal of pharmacology*. 158, 638-651.

Nakahara T, Uchi H, Urabe K, Chen Q, Furue M, Moroi Y (2004). Role of c-Jun N-terminal kinase on lipopolysaccharide induced maturation of human monocyte-derived dendritic cells. *Int Immunol*. 16, 1701-1709.

Nakano H, Yanagita M, Gunn MD (2001). CD11c(+)B220(+)Gr-1(+) cells in mouse lymph nodes and spleen display characteristics of plasmacytoid dendritic cells. *J Exp Med*. 194, 1171-1178.

Naldini L, Blomer U, Gage FH, Trono D, Verma IM (1996a). Efficient transfer, integration, and sustained long-term expression of the transgene in adult rat brains injected with a lentiviral vector. *Proc Natl Acad Sci U S A*. 93, 11382-11388.

Naldini L, Blomer U, Gallay P, Ory D, Mulligan R, Gage FH, Verma IM, Trono D (1996b). In vivo gene delivery and stable transduction of nondividing cells by a lentiviral vector. *Science*. 272, 263-267.

Napolitani G, Rinaldi A, Bertoni F, Sallusto F, Lanzavecchia A (2005). Selected Toll-like receptor agonist combinations synergistically trigger a T helper type 1-polarizing program in dendritic cells. *Nat Immunol*. 6, 769-776.

Negri DR, Michelini Z, Baroncelli S, Spada M, Vendetti S, Buffa V, Bona R, Leone P, Klotman ME, Cara A (2007). Successful immunization with a single injection of non-integrating lentiviral vector. *Mol Ther.* 15, 1716-1723.

Nielsen TT, Jakobsson J, Rosenqvist N, Lundberg C (2009). Incorporating double copies of a chromatin insulator into lentiviral vectors results in less viral integrants. *BMC Biotechnol.* 9, 13.

Norian LA, Rodriguez PC, O'Mara LA, Zabaleta J, Ochoa AC, Cella M, Allen PM (2009). Tumor-infiltrating regulatory dendritic cells inhibit CD8+ T cell function via L-arginine metabolism. *Cancer Res.* 69, 3086-3094.

O'Garra A, Vieira PL, Vieira P, Goldfeld AE (2004). IL-10-producing and naturally occurring CD4+ Tregs: limiting collateral damage. *J Clin Invest.* 114, 1372-1378.

O'Keeffe M, Hochrein H, Vremec D, Caminschi I, Miller JL, Anders EM, Wu L, Lahoud MH, Henri S, Scott B, Hertzog P, Tatarczuch L, Shortman K (2002). Mouse plasmacytoid cells: long-lived cells, heterogeneous in surface phenotype and function, that differentiate into CD8(+) dendritic cells only after microbial stimulus. *J Exp Med.* 196, 1307-1319.

Oki M, Ando K, Hagihara M, Miyatake H, Shimizu T, Miyoshi H, Nakamura Y, Matsuzawa H, Sato T, Ueda Y, Gansuvd B, Kato S, Hotta T (2001). Efficient lentiviral transduction of human cord blood CD34(+) cells followed by their expansion and differentiation into dendritic cells. *Exp Hematol.* 29, 1210-1217.

Pages G, Brunet A, L'Allemain G, Pouyssegur J (1994). Constitutive mutant and putative regulatory serine phosphorylation site of mammalian MAP kinase kinase (MEK1). *Embo J.* 13, 3003-3010.

Palmowski MJ, Lopes L, Ikeda Y, Salio M, Cerundolo V, Collins MK (2004). Intravenous injection of a lentiviral vector encoding NY-ESO-1 induces an effective CTL response. *J Immunol.* 172, 1582-1587.

Palucka K, Banchereau J, Mellman I Designing vaccines based on biology of human dendritic cell subsets. *Immunity.* 33, 464-478.

Pasare C, Medzhitov R (2003). Toll pathway-dependent blockade of CD4+CD25+ T cell-mediated suppression by dendritic cells. *Science.* 299, 1033-1036.

Pauwels K, Gijsbers R, Toelen J, Schambach A, Willard-Gallo K, Verheust C, Debyser Z, Herman P (2009). State-of-the-art lentiviral vectors for research use: risk assessment and biosafety recommendations. *Curr Gene Ther.* 9, 459-474.

Peng Y, Laouar Y, Li MO, Green EA, Flavell RA (2004). TGF-beta regulates in vivo expansion of Foxp3-expressing CD4+CD25+ regulatory T cells responsible for protection against diabetes. *Proc Natl Acad Sci U S A.* 101, 4572-4577.

Pichlmair A, Diebold SS, Gschmeissner S, Takeuchi Y, Ikeda Y, Collins MK, Reis e Sousa C (2007). Tubulovesicular structures within vesicular stomatitis virus G protein-pseudotyped lentiviral vector preparations carry DNA and stimulate antiviral responses via Toll-like receptor 9. *J Virol.* 81, 539-547.

Pincha M, Sundarasetty BS, Stripecke R (2010). Lentiviral vectors for immunization: an inflammatory field. *Expert Rev Vaccines.* 9, 309-321.

Polak L, Turk JL (1974). Reversal of immunological tolerance by cyclophosphamide through inhibition of suppressor cell activity. *Nature.* 249, 654-656.

Prechtel AT, Turza NM, Theodoridis AA, Steinkasserer A (2007). CD83 knockdown in monocyte-derived dendritic cells by small interfering RNA leads to a diminished T cell stimulation. *J Immunol*. 178, 5454-5464.

Pulendran B, Tang H, Denning TL (2008). Division of labor, plasticity, and crosstalk between dendritic cell subsets. *Curr Opin Immunol*. 20, 61-67.

Radhakrishnan S, Cabrera R, Bruns KM, Van Keulen VP, Hansen MJ, Felts SJ, Pease LR (2009). Indirect recruitment of a CD40 signaling pathway in dendritic cells by B7-DC cross-linking antibody modulates T cell functions. *PLoS ONE*. 4, e5373.

Raingeaud J, Whitmarsh AJ, Barrett T, Derijard B, Davis RJ (1996). MKK3- and MKK6-regulated gene expression is mediated by the p38 mitogen-activated protein kinase signal transduction pathway. *Mol Cell Biol*. 16, 1247-1255.

Randolph GJ, Inaba K, Robbiani DF, Steinman RM, Muller WA (1999). Differentiation of phagocytic monocytes into lymph node dendritic cells in vivo. *Immunity*. 11, 753-761.

Re F, Strominger JL (2001). Toll-like receptor 2 (TLR2) and TLR4 differentially activate human dendritic cells. *J Biol Chem*. 276, 37692-37699.

Reiner SL (2007). Development in motion: helper T cells at work. *Cell*. 129, 33-36.

Reiser J, Harmison G, Kluepfel-Stahl S, Brady RO, Karlsson S, Schubert M (1996). Transduction of nondividing cells using pseudotyped defective high-titer HIV type 1 particles. *Proc Natl Acad Sci U S A*. 93, 15266-15271.

Rescigno M, Granucci F, Ricciardi-Castagnoli P (2000). Molecular events of bacterial-induced maturation of dendritic cells. *J Clin Immunol*. 20, 161-166.

Rescigno M, Martino M, Sutherland CL, Gold MR, Ricciardi-Castagnoli P (1998). Dendritic cell survival and maturation are regulated by different signaling pathways. *J Exp Med*. 188, 2175-2180.

Rich RR, Pierce CW (1973). Biological expressions of lymphocyte activation. II. Generation of a population of thymus-derived suppressor lymphocytes. *J Exp Med*. 137, 649-659.

Romani N, Holzmann S, Tripp CH, Koch F, Stoitzner P (2003). Langerhans cells - dendritic cells of the epidermis. *APMIS*. 111, 725-740.

Romano G, Claudio PP, Tonini T, Giordano A (2003). Human immunodeficiency virus type 1 (HIV-1) derived vectors: safety considerations and controversy over therapeutic applications. *Eur J Dermatol*. 13, 424-429.

Rosenberg SA, Sherry RM, Morton KE, Scharfman WJ, Yang JC, Topalian SL, Royal RE, Kammula U, Restifo NP, Hughes MS, Schwartzentruber D, Berman DM, Schwarz SL, Ngo LT, Mavroukakis SA, White DE, Steinberg SM (2005). Tumor progression can occur despite the induction of very high levels of self/tumor antigen-specific CD8+ T cells in patients with melanoma. *J Immunol*. 175, 6169-6176.

Rossetti M, Gregori S, Hauben E, Brown BD, Sergi LS, Naldini L, Roncarolo MG HIV-1-Derived Lentiviral Vectors Directly Activate Plasmacytoid Dendritic Cells, Which in Turn Induce the Maturation of Myeloid Dendritic Cells. *Hum Gene Ther*. 22, 177-188.

Rothoeft T, Balkow S, Krummen M, Beissert S, Varga G, Loser K, Oberbanscheidt P, van den Boom F, Grabbe S (2006). Structure and duration of contact between dendritic cells and T cells are controlled by T cell activation state. *Eur J Immunol.* 36, 3105-3117.

Rowe HM, Lopes L, Brown N, Efklidou S, Smallie T, Karrar S, Kaye PM, Collins MK (2009). Expression of vFLIP in a lentiviral vaccine vector activates NF-{kappa}B, matures dendritic cells, and increases CD8+ T-cell responses. *J Virol.* 83, 1555-1562.

Rowe HM, Lopes L, Ikeda Y, Bailey R, Barde I, Zenke M, Chain BM, Collins MK (2006). Immunization with a lentiviral vector stimulates both CD4 and CD8 T cell responses to an ovalbumin transgene. *Mol Ther.* 13, 310-319.

Rusakiewicz S, Dosset M, Mollier K, Souque P, Charneau P, Wain-Hobson S, Langlade-Demoyen P, Adotevi O Immunogenicity of a recombinant lentiviral vector carrying human telomerase tumor antigen in HLA-B*0702 transgenic mice. *Vaccine.* 28, 6374-6381.

Rutella S, Danese S, Leone G (2006). Tolerogenic dendritic cells: cytokine modulation comes of age. *Blood.* 108, 1435-1440.

Sakaguchi S (2003). The origin of FOXP3-expressing CD4+ regulatory T cells: thymus or periphery. *J Clin Invest.* 112, 1310-1312.

Sakaguchi S, Yamaguchi T, Nomura T, Ono M (2008). Regulatory T cells and immune tolerance. *Cell.* 133, 775-787.

Sakuishi K, Apetoh L, Sullivan JM, Blazar BR, Kuchroo VK, Anderson AC (2010). Targeting Tim-3 and PD-1 pathways to reverse T cell exhaustion and restore anti-tumor immunity. *J Exp Med.* 207, 2187-2194.

Salio M, Cella M, Vermi W, Facchetti F, Palmowski MJ, Smith CL, Shepherd D, Colonna M, Cerundolo V (2003). Plasmacytoid dendritic cells prime IFN-gamma-secreting melanoma-specific CD8 lymphocytes and are found in primary melanoma lesions. *Eur J Immunol.* 33, 1052-1062.

Salio M, Palmowski MJ, Atzberger A, Hermans IF, Cerundolo V (2004). CpG-matured murine plasmacytoid dendritic cells are capable of in vivo priming of functional CD8 T cell responses to endogenous but not exogenous antigens. *J Exp Med.* 199, 567-579.

Sallusto F, Lanzavecchia A (1994). Efficient presentation of soluble antigen by cultured human dendritic cells is maintained by granulocyte/macrophage colony-stimulating factor plus interleukin 4 and downregulated by tumor necrosis factor alpha. *J Exp Med.* 179, 1109-1118.

Salmon P, Kindler V, Ducrey O, Chapuis B, Zubler RH, Trono D (2000). High-level transgene expression in human hematopoietic progenitors and differentiated blood lineages after transduction with improved lentiviral vectors. *Blood.* 96, 3392-3398.

Saraiva M, O'Garra A (2010). The regulation of IL-10 production by immune cells. *Nature reviews.* 10, 170-181.

Sato K, Nagayama H, Tadokoro K, Juji T, Takahashi TA (1999). Extracellular signal-regulated kinase, stress-activated protein kinase/c-Jun N-terminal kinase, and p38mapk are involved in IL-10-mediated selective repression of TNF-alpha-induced activation and maturation of human peripheral blood monocyte-derived dendritic cells. *J Immunol.* 162, 3865-3872.

Schaffer DV, Koerber JT, Lim KI (2008). Molecular engineering of viral gene delivery vehicles. *Annu Rev Biomed Eng*. 10, 169-194.

Schroers R, Sinha I, Segall H, Schmidt-Wolf IG, Rooney CM, Brenner MK, Sutton RE, Chen SY (2000). Transduction of human PBMC-derived dendritic cells and macrophages by an HIV-1-based lentiviral vector system. *Mol Ther*. 1, 171-179.

Segura E, Wong J, Villadangos JA (2009). Cutting edge: B220+CCR9- dendritic cells are not plasmacytoid dendritic cells but are precursors of conventional dendritic cells. *J Immunol*. 183, 1514-1517.

Sica GL, Choi IH, Zhu G, Tamada K, Wang SD, Tamura H, Chapoval AI, Flies DB, Bajorath J, Chen L (2003). B7-H4, a molecule of the B7 family, negatively regulates T cell immunity. *Immunity*. 18, 849-861.

Siegal FP, Kadowaki N, Shodell M, Fitzgerald-Bocarsly PA, Shah K, Ho S, Antonenko S, Liu YJ (1999). The nature of the principal type 1 interferon-producing cells in human blood. *Science*. 284, 1835-1837.

Silva G, Poirot L, Galetto R, Smith J, Montoya G, Duchateau P, Paques F (2011). Meganucleases and other Tools for Targeted Genome Engineering: Perspectives and Challenges for Gene Therapy. *Curr Gene Ther*. 11, 11-27.

Silvers RM, Smith JA, Schowalter M, Litwin S, Liang Z, Geary K, Daniel R (2010). Modification of integration site preferences of an HIV-1-based vector by expression of a novel synthetic protein. *Hum Gene Ther*. 21, 337-349.

Sirven A, Pflumio F, Zennou V, Titeux M, Vainchenker W, Coulombel L, Dubart-Kupperschmitt A, Charneau P (2000). The human immunodeficiency virus type-1 central DNA flap is a crucial determinant for lentiviral vector nuclear import and gene transduction of human hematopoietic stem cells. *Blood*. 96, 4103-4110.

Song XT, Evel-Kabler K, Shen L, Rollins L, Huang XF, Chen SY (2008). A20 is an antigen presentation attenuator, and its inhibition overcomes regulatory T cell-mediated suppression. *Nat Med*. 14, 258-265.

Soumelis V, Liu YJ (2006). From plasmacytoid to dendritic cell: morphological and functional switches during plasmacytoid pre-dendritic cell differentiation. *Eur J Immunol*. 36, 2286-2292.

Srivastava MK, Sinha P, Clements VK, Rodriguez P, Ostrand-Rosenberg S (2010). Myeloid-derived suppressor cells inhibit T-cell activation by depleting cystine and cysteine. *Cancer Res*. 70, 68-77.

Steinbrink K, Wolfl M, Jonuleit H, Knop J, Enk AH (1997). Induction of tolerance by IL-10-treated dendritic cells. *J Immunol*. 159, 4772-4780.

Steinman RM (2007). Dendritic cells: Understanding immunogenicity. *European Journal of Immunology*. 37, S53-60.

Steinman RM, Banchereau J (2007). Taking dendritic cells into medicine. *Nature*. 449, 419-426.

Steinman RM, Cohn ZA (1973). Identification of a novel cell type in peripheral lymphoid organs of mice. I. Morphology, quantitation, tissue distribution. *J Exp Med*. 137, 1142-1162.

Stephens GL, McHugh RS, Whitters MJ, Young DA, Luxenberg D, Carreno BM, Collins M, Shevach EM (2004). Engagement of glucocorticoid-induced TNFR family-related receptor on effector T cells by its ligand mediates resistance to suppression by CD4+CD25+ T cells. *J Immunol*. 173, 5008-5020.

Sumimoto H, Tsuji T, Miyoshi H, Hagihara M, Takada-Yamazaki R, Okamoto S, Ikeda Y, Takahashi T, Kawakami Y (2002). Rapid and efficient generation of lentivirally gene-modified dendritic cells from DC progenitors with bone marrow stromal cells. *J Immunol Methods*. 271, 153-165.

Takayama T, Nishioka Y, Lu L, Lotze MT, Tahara H, Thomson AW (1998). Retroviral delivery of viral interleukin-10 into myeloid dendritic cells markedly inhibits their allostimulatory activity and promotes the induction of T-cell hyporesponsiveness. *Transplantation*. 66, 1567-1574.

Tan PH, Beutelspacher SC, Xue SA, Wang YH, Mitchell P, McAlister JC, Larkin DF, McClure MO, Stauss HJ, Ritter MA, Lombardi G, George AJ (2005). Modulation of human dendritic-cell function following transduction with viral vectors: implications for gene therapy. *Blood*. 105, 3824-3832.

Taussig MJ (1974). Demonstration of suppressor T cells in a population of 'educated' T cells. *Nature*. 248, 236-238.

Toscano MG, Delgado M, Kong W, Martin F, Skarica M, Ganea D (2010). Dendritic cells transduced with lentiviral vectors expressing VIP differentiate into VIP-secreting tolerogenic-like DCs. *Mol Ther*. 18, 1035-1045.

Traver D, Akashi K, Manz M, Merad M, Miyamoto T, Engleman EG, Weissman IL (2000). Development of CD8alpha-positive dendritic cells from a common myeloid progenitor. *Science*. 290, 2152-2154.

Tseng JC, Daniels G, Meruelo D (2009). Controlled propagation of replication-competent Sindbis viral vector using suicide gene strategy. *Gene Ther*. 16, 291-296.

Tuyaerts S, Aerts JL, Corthals J, Neyns B, Heirman C, Breckpot K, Thielemans K, Bonehill A (2007a). Current approaches in dendritic cell generation and future implications for cancer immunotherapy. *Cancer Immunol Immunother*. 56, 1513-1537.

Tuyaerts S, Van Meirvenne S, Bonehill A, Heirman C, Corthals J, Waldmann H, Breckpot K, Thielemans K, Aerts JL (2007b). Expression of human GITRL on myeloid dendritic cells enhances their immunostimulatory function but does not abrogate the suppressive effect of CD4+CD25+ regulatory T cells. *J Leukoc Biol*. 82, 93-105.

Unutmaz D, KewalRamani VN, Marmon S, Littman DR (1999). Cytokine signals are sufficient for HIV-1 infection of resting human T lymphocytes. *J Exp Med*. 189, 1735-1746.

Valzasina B, Guiducci C, Dislich H, Killeen N, Weinberg AD, Colombo MP (2005). Triggering of OX40 (CD134) on CD4(+)CD25+ T cells blocks their inhibitory activity: a novel regulatory role for OX40 and its comparison with GITR. *Blood*. 105, 2845-2851.

van Duin D, Medzhitov R, Shaw AC (2006). Triggering TLR signaling in vaccination. *Trends Immunol*. 27, 49-55.

VandenDriessche T, Thorrez L, Naldini L, Follenzi A, Moons L, Berneman Z, Collen D, Chuah MK (2002). Lentiviral vectors containing the human immunodeficiency virus type-1 central polypurine tract can efficiently transduce nondividing hepatocytes and antigen-presenting cells in vivo. *Blood*. 100, 813-822.

Vence L, Palucka AK, Fay JW, Ito T, Liu YJ, Banchereau J, Ueno H (2007). Circulating tumor antigen-specific regulatory T cells in patients with metastatic melanoma. *Proc Natl Acad Sci U S A*. 104, 20884-20889.

Vereecke L, Beyaert R, van Loo G (2009). The ubiquitin-editing enzyme A20 (TNFAIP3) is a central regulator of immunopathology. *Trends Immunol*. 30, 383-391.

Verhasselt V, Vosters O, Beuneu C, Nicaise C, Stordeur P, Goldman M (2004). Induction of FOXP3-expressing regulatory CD4pos T cells by human mature autologous dendritic cells. *Eur J Immunol*. 34, 762-772.

Vu MD, Xiao X, Gao W, Degauque N, Chen M, Kroemer A, Killeen N, Ishii N, Chang Li X (2007). OX40 costimulation turns off Foxp3+ Tregs. *Blood*. 110, 2501-2510.

Wang B, He J, Liu C, Chang LJ (2006). An effective cancer vaccine modality: lentiviral modification of dendritic cells expressing multiple cancer-specific antigens. *Vaccine*. 24, 3477-3489.

Wang L, Pino-Lagos K, de Vries VC, Guleria I, Sayegh MH, Noelle RJ (2008). Programmed death 1 ligand signaling regulates the generation of adaptive Foxp3+CD4+ regulatory T cells. *Proc Natl Acad Sci U S A*. 105, 9331-9336.

Wanisch K, Yanez-Munoz RJ (2009). Integration-deficient lentiviral vectors: a slow coming of age. *Mol Ther*. 17, 1316-1332.

Warger T, Osterloh P, Rechtsteiner G, Fassbender M, Heib V, Schmid B, Schmitt E, Schild H, Radsak MP (2006). Synergistic activation of dendritic cells by combined Toll-like receptor ligation induces superior CTL responses in vivo. *Blood*. 108, 544-550.

Watts TH (2005). TNF/TNFR family members in costimulation of T cell responses. *Annu Rev Immunol*. 23, 23-68.

Wilson NS, El-Sukkari D, Villadangos JA (2004). Dendritic cells constitutively present self antigens in their immature state in vivo and regulate antigen presentation by controlling the rates of MHC class II synthesis and endocytosis. *Blood*. 103, 2187-2195.

Wing K, Sakaguchi S Regulatory T cells exert checks and balances on self tolerance and autoimmunity. *Nat Immunol*. 11, 7-13.

Wu L, D'Amico A, Winkel KD, Suter M, Lo D, Shortman K (1998). RelB is essential for the development of myeloid-related CD8alpha- dendritic cells but not of lymphoid-related CD8alpha+ dendritic cells. *Immunity*. 9, 839-847.

Wu L, Li CL, Shortman K (1996). Thymic dendritic cell precursors: relationship to the T lymphocyte lineage and phenotype of the dendritic cell progeny. *J Exp Med*. 184, 903-911.

Wu X, Wakefield JK, Liu H, Xiao H, Kralovics R, Prchal JT, Kappes JC (2000). Development of a novel trans-lentiviral vector that affords predictable safety. *Mol Ther*. 2, 47-55.

Xu Y, Darcy PK, Kershaw MH (2007). Tumor-specific dendritic cells generated by genetic redirection of Toll-like receptor signaling against the tumor-associated antigen, erbB2. *Cancer gene therapy*. 14, 773-780.

Yang L, Bailey L, Baltimore D, Wang P (2006). Targeting lentiviral vectors to specific cell types in vivo. *Proc Natl Acad Sci U S A*. 103, 11479-11484.

Yang L, Yang H, Rideout K, Cho T, Joo KI, Ziegler L, Elliot A, Walls A, Yu D, Baltimore D, Wang P (2008). Engineered lentivector targeting of dendritic cells for in vivo immunization. *Nat Biotechnol.* 26, 326-334.

Yang M, Sun L, Wang S, Ko KH, Xu H, Zheng BJ, Cao X, Lu L (2010). Novel function of B cell-activating factor in the induction of IL-10-producing regulatory B cells. *J Immunol.* 184, 3321-3325.

Yang Y, Huang CT, Huang X, Pardoll DM (2004). Persistent Toll-like receptor signals are required for reversal of regulatory T cell-mediated CD8 tolerance. *Nat Immunol.* 5, 508-515.

Zennou V, Petit C, Guetard D, Nerhbass U, Montagnier L, Charneau P (2000). HIV-1 genome nuclear import is mediated by a central DNA flap. *Cell.* 101, 173-185.

Zhang F, Thornhill SI, Howe SJ, Ulaganathan M, Schambach A, Sinclair J, Kinnon C, Gaspar HB, Antoniou M, Thrasher AJ (2007). Lentiviral vectors containing an enhancer-less ubiquitously acting chromatin opening element (UCOE) provide highly reproducible and stable transgene expression in hematopoietic cells. *Blood.* 110, 1448-1457.

Zhang XY, Kutner RH, Bialkowska A, Marino MP, Klimstra WB, Reiser J Cell-specific targeting of lentiviral vectors mediated by fusion proteins derived from Sindbis virus, vesicular stomatitis virus, or avian sarcoma/leukosis virus. Retrovirology. 7, 3.

Zhang XY, Kutner RH, Bialkowska A, Marino MP, Klimstra WB, Reiser J (2010). Cell-specific targeting of lentiviral vectors mediated by fusion proteins derived from Sindbis virus, vesicular stomatitis virus, or avian sarcoma/leukosis virus. *Retrovirology.* 7, 3.

Zhang Y, Yang H, Xiao B, Wu M, Zhou W, Li J, Li G, Christadoss P (2009). Dendritic cells transduced with lentiviral-mediated RelB-specific ShRNAs inhibit the development of experimental autoimmune myasthenia gravis. *Molecular immunology.* 46, 657-667.

Zufferey R, Donello JE, Trono D, Hope TJ (1999). Woodchuck hepatitis virus posttranscriptional regulatory element enhances expression of transgenes delivered by retroviral vectors. *J Virol.* 73, 2886-2892.

Zufferey R, Dull T, Mandel RJ, Bukovsky A, Quiroz D, Naldini L, Trono D (1998). Self-inactivating lentivirus vector for safe and efficient in vivo gene delivery. J Virol. 72, 9873-9880.

Zufferey R, Nagy D, Mandel RJ, Naldini L, Trono D (1997). Multiply attenuated lentiviral vector achieves efficient gene delivery in vivo. *Nat Biotechnol.* 15, 871-875.

Part 5

Other Types of Viral Vector

16

Development and Application of HIV Vectors Pseudotyped with HIV Envelopes

Koichi Miyake and Takashi Shimada
Department of Biochemistry and Molecular Biology, Division of Gene Therapy Research Center for Advanced Medical Technology, Nippon Medical School
Japan

1. Introduction

Retroviral vectors derived from the mouse moloney leukemia virus (MLV) are widely used for gene therapy of blood disorders because they are capable of permanently integrating a therapeutic gene into hematopoietic cells and achieving long-term expression. However, a limitation of MLV retroviral vectors is the inability to infect growth-arrested cells. It has been demonstrated that a passage through mitosis of infected cells is required for productive infection of MLV (Lewis & Emerman 1994). The breakdown of the nuclear membrane at mitosis may be necessary for nuclear transport of the oncoretroviral preintegration complex which is too large to enter a nuclear pore in the intact nuclear membrane. Because most of the target cells of gene therapy such as hematopoietic stem cells and lymphocytes are quiescent or rarely dividing, the requirement for cell division limits the use of MLV vectors for therapeutic gene transfer.

For clinical trial of gene therapy, the best-established therapeutic vector is a gamma retroviral vector. This retroviral vector system has successfully been used for gene transfer to hematopoietic cells to treat X-linked severe combined immunodeficiency (X-SCID) and adenosine deaminase deficiency (ADA-SCID). However, in these successful clinical trials, genotoxicity mediated by integrated vector proviruses has led to clonal expansion, and in 5 of 20 of these X-SCID patients have developed T-cell leukemia (Hacein-Bey-Abina et al. 2008; Hacein-Bey-Abina et al. 2003; Howe et al. 2008). Molecular analyses of the leukemia cases showed that these retroviral vectors were integrated into a small number of T-cell proto-oncogenes, especially LMO2, leading to its aberrant and high-level expression caused by the strong enhancer elements located in the U3 region of the MLV long-terminal repeat (LTR). Moreover, the 2 patients with X-linked chronic granulomatous disease (X-CGD) exhibited striking clonal dominance with most of their gene-corrected cells having insertions into or near of the MDS1-EVI1, PRDM16, or SETBP1 loci (Ott et al. 2006). These retroviral vector genotoxicity emphasize that next-generation vectors should further improve the safety and the genotoxicity of retroviral integration is a relevant factor to be considered in designing vectors for future clinical trials.

Human immunodeficiency virus type-1 (HIV-1), an etiological agent of acquired immunodeficiency syndrome (AIDS), is a member of lentivirinae which is a subfamily of retroviruses. We have previously established a packaging system which generates helper free recombinant HIV vectors (Shimada et al. 1991). Compared with widely used amphotrophic retroviral vectors, HIV vectors have several interesting features. First, since the major receptor for HIV infection is the CD4 molecules of helper T lymphocytes, the HIV vectors are capable of targeted gene transfer into $CD4^+$ cells (Miyake et al. 1996; Shimada et al. 1991). Second, since gene expression from the HIV-LTR is dependent upon the HIV encoded transacting factor TAT (Sodroski et al. 1984), in the presence of TAT, the HIV-LTR functions as a very strong promoter. However, because there is no TAT molecule in target cells, the HIV-LTR of the integrated provirus is inactive. Inactivation of the LTR of the retroviral vector is thought to be important to minimize the chance of insertional activation of cellular proto-oncogenes and promoter interference between the LTR and the internal promoter. Third, unlike oncoretroviruses, HIV and other lentiviruses have the ability to infect and integrate in non-dividing cells. Therefore, HIV based vectors can be used for gene transfer into non-dividing cells (Miyake et al. 1998). This possibility is particularly important, because none of the current vectors can efficiently integrate into chromosome of non-dividing cells.

In this chapter, we describe about HIV vector pseudotyped with HIV envelopes. Replication-incompetent HIV vectors pseudotyped with HIV envelopes (BH10 or SF162) were developed and were shown to be capable of targeted gene transfer into $CD4^+$ T cells and macrophages. This strict T cell tropism is important for the development of gene therapy of AIDS or adult T-cell leukemia (ATL). We also developed an improved strategy for preparation of high titer HIV vectors. Since primary un-stimulated T cells and terminally differentiated macrophages were transduced with high titer HIV vectors efficiently, HIV vectors are useful for the manipulation of gene expression in HIV infectable cells and the development of gene therapy targeting lymphocytes and macrophages. Finally, we present the application of HIV vectors for AIDS and ATL.

2. Production and concentration of HIV vectors

2.1 Plasmid construction

The first generation packaging plasmid (pCGPE) provided all gag and pol sequences, the viral regulatory genes tat and rev and the accessory genes vif, vpr and vpu from T-cell tropic HIV strain (BH10) (Ratner et al. 1987). To improve the safety, the single packaging plasmid (pCGPE) was divided into two plasmids. One is the pCAGgpR, which contains the CAG promoter and HIV gag, pol and RRE; another one is the T-cell tropic HIV env expression vector (penvBH10). We also developed macrophage tropic HIV env expression vector (penvSF162), which contains the macrophage tropic HIV env fragment from SF162 (Collman et al. 1989)(Figure 1A).

The transfer plasmid consists of an expression cassette and the HIV *cis*-acting factors necessary for packaging together with the packaging signal (Ψ). pHXN transfer vector plasmid contains the TK promoter and neomycin resistance gene (neoR). To improve the packaging efficiency and safety, we modified splicing donor (SD) site (TGGT -> TCGC) and initiation codon of gag gene (ATG -> ATC) (pHXNm). Since promoter activity of HIV-LTR is Tat dependent, we also developed Tat independent transfer vector by replacement of 5′ U3 region to CMV promoter (pCHXN). To improve the safety, self-inactivating (SIN) transfer vector was developed by deletion of 3′ U3 region (κB-κB-sp1-sp1-sp1-TATA) (pCHXNΔ) (Figure 1B).

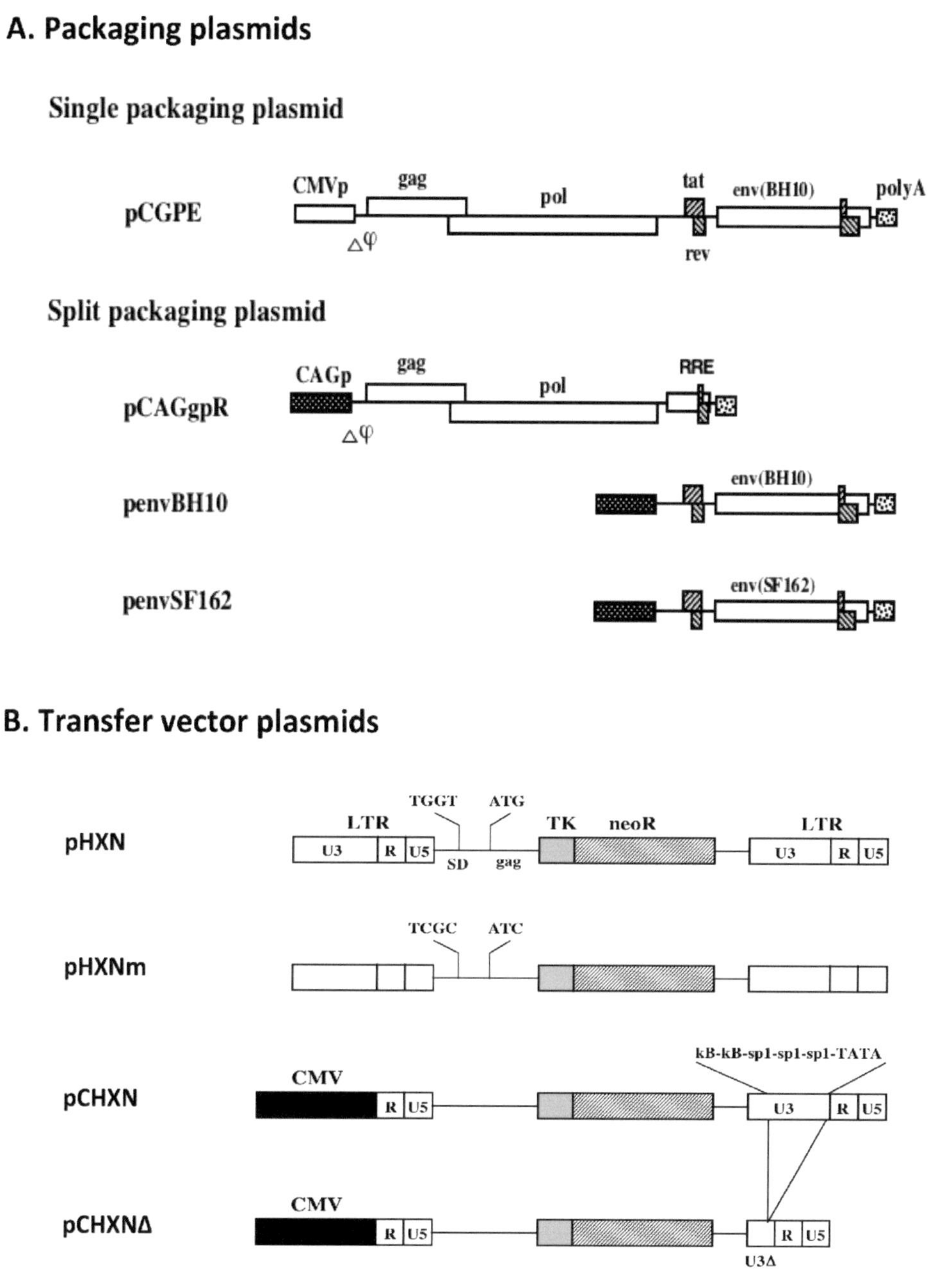

Fig. 1. Construction of recombinant HIV packaging (A) and transfer vector (B) plasmids.

2.2 Production of HIV vectors

Recombinant HIV vectors were prepared by transiently transfecting Cos cells ($2x10^6$ cells/10 cm dish) with 10 μg of packaging plasmid (pCGPE) and 10 μg of transfer vector plasmid (pHXN) using the $CaPO_4$ coprecipitation method described previously (Miyake et al. 1996; Shimada et al. 1991). For a separate packaging system, 7 μg of pCAGgpR, 7 μg of penvBH10 or penvSF162, and 7 μg of vector plasmids were used. After 48 h, the supernatant was collected, passed through a 45-μm filter to remove cell debris. The conditioned medium of transfected Cos cells were used as the HIV vector stock (Figure 2). To assess the transduction efficiency and cell specificity of the vectors, HeLa, CD4H ($CD4^+$ HeLa), and CD4H5 ($CD4^+$ and $CCR5^+$ HeLa) cells were incubated with various dilutions of the viral supernatants and cultured in the presence of 1,000 μg/ml active G418 for two weeks. G418 resistant colonies were calculated and the titer of HIV vector was presented as colony forming unit (cfu)/ml.

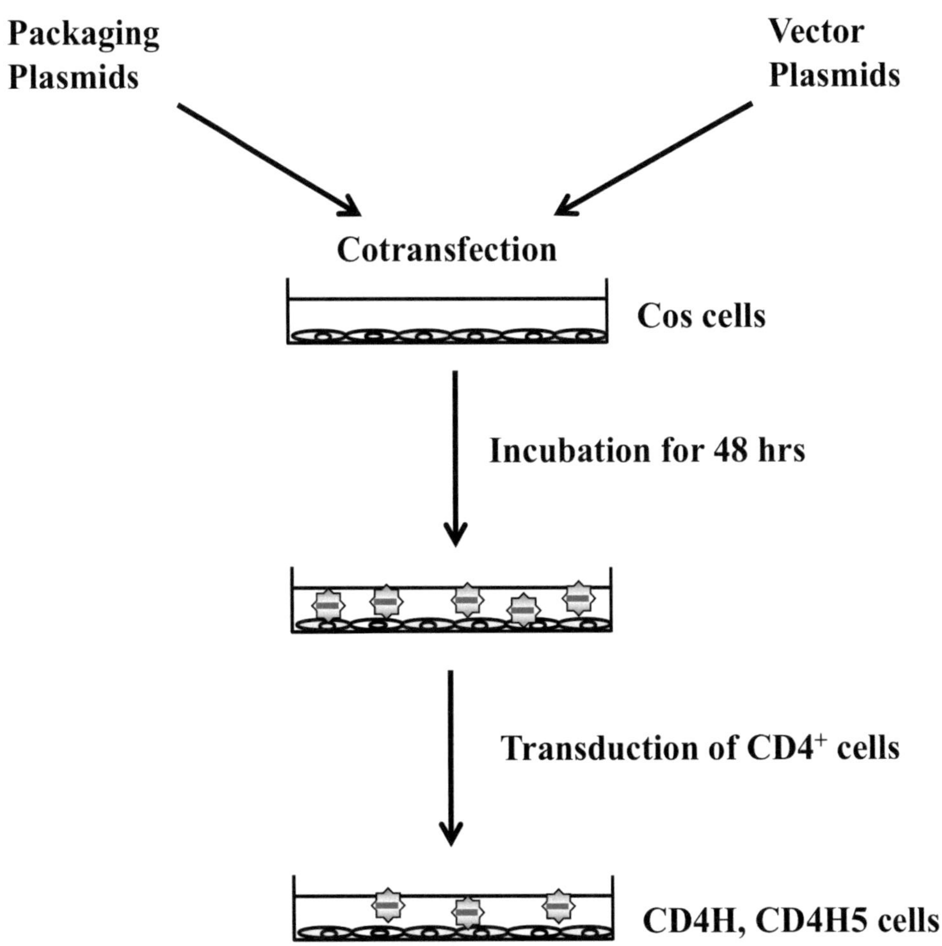

Fig. 2. Production of HIV vector pseudotyped with HIV envelope.

2.3 Concentration of HIV vectors

The titer of the HIV vector in Cos cell supernatants is approximately 10^4 cfu/ml when assayed on CD4H cells. This titer is too low to transduce primary $CD4^+$ cells. To overcome this problem, we concentrated HIV vectors using sulfonated cellulose column chromatography, thereby increasing the titer more than 20-fold (Matsuoka et al. 1998). For further improvement, among several possible procedures, we found that ultrafiltration using CENTRIPREP columns was highly effective to concentrate HIV particles (Miyake et al. 2007b). The titer could be increased four orders of magnitudes (Figure 3). The total recovery was more than 80 %. No replication competent cytopathic HIV was detected in concentrated vector preparation when assayed on MT2 cell-based syncytium formation assay, which is highly sensitive to the cytopathic effect of HIV.

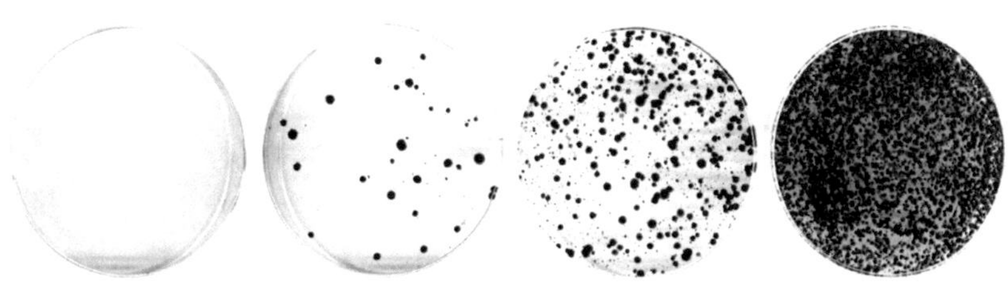

	Before conc.	1st column	2nd column	3rd column
Titer (cfu/ml)	$1.1x10^4$	$2.8x10^5$	$4.1x10^6$	$6.2x10^7$
Volume (ml)	120	4.0	0.32	0.02
Conc. rate (times)	1	25.4	372.7	5636.4

Fig. 3. Concentration of HIV vectors by ultrafiltration. By repeating the concentration step several times, we were able to obtain highly concentrated HIV vectors.

3. Characterization of HIV vectors

3.1 Targeted gene transfer into CD4-positive cells and macrophages

To examine the tissue specificity of the vectors, $CD4^-$ parental HeLa, CD4H, and CD4H5 ($CCR5^+$ CD4H) cells were incubated with the T-cell tropic HIV vector containing the neoR gene (HXN-T) or the macrophage tropic HIV vector (HXN-M). The T-cell tropic HIV vector selectively transduced $CD4^+$ and $CXCR4^+$ HeLa cells, while the macrophage tropic HIV vector transduced $CD4^+$ and $CCR5^+$ HeLa cells. Thus, the HIV vector has the same tissue specificity as wild type virus. The titer of HIV vectors generated from split packaging plasmids were slightly lower than those generated from single packaging plasmids (Table 1). Figure 4 shows the result of transduction of CD4H cells with MLV or HIV vector expressing enhanced green fluorescent protein (EGFP) gene (MLVG or HXG-T). Selective $CD4^+$ cells were transduced by HXG-T compared to MLVG vector.

	HeLa	CD4H	CD4H5
CD4	-	+	+
CXCR4	-	+	+
CCR5	-	-	+
pCGPE	0	$1.2x10^4$	$1.1x10^4$
pCAGgpR+penvBH10	0	$0.8x10^4$	$0.7x10^4$
pCAGgpR+penvSF162	0	0	$0.4x10^4$

Table 1. Selective transduction of CD4-positive HeLa cells by HIV vectors

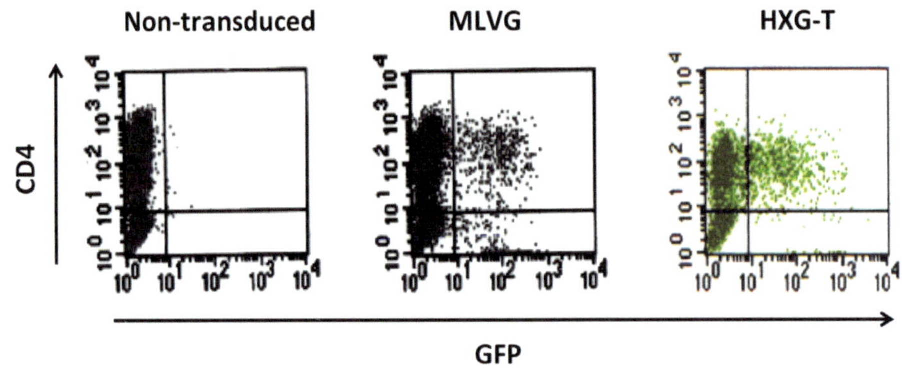

Fig. 4. Transduction of CD4-positive HeLa cells by MLV and HIV vectors expressing GFP.

We next attempted to transduce human primary cells using the high titer HIV vector carrying the EGFP gene. After enrichment of $CD4^+$ cells, the cells were stimulated with IL2 and PHA. Two days after stimulation, transduction was performed using the concentrated T-cell tropic HIV vector (HXG-T), and up to 84% of the stimulated T cells were found to be transduced. Samples of these transduced lymphocytes were analyzed to determine the duration of GFP expression, which was detected for more than one month with no decline in the percentage of GFP^+ cells (Miyake et al. 2007b). It thus appears that HIV vectors were integrated into the chromosomes, and the growth rate of vector-transduced cells was the same as that of non-transduced cells, making this highly concentrated HIV vector potentially useful for gene transfer into human primary lymphocytes.

We have reported that HIV vectors are capable of mediating gene transfer into non-dividing cells (Miyake et al. 1998). Therefore, we next attempted to transduce freshly isolated, un-stimulated $CD4^+$ T cells and terminally differentiated macrophages. The un-stimulated T cells were also efficiently transduced by HXG-T, with from 20 % to 54 % of the un-stimulated T cells being GFP positive, while these un-stimulated T cells could not transduced by MLV based retroviral vector. In addition, approximately 20 % of terminally differentiated, monocyte-derived macrophages were transduced using concentrated the macrophage tropic HIV vector expressing EGFP (HXG-M), indicating that macrophage trophic HIV vector should also be useful for targeted gene transfer into macrophages (Miyake et al. 2007b). We also construct HIV vectors containing LacZ gene and transduced with primary $CD4^+$ T cells and macrophages. Figure 5 shows the result of transduction of $CD4^+$ T cells and macrophages with HIV vector expressing LacZ gene. X-gal staining showed that both primary T cells and macrophages are efficiently transduced by HIV vectors.

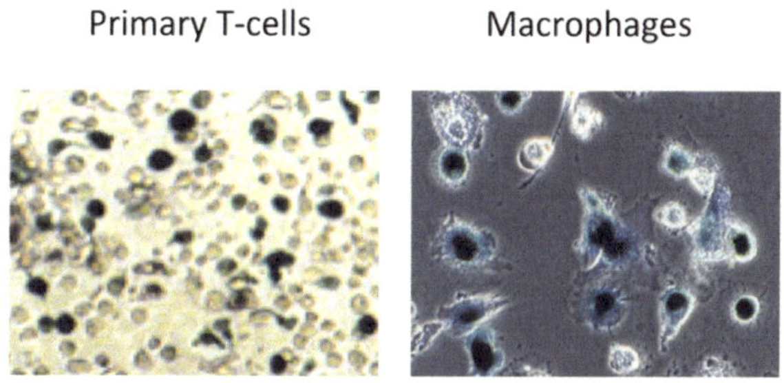

Fig. 5. Transduction of CD4+ T cells and macrophages with HIV vector expressing LacZ gene

3.2 *In vivo* targeted gene transfer

Targeted gene transfer is essential for safe and efficient gene therapy. Systemic injection of targeting vector is considered to be an ideal method of gene transfer. Since HIV vector was capable of targeted and efficient gene transfer into CD4+ human cells including non-stimulated primary CD4+ T-cells, it should be potentially useful for *in vivo* gene transfer into T lymphocytes. To analyze whether the HIV vector could be used for *in vivo* targeting gene transfer, Hu-PBL-NOD-scid mice were prepared by intraperitoneal injection of 1 x 10^7 human PBL into NK depleted NOD-scid mice. One ml of the HIV vector stock (HXG-T: 1 x 10^8 transduction unit (TU)/ml) was inoculated into the intraperitoneal cavity, and the mouse was sacrifices after 10 days. FACS analysis showed that 2-4 % of CD4+ T-cells recovered from the peritoneal cavity, peripheral blood, and spleen were transduced with the HXG-T vector (Figure 6).

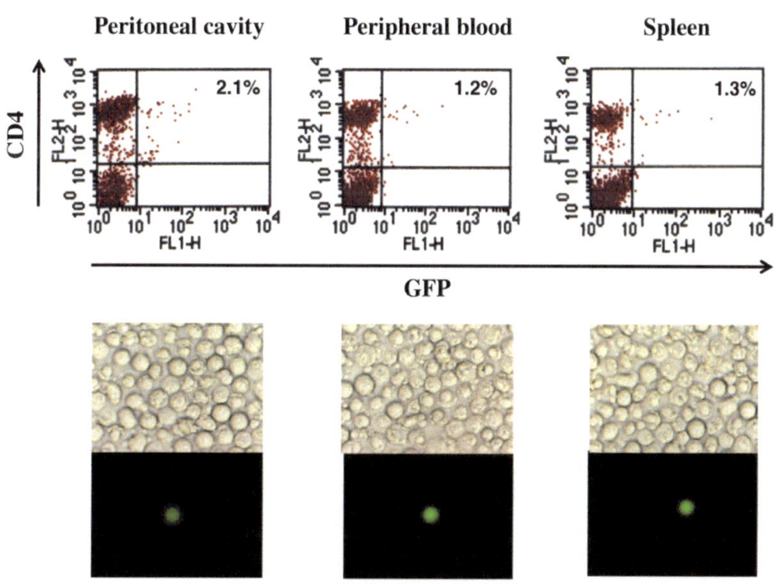

Fig. 6. *In vivo* targeted gene transfer by HIV vector. One ml of the HIV vector containing GFP stock (1 x 10^8 TU/ml) was inoculated into the intraperitoneal cavity of Hu-PBL-NOD-scid mice, and the mouse was sacrifices after 10 days. Expression of CD4 and GFP were analyzed by FACS.

These results indicate that HIV vector could be used for *in vivo* targeted gene transfer into $CD4^+$ T-cells. Lymphocytes are important target cells for gene therapy of various disorders. Targetable and injectable HIV vectors would greatly facilitate the development of such gene therapy strategies.

4. Applications of HIV vectors

4.1 Gene therapy for AIDS

A number of gene therapeutic strategies have been proposed for the treatment of AIDS. One approach, intracellular immunization (Baltimore 1988), entails rendering otherwise HIV-1-permissive cells resistant to HIV-1 infection by introducing such anti-HIV molecules as siRNA, antisense RNAs, ribozymes, RNA decoys, and trans-dominant negative mutants. A second approach entails vaccination using expression vectors for viral proteins, and a large scale clinical trial based on MLV vector-mediated transfer of the HIV-1 env and rev genes was examined. Finally, a third approach entails the use of a suicide gene to induce the death of HIV-1 infected cells, thereby preventing virus spread. The herpes simplex virus thymidine kinase (HSV-TK) gene is a most used typical suicide gene. HSV-TK acting in concert with cellular kinase specifically converts the prodrug gancyclovir (GCV) into highly toxic GCV-triphosphate, which causes DNA polymerase chain termination and eventually cell death. To minimize unwanted side effects, it is essential to develop a technique that enables tissue-specific gene transfer and expression only in targeted cells.

HIV vectors transduce only human $CD4^+$ lymphocytes and macrophages. Further, when used in conjunction with the HIV-LTR, an inducible promoter dependent on the virus encoded *trans*-activator Tat, HIV-based vectors pseudotyped with HIV envelope have the potential to mediate targeted gene transfer into HIV-1-permissive cells and for specific expression in HIV-1 infected cells. This would appear to make such vectors ideal for use in gene therapies against AIDS. Advantages of HIV vector for gene therapy of AIDS are summarized in Table 2.

1. Specific gene transfer into HIV infectable cells
2. Inducible expression on HIV infected cells
3. HIV vector sequences were packaged into newly synthesized virions
4. Useful for *in vivo* targeting gene transfer

Table 2. Advantages of HIV vector for gene therapy of AIDS

We constructed an HIV-based vector pseudotyped with HIV envelope containing the HSV-TK suicide gene under the control of the inducible HIV-LTR promoter (Figure 7A). This vector was selectively transferred into $CD4^+$ cells, and the HSVTK gene was subsequently expressed only in HIV-1-infected cells. Consequently, subsequent exposure to GCV selectively killed HIV-1 infected cells (Figure 7B). After transduction of H9 cells with HXTKN (HXTKN/H9), GCV-sensitivity was analyzed by MTT assay. Prior to HIV-1 infection, the GCV IC_{50} in HXTKN/H9 cells was approximately 100 μg/ml. On the other hand, HXTKN/H9 cells became highly sensitive to GCV after infection with HIV-1. The GCV IC_{50} of HIV-1-infected HXTKN/H9 cells were 0.1 μg/ml or about 1,000 times greater than in uninfected cells (Figure 7C). We next tested the extent to which HIV-1 replication was inhibited by the selective suicide of HIV-1-infected cells. In a model experiment,

HIV-1 infected HXTKN/H9 cells were mixed with uninfected HXTKN/H9 cells to a ratio of 1:100, and virus replication was studied by measuring p24 (Figure 7D). High levels of p24 were detected when the mixed cells were grown in the absence of GCV, but the amount of detected p24 declined dramatically following addition of 10 μg/ml GCV, indicating that selective suicide of HIV-infected cells effectively inhibited spread of the virus. In addition, on HIV-1 infection, HIV vector sequences were packaged into newly synthesized virions that were transferred into surrounding untransduced cells. These results support the rationale for treatment of HIV infection with HIV-based vectors (Miyake et al. 2001).

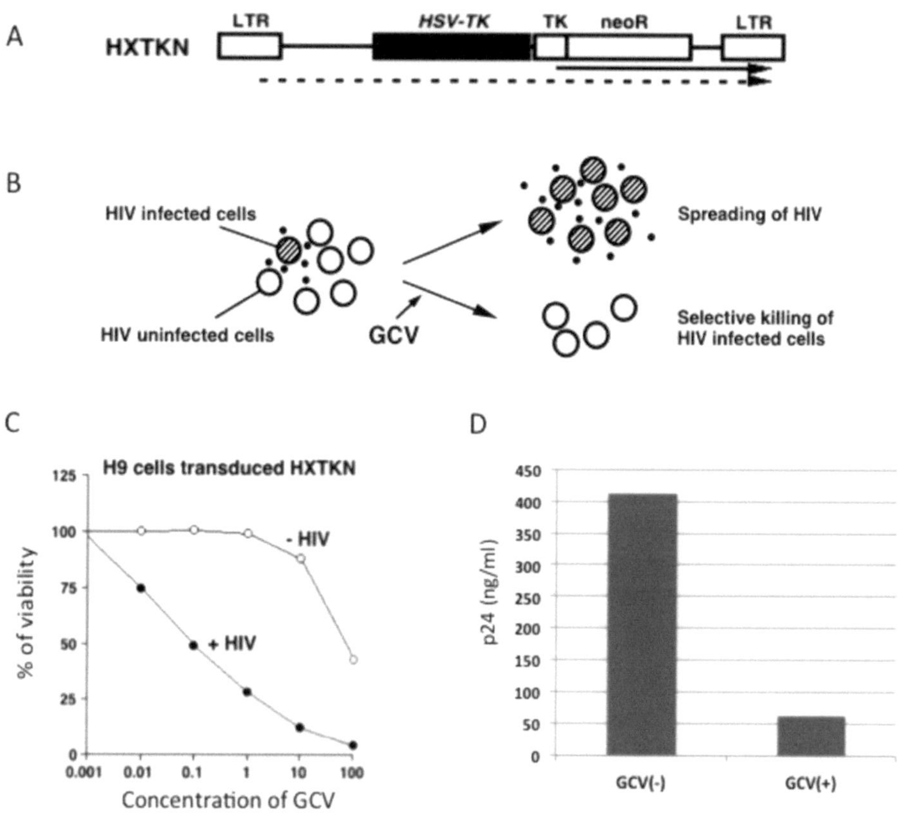

Fig. 7. Selective killing of HIV infected cells. (A) Inducible HIV vectors containing the HSV-TK suicide gene. (B) Rationale for treatment of HIV infection with HIV-based vectors. (C) HXTKN transduced H9 cells were incubated for 5 days with various concentrations of GCV (0.001-100 μg/mL), after which cell growth was estimated by MTT assay. (D) Effect of GCV on HIV-1 replication. A mixture of HIV-1-infected and uninfected HXTKN/H9 cells (1:100) were cultured with or without 10 μg/ml GCV. After 7 days, p24 levels in the culture supernatant were measured by ELISA.

We also investigated the utility of the HIV vector by intracellular immunization strategy. The chemokine receptors, CXCR4 and CCR5 (Alkhatib et al. 1996; Deng et al. 1996; Feng et al. 1996), have been identified as co-receptors for HIV-1 infection (Figure 8A). These cellular genes are attractive targets for intracellular immunization, because the mutation rate of the cellular gene is much less than that of the viral genome. We examined the feasibility of antisense inhibition of CXCR4 expression using HIV vector. We constructed the HIV vector containing the antisense sequence (738-429 nt) of CXCR4 driven by the CAG promoter and transduced CEM cells (Figure 8B). The level of CXCR4 in antisense expressing (HXCXAN-transduced) CEM cells was reduced up to 20 % of that in control (HXN-transduced) cells (Figure 8C). Inhibition of T-cell trophic HIV replication also observed in transduced CEM cells (Figure 8D). These results suggest that antisense inhibition of CXCR4 expression is effective to block HIV-1 infection at the early step and may be useful for gene therapy of HIV-1 infection.

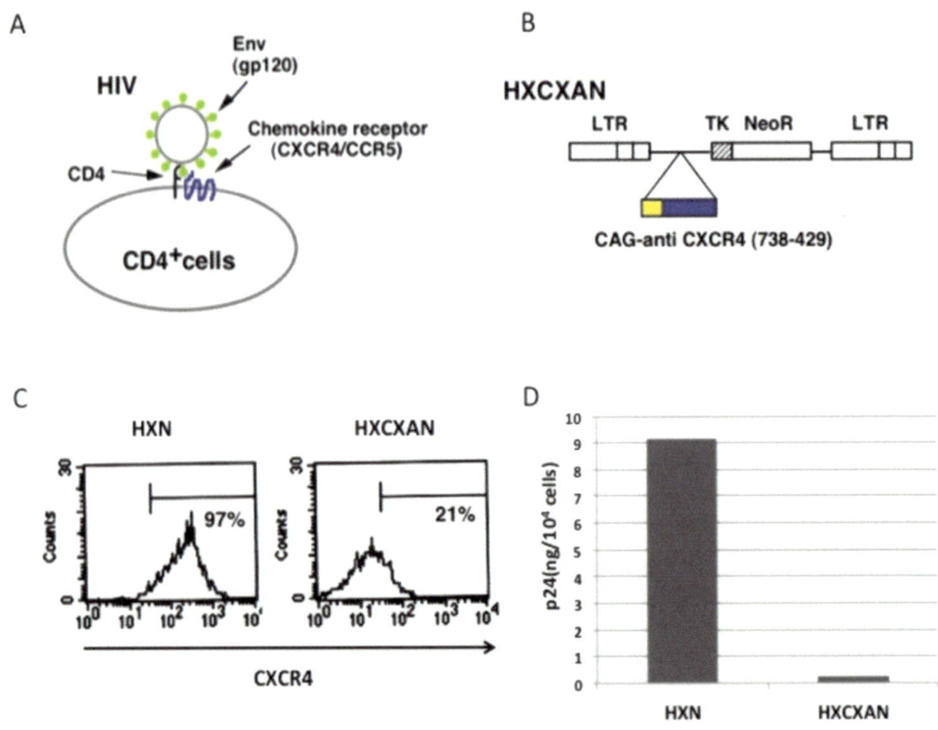

Fig. 8. Suppression of HIV-1 replication by HIV vector containing antisense CXCR4. (A) CXCR4 or CCR5 is a co-receptor of HIV-1 infection. (B) Construction of HIV vector expressing antisense CXCR4. (C) Expression of CXCR4 on HXN (control) or HXCXAN-transduced CEM cells. Expression of CXCR4 was analyzed by FACS. (D) Effect of antisense CXCR4 on HIV-1 replication. After HIV-1-infected HXN- or HXCXAN-transduced CEM cells were cultured for 7 days, p24 levels in the culture supernatant were measured by ELISA.

4.2 Development of selective transduction of HIV-1-infected cells

HIV based vectors bind specifically to the CD4 antigen and are capable of targeted gene transfer into CD4+ cells. The strict cell specificity of HIV vectors should be important for development of gene therapy of AIDS. However, HIV vectors may not be useful for gene transfer into cells already infected with HIV-1, because CD4 expression is usually down-regulated and in contrast, the HIV envelope glycoprotein (HIV-Env) is overexpressed in such cells (Hoxie et al. 1986; Maddon et al. 1986). Therefore, using a special feature of the HIV vectors, we have developed a novel strategy for targeted gene transfer into HIV-1 infected cells based on two-step gene transfer. Figure 9A shows the concept of two-step gene transfer. The first step involves the stable introduction of the HIV vector containing the ecotrophic MLV receptor (EcoRec) gene into human CD4+ T cells as a molecular switch.

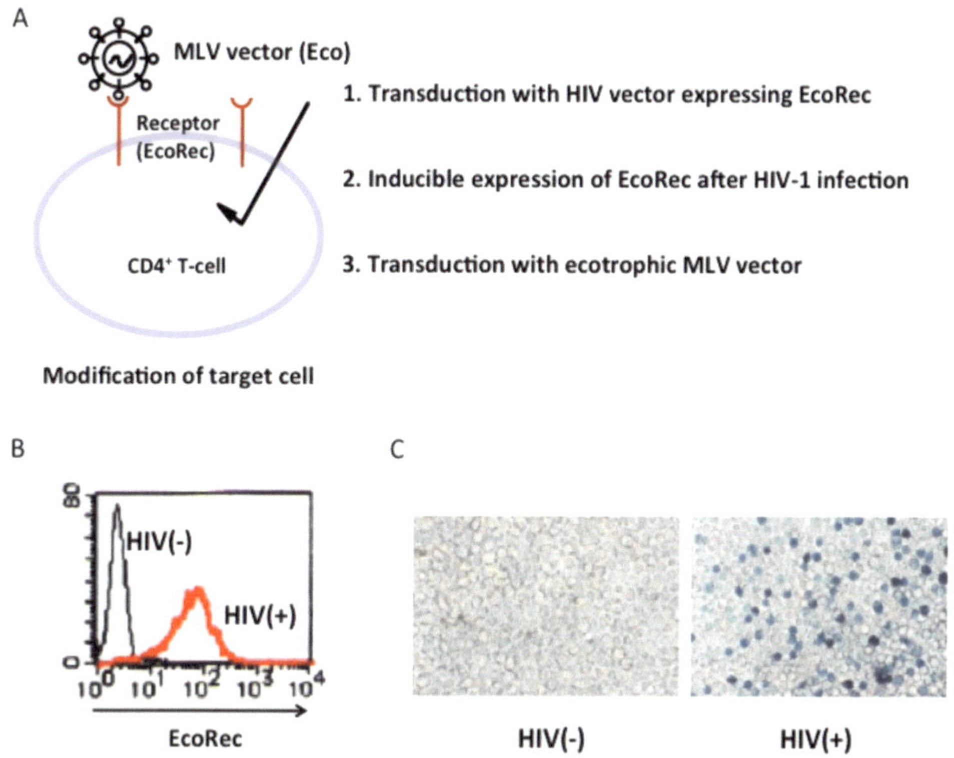

Fig. 9. Targeted gene transfer into HIV-1 infected cells. (A) Concept of two-step gene transfer for selective transduction of HIV-1 infected cells. (B) Inducible expression of EcoRec on HXERN transduced CEM cells. The cells were infected (HIV(+)) or uninfected (HIV(-)) with HIV-1. (C) HXERN transduced CEM cells were infected (HIV(+)) or uninfected (HIV(-)) with HIV-1 and then, transduced with the ecotrophic retroviral vectors containing LacZ gene. Expressions of β-galactosidase were assessed by X-gal staining.

Since the HIV-LTR is Tat-inducible, it is expected that EcoRec is expressed only after HIV-1 infection. High levels of EcoRec expression were observed only in HIV-1 infected cells.

These cells became highly susceptible to ecotrophic MLV infection and therefore, in the second step, HIV-1 infected cells were selectively transduced with ecotrophic MLV vectors. CEM cells were transduced with the HIV vector containing the EcoRec gene under the control of the HIV-LTR (HXERN). Inducible expression of EcoRec in transduced cells was studied by the virus binding assay. Prior to HIV-1 infection, no detectable EcoRec was observed on the cell surface. However, after HIV-1 infection, high levels of induced EcoRec expression were detected by FACS analysis (Figure 9B). These findings indicated that HXERN transduced cells were ecotrophic MLV non-permissive, but became highly sensitive to ecotrophic MLV infection, once infected with HIV-1. In the next step, HXERN transduced cells were incubated with the ecotrophic MLV vector containing the beta-galactosidase gene (MLVLacZ). X-gal staining showed that HXERN transduced cells were totally resistant to retroviral infection. However, HIV-1 infected HXERN transduced cells were selectively transduced with MLVLacZ (Figure 9C). These findings indicate that this two-step method can be used for efficient, selective and stable gene transfer into HIV-1 infected cells (Sakai et al. 2001).

A possible clinical application of this strategy is as follows. Targets should be HIV seropositive but disease free patients. Most $CD4^+$ T cells in these patients are HIV negative. HXERN is stably inserted into these T cells (1st step). After a variable asymptomatic period, the virus apparently starts replication and spreads within the whole body. During this stage, EcoRec is expressed on the surface of only HIV-1 infected cells. Therefore, HIV-1 infected cells can be selectively attacked with the ecotrophic MLV vector carrying the therapeutic gene.

4.3 Gene therapy for ATL

Adult T cell leukemia (ATL) is a malignant disease etiologically associated with human T cell leukemia virus type I (HTLV-I). The prognosis of acute- or lymphoma-type ATL is far worse than that of other lymphoid malignancies, and effective therapy has not been established. HIV based vectors are capable of targeted and highly efficient gene transfer into $CD4^+$ T cells regulated by the HIV envelope glycoprotein gp120 and CD4 interaction. Because almost all ATL cells express CD4, HIV based vectors are useful for targeting therapeutic genes to ATL cells. We investigated the potential efficacy of treating ATL cells using a gene therapeutic approach involving the use of an HSV-TK-mediated suicide system. HIV vectors containing the HSV-TK gene under the control of CMV promoter (Figure 10A) were constructed to achieve targeted gene transfer into $CD4^+$ ATL cells, after which the transduced cells were selectively killed by treatment with GCV. To examine the utility of HIV vectors *in vivo*, ATL-NOD-SCID mice were prepared by intraperitoneal injection of 1×10^7 MT2 cells into NK-depleted NOD-SCID mice. Thereafter, 1 ml of concentrated HIV vector expressing HSV-TK (HXCTKN) or GFP (HXG) stock was injected into the intraperitoneal cavity, and GCV was administered twice a day for 5 days (Figure 10B). After three weeks, plasma sIL2-Rα levels, which are indicator of growth of MT2 cells, were significantly lower in mice administered HXCTKN than in those administered control HXG. Moreover, HXCTKN-injected mice survived significantly longer than HXG-injected mice (Miyake et al. 2007a) (Figure 10C). Taken together, these findings suggest that HIV vectors could be used for *in vivo* targeted gene transfer into ATL cells and thus could serve as the basis for the development of effective new therapies for the treatment ATL.

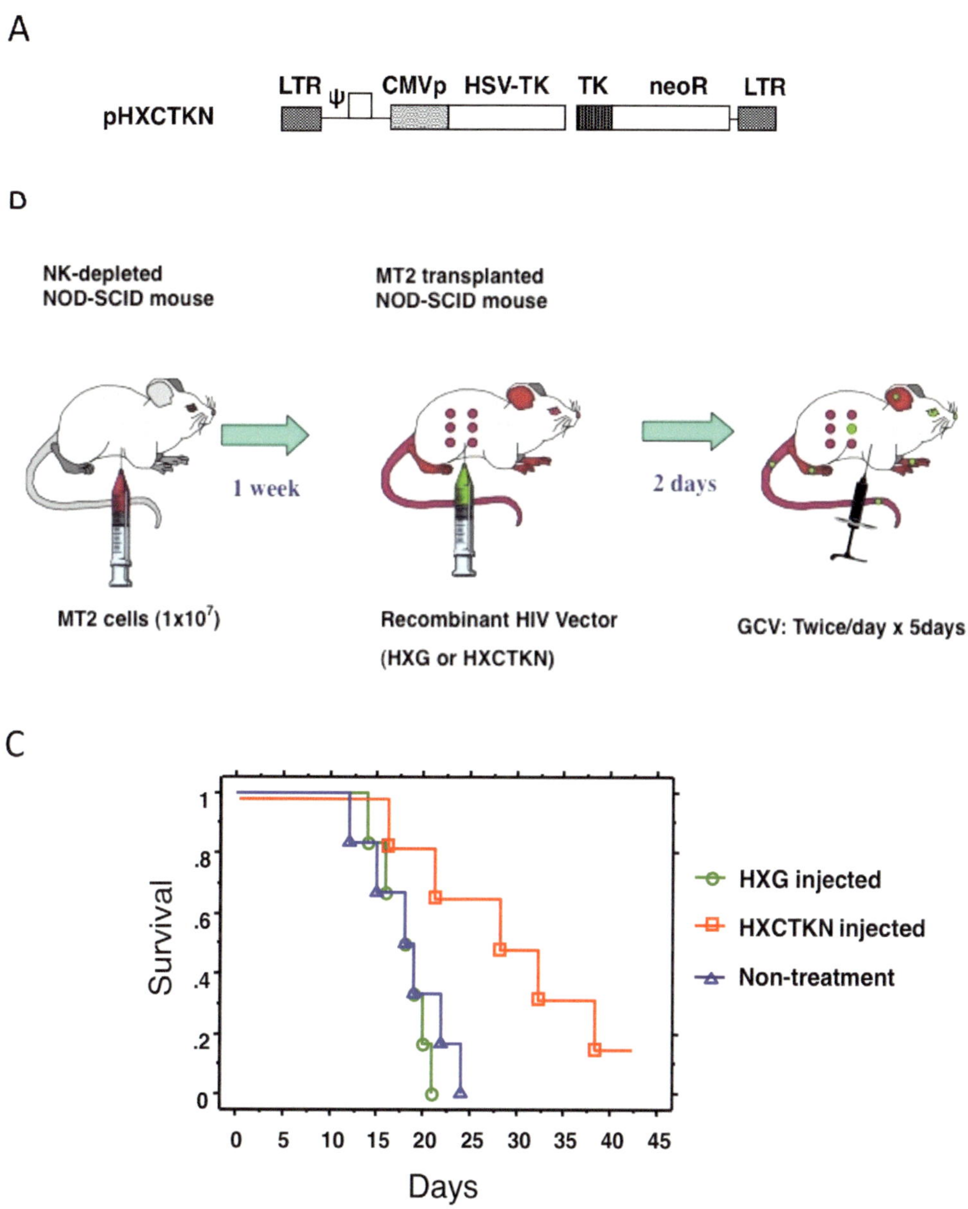

Fig. 10. Selective killing of ATL cells by HIV vector expressing HSV-TK gene. (A) Construction of HIV vector containing the HSV-TK suicide gene. (B) Experimental design of *in vivo* model for ATL. ATL model mice were prepared by intraperitoneal injection of 1×10^7 MT2 cells into NK-depleted NOD-SCID mice. Two days after treatment by HIV vectors (HXG or HXCTKN), GCV was administered twice a day for 5 days. (C) Survival curve of HIV vector treated ATL model mice. Mice administered HXCTKN-injected survived significantly longer than those injected with HXG ($p=0.002$).

5. Summary and future developments

Tissue-specific gene transfer and expression are crucial for the development of safe and effective gene therapy protocols. In that context, HIV-based retroviral vectors pseudotyped with HIV envelope have several advantages compared to MLV or VSV pseudotyped HIV vector. We succeeded in concentration of HIV vectors and primary $CD4^+$ cells were efficiently transduced with high titer HIV vectors. Moreover, HIV vector is potentially useful for *in vivo* gene transfer into T lymphocytes. These findings strongly suggest that concentrated HIV vectors should be useful in gene therapies targeting lymphocytes and macrophages.

HIV based retroviral vectors were originally designed for gene therapy in the treatment of AIDS. And HIV vector have a lot of advantages of for gene therapy of AIDS (Table. 2). Therefore, we developed novel gene therapy strategy for AIDS using our original HIV vectors. Tissue specific transduction into HIV-infectable cells and inducible expression of HIV-infected cells were achieved by using HIV vector. We used an HIV vector containing the HSV-TK gene to selectively kill HIV-1-infected cells and to inhibit HIV-1 replication. Although this system may not represent a complete cure for AIDS, combining gene therapy with other anti HIV-1 therapies may be useful for the long-term control of the disease.

Currently, recombinant HIV vectors were prepared by transiently transfecting Cos cells with packaging plasmid and transfer vector plasmid using the $CaPO_4$ coprecipitation method. Therefore, to make a high titer HIV vector, a large number of cell plate and a lot of plasmids are need. A stable packaging system for producing HIV vectors may be useful for future clinical applications using HIV vectors.

6. Acknowledgment

We thank Hiroki Matsuoka, Noriyasu Sakai, Noriko Miyake and Osamu Iijima for helpful discussion and technical assistance. This work was supported in part by grants from the Ministry of Health and Welfare of Japan and the Ministry of Education, Science and Culture of Japan.

7. References

Alkhatib G., Combadiere C., Broder C. C., Feng Y., Kennedy P. E., Murphy P. M. & Berger E. A. (1996). CC CKR5: a RANTES, MIP-1alpha, MIP-1beta receptor as a fusion cofactor for macrophage-tropic HIV-1. Science 272,1955-1958.

Baltimore D. (1988). Gene therapy. Intracellular immunization. Nature 335,395-396.

Collman R., Hassan N. F., Walker R., Godfrey B., Cutilli J., Hastings J. C., Friedman H., Douglas S. D. & Nathanson N. (1989). Infection of monocyte-derived macrophages with human immunodeficiency virus type 1 (HIV-1). Monocyte-tropic and lymphocyte-tropic strains of HIV-1 show distinctive patterns of replication in a panel of cell types. J Exp Med 170,1149-1163.

Deng H., Liu R., Ellmeier W., Choe S., Unutmaz D., Burkhart M., Di Marzio P., Marmon S., Sutton R. E., Hill C. M., Davis C. B., Peiper S. C., Schall T. J., Littman D. R. & Landau N. R. (1996). Identification of a major co-receptor for primary isolates of HIV-1. Nature 381,661-666.

Feng Y., Broder C. C., Kennedy P. E. & Berger E. A. (1996). HIV-1 entry cofactor: functional cDNA cloning of a seven-transmembrane, G protein-coupled receptor. Science 272,872-877.

Hacein-Bey-Abina S., Garrigue A., Wang G. P., Soulier J., Lim A., Morillon E., Clappier E., Caccavelli L., Delabesse E., Beldjord K., Asnafi V., MacIntyre E., Dal Cortivo L., Radford I., Brousse N., Sigaux F., Moshous D., Hauer J., Borkhardt A., Belohradsky B. H., Wintergerst U., Velez M. C., Leiva L., Sorensen R., Wulffraat N., Blanche S., Bushman F. D., Fischer A. & Cavazzana-Calvo M. (2008). Insertional oncogenesis in 4 patients after retrovirus-mediated gene therapy of SCID-X1. J Clin Invest 118,3132-3142.

Hacein-Bey-Abina S., Von Kalle C., Schmidt M., McCormack M. P., Wulffraat N., Leboulch P., Lim A., Osborne C. S., Pawliuk R., Morillon E., Sorensen R., Forster A., Fraser P., Cohen J. I., de Saint Basile G., Alexander I., Wintergerst U., Frebourg T., Aurias A., Stoppa-Lyonnet D., Romana S., Radford-Weiss I., Gross F., Valensi F., Delabesse E., Macintyre E., Sigaux F., Soulier J., Leiva L. E., Wissler M., Prinz C., Rabbitts T. H., Le Deist F., Fischer A. & Cavazzana-Calvo M. (2003). LMO2-associated clonal T cell proliferation in two patients after gene therapy for SCID-X1. Science 302,415-419.

Howe S. J., Mansour M. R., Schwarzwaelder K., Bartholomae C., Hubank M., Kempski H., Brugman M. H., Pike-Overzet K., Chatters S. J., de Ridder D., Gilmour K. C., Adams S., Thornhill S. I., Parsley K. L., Staal F. J., Gale R. E., Linch D. C., Bayford J., Brown L., Quaye M., Kinnon C., Ancliff P., Webb D. K., Schmidt M., von Kalle C., Gaspar H. B. & Thrasher A. J. (2008). Insertional mutagenesis combined with acquired somatic mutations causes leukemogenesis following gene therapy of SCID-X1 patients. J Clin Invest 118,3143-3150.

Hoxie J. A., Alpers J. D., Rackowski J. L., Huebner K., Haggarty B. S., Cedarbaum A. J. & Reed J. C. (1986). Alterations in T4 (CD4) protein and mRNA synthesis in cells infected with HIV. Science 234,1123-1127.

Lewis P. F. & Emerman M. (1994). Passage through mitosis is required for oncoretroviruses but not for the human immunodeficiency virus. J Virol 68,510-516.

Maddon P. J., Dalgleish A. G., McDougal J. S., Clapham P. R., Weiss R. A. & Axel R. (1986). The T4 gene encodes the AIDS virus receptor and is expressed in the immune system and the brain. Cell 47,333-348.

Matsuoka H., Miyake K. & Shimada T. (1998). Improved methods of HIV vector mediated gene transfer. Int J Hematol 67,267-273.

Miyake K., Iijima O., Suzuki N., Matsukura M. & Shimada T. (2001). Selective killing of human immunodeficiency virus-infected cells by targeted gene transfer and inducible gene expression using a recombinant human immunodeficiency virus vector. Hum Gene Ther 12,227-233.

Miyake K., Inokuchi K., Miyake N., Dan K. & Shimada T. (2007a). HIV vector-mediated targeted suicide gene therapy for adult T-cell leukemia. Gene Ther 14,1662-1667.

Miyake K., Miyake N. & Shimada T. (2007b). Development of targeted gene transfer into human primary T lymphocytes and macrophages using high-titer recombinant HIV vectors. J Biotechnol 129,532-538.

Miyake K., Suzuki N., Matsuoka H., Tohyama T. & Shimada T. (1998). Stable integration of human immunodeficiency virus-based retroviral vectors into the chromosomes of nondividing cells. Hum Gene Ther 9,467-475.

Miyake K., Tohyama T. & Shimada T. (1996). Two-step gene transfer using an adenoviral vector carrying the CD4 gene and human immunodeficiency viral vectors. Hum Gene Ther 7,2281-2286.

Ott M. G., Schmidt M., Schwarzwaelder K., Stein S., Siler U., Koehl U., Glimm H., Kuhlcke K., Schilz A., Kunkel H., Naundorf S., Brinkmann A., Deichmann A., Fischer M., Ball C., Pilz I., Dunbar C., Du Y., Jenkins N. A., Copeland N. G., Luthi U., Hassan M., Thrasher A. J., Hoelzer D., von Kalle C., Seger R. & Grez M. (2006). Correction of X-linked chronic granulomatous disease by gene therapy, augmented by insertional activation of MDS1-EVI1, PRDM16 or SETBP1. Nat Med 12,401-409.

Ratner L., Fisher A., Jagodzinski L. L., Mitsuya H., Liou R. S., Gallo R. C. & Wong-Staal F. (1987). Complete nucleotide sequences of functional clones of the AIDS virus. AIDS Res Hum Retroviruses 3,57-69.

Sakai N., Miyake K., Suzuki N. & Shimada T. (2001). Selective transduction of HIV-1-infected cells by the combination of HIV and MMLV vectors. Int J Hematol 73,476-482.

Shimada T., Fujii H., Mitsuya H. & Nienhuis A. W. (1991). Targeted and highly efficient gene transfer into CD4+ cells by a recombinant human immunodeficiency virus retroviral vector. J Clin Invest 88,1043-1047.

Sodroski J. G., Rosen C. A. & Haseltine W. A. (1984). Trans-acting transcriptional activation of the long terminal repeat of human T lymphotropic viruses in infected cells. Science 225,381-385.

17

Highly Efficient Retrograde Gene Transfer for Genetic Treatment of Neurological Diseases

Shigeki Kato[1], Masahito Kuramochi[1], Kenta Kobayashi[1], Ken-ichi Inoue[2], Masahiko Takada[2] and Kazuto Kobayashi[1]
[1]*Department of Molecular Genetics, Institute of Biomedical Sciences, Fukushima Medical University School of Medicine, Fukushima,*
[2]*Systems Neuroscience Section, Primate Research Institute, Kyoto University, Inuyama,*
Japan

1. Introduction

Gene transfer vectors derived from neurotropic viruses provide a powerful tool for gene therapy of a variety of neurological diseases. The lentiviral vector system permits the efficient transfer of genes into non-dividing cells in the central nervous system and sustains long-term expression of the genes (Naldini et al., 1996; Reiser et al., 1996; Mochizuki et al., 1998; Mitrophanous et al., 1999). This vector system has been used for gene therapy trials in animal models for neurological diseases (for reviews, see Azzouz et al., 2004a; Wong et al., 2006; Lundberg et al., 2008). Axonal transport in the retrograde direction, as observed in the case of some viral vectors, has a considerable advantage for transferring genes into neuronal cell bodies situated in regions remote from the injection sites of the vectors (see Fig. 1). These viral vectors, when injected into the striatum, deliver the genes through retrograde transport into nigrostriatal dopamine neurons that are the major target for gene therapy of Parkinson's disease (Zheng et al., 2005; Barkats et al., 2006). Intramuscular injection of the vectors also delivers retrogradely the genes into motor neurons that are the target for gene therapy of motor neuron diseases (Baumgartner & Shine, 1998; Perrelet et al., 2000; Mazarakis et al., 2001; Sakamoto et al., 2003; Azzouz et al., 2004b).

To enhance the gene transfer of a human immunodeficiency virus type-1 (HIV-1)-based vector via retrograde transport, we have previously generated the HIV-1 vector pseudotyped with a selective variant of rabies virus glycoprotein (RV-G) (Kato et al., 2007). Injection of this RV-G-pseudotyped vector into the mouse striatum yields an increase in gene transfer into neuronal populations in the cerebral cortex, thalamus, and ventral midbrain, each of which innervates the striatum. Injection of the RV-G pseudotype into the monkey striatum (caudate and putamen) results in increased gene transfer into the nigrostriatal dopamine neurons. The RV-G pseudotyping of the HIV-1 vector enhances the efficiency of gene transfer through retrograde axonal transport in the rodent and nonhuman primate brains. However, because large-scale application of gene therapy trials requires

high-titer stocks of the vector, a lentiviral vector system that produces more efficient retrograde gene transfer is needed.
Recently, we developed a novel vector system for highly efficient retrograde gene transfer (designated as HiRet vector) by pseudotyping the HIV-1 vector with fusion glycoprotein B type (FuG-B), in which the cytoplasmic domain of RV-G was substituted by the corresponding part of the vesicular stomatitis virus glycoprotein (VSV-G) (Kato et al., 2011). The HiRet vector shifts the transducing property of the lentiviral vector and promotes the retrograde gene transfer into different brain regions innervating the striatum with greater efficiency than that of the RV-G pseudotype in both rodent and nonhuman primate brains. In the present chapter, we describe the development and property of the HiRet vector as well as the retrograde gene transfer of the vector into target neurons for gene therapy of neurological diseases, such as Parkinson's and motor neuron diseases.

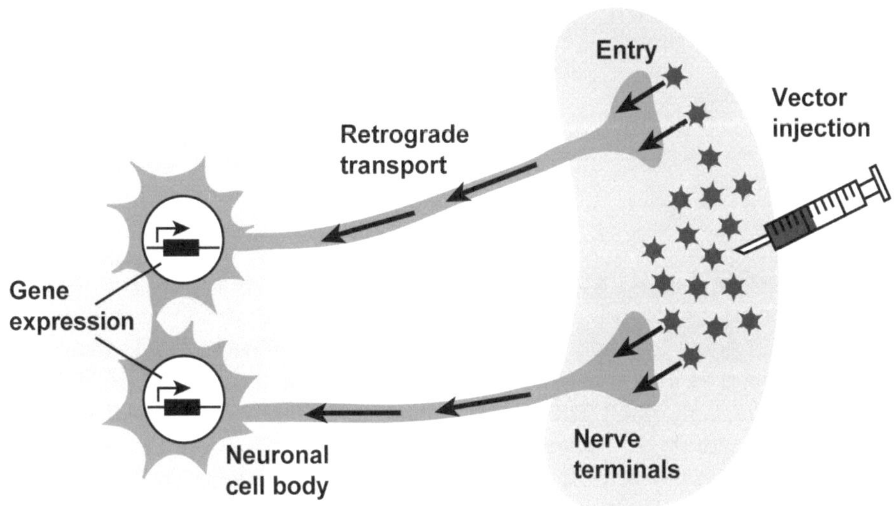

Fig. 1. **Schematic illustration of gene transfer process through retrograde axonal transport.** The viral vectors enter synaptic terminals and are transported within axons in the retrograde direction to neuronal cell bodies where transgene expression is induced.

2. Development and characterization of HiRet vector

2.1 Pseudotyping with fusion envelope glycoprotein

To develop the HiRet vector, we tested two kinds of fusion glycoprotein (termed FuG-A and FuG-B), both of which are composed of the RV-G and VSV-G segments, for the pseudotyping of the HIV-1 vector. FuG-A contains the extracellular domain of RV-G fused to the transmembrane and cytoplasmic domains of VSV-G, whereas FuG-B contains the extracellular and transmembrane domains of RV-G connected to the VSV-G cytoplasmic domain (Fig. 2A). HIV-1-based lentiviral vectors carrying transgene encoding green fluorescent protein (GFP) were produced by pseudotyping with RV-G, FuG-A, or FuG-B. When the functional titer (transducing unit) in HEK293T cells was measured by flow cytometry, the titer of the FuG-B pseudotype was 13 times greater than that of the RV-G pseudotype, whereas the titer of the FuG-A pseudotype in this cell line showed only a moderate increase compared with the RV-G vector titer (Fig. 2B). The functional titer of the FuG-B pseudotype, when measured in neuronal cell lines (Neuro2A and N1E-115 cells), was also the highest among the three vector pseudotypes (Fig. 2B). In contrast, the concentration of physical particles (or RNA copy number) of the vectors, when estimated by quantitative reverse transcription-PCR analysis, showed no remarkable change among the three pseudotypes (data not shown). Therefore, the HIV-1 vector pseudotyped with FuG-B exhibited a greatly increased efficacy of transduction into cultured cells.

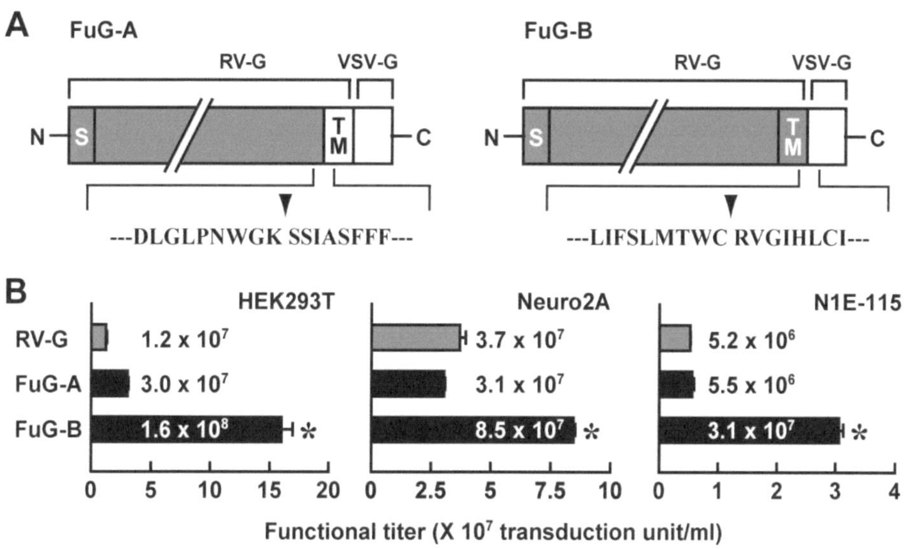

Fig. 2. **Production of vector pseudotypes with fusion glycoproteins.**
(**A**) Structure of the fusion glycoproteins FuG-A and FuG-B composed of different combinations of the N-terminal and C-terminal segments from RV-G and VSV-G. Amino acid sequences around the junction (arrowhead) between the RV-G and VSV-G segments are indicated. S, signal peptide; TM, transmembrane domain. (**B**) Functional titer of the vector pseudotypes. HEK293T cells (eighteen 10-cm-diameter tissue culture dishes) were transfected, and the conditioned medium was collected. Vector particles were pelleted by ultracentrifugation and resuspended in PBS (1 ml). HEK293T, Neuro2A, and N1E-115 cells were transduced with viral vectors, and the functional titer was determined by flow cytometry. Values were obtained from four independent experiments. *$p < 0.001$, significant difference from the titer of the RV-G or FuG-A pseudotype (ANOVA, Tukey HSD test). (Data from Kato et al., 2011)

2.2 Promoted efficiency of retrograde gene transfer

To characterize the *in vivo* gene transfer of the pseudotyped lentiviral vectors, we injected the vectors into the dorsal striatum of mice, and studied gene expression in the brain regions that innervate the striatum, including the primary motor cortex (M1), primary somatosensory cortex (S1), parafascicular thalamic nucleus (PF), and substantia nigra pars compacta (SNc). The number of GFP-positive cells in each brain region was prominently increased in the FuG-B vector-injected mice over that in the RV-G vector-injected mice (Fig. 3A); and the increases in the cell number were 12-, 12-, 8-, and 14-fold in the M1, S1, PF, and SNc, respectively (Fig. 3B). In contrast, the cell number in each brain region was comparable between the FuG-A and RV-G vector-injected animals (Fig. 3A, B). Therefore, the FuG-B pseudotyping of the HIV-1 vector greatly enhanced the efficiency of retrograde gene transfer into the brain regions innervating the dorsal striatum. Based on these *in vivo* data, we designated the FuG-B pseudotype as the HiRet vector.

In the HiRet vector, the cytoplasmic domain of RV-G was substituted by the corresponding part of VSV-G, which resulted in the enhancement of transduction of cell lines and

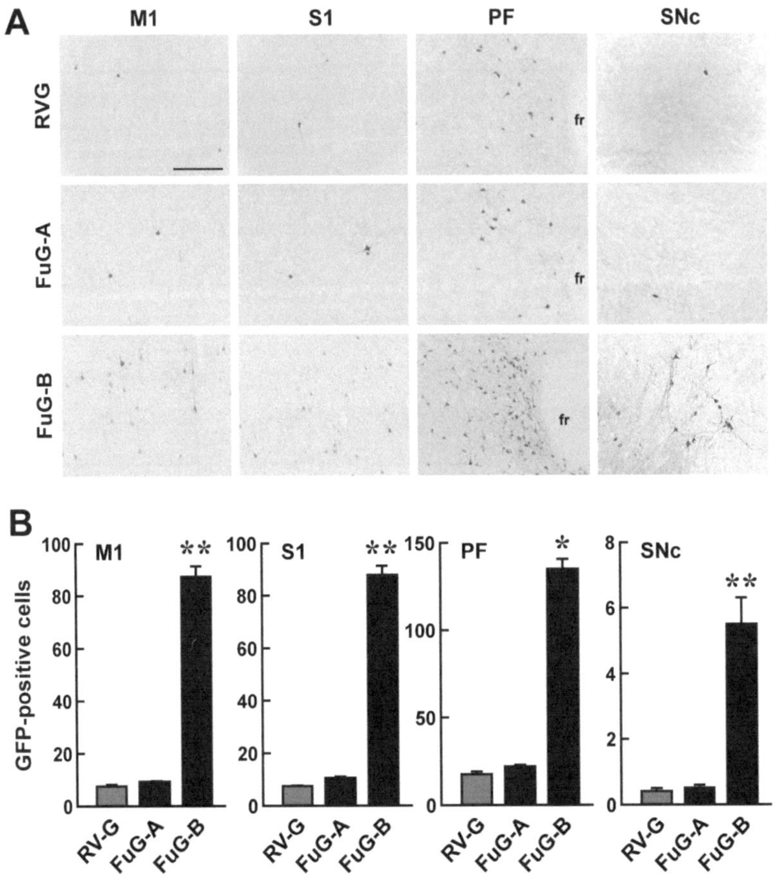

Fig. 3. **Efficiency of retrograde gene transfer by the pseudotyped vectors.**
Lentiviral vectors pseudotyped with RV-G, FuG-A or FuG-B with equivalent copy numbers of viral RNA (1.2 x 10^{10} copies/ml, 1.0 µl x 2 sites) were injected into the mouse striatum, and four weeks later sections were used for GFP immunostaining. (**A**) Transgene expression through retrograde transport in the primary motor cortex (M1), primary somatosensory cortex (S1), parafascicular thalamic nucleus (PF), and substantia nigra pars compacta (SNc). fr, fasciculus retroflexus. Scale bars: 200 µm. (**B**) The cell number in the various brain regions. The number of GFP-positive cells per section was counted (n = 4). $^{*}p < 0.01$, $^{**}p < 0.001$, significant differences from the RV-G or FuG-A pseudotype (ANOVA/Tukey HSD test). (Data from Kato et al., 2011)

retrograde gene transfer. The cytoplasmic domain differs in length between RV-G (44 amino acids) and VSV-G (29 amino acids), and their amino acid sequences do not show any particular homology (Rose et al., 1982). To test whether the length of the cytoplasmic sequence may be involved in the enhancement of retrograde gene transfer, we constructed deletion mutants of the RV-G cytoplasmic domain consisting of 10 or 20 amino acids, and used them for the pseudotyping of the HIV-1 vector. Analysis of the *in vivo* gene transfer indicated that shorter cytoplasmic domain of RV-G increased the efficiency of gene transfer through retrograde transport, but that the VSV-G cytoplasmic domain induced most efficiently the retrograde gene transfer (data not shown). The results suggest the importance of both the length and sequence of the glycoprotein cytoplasmic domain in the retrograde gene transfer of the HiRet vector. Based on our titration experiments using the pseudotyped vectors, the viral RNA titration displayed no significant change in the yield of physical particles between the pseudotyped vectors. Modification of the cytoplasmic domain of a viral glycoprotein thus seemed to shift the property of gene transduction of the pseudotyped vectors into the host cells, although the efficacy of formation or budding of the particles appeared to be unaffected.

The host range of lentiviral vectors is altered by pseudotyping with distinct envelope glycoproteins (for review, see Cronin et al., 2005). RV-G interacts with certain neuronal receptors, such as the nicotinic acetylcholine receptor α-subunit, low-affinity nerve growth factor receptor, and neural cell adhesion molecule (Hanham et al., 1993; Gastka et al., 1996; Thoulouze et al., 1998; Tuffereau et al., 1998). Substitution of the cytoplasmic domain of a viral glycoprotein may influence incorporation of the glycoprotein into vector particles or cause conformational changes in the glycoprotein structure involved in binding to receptor molecules or membrane fusion of the pseudotyped vector. These changes may affect the mechanism involved in vector entry into synaptic terminals or the transduction level of the vector, resulting in the enhanced retrograde gene transfer.

3. Retrograde gene delivery by HiRet vector into target neurons for gene therapy

3.1 Nigrostriatal dopamine neurons

We investigated the capability of the HiRet vector to introduce retrograde gene transfer into target neurons for gene therapy of neurological diseases. Nigrostriatal dopamine neurons are the major target for the therapy of Parkinson's disease (Zheng et al., 2005; Barkats et al., 2006). Retrograde gene transfer of the HiRet vector into the dopamine neurons in the mouse SNc was less efficient, although transfer of the vector into cortical and thalamic neurons was greatly increased (see Fig. 3). We thus tested the retrograde gene transfer of the HiRet vector into the SNc of the monkey. The pseudotyped vectors were injected into the striatum (caudate nucleus and putamen) of crab-eating monkeys, and sections through the SNc were stained immunohistochemically for GFP. Injection of the HiRet vector (FuG-B pseudotype) resulted in the appearance of a larger number of GFP-positive cells in the SNc as compared with that of the RV-G pseudotype (Fig. 4A), and the increase was 10-fold of the RV-G pseudotype control (Fig. 4B). The GFP transgene was expressed in a majority of the dopamine neurons (74.8%, n = 2), which were identified by immunostaining for tyrosine hydroxylase (TH), a key enzyme of dopamine biosynthesis (Fig. 4C). The HiRet vector thus achieved highly efficient delivery of genes through retrograde transport into the nigrostriatal dopamine system in the nonhuman primate brain.

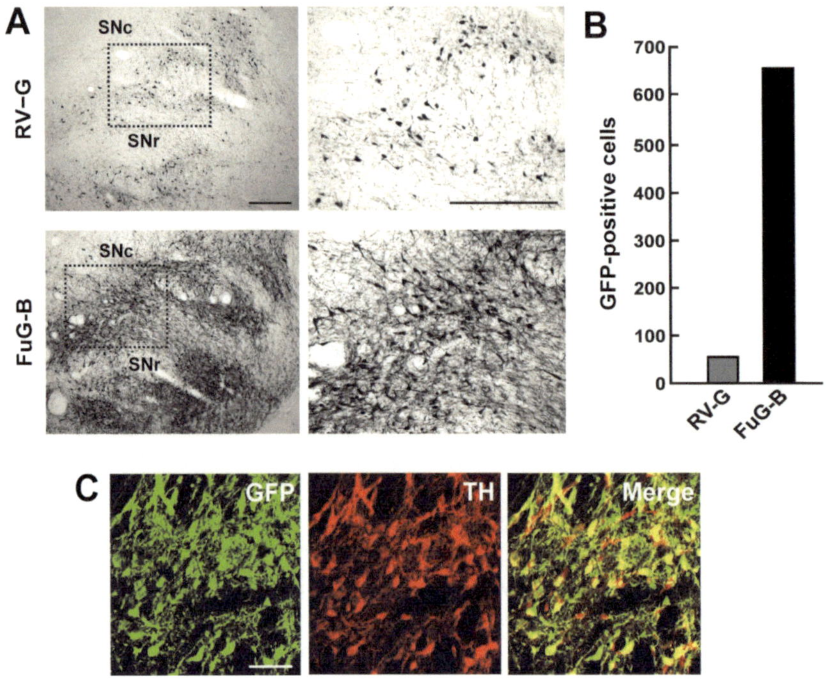

Fig. 4. **Retrograde gene transfer into nigrostriatal dopamine neurons.**
Lentiviral vectors pseudotyped with RV-G or FuG-B with equivalent copy numbers of viral RNA (8.5×10^9 copies/ml, 7.5 µl x 14 sites) were stereotaxically injected into the caudate and putamen, and four weeks later a series of sections were used for histological analysis. (**A**) GFP staining of sections through the SNc. Photos at the right denote magnified views of the rectangular boxes in the left ones. (**B**) Average number of GFP-positive cells per SNc section (n = 2). (**C**) Double immunofluorescence staining for GFP and TH in the SNc. GFP-positive signals, TH-positive signals, and merged images are presented in green, red, and yellow, respectively. SNr, substantia nigra pars reticulata. Scale bars, 1 mm (**A**) and 50 µm (**C**). (Data from Kato et al., 2011)

3.2 Hindbrain/spinal motor neurons

Motor neurons are the target for gene therapy of motor neuron diseases (Baumgartner & Shine, 1998; Perrelet et al., 2000; Mazarakis et al., 2001; Sakamoto et al., 2003; Azzouz et al., 2004b). Therefore, we studied retrograde gene transfer of the HiRet vector into motor neurons in the hindbrain and spinal cord. The vector was injected into the tongue or hindlimb muscles in mice, and sections through the hindbrain (hypoglossal nerve) or spinal cord (lumbar level) were stained for GFP immunohistochemistry. Such injections labeled cells in the hypoglossal nucleus of the posterior hindbrain and in the ventral horn of the spinal cord at the lumbar level (Fig. 5A). Double immunofluorescence histochemistry for GFP and the motor neuronal marker choline acetyltransferase confirmed GFP expression in the hypoglossal and spinal motor neurons that innervate the injected muscles (Fig. 5B). The HiRet vector thus enabled us to induce retrograde gene delivery into motor neurons. The extent of motor neuron transfer of the HiRet vector will be compared with that of the RV-G pseudotype elsewhere.

4. Conclusion

The lentiviral vector system based on HIV-1 has been extensively applied to gene therapy trials for neurological diseases. Retrograde axonal transport of viral vectors offers a great advantage to the delivery of genes into neuronal cell bodies that are located in brain areas distant from the injection site. The pseudotyping of HIV-1-based vectors with selective variants of RV-G increases gene transfer via retrograde transport into the central nervous system. Since the large-scale application for gene therapy trials requires high-titer stocks of the vector, the pseudotyping of a lentiviral vector that generates a greater efficiency of retrograde transport was needed. Therefore, we developed the HiRet vector for highly efficient retrograde gene transfer by pseudotyping an HIV-1 vector with a fusion envelope glycoprotein FuG-B, in which the cytoplasmic domain of RV-G was substituted by the corresponding part of VSV-G. The HiRet vector shifted the transducing property of the

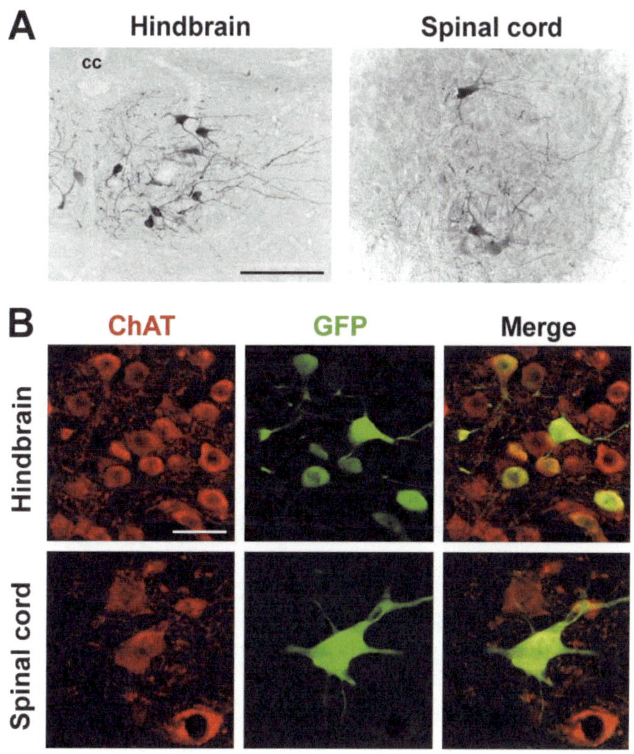

Fig. 5. **Retrograde gene transfer into motor neurons.**
(**A**) GFP expression in the hindbrain and spinal cord after the FuG-B vector injection (2.4×10^9 transduction units/ml). Sections through the posterior hindbrain containing the hypoglossal nucleus and the lumbar spinal cord were prepared from the injected animals and stained by using GFP immunohistochemistry. (**B**) GFP expression in motor neurons. The sections were used for double immunofluorescence staining for GFP and choline acetyltransferase (ChAT), a marker of motor neurons. GFP-positive signals, ChAT-positive signals, and merged images are shown in green, red, and yellow, respectively. cc, central canal. Scale bar: 50 μm.

lentiviral vector and enhanced the retrograde transport-mediated gene transfer into different brain regions. In particular, its transfer efficiency into the brain regions innervating the striatum attained 8- to 14-fold increases over the efficiency of the RV-G pseudotype. In addition, intrastriatal injection of the HiRet vector in the monkey brain resulted in gene transfer into a large number of nigrostriatal dopamine neurons that are the major target for gene therapy of Parkinson' disease. Furthermore, intramuscular injection of the HiRet vector achieved gene transfer into motor neurons in the hindbrain and spinal cord that are the target for gene therapy of motor neuron diseases. Our strategy with the HiRet vector provides a powerful tool for the treatment of certain neurological diseases by promoting retrograde gene delivery of this viral vector.

5. Acknowledgements

This work was supported by grants-in aid from Core Research for Evolutional Science and Technology of Japan Science and Technology Agency. A part of this work was supported by "Highly Creative Animal Model Development for Brain Sciences" carried out under the Strategic Research Program for Brain Sciences by the Ministry of Education, Culture, Sports and Technology of Japan. We thank St. Jude Children's Research Hospital (Dr. A. Nienhuis) and the George Washington University for providing the HIV-1-based vector system, Drs. T. Okada and H. Yaginuma for the analysis of gene transfer into motor neurons, Dr. H. Mizukami for critical reading of the manuscript. We are also grateful to M. Kikuchi, N. Sato, M. Watanabe, and T. Kobayashi for their technical support in the animal experiments.

6. References

Azzouz, M., Kingsman, S.M. & Mazarakis, N.D. (2004a). Lentiviral Vectors for Treating and Modeling Human CNS Disorders. The *Journal of Gene Medicine,* Vol.6, No.6, (September), pp. 951-962.

Azzouz, M., Ralf, G.S., Storkebaum, E., Walmsley, L.E., Mitrophanous, K.A., Kingsman, S.M., Carmellet, P. & Mazarakis, N.D. (2004b). VEGF Delivery with Retrogradely Transported Lentivector Prolongs Survival in a Mouse ALS Model. *Nature,* Vol.429, No. , (May), pp.413-417.

Barkats, M., Horellou, P., Colin, P., Millecamps, S., Faucon-Biguet, N. & Mallet, J. (2006). 1-Methyl-4-phenylpyridinium Neurotoxicity Is Attenuated by Adenoviral Gene Transfer of Human Cu/Zn Superoxide Dismutase. *Journal of Neuroscience Research,* Vol.83, No.1, (February), pp. 233-242.

Baumgartner, B.J. & Shine, H.D. (1998). Permanent Rescue of Lesioned Neonatal Motoneurons and Enhanced Axonal Regeneration by Adenovirus-Mediated Expression of Glial Cell Line-Derived Neurotrophic Factor. *Journal of Neuroscience Research,* Vol.54, No.6, (December), pp.766-777.

Cronin, J., Zhang, X.-Y. & Reiser, J. (2005). Altering the Tropism of Lentiviral Vectors through Pseudotyping. *Current Gene Therapy,* Vol. 5, No.4, (August), pp.387-398.

Gastka, M., Horvath, J. & Lentz, T.L. (1996). Rabies Virus Binding to the Nicotinic Acetylcholine Receptor α Subunit Demonstrated by Virus Overlay Protein Binding Assay. *Journal of General Virology,* Vol.77, No.10, (October), pp. 2437-2440.

Hanham, C.A., Zhao, F. & Tignor, G.H. (1993). Evidence from the Anti-Idiotypic Network That the Acetylcholine Receptor Is a Rabies Virus Receptor. *Journal of Virology*, Vol. 67, No.1, (January), pp.530-542.

Kato, S., Inoue, K., Kobayashi, K., Yasoshima, Y., Miyachi, S., Inoue, S., Hanawa, H., Shimada, T., Takada, M. & Kobayashi, K. (2007). Efficient Gene Transfer via Retrograde Transport in Rodent and Primate Brains Using a Human Immunodeficiency Virus Type 1-Based Vector Pseudotyped with Rabies Virus Glycoprotein. *Human Gene Therapy*, Vol.18, No.11, (November), pp.1141-1151.

Kato, S., Kobayashi, K., Inoue, K., Kuramochi, M., Okada, T., Yaginuma, H., Morimoto, K., Shimada, T., Takada, M. & Kobayashi, K. (2011). A Lentiviral Strategy for Highly Efficient Retrograde Gene Transfer by Pseudotyping with Fusion Envelope Glycoprotein. *Human Gene Therapy*, Vol.22, No.2, (February), pp.197-206.

Lundberg, C., Björklund, T., Carlsson, T., Jakobsson, J., Hantraye, P., Déglon, N. & Kirik, D. (2008). Applications of Lentiviral Vectors for Biology and Gene Therapy of Neurological Disorders. *Current Gene Therapy*, Vol.8, No.6, (December), pp. 461-473.

Mazarakis, N.D., Azzouz, M., Rohll, J.B., Ellard, F.M., Wilkes, F.J., Olsen, A.L., Carter, E.E., Barber, R.D., Baban, D.F., Kingsman, S.M., Kingsman, A.J., O'Malley, K. & Mitrophanous, K.A. (2001). Rabies Virus Glycoprotein Pseudotyping of Lentiviral Vectors Enables Retrograde Axonal Transport and Access to the Nervous System after Peripheral Delivery. *Human Molecular Genetics*, Vol.10, No.19, (September), ppt.2109-2121.

Mitrophanous, K.A., Yoon, S., Rohll, J.B., Patil, D., Wilkes, F.J., Kim, V.N., Kingsman, S.M., Kingsman, A.J., & Mazarakis, N.D. (1999). Stable Gene Transfer to the Nervous System Using a Non-Primate Lentiviral Vector. *Gene Therapy*, Vol.6, No.11, (November), pp.1808-1818.

Mochizuki, H., Schwartz, J.P., Tanaka, K., Brady, R.O. & Reiser, J. (1998). High-Titer Human Immunodeficiency Virus Type 1-Based Vector Systems for Gene Delivery into Nondividing Cells. *Journal of Virology*, Vol.72, No.11, (November), pp.8873-8883.

Naldini, L., Blömer, U., Gage, F.H., Trono, D. & Verma, I.M. (1996). Efficient Transfer, Integration, and Sustained Long-Term Expression of the Transgene in Adult Rat Brains Injected with a Lentiviral Vector. *Proceedings of the National Academy of Sciences of the United States of America*, Vol.93, No.21, (October), pp.11382-11388.

Perrelet, D., Ferri, A., MacKenzie, A.E., Smith, G.M., Korneluk, R.G., Liston, P., Sagot, Y., Terrado, J., Monnier, D. & Kato, A.C. (2000). IAP Family Proteins Delay Motoneuron Cell Death *In Vivo*. *European Journal of Neuroscience*, Vol.12, No.6, (June), pp.2059-2067.

Reiser, J., Harmison, G., Kluepfel-Stahl, S., Brady, R.O., Karlsson, S. & Schubert, M. (1996). Transduction of Nondividing Cells Using Pseudotyped Defective High-Titer HIV Type 1 Particles. *Proceedings of the National Academy of Sciences of the United States of America*, Vol.93, No.26, (December), pp.15266-15271.

Rose, J.K., Doolitttle, R.F., Anilionis, A., Curtis, P.J. & Wunner, W.H. (1982). Homology between the Glycoproteins of Vesicular Stomatitis Virus and Rabies Virus. *Journal of Virology*, Vol.43, No.1, (July), pp.361-364.

Sakamoto, T., Kawagoe, Y., Shen, J.-S., Takeda, Y., Arakawa, Y., Ogawa, J., Oyanagi, K., Ohashi, T., Watanabe, K., Inoue, K., Eto, Y. & Watabe, K. (2003). Adenoviral Gene Transfer of GDNF, BDNF and TGFβ, but not CNTF, Cardiotrophin-1 or IGF1,

Protects Injured Adult Motoneurons after Facial Nerve Avulsion. *Journal of Neuroscience Research*, Vol.72, No.1, (April), pp.54-64.

Thoulouze, M.-I., Lafage, M., Schachner, M., Hartmann, U., Cremer, H. & Lafon, M. (1998). The Neural Cell Adhesion Molecule Is a Receptor for Rabies Virus. *Journal of Virology*, Vol.72, No.9, (September), pp.7181-7190.

Tuffereau, C., Bënëjean, J., Blondel, D., Kieffer, B. & Flamand, A. (1998). Low-Affinity Nerve-Growth Factor Receptor (P75NTR) Can Serve as a Receptor for Rabies Virus. *The EMBO Journal*, Vol.17, No.24, (December), pp.7250-7259.

Wong, L.F., Goodhead, L., Prat, C., Mitrophanous, K.A., Kingsman, S.M. & Mazarakis, N.D. (2006). Lentivirus-Mediated Gene Transfer to the Central Nervous System: Therapeutic and Research Applications. *Human Gene Therapy*, Vol.17, No.1, (January), pp.1-9.

Zheng, J.S., Tang, L.L., Zheng, S.S., Zhan, R.Y., Zhou, Y.Q., Goudreau, J., Kaufman, D. & Chen, A.F. (2005). Delayed Gene Therapy of Glial Cell Line-Derived Neurotrophic Factor is Efficacious in a Rat Model of Parkinson's Disease. *Molecular Brain Research*, Vol.134, No.1, (March), pp.155-161.

18

Herpes Simplex Virus Type 1 for Use in Cancer Gene Therapy: Looking Backward to Move Forward

Cuddington, Breanne and Mossman, Karen
McMaster University
Canada

1. Introduction

Herpes simplex virus type 1 (HSV-1) belongs to the *Herpesviridae* family, *Alphaherpesvirinae* subfamily. HSV-1 is a human pathogen associated with keratitis and cold sores, the formation of which is exacerbated by periods of elevated stress, corticosteroid use and immunosuppression. HSV-1 is an enveloped double stranded DNA (dsDNA) virus which following primary infection in epithelial cells follows a retrograde course to establish latency in sensory nerves of the sacral ganglia. Upon reactivation, HSV-1 travels anterograde from latently infected neurons to epithelial cells at the site of primary infection. Antiherpetic drugs such as Acyclovir (ACV) and Gancyclovir (GCV) are used to control herpes virus infection by inhibiting virus replication.

The mature HSV-1 virion consists of an envelope containing 13 different glycoproteins embedded in a lipid bilayer. An icosahedral nucleocapsid encases the dsDNA genome and consists of three different proteins; VP5 forms both hexameric and pentameric complexes that are supported by VP19C/VP23 trimers. The tegument lies between the envelope and capsid and contains viral and cellular proteins, some of which are essential for virus replication. Following cellular entry, capsids dock at the nuclear pore and the genome exits the capsid via channels, which are controlled by tegument proteins.

The HSV-1 genome is ~152 kbp and consists of long and short regions which are covalently linked (Figure 1). Each region is comprised of unique and repeated sequences. Terminal repeat sequences with single nucleotide overhangs allow for circularization during replication and latency. Homologous recombination between these regions produces four isomers in equimolar concentrations (Shen & Nemunaitis, 2006). Overall, the HSV-1 genome codes for approximately 90 proteins, some of which are dispensable for virus replication *in vitro* and some of which are present in more than once copy, making HSV-1 diploid for genes such as infected cell protein 0 (ICP0), ICP4 and ICP34.5.

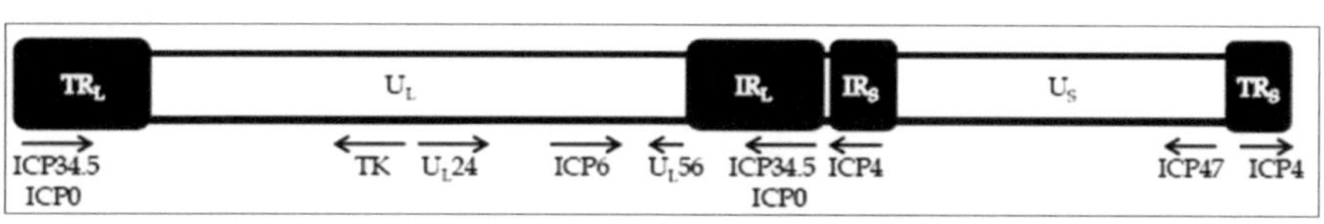

Fig. 1. Schematic of the HSV Genome (TR$_L$: terminal repeat long, U$_L$: unique long, IR$_L$: internal repeat long, IR$_S$: internal repeat short, U$_S$: unique short, TR$_S$: terminal repeat short)

1.1 Cellular entry

Initial attachment of HSV-1 involves binding of glycoprotein B (gB) and/or gC to heparin sulphate proteoglycans on the cellular surface in a low-affinity interaction. This interaction induces a conformational change in gD, relieving steric hindrance of its N-terminal domain and exposing a flexible hairpin loop which binds Herpesvirus entrance mediators (HVEMs) in a high-affinity interaction (Heldwein & Krummenacher, 2008). Members of the immunoglobulin superfamily, nectin-1 and nectin-2, bind via a separate site at tyrosine 28 of gD (Heldwein & Krummenacher, 2008). The binding sites of HVEM and nectin do not overlap and thus require different conformations of gD for binding to occur. Downstream signalling cascades induce a conformational change in gB and/or gC and the gH/gL complex to bring about full fusion of the virus envelope with the cellular membrane. The viral capsid is released into the cytoplasm, and along with several tegument proteins, travels to the nucleus via the microtubular network (Shen & Nemunaitis, 2006). The HSV-1 genome enters the nucleus via nuclear pores to initiate virus replication. While HSV-1 has also been shown to enter cells via endocytosis, the factor(s) which dictate this method of entry remain uncertain.

1.2 Virus replication

Upon entry into the nucleus the HSV-1 genome is transcribed in a highly regulated cascade proceeding from immediate early (IE) genes, to early (E), then late (L) genes. Each gene functions as an independent transcriptional unit through a separate promoter. In general, genes are clustered based on function, not on the order in which they are transcribed. For a comprehensive review, please refer to Roizman & Sears (1996).

Transcription is initiated through association of VP16, a L gene product which resides in the tegument, with the cellular DNA-binding protein Oct-1, which binds the "TATGARAT box" within the enhancer region of IE promoters. The C-terminus of VP16 is a potent transcriptional activating domain which enhances RNA polymerase II (RNA Pol II) activity. There are five IE genes, ICP0, ICP4, ICP22, ICP27 and ICP47, four of which have functions as regulatory factors to initiate lytic infection, while the fifth, ICP47, functions in immune evasion. ICP4 is a major transcriptional activator essential to viral replication. ICP0 acts along with ICP4 to enhance E gene transcription and is also involved in countering the host antiviral response. In addition, ICP22 and ICP27 enhance viral gene transcription by regulating activation of RNA Pol II and modulating post-transcriptional events, respectively. When sufficient levels of IE genes have been transcribed, ICP4 inhibits IE gene expression and activates E gene expression. This switch is mediated by the activation of host RNA Pol II by IE gene products and results in the expression of proteins essential for viral replication such as DNA polymerase, single-strand DNA binding proteins, helicase-primase complex and ori-binding proteins. The accumulation of E gene products results in viral DNA replication at replication compartments located in the nucleus. Lastly, L genes are transcribed following DNA replication and code for structural proteins such as those included in the nucleocapsid and viral envelope. Rolling circle replication produces concatemers which are cleaved by pac1/2 enzymes at specific sequences forming monomers which are then packaged into a nucleocapsid. At this time several tegument proteins associate with the newly formed nucleocapsid and help direct budding through the inner nuclear membrane, resulting in acquisition of an immature envelope. The immature envelope is lost and a new one is formed as the virion fuses and passes through the outer nuclear membrane into the cytoplasm. Additional tegument proteins, such as VP16, associate with the nucleocapsid to direct formation of the mature envelope, which is acquired as the virion passes through the Golgi complex to the cellular membrane. Incorporation of glycoproteins into the envelope occurs at the Golgi and functions to direct the virus to the cellular membrane from which the new virion will bud.

1.3 Latency

HSV-1 is a neurotropic virus which establishes life-long latency within the neurons of its host. Primary infection occurs in epithelial cells after which the nucleocapsid and tegument are transported retrograde along sensory neurons at the site of infection. During latency, viral DNA associates with histones to form an episome and active replication does not occur (Shen & Nemunaitis, 2006). However, latency-associated transcripts (LATs) are abundantly transcribed during latency and are antisense (in part) to the gene transcript which encodes ICP0, suggesting it may interfere with ICP0 synthesis to prevent productive gene expression from occurring in latently infected neurons. Furthermore, LATs do not code for protein products but rather are alternatively spliced RNA species forming two different transcripts (2 and 1.5 kb) of varying abundance (Shen & Nemunaitis, 2006). LATs have also been shown to protect neuronal cells from apoptosis by inhibiting both extrinsic and intrinsic apoptosis pathways by blocking caspase 8 and 9 activity, respectively (Ahmed et al., 2002; Henderson et al., 2002). Reactivation from latency occurs following cellular stress, increases in corticosteroid and/or hormone levels and immunosuppression, resulting in limited productive gene expression and viral replication. Newly formed virus travels anterograde to re-infect epithelial cells within the site of primary infection.

1.4 Host defense mechanisms

From the moment HSV-1 infects host cells at the site of primary infection, viral mechanisms are in place to counteract host immune responses. The innate immune response is the first line of defense against HSV-1 infection followed by high-affinity adaptive responses. HSV-1 encodes proteins which function to evade the host interferon (IFN) response (Paladino & Mossman, 2009), elude complement system opsonisation (Wakimoto et al., 2003), inhibit antigen presentation on MHC I molecules (Hill et al., 1995), block synthesis of host proteins (Shen & Nemunaitis, 2006), hinder apoptosis, and impede maturation of dendritic cells (DCs) (Kobelt et al., 2003).

Innate cytokines including IFN are produced in response to HSV-1 infection. There are three types of IFN, type I, II and III, with type I and III comprising multiple species. Type I and III IFN are expressed by many different cell types, however type II IFN is primarily produced by activated T cells and natural killer (NK) cells. The effects of IFN are pleiotropic and include antiproliferative, antiviral and immunoregulatory functions executed through the expression of interferon stimulated genes (ISGs) (Sen & Sarkar, 2007). Overall, IFN signalling serves to expand the repertoire of immune effectors involved in the antiviral response and thereby regulates viral replication and spread. The production of IFN in most cell types occurs in three phases: sensitization, induction and amplification. During the sensitization phase, pathogen-associated molecular patterns are recognized by pattern recognition receptors including members of the toll-like receptor (TLR) and retinoic acid-inducible gene-I receptor families. Recognition results in the activation of several cellular transcription factors, including interferon regulatory factor 3 (IRF3) and nuclear factor kappa-light-chain-enhancer of activated B cells (NFκB), and the subsequent expression of

IFNβ. During the inductive phase, secreted IFNβ functions in a positive feedback mechanism by binding its cognate receptor. This leads to expression of additional ISGs via the Janus-activated kinase and signal transducer and activator of transcription (STAT) pathway. The interferon stimulated gene factor 3 (ISGF3) complex, consisting of STAT1, STAT2 and IRF9, translocates to the nucleus and binds the promoter of ISGs, including IRF7. Once activated, the IRF3-IRF7 heterodimer induces expression of additional ISGs including IFNα species. Lastly, during the amplification phase IFNα/β stimulate the production of ISGs such as dsRNA-dependent protein kinase receptor (PKR) and oligoadenylate synthetase (OAS) pathways, which function to inhibit viral protein synthesis and degrade viral RNA, respectively. Due to the pleiotropic effects of IFN during infection, HSV-1 has evolved mechanisms by which to inhibit this potent antiviral response.

Infected cell protein 0 (ICP0) is an IE gene product which is pivotal in counteracting the IFN response. HSV-1 ICP0-null mutants are hypersensitive to IFN such that production of viral mRNA and resultant protein is diminished, leading to reduced plaque forming ability (Mossman et al., 2000). The diverse mechanisms by which ICP0 counteracts the IFN response include inhibition of IRF3, IRF7, and STAT1 activation, and degradation of promyelocytic leukemia protein (PML) (Paladino & Mossman, 2009; Lin et al., 2004; Halford et al., 2006; Everett et al., 1998; Sobol & Mossman, 2006). Although the E3 ubiquitin ligase activity of the RING finger domain of ICP0 has been implicated in the inhibition of cytoplasmic IRF3, this mechanism has been shown to be proteasome-independent (Paladino et al., 2010). In addition to ICP0, the IE gene ICP27 functions in IFN evasion by repressing host transcription, translation, mRNA splicing and induces mRNA degradation. Through these mechanisms ICP27 inhibits IRF3 and STAT1 activation (Melchjorsen et al., 2006; Lin et al., 2004; Melroe et al., 2004; Johnson et al., 2008). However, it should be noted that the ability of ICP27 to inhibit IRF3 may be cell type specific. Deletion of ICP27 does not result in an increase in ISG production in primary human fibroblasts, while the opposite was observed in human macrophages (Melroe et al., 2004; Melchjorsen et al., 2006).

Furthermore, several L proteins including ICP34.5, Us11, virion host shutoff (vhs) and Us3 inhibit the IFN response. ICP34.5 acts in concert with the IRF3 kinase TBK-1 to inhibit IRF3 activation (Verpooten et al., 2009) and with the cellular phosphatase PP1 to reverse PKR-induced inhibition of viral protein synthesis (Chou et al., 1995; He et al., 1997). Us11 inhibits PKR activation by binding PKR itself, or activators of PKR such as dsRNA and PACT (Peters et al., 2002). Us11-mediated inhibition of PKR has been found to enhance the growth of ICP34.5-null HSV-1 (Poppers et al., 2000). Conversely, PKR activation levels in Us11-null HSV-1 infected cells are reduced in comparison to levels in wild type HSV-1 infected cells (Mulvey et al., 2003). Together these data demonstrate an additive effect of Us11 in PKR inhibition. The ability of Us11 to bind dsRNA at late phases of infection prevents the synthesis of 2′-5′ oligoadenylates by inhibiting OAS activation (Cayley et al., 1984; Sanchez & Mohr, 2007). It has been shown that Us11 and OAS directly interact at RNA-containing complexes and can bind the same RNA molecules (Sanchez & Mohr, 2007). The vhs protein is integral in counteracting the host antiviral response, in particular the type I and II IFN signalling cascades. In addition to its roles in inhibiting host protein synthesis by degrading mRNA and disrupting polyribosomes, vhs regulates the expression of ISG transcripts. A study by Leib et al. (1999) found that vhs-null HSV-1 replication was severely reduced in non-dividing cells *in vitro* as well as *in vivo*, resulting in viral clearance within 24 hours. Moreover, vhs mutants are hypersensitive to IFN (Pasieka et al., 2008) and in comparison to wild type HSV-1 show a marked increase in

ISG accumulation (Lin et al., 2004). vhs has also been shown to induce the degradation of IFNγ-specific transcripts, thereby inhibiting type II IFN signalling. Furthermore, vhs inhibits STAT-1 activation and formation of the ISGF3 complex following IFNγ treatment of human DCs (Eisemann et al., 2007; Chee & Roizman, 2004). Lastly, Us3 functions as a protein kinase to impede apoptosis thereby promoting viral gene expression (Leopardi et al., 1997). With respect to the type I and II IFN response, Us3 alters TLR3-mediated signalling by decreasing TLR3 mRNA expression, resulting in depleted IRF3 homodimerization (Peri et al., 2008). Additionally, Us3 post-translationally modifies type II IFN receptors via phosphorylation, resulting in decreased expression of IFNγ-dependent genes (Liang & Roizman, 2008).

The complement system is activated in response to HSV-1 infection leading to formation of a membrane attack complex and lysis of the infected cell. By-products of the complement system recruit inflammatory cells to the site of infection resulting in opsonisation by macrophages. To evade the complement system, HSV-1 gC binds to and inactivates C3, the central convertase in the complement cascade, as well as other components such as C5 and properdin (Wakimoto et al., 2003). This response is variable due to differences in the binding efficiency of gC to its' targets between different strains of virus (Wakimoto et al., 2003). In addition, activity of virus-specific antibodies has been shown to enhance the antiviral activity of the complement system by aiding in activation of the classical pathway (Wakimoto et al., 2003).

Activation of cellular immune effectors is critical to controlling infection, as well as determining the type and strength of the adaptive immune response. Macrophages, NK, DC, cytokines and chemokines control the initial infection and prevent its spread to other tissues (Wakimoto et al., 2003). Persistence of CD8+ T cells in infected neuronal tissue has been implicated in controlling HSV-1 during latency and reactivation (Knickelbein et al., 2008). DCs are potent antigen presenting cells as they are able to induce naïve T cells which in turn stimulate maturation of B cells resulting in production of HSV-1-specific antibodies. HSV-1 is able to infect DCs and thereby block maturation via the IE protein ICP27 (Kobelt et al., 2003). This results in the inability of DCs to induce a potent immune response and antiviral T cell stimulation. HSV-1 ICP47 blocks transporter associated with antigen processing (TAP) preventing translocation of peptides to the endoplasmic reticulum (ER) and thus MHC I formation, ultimately leading to a decrease in activation of CD8+ T cells. Furthermore, vhs reduces expression of MHC I & II, IL-1β and IL-8 and activation of DCs (Eisemann et al., 2007; Chee & Roizman, 2004; Suzutani et al., 2000). Due to repressed CD8+ T cell activity, CD4+ T cells migrate to the area of infection where they secrete cytokines to activate NK cells. This culminates in secretion of IFNγ which increases MHC I production and thus CD8+ T cell activation.

2. Oncolytic virotherapy

The use of viruses to target and lyse cancer cells is a novel approach to cancer therapy that lacks the toxic side effects of many cancer treatments that are currently used. Furthermore, virotherapy has been used in cases where cancer cells have become apoptosis-resistant and are refractory to common treatment modalities. Although the safety and potential benefit of using viruses has been addressed in phase I and II clinical trials, the efficacy remains poor (Ries & Brandts, 2004). Thus, the search for new cancer therapy approaches with a high therapeutic index but limited pathogenicity continues.

Oncolytic virotherapy is based on the observation that some viruses preferentially replicate in and kill cancer cells while having minimal detrimental effects on normal cells (Cervantes-García et al., 2008). It holds potential as a successful avenue of gene therapy given its two-pronged approach, the destruction of cancer cells as a direct result of viral replication, and induction of tumour-specific immunity (Vaha-Koskela et al., 2007). Oncolytic viruses lack the widespread toxicity of chemotherapeutics with local replication of the virus amplifying the input dose and resulting in spread to adjacent tumor cells.
Oncolytic viruses can be divided into two groups, wild type viruses that are naturally oncolytic and do not require mutations to render them oncotropic and those that require genetic modification for selective oncolysis. HSV-1 was the first virus used to demonstrate that a genetic mutation can render a virus oncolytic (Jia & Zhou, 2005, Shen & Nemunaitis, 2006). In fact, HSV-1 has been studied extensively as an oncolytic virus due to the many advantages it possesses for use in virotherapy. A brief section on natural oncolytic viruses has been included and will be followed by a detailed discussion of genetically modified HSV-1 vectors.

2.1 Natural oncolytic viruses

Wild type viruses including, but not limited to, reovirus, measles virus (MV), Newcastle disease virus (NDV), myxoma virus (MYXV), vesicular stomatitis virus (VSV), and Bovine herpesvirus type 1 (BHV-1) do not require a mutation to selectively replicate in tumor cells. These viruses exploit biochemical differences between normal and tumour cells to allow for preferential replication in cancer cells (Vaha-Koskela et al., 2007). In addition, species-specific viruses have gained popularity for use in oncolytic virotherapy due to the absence of pre-existing immunity to these viruses. This lack of immunity prevents premature neutralization through antibody-mediated opsonisation and may also allow for systemic delivery of the virus, therefore improving the therapeutic potential against metastatic lesions.
The selective replication of oncolytic viruses is the result of a collection of gain- or loss-of-function mutations in a given cancer type (Vaha-Koskela et al., 2007). An example of one essential modification and hallmark of most malignant cancer types is the evasion of apoptosis (Hanahan & Weinberg, 2000). This is often the result of gain-of-function mutations in cellular signalling pathways, such as in constituents of the Ras signalling cascade (Ayllon & Rebollo, 2000). Activating mutations in Ras inhibit autophosphorylation of PKR, an important effector molecule in the IFN-mediated antiviral and apoptotic response (Everts & van der Poel, 2005). Wild type viruses that are sensitive to the effects of PKR, such as reovirus and NDV, can infect and replicate in cells with a Ras activating mutation, such as in cancer cells, while remaining inhibited in normal cells (Strong et al., 1998). In addition to its function as a cell cycle and apoptosis regulatory protein, p53 also functions as a potent tumor suppressor. In fact, p53 is the most commonly mutated oncogene in human cancers with over 50% of tumor cells carrying a mutation in p53 (Morris et al., 2002). Furthermore, p53 amplifies innate immune responses to virus infection through such mechanisms as enhancing IFN-dependent responses and increasing IRF9 gene transcription (Muñoz-Fontela et al., 2008). Therefore, disruption of p53 is thought to dampen antiviral defense mechanisms conferring heightened sensitivity of cells to infection (Carroll, P.E. et al., 1999). Reovirus and MYXV replicate to higher levels in cancer cells with reduced expression of p53, and although this is not the major determinant dictating their selective replication in tumor cells, it enhances efficiency of infection (Kim et al., 2010).

Another feature of cancer cells that is often exploited by oncolytic viruses is an impaired IFN response. Upon binding to cellular receptors, IFN induces the expression of ISGs, many of which function to block viral replication (Platanias, 2005; Everts & van der Poel, 2005). A well characterized ISG involved in blocking viral replication is PKR, as discussed previously (Sadler & Williams, 2008; Everts & van der Poel, 2005). In addition to antiviral functions, many ISGs have been identified as tumour suppressors, including PML, ribonuclease (RNase) L, and ISG15 (Everts & van der Poel, 2005; Bernardi & Pandolfi, 2003; Salomoni & Pandolfi, 2002). Furthermore, IRFs have been shown to possess tumour suppressive functions (Pitha et al., 1998; Taniguchi et al., 2001; Shen & Nemunaitis, 2006). For example, IRF-1 has been implicated in cell cycle regulation and apoptosis (Tamura et al., 2008), and the development of some cancers, such as breast (Connett et al., 2005) and hepatocellular carcinoma (Moriyama et al., 2001), is correlated with decreases or loss of IRF-1 expression. Other pathways involved in IFN production, such as NFκB, have been implicated in tumour suppression (Everts & van der Poel, 2005; Chen & Castranova, 2007). Given the diverse antitumorigenic functions of IFN signalling it is common for tumour cells to harbour defects in these pathways, and oncolytic viruses that are sensitive to IFN, such as VSV and NDV, preferentially replicate in tumor cells over normal cells (Jia & Zhou, 2005; Ries & Brandts, 2004; Everts & van der Poel, 2005).

2.1.1 Reovirus

Reovirus is a non-enveloped dsRNA virus which has minimal pathogenicity in humans but can cause gastrointestinal and respiratory symptoms. Selective replication of reovirus occurs in tumor cells harbouring activating mutations in the Ras pathway (Strong et al., 1998; Coffey et al., 1998), as outlined above. Reovirus has shown promise in pre-clinical studies with selective replication in tumors of breast (Strong et al., 1996; Norman et al., 2002; Hirasawa et al., 2002), colon (Kinzler & Vogelstein, 1996), ovarian (Hirasawa et al., 2002), and lymphoid (Alain et al., 2002) origins. Combination therapy involving the immunosuppressant cyclosporine A or anti-CD4+/CD8+ antibodies enhances the oncolytic ability of reovirus in systemic treatment of metastatic malignancies (Hirasawa et al., 2002). A phase I open-label dose-escalation trial with reovirus type 3 Dearing (RT3D) in combination with radiotherapy was performed on twenty-three patients with advanced or metastatic solid tumors (Harrington et al., 2010a). Patients received intralesional injections of RT3D ($1x10^8$ pfu up to $1x10^{10}$ pfu) and were monitored for tumor regression and adverse events. Treatment was well tolerated with no adverse effects associated with virus treatment. Overall, seven patients achieved partial response and seven achieved stable disease. Results of this and other clinical trials using reovirus for the treatment of malignancies support development of this virus as a therapeutic option.

2.1.2 Measles virus

Measles virus (MV) is an enveloped (-)ssRNA virus that causes rash, fever, cough and conjunctivitis in infected humans. Several cases of spontaneous tumor regression have occurred in individuals with MV infection, suggesting an oncolytic attribute for the virus. However, the cellular receptor SLAM, which is used by wild type MV for cellular entry, is not commonly expressed on tumor cells. A live attenuated measles strain with no pathogenicity in humans has been generated by serially passaging the virus in tissue culture. This virus has adapted to use CD46, an inhibitor of complement activation, for cellular entry (Peng et al., 2003a). The CD46 receptor is expressed in higher abundance on human tumor cells than on their non-transformed counterparts, rendering the attenuated strain oncolytic. Attenuated MV has been used to treat B cell malignancies such as non-Hodgkin's lymphoma and myeloma (Grote et al., 2001; Peng et al., 2001). In these studies the formation of multinucleated syncytia increased viral spread and thus the efficacy of virus treatment. In addition, a MV expressing an antibody against CD38, a cell marker highly expressed on myeloma cells, induced cell-cell fusion and cytopathic effects in mouse xenografts resulting in inhibition of tumor growth and prolonged survival (Peng et al., 2003b).

2.1.3 Newcastle disease virus

Newcastle disease virus (NDV) is an enveloped (-)ssRNA avian paramyxovirus that is non-pathogenic to humans. Like reovirus, NDV is unable to counter the effects of PKR and thus requires activated Ras to replicate in tumor cells. While Ras is the main factor determining NDV tropism, mutations in the IFN signalling pathway also confer sensitivity to NDV. Live attenuated strains of NDV have shown efficacy in mouse models of fibroblastoma (Lorence et al., 1994a), neuroblastoma (Lorence et al., 1994b; Reichard et al., 1993), colon (Schulze et al., 2009), prostate (Phuangsab et al., 2001), melanoma (Zamarin et al., 2009), large cell lung (Phuangsab et al., 2001) and breast carcinoma (Zhao et al., 2008; Janke et al., 2007). Moreover, live attenuated NDV strains MTH-68/H and PV701 are currently in clinical trials for high-grade gliomas (HGG) and advanced solid cancer, respectively (Csatary et al., 2004; Pecora et al., 2002).

2.1.4 Vesicular stomatitis virus

Vesicular stomatitis virus (VSV) is an enveloped (-)ssRNA virus that is non-pathogenic to humans. VSV is exquisitely sensitive to the effects of IFN signalling and as such selectively replicates in tumor cells harbouring mutations in IFN and its signalling effectors (Stojdl et al., 2000). The oncolytic ability of VSV has been demonstrated in *in vivo* models of melanoma (Luo et al., 2010; Galivo et al., 2010), colon, and hepatocellular carcinoma (Shinozaki et al., 2004). In a recent study, recombinant VSV expressing human dopachrome tautomerase (hDCT) was used as an immune boost resulting in enhanced efficacy in the B16-F10 model of melanoma. Results indicate the efficacy of VSV in augmenting the antitumor immune response (Bridle et al., 2009).

2.1.5 Myxoma virus

Myxoma virus (MYXV) is an enveloped dsDNA virus that is non-pathogenic in humans. It causes Myxomatosis in European rabbits, which is uniformly fatal due to immunomodulation by several virus-encoded proteins (Stanford et al., 2007). Even in cases of routine exposure to the virus humans do not seroconvert (Stanford & McFadden, 2007). MYXV is restricted from normal mouse cells due to the IFN response, and from normal human cells due to IFN and tumour necrosis factor (TNF) responses (Lun et al., 2005). MYXV has been shown to selectively replicate in human cancer cells of various histological origins (Sypula et al., 2004; Lun et al., 2005, Wang et al., 2008). The cellular tropism of MYXV for human tumor cells largely depends on the interaction of a viral host range factor (M-T5) and cellular Akt, a protein kinase with roles in cellular proliferation, migration, transcription and apoptosis (Wang et al., 2006). This interaction has been shown to induce the kinase activity of Akt resulting in MYXV replication. In a xenograft model of human glioma in immunocompromised mice, intracranial injection of MYXV was well-tolerated and caused regression of the injected tumor. Regression in distal tumors was not observed but virus replication was sustained long term (Lun et al., 2005). Combination therapy trials using rapamycin, an immune and tumor suppressant which upregulates Akt activation via the mTOR pathway, resulted in increased MYXV replication in select tumor types (Werden et al., 2010).

2.1.6 Bovine herpesvirus type 1

Bovine herpesvirus type 1 (BHV-1) is a member of the Herpesviridae family, and Alphaherpesviridae subfamily. BHV-1 causes infectious bovine rhinotracheitis (IBR) in cattle, manifesting in symptoms such as ocular and nasal secretions, lesions on mucosal surfaces, anorexia, dyspnoea, conjunctivitis, and abortions (Turin et al., 1999, Hushur et al., 2003). In approximately 10% of affected animals bacterial superinfection occurs, resulting in bronchopneumonia (Turin et al., 1999). However, in the absence of bronchopneumonia the infection is self-limiting due to the immune response, and recovery occurs within 1 to 2 weeks (Turin et al., 1999). BHV-1 is a neurotropic virus which establishes life-long latency in neurons, with reactivation of the virus resulting from parturition, pregnancy, transport, entrance into a new herd, concomitant bacterial or viral infections, poor living conditions, deficient diet and increases in corticosteroids (Turin et al., 1999, Jones & Chowdhury, 2007).

The structure of BHV-1 is similar to that of HSV-1, however some important differences exist. BHV-1 binds attachment and entry receptors used by HSV-1, such as heparan sulfate and nectin-1 (Campadelli-Fiume et al., 2000). However, it is unable to bind nectin-2, but binds CD155 instead (Campadelli-Fiume et al., 2000). CD155 is a poliovirus receptor associated with tumour cell migration and invasion, and has been shown to be up-regulated in human cancers (Merrill et al., 2004; Pende et al., 2005). Genes expressed by BHV-1 are generally named after the coinciding HSV-1 gene, which often have similar activities although there are some functional differences. For example, bICP0 is similar to HSV-1 ICP0 in that it is an IE gene product which acts as a transcriptional activator and possesses E3 ubiquitin ligase activity inherent to the RING-finger domain. However, bICP0 differs from HSV-1 ICP0 in that it promotes proteasomal-dependent degradation of IRF-3 (Henderson et al., 2005, Saira et al., 2007). Furthermore, while ICP0 induces disruption of PML nuclear bodies (PML-NB) by degrading SUMO-modified forms of PML, bICP0 does not decrease steady-state levels of PML but rather degrades sp100, another major component of PML-NBs (Everett et al., 2010).

Of particular interest is the narrow host range of BHV-1, as it is unable to productively infect mice and normal human cells (Hushur et al., 2003). Also, cattle farmers whom are routinely exposed to the virus do not seroconvert. Rodrigues et al. (2010) showed that human transformed and phenotypically normal immortalized cell types are permissive to BHV-1, while normal primary cell types are relatively resistant to BHV-1 infection (Figure 2). BHV-1 induces cytopathic effects (CPE) and decreases cellular metabolism in immortalized and transformed cells from the lung, mammary, bone and prostate origins with varying efficiency.

Naturally occurring oncolytic viruses such as VSV, MYXV and NDV are sensitive to the effects of type I IFN signalling. However, this is not the case for BHV-1 as cellular IFN-responsiveness does not correlate with sensitivity to BHV-1 (Table 1) (Rodriguez et al.,

2010). IFN production was also absent in BHV-1 infected cells. These observations suggest that a broader factor, or group of factors, limit BHV-1 replication in normal cells.

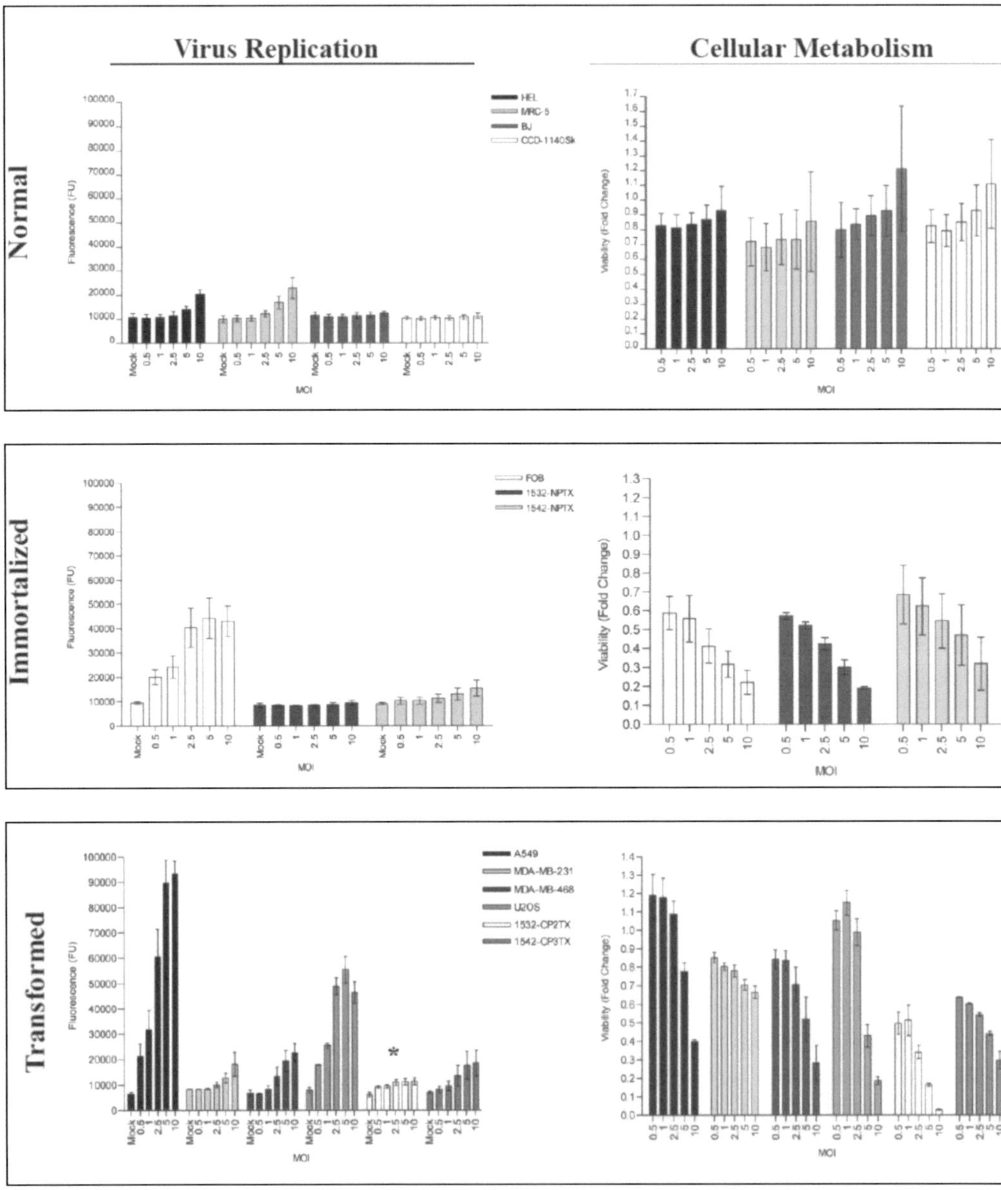

Fig. 2. BHV-1gfp replication and cellular viability in normal, immortalized and transformed human cells. Virus replication, as a function of GFP fluorescence, was quantified two days post infection using a Typhoon Bioanalyzer (Amersham Biosciences). Virus replication is represented in absolute fluorescence units (FU). Cellular metabolism was measured using Alamar blue and is represented as a fold change over uninfected controls. (*) indicates loss of fluorescence due to the absence of viable cells. Data is expressed as the mean from three independent experiments. (Rodriguez et al., 2010)

State	Tissue Type	Cell Line	EC_{50} (U ml^{-1})	CPE
Normal	Lung	HEL	1.499	-
		Ronald	0.538	-
		Ventressca	0.705	-
	Skin	CCD-1140Sk	0.362	-
Immortalized	Mammary	MCF-10A	0.500	++
		HME-1	1.198	+++
	Bone	FOB	1.215	+++
	Prostate	RWPE-1	0.680	+++
		1542-NPTX	0.769	+
Transformed	Lung	A549	3.554	+++
	Mammary	MDA-MB-231	1.317	+
		MDA-MB-468	3.548	+++
	Bone	U2OS	41.249	+++
	Bone metastasis of prostate origin	PC-3	7.226	++
		PC-3M	2.867	++
		PC-3M-M2	10.327	++
		PC-3M-Pro4	8.303	++
		PC-3M-LN4	10.047	+

Table 1. IFN responsiveness for normal, immortalized and transformed cells from a variety of histological origins. Cells were treated with human IFNα for 24 hours prior to infection with VSV-GFP. VSV replication was used to assess the IFN responsiveness of each cell line, as cells responsive to IFN will be unable to support VSV replication. The effective concentration of IFN required to inhibit 50% of GFP fluorescence (EC_{50}) was calculated to compare IFN responsiveness between cell lines. Cytopathic effect (CPE) scoring was performed by infecting cells with BHV-1 at an MOI 0.5, 1. 2.5, 5 or 10. Three days pi cell monolayers were stained with Giemsa to evaluate CPE. (- indicates a non-permissive cell type, no visible CPE; + indicates a cell type that is not very permissive, 50% CPE at MOI >2.5; ++ indicates a moderately permissive cell type, 50% CPE between MOI 1 and 2.5; +++ indicates a highly permissive cell, 50% CPE at MOI <1) (Rodriguez et al., 2010).

These data suggest that BHV-1 holds promise for use in broad spectrum oncolytic virotherapy. The non-pathogenic nature of BHV-1 and lack of pre-existing immunity in humans, as well as the potential for systemic treatment with increased safety offers an advantage over current HSV-1 vectors.

2.2 Engineered oncolytic viruses: HSV-1 vectors

Genetically modified tumor-selective oncolytic viruses are often generated from the deletion of genes that are required for replication in normal cells, but are dispensable in tumor cells. A wide variety of viruses have been engineered for oncolytic virotherapy, including but not limited to, HSV-1, adenovirus, vaccinia virus, poliovirus, and influenza virus. Pathways commonly mutated in tumor cells, such as those involved in regulation of cell cycle and proliferation, are often those exploited by viruses. For example, cell cycle checkpoint proteins p53 and retinoblastoma (Rb), and the Ras family of proteins and their downstream effectors, are commonly mutated in solid and hematologic cancers (Ayllon & Rebollo, 2000). Thus, oncolytic viruses have been generated to selectively replicate in tumor cells possessing these and other mutations. This section will focus on discussion of engineered HSV-1 oncolytic viruses.

2.2.1 First generation vectors

HSV-1 was the first virus used to demonstrate that a genetic mutation can render a virus oncolytic (Jia & Zhou, 2005; Shen & Nemunaitis, 2006). In fact, HSV-1 has been studied extensively as an oncolytic virus due to the many advantages it possesses for use in virotherapy. Its large dsDNA genome (~150 kbp) allows for the insertion of multiple transgenes, up to 30 kbp in length (Everts & van der Poel, 2005; Shen & Nemunaitis, 2006). HSV-1 has been shown to infect a broad number of cell types due to the ubiquitous expression of its receptor in human tissues. The virus is able to kill infected cells as a result of lytic replication and does not insert its DNA into the host genome, reducing the risk of insertional mutagenesis (Varghese & Rabkin, 2002; Shen & Nemunaitis, 2006). Moreover, HSV-1 rarely causes severe illness in immunocompetent adults (Varghese & Rabkin, 2002; Shen & Nemunaitis, 2006) and antiherpetic drugs, such as ACV and GCV, can be used to control viral replication.

Common mutations in HSV-1 oncolytic viruses are in the genes that encode for thymidine kinase (tk) and ribonucleotide reductase, also known as ICP6. These genes are responsible for synthesis of deoxynucleotide triphosphates (dNTPs) and are required for virus replication. Cellular synthesis of dNTPs is upregulated during G1 and S phases of the cell cycle but otherwise remain low. Thus, mutation of the genes encoding tk and ICP6 restrict replication to rapidly proliferating tumor cells. However, studies of the tk-null mutant dlsptk (Table 1) in severe combined immunodeficient (SCID) mice indicated the spread of the virus to normal tissue (Valyi-Nagy et al., 1994). Presence of an intact tk gene can serve as a safe guard against unwanted replication through the use of antiherpetic drugs, such as ACV and GCV. The HSV-1 recombinant hrR3 (Table 1), which is deleted for ICP6, selectively replicates in tumor cells with active ribonucleotide reductase due to their high rate of proliferation. ICP6-null mutants retain sensitivity to ACV and GCV, adding to their safety profile. This mutant has shown promising antitumor effects in animal models of brain (Mineta et al., 1994), pancreas (Kasuya et al., 1999), colon (Yoon et al., 2000; Carroll, N.M. et al., 1996), and liver (Pawlik et al., 2000) carcinoma. In combination therapy trials, co-administration of cyclophosphamide (CPA) or cobra venom factor (CVF) and hrR3 resulted in enhanced antineoplastic effects (Ikeda et al., 2000).

The leaky L gene ICP34.5 is a neurovirulence factor, which when deleted inhibits virus replication in neurons and other cells with a slow doubling time. ICP34.5 also functions to reverse PKR-mediated inhibition of viral protein synthesis. A wide variety of ICP34.5-null HSV-1 mutants have been described which preferentially replicate in cancer cells with Ras gain-of-function mutations (Davis & Fang, 2005; Farassati et al., 2001; Shen & Nemunaitis, 2006). The HSV-1 mutant HSV1716 (Table 1), deleted for both copies of ICP34.5, has shown promise in animal models of glioma (Andreansky et al., 1996), mesothelioma (Kucharczuk et al., 1997), melanoma (Randazzo et al., 1995; Randazzo et al., 1997), and lung carcinoma (Lambright et al., 1999). HSV1716 treatment caused significant tumor regression and prolonged survival. Clinical trials have been initiated for many ICP34.5-null HSV-1 vectors including HSV1716, the details of which will be discussed in section 3.

Virus	Gene(s) Mutated	Transgene	Description	Reference
First Generation				
dlsptk	TK		TK gene deletion	Martuza et al., 1991
hrR3	ICP6	LacZ	LacZ gene insertion within ICP6 coding region	Mineta et al., 1994
HSV1716	ICP34.5 (2)		deletion of both copies of ICP34.5	Randazzo et al., 1995
Second Generation				
NV1020	U_L24, ICP34.5, U_L56	TK	deletion of U_L24, U_L56, one copy of ICP34.5 exogenous TK under control of ICP4 promoter	Advani et al., 1999
G207	ICP34.5 (2), ICP6	LacZ	deletion of both copies of ICP34.5 LacZ gene insertion within ICP6 coding region	Mineta et al., 1995
G47Δ	ICP47, ICP34.5 (2)	LacZ	deletion of ICP47 and both copies of ICP34.5 LacZ gene insertion within ICP6 coding region	Todo et al., 2001b
Transcriptional Targeting				
G92A	TK, U_S3, U_L24	LacZ Alb-ICP4	based on HSV-1 d120 backbone LacZ gene insertion within TK coding regioninsertion of albumin promoter-ICP4 transgene within TK coding region	Miyatake et al., 1999
d12.CALP	TK, U_S3, U_L24	LacZ Cal-ICP4	based on HSV-1 d120 backbone E. coil LacZ gene insertion within TK coding region insertion of the CALP promoter-ICP4 transgene within TK coding region	Yamamura et al., 2001
DF3γ34.5	ICP34.5 (2)	DF3/Muc1 -ICP34.5	deletion of both copies of ICP34.5 insertion of exogenous ICP34.5 gene under control of DF3-MUC1 promoter	Chung et al., 1999
Transgene-expressing/Immunostimulatory				
rRp450	ICP6	CYP2B1	cytochrome p450 oxidase gene insertion within ICP6 coding region	Pawlik et al., 2001
HSV1γCD	ICP6	CD AFP	CD gene insertion within ICP6 coding region AFP gene insertion within ICP6 coding region	Nakamura et al., 2001
dvB7Ig	ICP34.5 (2), ICP6	LacZ B7-1	deletion in both copies of ICP34.5 LacZ gene insertion within ICP6 coding region B7-1Ig inserted within the ICP6 coding region	Ino et al., 2006
NV1034	ICP47, U_L56	LacZ GM-CSF	deletion of ICP47 and U_L56 LacZ gene insertion within ICP47 coding region GM-CSF under control of ICP6-TK hybrid promoter	Wong et al., 2001
NV1042	ICP47, U_L56, ICP34.5	LacZ TK IL-12	deletion of ICP47, U_L56, and one copy of ICP34.5 LacZ gene insertion within ICP47 coding region Rescue of TK expression through insertion of a 5.2kb sequence of HSV-2 origin at the L-S junction mIL-12 under control of the ICP6 promoter	Wong et al., 2001
OncoVEX GM-CSF	ICP47, ICP34.5 (2)	GM-CSF	deletion of ICP47 deletion of both copied of ICP34.5 GM-CSF expressed under control of the ICP47 promoter	Hu et al., 2006

Table 2. Oncolytic HSV-1 Vectors and their corresponding mutations (ICP: infected cell protein, CALP: calponin, MUC1: mucin-1, CD: cytosine deaminase, AFP: alphafetoprotein, GM-CSF: granulocyte macrophage colony-stimulating factor, IL: interleukin, TK: thymidine kinase)

Concerns over safety of using single gene deletion mutants are centered on observations of residual replication and toxicity in normal cells. The development of HSV-1 oncolytic viruses containing mutations in multiple genes increases their safety profile while also decreasing the risk of reversion to wild type. These viruses are referred to as second generation oncolytic vectors.

2.2.2 Second generation vectors

The second generation mutant G207 (Table 1) is at the forefront of oncolytic virotherapy. G207 contains deletions in both copies of ICP34.5 and a lacZ gene insertion within the ICP6 coding region. This virus selectively replicates in human tumor cells over normal cells while retaining sensitivity to antiherpetic drugs. Also, the lacZ gene insertion encodes an easily detectible histochemical maker for virus replication and spread. The safety of G207 has been demonstrated in animal models of liver (Kooby et al., 1999), ovarian (Coukos et al., 2000), melanoma (Todo et al., 2002), breast (Toda et al., 1998), colon, gallbladder, gastric (Todo et al., 2002), head and neck (Wong et al., 2001), pancreatic, prostate (Todo et al., 2002) and cervical carcinoma (Blank et al., 2002). G207 is currently in clinical trials for treatment of malignant glioma (Markert et al., 2000). Another second generation mutant, NV1020 (Table 1), is deleted for tk and one copy of ICP34.5. TK function is provided by insertion of a 5.2 kb fragment of HSV-2 DNA under the control of the ICP4 promoter (Shen & Nemunaitis, 2006). Therefore, NV1020 retains sensitivity to ACV and GCV. The efficacy of NV1020 has been demonstrated in animal models of pancreatic (McAuliffe et al., 2000), head and neck (Wong et al., 2001), and hormone-resistant prostate carcinoma (Advani et al., 1999) with the virus replicating to higher levels in comparison to mutants deleted for both copies of ICP34.5 (Bennett et al., 2002; McAuliffe et al., 2000; Advani et al., 1999). Clinical trials are currently underway using NV1020 to treat colon carcinoma liver metastases via intrahepatic arterial delivery (Kemeny et al., 2006). Furthermore, immunostimulatory HSV-1 vectors and mutants deleted for viral proteins involved in counteracting the immune response have been developed to augment antiviral and antitumor immune responses aiding in tumor regression. G47Δ (Table 1) is a derivative of G207 with an additional deletion in ICP47. Since ICP47 decreases expression of MHC I molecules through inhibition of TAP, its absence promotes tumor antigen presentation and increased antitumor immune responses (Todo et al., 2001b). In comparison to G207, G47Δ conferred enhanced inhibition of tumor growth in both immunodeficient and immunocompetent animal models while retaining the same safety profile (Todo et al., 2001b).

2.3 Transcriptional targeting

Another method of restricting virus replication to tumor cells involves insertion of tissue and/or tumor-specific promoters to drive the expression of genes which are essential to virus replication in tumor cells. This is referred to as transcriptional targeting and has shown promise as an efficient restriction mechanism. The HSV-1 mutant G92A (Table 1) places expression of the IE gene ICP4 under the control of the albumin-enhancer promoter to direct tropism to the liver and hepatocellular carcinomas (Miyatake et al., 1999). Another HSV-1 vector, d12.CALP (Table 1) expresses ICP4 under the control of the calponin promoter and selectively replicates in smooth muscle and bone tumors (Yamamura et al., 2001). In addition, a similar virus DF3γ34.5 (Table 1) expresses ICP34.5 under the control of the DF3/MUC1 enhancer/promoter and is limited to tumors expressing the DF3/MUC1 antigen, such as breast carcinomas (Kasuya et al., 2004). In an effort to direct the tropism of oncolytic herpesvirus KeM34.5 to gliomas, Kanai et al. (2007) used the musashi1 promoter to control expression of ICP34.5. Musashi1 is a neural RNA-binding protein which is used as a molecular marker for malignant glioma. In comparison to its parental vector G207, KeM34.5 showed enhanced cytotoxic ability *in vitro* as well as increased tumor regression in a murine glioma model. Recently, an oncolytic HSV-1 vector (oHSV-MDK-34.5) was developed to treat malignant peripheral nerve sheath tumors (MPNST) by fusing the human midkine (MDK) promoter to the ICP34.5 gene (Maldonado et al., 2010). Selective replication of oHSV-MDK-34.5 in MDK-positive MPNSTs resulted in antitumor effects and prolonged survival of MPNST-bearing nude mice. Oncolytic adenoviruses have been engineered with restricted expression of E1A and E1B genes by placing them under the control of the prostate-specific antigen (PSA) and probasin promoters in CV706 and CV787 respectively (Chen et al., 2001; Yu et al., 1999). For instance, the replication of CV706 was found to be highest in PSA-producing tissues and was able to induce cytotoxic effects in infected tumor cells (Rodriguez et al., 1997).

The differential expression of micro-RNAs (miR) between normal and tumor cell types has been exploited to generate oncolytic HSV-1 vectors which selectively replicate in the absence of select miRs. The expression of miR-143 and miR-145 is significantly down-regulated in prostate carcinomas in comparison to normal healthy tissue. Target sequences for miR-143 or miR-145 were incorporated into the 3′-untranslated region of ICP4 to generate the oncolytic HSV-1 vectors CMV-ICP4-143T and CMV-ICP4-145T (Lee et al., 2009). Tumor-specific replication resulted in significant reductions in tumor volume and enhanced survival in mice bearing LNCaP human prostate tumors.

2.4 Cellular targeting

Modification of viral entry proteins, referred to as cellular targeting, is another method by which the replication of oncolytic vectors can be restricted to certain tissues and tumor cells. The recombinant HSV-1 virus, R5141, was engineered to enter cells solely via the IL-13Rα2 receptor (Zhou et al., 2006). Briefly, the natural binding sites for HSPGs in gB and gC were replaced with the amino acid sequences encoding IL-13. Multiple amino acid substitutions were made in and around the HveA and nectin-1 binding sites to abolish their interaction with gD. An additional vector developed by the same group, R5181, enters cells via the urokinase plasminogen activator receptor. These studies demonstrate the application of this method to multiple receptor classes (Kamiyama et al., 2006). Although the mechanism of HSV-1 entry has not been fully elucidated, the upregulation of receptors on cancer cells, such as epidermal growth factor receptor (EGFR), folate receptor, CD44, CD38 and others, provides the basis for this approach but requires further study to achieve full tumor selectivity.

2.5 Armed oncolytic vectors

Although oncolytic vectors show promise as novel cancer therapeutics, studies indicate that in the majority of cases virus replication on its own is insufficient to induce full tumor regression. Thus, enhanced cytotoxic effects are desired and have been achieved through the expression of 'suicide' and immunostimulatory genes.

Introduction of genes encoding immunostimulatory molecules and prodrug-converting enzymes have been used to enhance the cytolytic ability of oncolytic viruses and augment the antitumor immune response leading to increased tumor regression and survival. Initial 'suicide' gene therapy vectors focused on expressing HSV-1 tk to infer sensitivity to GCV. However, this method inhibited virus replication at early stages and therefore was not efficient. As a result, expression of therapeutic genes are generally placed under the control of a late viral promoter to allow for sufficient virus replication to occur before induction of cytolytic effects that would otherwise halt replication prematurely.

Studies in immunocompetent animals have highlighted a bimodal mechanism of tumor clearance: tumor cell lysis as a result of oncolytic virus replication and induction of an antitumor immune response. Direct injection or use of oncolytic vectors expressing immunostimulatory cytokines has been used to induce inflammatory and tumor antigen-specific responses. Several studies describe vectors expressing granulocyte-macrophage colony-stimulating factor (GM-CSF) as an immunostimulant. GM-CSF induces myeloid precursor cell activation, recruits DCs, and has been used in tumor cell vaccines resulting in increased therapeutic benefits (Toda et al., 2000; Nemunaitis, 2005; Eager et al., 2005). For example, treatment with OncoVEX$^{GM\text{-}CSF}$ (Table 1), a second generation HSV-1 vector, resulted in tumoristatic effects on injected and distal tumors in patients with cutaneous or subcutaneous breast, head and neck, gastrointestinal and malignant melanoma (Hu et al., 2006). HSV-1 constructs NV1034 and NV1042 (Table 1) , expressing GM-CSF or IL-12 respectively, prolonged survival and caused tumor regression in murine models of squamous cell carcinoma (Wong et al., 2001). NV1042 treatment resulted in an enhanced antitumor effect in comparison to NV1034 and a control vector NV1023, which does not express cytokines (Wong et al., 2001). Oncolytic virus treatment was accompanied by the induction of a strong inflammatory response, including accumulation of CD4+ and CD8+ T cells (Wong et al., 2001) and inhibition of tumor angiogenesis (Wong et al., 2004). Overall, 57% of mice treated with NV1042 were refractory to tumor re-challenge, in comparison to 14% of NV1034 and NV1023-treated animals (Wong et al., 2001). These results suggest the establishment of an antitumor memory immune response. The B7 family of membrane proteins, B7-1 (CD80) and B7–2 (CD86), are potent co-stimulatory molecules and interact with CD28 and CTLA-4 (CD152) on the T-cell surface. A HSV-1 vector expressing the B7-1-immunoglobulin (B7-1-Ig) fusion transgene (dvB7Ig) (Table 1) has been studied in a murine model of neuroblastoma (Todo et al., 2001a). Intraneoplastic inoculation of dvB7Ig inhibited tumor growth and prolonged the survival of mice bearing intracerebral tumors. A significant CD4+ and CD8+ T-cell response was observed, with immunodepletion studies indicating that CD8+ T cells play a key role in the antitumor response. Cured animals were refractory to tumor re-challenge indicating establishment of an antitumor memory immune response.

Prodrug-converting enzymes such as cytosine deaminase (CD) and cytochrome p450 oxidase have been used to induce the expression of noxious compounds to enhance oncolytic cytotoxicity. Yeast CD converts the prodrug 5-fluorocytosine to 5-fluorouracil, which inhibits DNA synthesis. HSV1γCD (Table 1), in which ICP6 is inactivated by insertion of CD, has shown promise in murine models of liver metastases (Nakamura et al., 2001). Expression of CD prolonged survival and enhanced tumor regression without significantly affecting virus replication and oncolysis. Furthermore, similar results were obtained using rRp450 (Table 1) a HSV-1 mutant expressing the CYP2B1 transgene which codes for cytochrome p450 oxidase and converts cyclophosphoramide (CPA) into phosphoramide mustard. Despite the immunosuppressive activity of CPA, its expression enhanced the cytolytic effect of rRp450 against hepatocellular carcinoma both *in vitro* and *in vivo* without prematurely inhibiting HSV-1 replication (Pawlik et al., 2002).

3. Clinical trials

The antitumor efficacy of oncolytic herpesviruses has been demonstrated in preclinical animal models. However, evaluation of tumor-selectivity, virus replication and spread must be evaluated in humans. Clinical trials have been completed, or are in progress, for NV1020, HSV1716, G207, OncoVEX$^{GM\text{-}CSF}$ and HF10 (Table 2).

3.1 NV1020 clinical trials

The liver is the most common site of colorectal metastases. It has been estimated that 60% of patients with metastatic colorectal cancer have liver-predominant disease which is the limiting factor determining patient survival (Kemeny et al., 1994; Rosen et al., 1995). Currently, chemotherapy is the first line of treatment prescribed to patients, but rarely produces significant antitumor results (Meyers et al., 2003). Second line therapies are thus pivotal in the treatment of colorectal liver metastases.

In a phase I dose-escalating study twelve patients were divided equally into four cohorts receiving $3x10^6$ plaque forming units (pfu), $1x10^7$ pfu, $3x10^7$ pfu or $1x10^8$ pfu NV1020 via hepatic arterial infusion (Kemeny et al., 2006). NV1020 treatment was well tolerated; however, adverse events associated with virus administration occurred and included pyrexia, headache and rigors. Within the first forty-eight hours, minor elevations in liver enzymes occurred but were self-limiting without intervention and normalized shortly thereafter. Hepatic artery samples indicated viral clearance in all participants, including those receiving a dose of $1x10^8$ pfu. With the exception of one patient, PCR analysis did not detect HSV DNA in saliva, urine, conjunctiva, vaginal, and serum samples. The HSV-positive patient did not experience any HSV-specific adverse effects during the course of the study. Furthermore, levels of serum cytokines, including IL-1, IL-2, IFNγ, and TNFα, as well as cytotoxic T cell counts were measured one week following NV1020 treatment. Minor increases in serum IL-1, IL-2, IFNγ and TNFα occurred but with no apparent relationship to virus administration. Variations in cytotoxic T cell counts were minor and inconsistent among patients. Overall, at twenty-eight days post-treatment two patients exhibited 39% and 20% reductions in tumor size. Of the remaining patients, three showed tumor progression while seven achieved tumor stabilization. This study established that hepatic arterial infusion of NV1020 holds potential as a treatment for colorectal liver metastases.

The phase I study by Kemeny et al. (2006) was used as the foundation for a multicentre phase I/II study evaluating the safety and antitumor effects of multiple doses of NV1020 in patients with colorectal liver metastases (Geevarghese et al., 2010). A total of thirteen and nineteen patients were enrolled in the phase I and II trials respectively. Each patient received four doses of NV1020 via hepatic arterial infusion followed by chemotherapy. The phase I cohort received doses of $3x10^6$ pfu, $1x10^7$ pfu, $3x10^7$ pfu, and $1x10^8$ pfu to determine the optimal dose for use in phase II trials. Adverse events associated with virus treatment were mild and did not involve altered liver function. PCR analysis failed to detect NV1020 DNA in the serum, genital swabs, and saliva of patients. However, HSV-1 DNA was present in the samples of two patients but no HSV-related symptoms were observed. Moreover, serological levels of IL-6, TNFα and IFNγ transiently increased in a dose-dependent manor. Following NV1020 administration, 50% of patients exhibited stable disease and after subsequent chemotherapy 68% maintained this status. The one year survival was 47.2%, a significant increase compared to conventional outcomes. A phase III trial is currently underway for NV1020 treatment of colorectal liver metastases.

Virus	Cancer Type	Phase	Participants	Delivery	Reference
NV1020	Colorectal liver metastases	I	12	hepatic artery	Kemeny et al., 2006
	Colorectal liver metastases	I	13	hepatic artery	Geeverghese et al., 2010
	Colorectal liver metastases	II	19	hepatic artery	Geeverghese et al., 2010
HSV1716	Recurrent glioma	I	9	intratumoral	Rampling et al., 2000
	High-grade glioma	I	12	intratumoral	Papanastassiou et al., 2002
	Recurrent glioma	I	12	intratumoral	Harrow et al., 2004
	Malignant Melanoma	I	5	intratumoral	MacKie et al., 2001
	HNSCC	I	20	intratumoral	Mace et al., 2008
G207	Malignant glioma	I	21	intratumoral	Markert et al., 2000
	Malignant glioma	Ib	6	intratumoral	Markert et al., 2009
	Recurrent glioma	I	9	intratumoral	Karrasch et al., 2009
OncoVEX^{GM-CSF}	Solid tumors	I	30	intratumoral	Hu et al., 2006
	HNSCC	I/II	17	intratumoral	Harrington et al., 2010b
	Metastatic melanoma	II	50	intratumoral	Senzer et al., 2009
HF10	Reccurent breast carcinoma, pancreatic carcinoma	I	9	intratumoral	Nakao et al., 2007
	pancreatic carcinoma	I	6	intratumoral	Nakao et al., 2011

Table 2. Clinical Trials with Oncolytic Herpes Simplex Viruses (HNSCC; head and neck squamous cell carcinoma)

3.2 HSV1716 clinical trials

The use of HSV1716 in the treatment of patients with recurrent glioma and high grade glioma (HGG) has been evaluated in clinical trials. Current therapies for malignant glioma, including radiotherapy and chemotherapy, provide a median survival time of only 1 year following diagnosis (Rampling et al., 1997; Rampling et al., 1998; Subach et al., 1999). Patient survival following primary therapy is a staggering 5 months (Rajan et al., 1994), warranting development of novel treatments which will prolong survival and improve patient outcomes. Preclinical data indicates the ability of HSV1716 to replicate in a wide variety of tumor types including those of central nervous system (CNS) origin (Brown et al., 1994; Randazzo et al., 1995). In murine models of malignant glioma HSV1716 induced significant tumor regression with minimal effect on normal CNS tissue (McKie et al., 1998).

In a phase I dose escalation study nine patients with recurrent malignant glioma received an intratumoral injection of HSV1716 at doses ranging from $1x10^3$-$1x10^5$ pfu (Rampling et al., 2000). All patients had previously undergone radiotherapy and/or surgery and had since relapsed. Virus treatments were well tolerated with no adverse effects. In addition, PCR analysis failed to detect shed HSV1716 or HSV-1 DNA in patient buccal and serum samples. Furthermore, HSV-1 reactivation in the form of skin lesions did not occur. After 14 months, four patients remained alive with two in complete remission. This study demonstrated the feasibility and safety of HSV1716 for treatment of recurrent malignant glioma and constituted the framework for subsequent phase II clinical trials.

An additional proof of principle study evaluated the toxicity and replication of HSV1716 in patients with HGG (Papanastassiou et al., 2002). Twelve patients with HGG received an intratumoral injection of HSV1716 at $1x10^5$ pfu. No adverse effects were observed following injection of the virus or throughout the duration of the study. At four to nine days post-injection, tumors were removed and assayed for the presence of virus. The tumors removed from two participants contained a higher concentration of virus than was injected and contained HSV-specific antigens. It should be noted that these patients were seronegative at the time of injection and subsequently seroconverted. Furthermore, virus replication was not detected in tumors of seropositive patients which could be the result of virus neutralization during the tumor resection process. However, PCR analysis detected HSV1716 DNA at the injection site of ten patients and at distal sites in four, including seropositive individuals. Together these data demonstrate that HSV1716 was able to selectively replicate in patient gliomas and spread to distal tumor sites despite the presence of pre-existing immunity in seropositive individuals. Further to the first study, this clinical trial added to the safety profile of HSV1716 for use in the treatment of malignant glioma.

In the third clinical trial with HSV1716 for treatment of HGG, the virus was used to clear residual tumor cells after resection (Harrow et al., 2004). Following tumor resection, residual tumor cells remain within the resection cavity and ultimately divide to form a new tumor mass. A total of twelve patients were enrolled in the trial, six with recurrent disease and six newly diagnosed. Following tumor resection patients were injected with $1x10^5$ pfu HSV17161 into adjacent brain tissue. In addition, eight to ten sites adjacent to the tumor bed were also injected. All patients received subsequent radiotherapy or chemotherapy. Magnetic resonance imaging (MRI) or computed tomography (CT) scans were taken pre- and postoperatively to monitor tumor regression and the structural anatomy of the surrounding brain tissue. Patients also underwent single photon emission computed tomography (SPECT) to identify HGG growth as indicated by areas of high cellular metabolic activity. At the time of tumor resection, patient tumor cells were collected for *ex vivo* HSV1716 replication analysis. Results indicate the ability of HSV1716 to replicate in HGG tumor cells. No significant adverse effects or toxicity associated with HSV1716

treatment was observed. Overall, three patients were clinically stable up to twenty-two months post-treatment. Tumor regression was evident in the patient alive after twenty-two months as indicated by imaging analysis. The lack of viral-mediated toxicity post-HSV1716 injection into normal brain tissue demonstrates the utility of this virus for use in combination therapy for patients with HGG.
Preclinical studies indicate the ability of HSV1716 to selectively replicate in human melanoma cells *in vitro* and cause tumor regression in murine models of melanoma (MacKie et al., 2001). In a pilot study to ascertain the efficacy of HSV1716 treatment for melanoma, five HSV-1 seropositive patients with stage four melanoma received intratumoral injections of HSV1716 at $1x10^3$ pfu (MacKie et al., 2001). Two patients received one injection, two received two injections and one received four injections. No adverse effects were observed and anti-HSV antibody titres did not significantly increase with treatment. Injected nodules were excised at fourteen (single injection) or twenty one (multiple injections) days post-injection for assessment of pathology and virus replication. One patient showed flattening of tumor nodules twenty-one days post-injection while all participants had evidence of tumor necrosis. There was no indication of pathogenesis or necrosis in adjacent normal melanocytes. This study established the utility of HSV1716 as a treatment for melanoma, with replication and associated pathology restricted to tumor cells.
Comparable to malignant glioma, the five year survival rates for patients with head and neck squamous cell carcinoma (HNSCC) ranges from 0-40% depending on localization of the tumor (Forastiere et al., 1998). Patient relapse rates and the high incidence of distant metastases makes HNSCC a formidable challenge requiring novel therapeutic options. A total of twenty patients with oral HNSCC received intratumoral injections of $1x10^5$ pfu (five patients) or $5x10^5$ pfu (fifteen patients) HSV1716 (Mace et al., 2008). Injections were well tolerated with no adverse effects associated with virus treatment. Of the patients enrolled in the study two were seronegative, but both seroconverted within a week of HSV1716 injection. However, the seropositive cohort did not experience changes in anti-HSV antibody levels post-injection. Interestingly, PCR analysis detected HSV DNA in the blood of all patients receiving the lower dose of $1x10^5$ pfu; however, no infectious virus was recovered from any tissue sample as determined by an infectious plaque assay. Tumor histology was negative for inflammation and necrosis at injection sites but infiltration of inflammatory lymphocytes was apparent. Although significant tumor regression was not observed in this trial, results warrant a dose escalation study due to the established safety profile of HSV1716 for treatment of HNSCC.

3.3 G207 Cclinical trials

The HSV-1 mutant G207 has shown exceptional promise in clinical trials for the treatment of malignant glioma. Preclinical data shows that G207 is able to selectively replicate in tumor cells from a variety of histological origins including gliomas (Mineta et al., 1995). Furthermore, the non-pathogenic nature of G207 was confirmed through intracerebral injection of the virus into HSV-susceptible mice and simian primates (Hunter et al., 1999; Mineta et al., 1995). These data led to evaluation of G207 in a phase I dose escalation trial for the treatment of malignant glioma (Markert et al., 2000). Twenty one patients were enrolled in the study and received one of three intratumoral dosing regimens. Patients in the first cohort received doses ranging from $1x10^6$ to $1x10^8$ pfu, the second cohort received a single dose of $1x10^9$ pfu, and the third cohort received a dose of $3x10^9$ pfu at five distinct sites within the tumor mass. Three patients were included in each dose cohort and injection sites were determined by contrast enhanced areas indicated on CT scans. All doses of G207 were well tolerated with no serious adverse effects associated with virus inoculation. Tumor biopsies were performed post-injection on six patients, and brains were obtained upon autopsy from five deceased patients. PCR analysis indicated the presence of G207 DNA in resected tumors obtained from patients at 56 and 157 days post-injection. However, viral shedding was absent from all patient saliva samples. Tumor regression was seen in eight patients ranging from four days to one month post-injection. Two patients have survived over four years and one patient died from causes unrelated to G207 treatment. The promising results borne from this trial are the cornerstones for design of a phase 1b trial involving G207 treatment of recurrent malignant glioma followed by tumor resection and tumor bed inoculation.

Objectives of the phase 1b clinical trial were four fold (Markert et al., 2009). The safety of two intratumoral injections within a one week period was ascertained as well as the safety associated with direct injection of G207 into normal brain tissue. Furthermore, virus replication and the presence of anti-HSV immune effectors were measured in inoculated tumors. Six patients were enrolled in the study, each receiving two doses of G207 totalling 1.5×10^9 pfu. Specifically, an initial intratumoral injection of 1.5×10^8 pfu was delivered via catheter followed by tumor resection two to five days later. Subsequent injections of G207 were administered into brain tissue surrounding the resection cavity. Treatment was well tolerated with most adverse effects unrelated to G207 inoculation. PCR analysis did not detect HSV DNA in patient saliva, urine, conjunctiva and serum samples despite the presence of virus replication in resected tumor samples from three patients. Inflammation was not present at the inoculation site as determined through patient MRIs, and no patients developed viral encephalitis, even after two injections of G207. Tumor samples were obtained from one patient pre- and post-G207 treatment for immunohistochemical analysis. Prior to treatment only a small population of immune effectors, including lymphocytes and macrophages, were present in the tumor. However, two days post G207 injection there was significant infiltration of mature T cells including cytotoxic T cells, monocytes, macrophages, microglia, and NK cells (Figure 3). The presence of B cells was also detected in the tumor sample but at much lower levels. All seronegative patients subsequently seroconverted following G207 treatment and half of seropositive participants experienced an increase in anti-HSV antibody titres. Due to the small sample size no conclusions regarding the efficacy of G207 treatment can be drawn. However, according to MRI analysis no participants achieved a complete or partial response, defined as a 50% decrease in contrast enhancing tumor volume following G207 administration. Results from this study warrant the progression of G207 therapy for malignant glioma to phase II clinical trials.

A combination therapy study for the treatment of recurrent malignant glioma demonstrated an additive effect of G207 and radiotherapy (Karrasch et al., 2009). In a phase I clinical trial, nine patients received intratumoral injections of 1×10^9 pfu G207 followed by focal radiotherapy (5 Gray) twenty four hours later. Combination therapy was well tolerated and dose-limiting toxicities were not reached. Patients achieving a partial response were re-treated with G207 and radiotherapy one month following initial treatment due to tumor recurrence. The median survival times for patients suffering from relapsed gliomablastoma multiforme and anaplastic astrocytoma was 7.4 and 9.25 months, respectively. HSV DNA was detected within tumors indicating intratumoral G207 replication. Overall, G207 combination therapy prolonged patient survival over traditional treatment modalities.

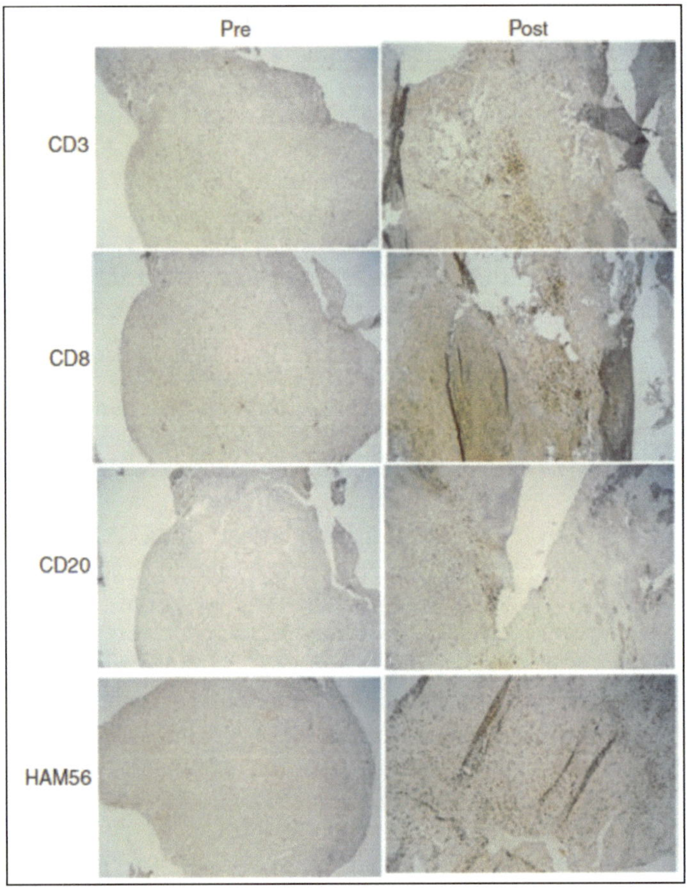

Fig. 3. Tumor-infiltrating lymphocytes and macrophages in patient tumor tissue pre- and post-G207 treatment. Immunohistochemical staining was performed on paraffin blocks of patient tumor samples pre- and post-G207 treatment using antibodies against CD3 (infiltrating T cells), CD8 (cytotoxic and suppressor T cells), CD20 (B cells), and HAM56 (monocyte/macrophage).

3.4 OncoVEX^{GM-CSF} clinical trials

Generation of OncoVEX^{GM-CSF} was prompted by the success of other HSV vectors as well as the need for increased antitumor immune activity during therapy.

A phase I study involving thirty patients with breast, head and neck, gastrointestinal, and melanoma malignancies evaluated the safety and antitumor activity of OncoVEX^{GM-CSF} (Hu et al., 2006). Participants were divided into two cohorts, thirteen received a single intratumoral injection at one of three dose levels ($1x10^6$ pfu, $1x10^7$ pfu and $1x10^8$ pfu), and the remaining seventeen were placed in a multi-dose group and received escalating doses of virus every one to three weeks. All doses were well tolerated with no adverse events associated with virus treatment occurring in either the single or multi-dose groups. However, seronegative participants experienced more pronounced injection site irritation which eventually cleared without intervention. It was also observed that all seronegative individuals seroconverted within three to four weeks of their first injection of OncoVEX^{GM-CSF}. Transient elevations in anti-HSV antibody titres occurred in seropositive patients but did not limit therapeutic efficacy. PCR analysis detected HSV DNA in the blood of two patients in the single dose cohort (eight hours and one week post-injection) and in eight patients in the multi-dose cohort (one and eight hours post-injection). Low levels of HSV DNA were detected in the urine of two patients in the single dose cohort (eight hours and one week post-injection), and no patients tested positive in the multi-dose cohort. Viral DNA was not detected at any other time points during the study. Tumor biopsies indicated the infiltration of immune effectors following OncoVEX^{GM-CSF} injection, including increases in T cell and macrophage populations. Areas of tumor necrosis were found to correspond to sites of virus injection, while normal tissue showed no evidence of necrosis. Stable disease was detected in three patients, two with melanoma and one with breast cancer. Furthermore, the injected tumors of several patients with metastatic melanoma regressed or were cleared but other metastatic lesions appeared at distal sites. No partial or complete responses were reached in this study but the safety and tumoristatic effects of OncoVEX^{GM-CSF} treatment on injected and distal tumors was established.

The phase I trial by Hu et al. (2006) established the safety and efficacy of OncoVEX^{GM-CSF} for the treatment patients with metastatic melanoma, laying the ground work for a phase II clinical trial (Senzer et al., 2009). A total of fifty patients with stage IIIc (10) or stage IV (40) metastatic melanoma received an initial intratumoral injection of OncoVEX^{GM-CSF} at $1x10^6$ pfu to seroconvert patients who were seronegative and to reduce adverse effects associated with virus injection, as primarily seen in seronegative patients. Three weeks later patients received another intratumoral injection at $1x10^8$ pfu, which was repeated every two weeks thereafter. Tumors were injected based on size with a maximum of ten treated per visit. The adverse effects associated with OncoVEX^{GM-CSF} administration were primarily mild in nature. However, ten patients experienced fatigue, dyspnea, and pain which was possibly disease related. Injection site swabs and urine were collected from patients and analyzed for the presence of HSV DNA by PCR. Analysis detected HSV DNA from the swab of one patient at very low levels, while no urine contained viral DNA. Local effects on OncoVEX^{GM-CSF}-injected tumors were apparent after as few as two treatments, but regression of distal tumors typically occurred twelve months after the first treatment. Overall, ten patients achieved complete response without additional surgery and thirteen did not have evidence of disease after further surgical tumor resection. Interestingly, HSV serostatus did not seem to play a role in response to OncoVEX^{GM-CSF} therapy. The prolonged survival (>1 year) of patients enrolled in this study and the antitumor activity of OncoVEX^{GM-CSF} prompted approval of a phase III study, which is currently underway.

A study by Kaufman et al. (2010) evaluated local and distal immune responses in patients enrolled in the phase II Senzer et al. (2009) clinical trial. Peripheral blood and tumor samples were analyzed for the presence of myeloid-derived suppressive cells (MDSC), regulatory T cells (Treg, CD4+ FOXP3+) and suppressor T cells (Ts, CD8+ FOXP3+). Significant increases in the level of peripheral and tumor-associated antigen-specific T cells (MART-1) were observed following OncoVEX^{GM-CSF} injection. Notable decreases in Treg and Ts cell populations occurred in injected tumors in comparison to non-injected distal tumors. This may be due to decreases in MDSCs which have been shown to negatively regulate activator T cell activity by diverting them to a regulatory phenotype.

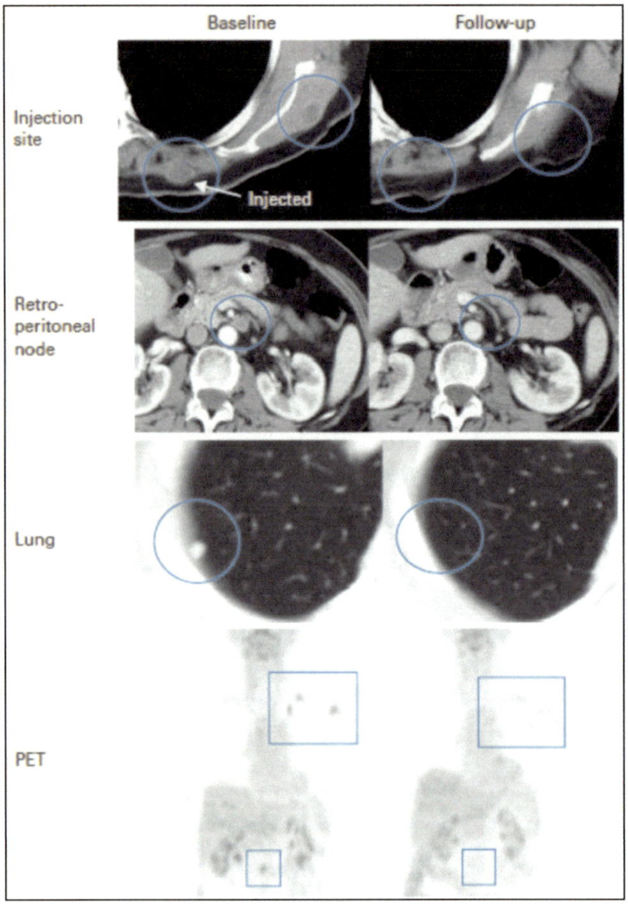

Fig. 4. Patient 703 Response to OncoVEX^{GM-CSF} Therapy. CT images of injections sites in the left shoulder, retroperitoneal lymph node, and lungs at baseline (left) and three months (right). Positron emission tomography (PET) image at baseline (left) and at eight months (right). Highlighted areas indicate lesions before and after OncoVEX^{GM-CSF} injection.

A combination therapy phase I/II trial for the treatment of stage III/IVA head and neck squamous cell carcinoma demonstrated an additive effect of OncoVEX^{GM-CSF} and chemo radiotherapy (CRT) (Harrington et al., 2010b). Seventeen patients were enrolled in the study and received dose escalating OncoVEX^{GM-CSF} (cohort one: four injections at $1x10^6$ pfu; cohort two: $1x10^6$ pfu followed by three injections at $1x10^7$ pfu; cohort three: $1x10^6$ pfu followed by three injection at $1x10^8$ pfu) intratumoral injections on days one, twenty two, forty three and sixty four. Patients were treated with full-dose radical CRT comprised of radiotherapy (70 Gray) in thirty five daily fractions over seven weeks with cisplatin administered on days one, twenty one and forty two at 100 mg/m^2 body surface area. Treatment was well tolerated and dose-limiting toxicities were not identified in any cohorts. Viral shedding was detected at transient low levels in three patients. HSV DNA was detected at levels higher than the input dose in injected and adjacent uninjected tumors by immunohistochemistry and PCR analysis. All seronegative patients seroconverted and increased antibody titres were measured in all patients in a dose-dependent manor. Overall, thirteen patients achieved partial or complete response including five whom achieved complete response following only two or three doses of OncoVEX$^{GM\text{-}CSF}$. All patients achieved loco-regional control with 70.5% remaining alive and in complete remission at the time of publication. A phase III study is currently underway.

3.5 HF10 clinical trials

The HF10 oncolytic vector is a naturally mutated clonal derivative of patient strain HF which contains inactivating mutations in U_L43, $U_L49.5$, U_L55, U_L56 and LAT coding sequences (Takakuwa et al., 2003). Although the function of U_L56 is unknown, U_L43, $U_L49.5$ and U_L55, encode membrane, envelope and tegument proteins, respectively. Preclinical data has shown that HF10 therapy causes significant tumor regression and prolongs survival in animal models of breast and colon carcinoma (Kimata et al., 2003; Teshigahara et al., 2004). Furthermore, cured mice were refractory to tumor re-challenge indicating that an antitumor immune response was established.

A phase I trial to evaluate the safety and antitumor activity of HF10 was performed on six patients with recurrent breast carcinoma (Nakao et al., 2007). Patients were chosen with metastatic skin lesions to facilitate administration of the virus subcutaneously. Patients received $1x10^4$ pfu, $1x10^5$ pfu or $1x10^5$ pfu for three days, $5x10^5$ pfu or $5x10^5$ pfu for three days. Tumor nodules were excised fourteen days post-injection for evaluation of virus pathology and replication. The same treatment regimen was adopted for three patients with non-resectable pancreatic carcinoma except HF10 was delivered via intratumoral catheter. HF10 therapy was well tolerated with no adverse events associated with virus administration in either the breast or pancreatic carcinoma participants. Analysis of excised tumor samples revealed significant decreases in tumor cell viability (30-100%) associated with virus replication. Tumor regression was evident in the skin nodule of one patient with recurrent breast carcinoma, but no other significant decreases in tumor volume were noted.

An additional phase I clinical trial was performed on six patients with non-resectable pancreatic tumors caused by liver metastases and invasion of lymph nodes surrounding the aorta (Nakao et al., 2011). Intratumoral injection of HF10 ($1x10^6$ pfu) was performed at four sites during laparotomy or with the aid of CT imaging. An intratumoral catheter was inserted during surgery for subsequent delivery of three daily doses of HF10 for three days. No adverse effects associated with HF10 treatment were observed during the trial. PCR analysis failed to detect HSV DNA in blood samples and abdominal cavities of patients, but prolonged viral expression was evident in several patient tumors up to 318 days post-injection. Moreover, analysis of resected tumor samples indicated significant infiltration of macrophages, CD4+ and CD8+ T cells into HF10-injected tumor tissue. Upon completion of this trial four patients achieved partial response while the remaining two maintained progressive disease status. Together, these studies demonstrate the efficacy of HF10 for use in oncolytic virotherapy for the treatment of patients with breast and pancreatic carcinoma.

4. Challenges with oncolytic virotherapy

The safety and antitumor efficacy of HSV-1 vectors in clinical trials has inspired the development of treatment platforms using engineered and natural oncolytic viruses, as well as combination therapy trials. Despite promising results in preclinical studies, *in vitro* assays do not always predict *in vivo* outcomes. These discrepancies can be attributed to the challenges of adapting therapy from cell culture to *in vivo* tumors which contain a plethora of hurdles to both virus replication and tumor clearance.

4.1 The tumor microenvironment

The heterogeneity of the tumor mass, including necrotic foci, normal stroma, the basal membrane and extracellular matrix (ECM), presents a formidable road block to virus penetration. Furthermore, viral infection often elicits host inflammatory responses resulting in increased recruitment of immune effectors. Overall, the effects of the tumor microenvironment may counteract the antitumor effects of oncolytic virotherapy.

The ECM forms a complex molecular sieve which regulates cell signalling processes between tumor and normal stromal cells. Modifications to the ECM impact tumor biology and accessibility, and therefore the response to therapy. McKee et al. (2006) demonstrated that fibrillar collagen acts as a barrier to HSV-1 vector MGH2 spread within melanoma. Viral particles localized to collagen-free areas of the tumor with limited spread to collagen-rich regions. Co-treatment of tumors with MGH2 and collagenase enhanced virus spread and tumor regression. In addition, viruses expressing enzymes such as matrix metalloproteinases (MMPs), which degrade ECM components, could be used. Chondroitinase ABC (Chase-ABC) is a bacterial enzyme which cleaves chondroitin sulphate glycosaminoglycans from proteoglycans. In comparison to the control (rHsvQ), the oncolytic HSV-1 vector expressing Chase-ABC (OV-Chase) enhanced viral spread, inhibited tumor growth, and prolonged survival of animals with subcutaneous and intracranial glioma xenografts (Dmitrieva et al., 2011). Furthermore, the ectopic expression of MMP-9 on murine malignant glioma xenografts has been shown to increase spread of the oncolytic HSV-1 vector JD0G through degradation of collagen type IV, a major component of the ECM and basal membrane.

Angiogenesis is crucial to tumor growth as vasculature provides a network from which cells obtain oxygen, metabolites and dispose of waste. Disruption of the balance between pro- and anti-angiogenic factors is caused by changes in the tumor microenvironment such as hypoxia, acidosis, inflammation and gene mutations. Ultimately, an 'angiogenic switch' occurs which leads to increased synthesis of vasculature supporting rapid tumor growth. Necrotic, acidotic, and hypoxic areas result, in part, from abnormalities in tumor vasculature such as aberrations in the morphology of endothelial cells and mechanical stress on developing vessels from rapidly proliferating tumor cells. Infection of tumor cells with oncolytic viruses can have both pro- and anti-angiogenic effects. Infection of ovarian tumor endothelial cells with HSV1716 has been shown to disrupt tumor vasculature (Benencia et al., 2005). Conversely, infection of human glioma cells with G207 reduces expression of thrombospondin, resulting in increased vasculature (Aghi et al., 2007). This effect can be countered through the administration of thrombospondin-derived peptides. In models of glioblastoma, cases where oncolytic virus infection results in an anti-angiogenic response, adjacent virus-free areas have been shown to upregulate angiogenesis (Huszthy et al., 2010). Furthermore, increases in tumor angiogenesis can facilitate virus-induced inflammatory responses. The resultant changes in vascular perfusion can lead to hypoxia-mediated killing of uninfected tumor cells (Breitbach et al., 2007) and increased vascular leakage due to vascular shutdown and hyperpermeability, respectively (Kurozumi et al., 2007). The impact of vascularity on oncolytic virotherapy and vice versa has inspired combination therapy trials using anti-angiogenic drugs such as Bevacizumab (Willett et al., 2004), Trichostatin A (Liu et al., 2008) and Cilengitide (Kurozumi et al., 2007). In addition, oncolytic vectors expressing anti-angiogenic genes have been engineered to modulate the activity of factors such as vascular epithelial growth factor (VEGF), MMPs, fibroblast growth factors (FGF), and interleukins. Rapid anti-angiogenesis mediated by oncolytic virus (RAMBO), a novel HSV-1 vector expressing vasculostatin, a brain-specific angiostatic peptide, has been used in the treatment of subcutaneous and intracranial gliomas. Compared to a control virus, intratumoral injection of RAMBO resulted in tumor regression and enhanced antitumor effects including decreased tumor vascularity, microvessel density, and angiogenesis (Hardcastle et al., 2010).

4.2 Virus delivery

The importance of diffuse inoculation has been illustrated in mathematical models of virus replication. Three methods of intratumoral inoculation including injection into the entire tumor, the tumor core and the tumor rim were analyzed for their ability to eradicate the entire tumor in the presence of necrosis and an innate immune response (Wein et al., 2003). Data from preclinical and clinical trials were used to design the model and identify parameter values. Even in the absence of an innate immune response, complete tumor regression requires widespread distribution of the virus achieved by multiple injections into the entire tumor. However, an antiviral innate immune response can prevent tumor eradication, warranting methods for immune evasion to ensure efficient virus spread. While intratumoral injection is feasible for easily accessible and solid tumors, systemic delivery options are necessary for the treatment of metastatic disease and non-accessible tumors. Virus inactivation by neutralizing antibodies, innate immune responses, complement-mediated opsonisation, and insufficient adsorption limit the efficacy of systemic delivery options. Delivery of oncolytic vectors within a collagen matrix or liposomes could be used to minimize premature inactivation by immune surveillance mechanisms. Alternatively, transient immunosuppression using antibody neutralizing compounds, inhibiting B cell maturation or antibody-receptor interactions may allow for efficient vector delivery. Administration of anti-CD20 antibodies, CPA, and plasmapheresis has been used to inhibit immunoglobulin production by B cells and counteract the neutralizing activity of antiviral antibodies (Ikeda et al., 2000; Vile et al., 2002). For instance, pretreatments of cobra venom factor (CVF) and CPA followed by intravascular injection of hrR3 leads to increased viral spread and prolonged survival in a rat model of malignant glioma (Ikeda et al., 2000). Although studies have indicated that pre-existing antibodies to HSV-1 do not limit antitumor efficacy of oncolytic virus treatment, seronegative patients have a higher incidence of adverse effects from virus inoculation (Chahlavi et al., 1999; Lambright et al., 2000; Hu et al., 2006). In a phase II study for the treatment of metastatic melanoma, seronegative participants received an initial intratumoral injection of OncoVEX$^{GM\text{-}CSF}$ to induce seroconvertion (Senzer et al., 2009). This pre-treatment reduced adverse effects associated with virus injection.

Although increasing input dose is a tempting strategy to augment low infectivity from vector loss during systemic delivery, current manufacturing processes limit attainable HSV titres to $3x10^9$ pfu/mL (Varghese & Rabkin, 2002). The use of a wild type virus, which does not require attenuation to achieve selective oncolysis, could facilitate manufacturing processes and yield higher titres. The use of replication-competent vectors is another method by which the input dose can be amplified. However, care should be taken to direct the tropism of such viruses to preclude unwanted replication within normal healthy tissue.

4.3 The immune response

The infiltration of host immune cells into the tumor microenvironment is an important factor modulating the success of oncolytic virotherapy. Innate and adaptive immune responses can limit virus spread resulting in suboptimal tumor clearance and persistence of residual tumor cells. Treatment of metastatic glioma using oncolytic HSV-1 vectors results in an inflammatory response and increased vasodilation induced by expression of IFNγ and ISGs (Kurozumi et al., 2007). This prompts the infiltration of innate and adaptive immune cells causing a decrease in virus replication and spread. Controlling the entry of immune cells into the tumor microenvironment can be used to increase virus replication. Analysis of glioma tissue samples treated with hrR3 indicates acute depletion of virus particles due to infiltration of CD68+ and CD163+ monocytes, microglia and macrophages (Fulci et al., 2006). Depletion of these cell populations in intracranial gliomas through systemic delivery of CPA decreased intratumoral infiltration resulting in increased hrR3 titres, viral persistence within the tumor and prolonged survival (Fulci et al., 2007). Alternatively, viruses which spread by intracellular methods evade virus-specific antibodies and the complement system. HSV-1 vectors expressing the fusogenic membrane glycoprotein (FMG) have shown that the formation of multinucleated syncytia can aid in viral spread and enhance the antitumor response (Galanis et al., 2001; Nakamori et al., 2003).

In a seemingly contradictory paradigm, immunostimulatory vectors can augment the efficacy of oncolytic virotherapy by inducing an immune response against the virus as well as the tumor. It has been well established that induction of an antitumor immune response is vital to achieving complete and lasting tumor regression. The HSV-1 vector G47Δ contains a deletion in the ICP47 gene, which functions to block antigen presentation via MHC class I molecules. Accordingly, tumor cells infected with G47Δ show enhanced stimulation of tumor-associated T cells due to increased expression of MHC class I molecules compared to cells infected with G207 which expresses functional ICP47 (Todo et al., 2001b). In an immunocompetent model of neuroblastoma, G47Δ treatment enhanced tumor regression and prolonged survival compared to G207, which elicited tumor regression but did not significantly affect survival (Todo et al., 2001b). Furthermore, a combination therapy trial involving co-administration of G47Δ with immature DCs resulted in significant reductions in tumor volume and increased survival attributed to substantial lymphocyte infiltration and robust antitumor immunity (Farrell et al., 2008). The expression of peptides derived from the epitopes of tumor-associated antigens (TAAs) has been incorporated into replication-defective vectors to amplify cytotoxic T lymphocyte (CTL) responses (Rosenberg et al., 2004). However, the antitumor effects of these vectors are meagre due to immune tolerance which inhibits efficacy of the CTL response (Rosenberg et al., 2004; Frey et al., 2006). Replication-competent vectors expressing immunogenic model antigens circumvent tolerance and allow for sustained CTL responses against the bulk of the tumor due to virus spread. In a dual vaccination strategy Zhang et al. (2009) injected murine ovarian surface epithelial carcinomas (MOSECs) with vaccinia virus expressing ovalbumin (VV-OVA) followed by Semliki Forest Virus also expressing ovalbumin (SFV-OVA), or vice versa. Immune tolerance was not established and an enhanced OVA-specific CTL response and antitumor effect was observed in comparison to treatment with the wild type viruses. This demonstrates the efficacy of the bimodal approach of oncolytic virotherapy, including viral oncolysis and tumor-specific immune responses.

4.4 Safety

Concerns regarding the use of oncolytic HSV vectors in cancer therapy focus on the risk of unwanted replication in normal healthy tissue. HSV-1 is able to infect a wide variety of cell types due to the ubiquitous expression of its cellular receptor in multiple human tissues. This presents a danger for wide-spread replication, especially when patients receiving oncolytic virotherapy are most likely immunosuppressed and highly susceptible to viral infection. Therefore, mechanisms to ensure accurate viral targeting and methods to control unwanted replication are required. Use of tissue and tumor-specific promoters, or cellular receptor-mediated targeting can be used to direct tumor-specific infection. Furthermore, Tet-off, Cre-recombinase, HSV-tk/gancyclovir regulation systems, and incorporation of suicide genes into oncolytic vectors provide a safeguard to restrict unwanted replication, should it occur. Safety evaluations in preclinical studies should include careful considerations of dose limiting toxicity, potential of reversion or acquisition of virulent phenotypes, altered tropism, and the effect of transgene expression on the host. Choosing an appropriate animal model is imperative to accurately evaluate vectors for clinical use.

Results from clinical trials using oncolytic HSV-1 vectors are promising. Adverse effects are non-life threatening, including moderate to mild flu-like symptoms and injection site irritation demonstrating the safety profile of this treatment modality. In many cases complete responses were observed resulting in prolonged patient survival and therefore, initiation of subsequent clinical trials. Oncolytic vectors, especially HSV-1-based, are rookies in the field of cancer therapy. However, with careful coaching they have the potential to achieve all-star status.

5. References

Advani, S.J. *et al.* Replication-competent, nonneuroinvasive genetically engineered herpes virus is highly effective in the treatment of therapy-resistant experimental human tumors. *Cancer Res.* 1999; 59(9): 2055-2058.

Aghi, M. *et al.* Angiogenic response caused by oncolytic herpes simplex virus-induced reduced thrombospondin expression can be prevented by specific viral mutations or by administering a thrombospondin-derived peptide. *Cancer Res.* 2007; 67(2): 440-444.

Ahmed, M. *et al.* Regions of the herpes simplex virus type 1 latency-associated transcript that protect cells from apoptosis in vitro and protect neuronal cells in vivo. *J Virol.* 2002; 76(2): 717-729.

Alain, T. *et al.* Reovirus therapy of lymphoid malignancies. *Blood.* 2002; 100(12): 4146-4153.

Andreansky, S.S. *et al.* The application of genetically engineered herpes simplex viruses to the treatment of experimental brain tumors. *Proc Natl Acad Sci USA.* 1996; 93(21): 11313-11318.

Ayllón, V. & Rebollo, A. Ras-induced cellular events (review). *Mol Membr Biol.* 2000; 17(2): 65-73.

Benencia, F. *et al.* Oncolytic HSV exerts direct antiangiogenic activity in ovarian carcinoma. *Human Gene Ther.* 2005; 16(6): 765-778.

Bennett, J.J. *et al.* Comparison of safety, delivery, and efficacy of two oncolytic herpes viruses (G207 and NV1020) for peritoneal cancer. *Cancer Gene Ther.* 2002; 9(11): 935-945.

Bernardi, R. & Pandolfi, P.P. Role of PML and the PML-nuclear body in the control of programmed cell death. *Oncogene.* 2003; 22(56): 9048-9057.

Blank, S.V. *et al.* Replication-selective herpes simplex virus type 1 mutant therapy of cervical cancer is enhanced by low-dose radiation. *Hum Gene Ther.* 2002; 13(5): 627-639.

Breitbach, C.J. *et al.* Targeted inflammation during oncolytic virus therapy severely compromises tumor blood flow. *Mol Ther.* 2007; 15(9):1686–93.

Bridle, B.W. *et al.* Vesicular stomatitis virus as a novel cancer vaccine vector to prime antitumor immunity amenable to rapid boosting with adenovirus. *Mol Ther.* 2009; 17(10): 1814-1821.

Brown, S.M. *et al.* Cell type and cell state determine differential *in vitro* growth of non-virulent ICP34.5 negative herpes simplex virus. *J Gen Virol.* 1994; 75 (Pt 9): 2367–2377.

Campadelli-Fiume, G. *et al.* The novel receptors that mediate the entry of herpes simplex viruses and animal alphaherpesviruses into cells. *Rev Med Virol.* 2000; 10(5), 305-319.

Carroll, N.M. *et al.* Enhancement of gene therapy specificity for diffuse colon carcinoma liver metastases with recombinant herpes simplec virus. *Ann Surg.* 1996; 224(3): 323-329.

Carroll, P.E. *et al.* Centrosome hyperamplification in human cancer: chromosome instability induced by p53 mutation and/or Mdm2 overexpression. *Oncogene.* 1999; 18(11): 1935-1944.

Cayley, P.J. *et al.* Activation of the ppp(A2'p)nA system in interferon-treated, herpes simplex virus-infected cells and evidence for novel inhibitors of the ppp(A2'p)nA-dependent RNase. *Eur J Biochem.* 1984; 143(1): 165-174.

Cervantes-García, D. *et al.* Oncolytic virotherapy. *Ann Hepatol.* 2008; 7(1): 34-45.

Chahlavi, A. *et al.* Effect of prior exposure to herpes simplex virus 1 on viral vector-mediated tumor therapy in immunocompetent mice. *Gene Ther.* 1999; 6(10): 1751-1758.

Chee, A.V. & Roizman, B. Herpes simplex virus 1 gene products occlude the interferon signalling pathway at multiple sites. *J Virol.* 2004; 78(8): 4185-4196.

Chen, F. & Castranova, V. Nuclear factor-kappaB, an unappreciated tumor suppressor. *Cancer Res.* 2007; 67(23): 11093-11098.

Chen, Y. *et al.* Pre-existent adenovirus antibody inhibits systemic toxicity and antitumor activity of CN706 in nude mouse LNCaP xenograft model: implications and proposals for human therapy. *Hum Gene Ther.* 2000; 11(11): 1553-1567.

Chen, Y. *et al.* CV706, a prostate cancer-specific adenovirus variant, in combination with radiotherapy produces synergistic antitumor efficacy without increasing toxicity. *Cancer Res.* 2001; 61(14): 5453-5460.

Chou, J. *et al.* Association of a M(r) 90,000 phosphoprotein with protein kinase PKR in cells enhanced phosphorylation of translation initiation factor eIF-2 alpha and premature shutoff of protein synthesis after infection with gamme 34.5-mutants of herpes simplex virus 1. *Proc Natl Acad Sci USA.* 1995; 92(23): 10516-10520.

Coffey, M.C. *et al.* Reovirus therapy of tumors with activated Ras pathway. *Science.* 1998; 282(5392): 1332-1334.

Connett, J.M. *et al.* Interferon regulatory factor 1 (IRF-1) and IRF-2 expression in breast cancer tissue microarrays. *J Interferon Cytokine Res.* 2005; 25(10): 587-594.

Coukos, G. *et al.* Multi-attenuated herpes simplex virus-1 mutant G207 exerts cytotoxicity against epithelial ovarian cancer but not normal mesothelium and is suitable for intraperitoneal oncolytic therapy. *Cancer Gene Ther.* 2000; 7(2): 275-283.

Csatary, L.K. *et al.* MTH-68/H oncolytic viral treatment in human high-grade gliomas. *J Neurooncol.* 2004; 67(1-2): 82-93.

Davis, J.J. & Fang, B. Oncolytic virotherapy for cancer treatment: challenges and solutions. *J Gene Med.* 2005; 7(11): 1380-1389.

Dmitrieva, N. *et al.* Chondroitinase ABC I-mediated enhancement of oncolytic virus spread and antitumor efficacy. *Clin Cancer Res.* 2011; 17(6): 1362-1372.

Eager, R. & Nemunaitis, J. GM-CSF gene-transduced tumor vaccines. *Mol Ther.* 2005; 12(1): 18-27.

Eisemann, J. *et al.* Infection of mature dendritic cells with herpes simplex virus type 1 interferes with the interferon signalling pathway. *Immunobiology.* 2007; 212(9-10): 877-886.

Everett, R.D. *et al.* The disruption of ND10 during herpes simplex virus infection correlates with the Vmw110- and proteasome-dependent loss of several PML isoforms. *J Virol.* 1998; 72(8): 6581-6591.

Everett, R.D. *et al.* Comparison of the biological and biochemical activities of several members of the alphaherpesvirus ICP0 family of proteins. *Journal of Virol.* 2010; 84(7): 3476-3487.

Everts, B., & van der Poel, H.G. Replication-selective oncolytic viruses in the treatment of cancer. *Cancer Gene Ther.* 2005; 12(2): 141-161.

Farassati, F. *et al.* Oncogenes in Ras signalling pathway dictate host-cell permissiveness to herpes simplex virus 1. *Nat Cell Biol.* 2001; 3(8): 745-750.

Forastiere, A.A. *et al.* Final report of a phase II evaluation of paclitaxel in patients with advanced squamous cell carcinoma of the head and neck: an Eastern Cooperative Oncology Group trial (PA390). *Cancer.* 1998; 82(11): 2270-2274.

Frey, A.B. *et al.* Effector-phase tolerance: another mechanism of how cancer escapes antitumor immune response. *J Leukoc Biol.* 2006; 79(4): 652–662.

Fulci, G. *et al.* Cyclophosphamide enhances glioma virotherapy by inhibiting innate immune responses. *Proc Natl Acad Sci U S A.* 2006; 103(34): 12873–12878.

Fulci, G. *et al.* Depletion of peripheral macrophages and brain microglia increases brain tumor titers of oncolytic viruses. *Cancer Res.* 2007; 67(19): 9398–406.

Galanis, E. *et al.* Use of viral fusogenic membrane glycoproteins as novel therapeutic transgenes in gliomas. *Hum Gene Ther.* 2001; 12(7): 811-821.

Galivo, F. *et al.* Single-cycle viral gene expression, rather than progressive replication and oncolysis, is required for VSV therapy B16 melanoma. *Gene Ther.* 2010; 17(2): 158-170.

Geevarghese, S.K. *et al.* Phase I/II clinical study of oncolytic herpes simplex virus NV1020 in patients with extensively pre-treated refractory colorectal cancer metastatic to the liver. *Human Gene Ther.* 2010; 21(9): 1119-1128.

Grote, D. *et al.* Live attenuated measles virus induces regression of human lymphoma xenografts in immunodeficient mice. *Blood.* 2001; 97(12): 3746–3754.

Halford, W.P. *et al.* ICP0 antagonizes Stat 1-dependent repression of herpes simplex virus: implications for the regulation of viral latency. *Virol J.* 2006; 3: 44.

Hanahan, D. & Weinberg, R.A. The hallmarks of cancer. *Cell.* 2000; 100(1): 57-70.

Hardcastle, J. *et al.* Enhanced antitumor efficacy of vasculostatin (Vstat120) expressing oncolytic HSV-1. *Mol Ther.* 2010; 18(2): 285–294.

Harrington, K.J. *et al.* Two-Stage phase I dose-escalation study of intratumoral reovirus type 3 Dearing and palliative radiotherapy in patients with advanced cancers. *Clin Cancer Res.* 2010a; 16(11): 3067-3077.

Harrington, K.J. *et al.* Phase I/II study of oncolytic HSVGM-CSF in combination with radiotherapy and cisplatin in untreated stage III/IV squamous cell cancer of the head and neck. *Clin Cancer Res.* 2010b; 16: 4005-4015.

Harrow, S. *et al.* HSV1716 injection into the brain adjacent to tumor following surgical resection of high-grade glioma: safety data and long-term survival. *Gene Ther.* 2004; 11(22): 1648-1658.

He, B. *et al.* The gamma(1)34.5 protein of herpes simplex virus 1 complexes with protein phosphatase 1alpha to dephosphorylate the alpha subunit of the eukaryotic translation initiation factor 2 and preclude the shutoff of protein synthesis by double-stranded RNA-activated protein kinase. *Proc Natl Acad Sci USA.* 1997; 94(3): 843-848.

Heldwein, E. E. & Krummenacher, C. Entry of herpesvirus into mammalian cells. *Cell. Mol. Life. Sci.* 2008; 65(11), 1653-1668.

Henderson, G. *et al.* Regulation of caspase 8- and caspase 9-induced apoptosis by the herpes simplex virus type 1 latency-associated transcript. *J Neurovirol.* 2002; 8:103-111.

Henderson, G. *et al.* The Bovine herpesvirus 1 gene encoding infected cell protein 0 (bICP0) can inhibit interferon-dependent transcription in the absence of other viral genes. *J Gen Virol.* 2005; 86(Pt 10), 2697-2702.

Hill, A. *et al.* Herpes simplex virus turns off the TAP to evade host immunity. *Nature.* 1995; 375(6530): 411-415.

Hirasawa, K. *et al.* Oncolytic reovirus against ovarian and colon cancer. *Cancer Res.* 2002; 62(6): 1696-1701.

Hu, J. *et al.* A phase I study of OncoVEXGM-CSF, a second generation oncolytic herpes virus expressing granulocyte macrophage colony-stimulating factor. *Clin Cancer Res.* 2006; 12(22): 6737-6747.

Hunter, W.D. *et al.* Attenuated, replication-competent herpes simplex virus type 1 mutant G207: safety evaluation of intracerebral injection in nonhuman primates. *J Virol* . 1999; 73(8): 6319–6326.

Hushur, O. *et al.* Restriction of bovine herpesvirus 1 (BHV-1) growth in non-permissive cells beyond the expression of immediate early genes. *J Vet Med Sci.* 2004; 66(4), 453-5.

Huszthy, P.C. *et al.* Cellular effects of oncolytic viral therapy on the glioblastoma microenvironment. *Gene Ther.* 2010; 17(2): 202-216.

Ikeda, K. *et al.* Complement depletion facilitates the infection of multiple brain tumors by an intravascular, replication-conditional herpes simplex virus mutant. *J Virol.* 2000; 74(10): 4765-4775.

Janke, M. *et al.* Recombinant Newcastle disease virus (NDV) with inserted gene coding for GM-CSF as a new vector for cancer immunogene therapy. *Gene Ther.* 2007; 14(23): 1639-1649.

Jia, W. & Zhou, Q. Viral vectors for cancer gene therapy: viral dissemination and tumor targeting. *Curr Gene Ther.* 2005; 5(1): 133-142.

Johnson, K.E. *et al.* Role for herpes simplex virus 1 ICP27 in the inhibition of type I interferon signalling. *Viology.* 2008; 374(2): 487-494.

Jones, C. & Chowdhury, S. A review of the biology of bovine herpesvirus type 1 (BHV-1), its role as a cofactor in the bovine respiratory disease complex and development of improved vaccines. *Animal health research reviews / Conference of Research Workers in Animal Diseases.* 2007; 8(2), 187-205.

Kamiyama, H. *et al.* Herpes simplex virus 1 recombinant virions exhibiting the amino terminal fragment of urokinase-type plasminogen activator can enter cells via the cognate receptor. *Gene Ther.* 2006; 13(7): 621-629.

Kanai, R. *et al.* Augmented therapeutic efficacy of an oncolytic herpes simplex virus type 1 mutant expressing ICP34.5 under the transcriptional control of *musashi1* promoter in the treatment of malignant glioma. *Human Gene Ther.* 2007; 18(1): 63-73.

Karrasch, M. *et al.* Treatment of recurrent malignant glioma with G207, a genetically engineered herpes simplex virus-1, followed by irradiation: Phase I study results. *J Clin Oncol ASCO Annual Meeting Proceedings.* 2009; 27(15S): 2042.

Kasuya, H. *et al.* Intraperitoneal delivery of hrR3 and ganciclovir prolongs survival in mice with disseminated pancreatic cancer. *J Surg Oncol.* 1999; 72(3): 136-141.

Kasuya, H. *et al.* Selectivity of an oncolytic herpes simplex virus for cells expressing the DF3-MUC1 antigen. *Cancer Res.* 2004; 64(7): 2561-2567.

Kaufman, H. *et al.* Local and distal immunity induced by intralesional vaccination with an oncolytic herpes virus encoding GM-CSF in patients with stage IIIc or stage IV melanoma. 2010; 17(3): 718-730.

Kemeny, N. *et al.* Phase II study of hepatic arterial floxuridine, leucovorin, and dexamethasone for unresectable liver metastases from colorectal carcinoma. *J. Clin. Oncol.* 1994; 12(11): 2288–2295.

Kemeny, N. *et al.* Phase I, open-label, dose-escalating study of a genetically engineered herpes simplex virus, NV1020, in subjects with metastatic colorectal carcinoma to the liver. *Human Gene Ther.* 2006; 17(12): 1214-1224.

Kim, M. *et al.* The viral tropism of two distinct oncolytic viruses, reovirus and myxoma virus, is modulated by cellular tumor suppressor gene status. *Oncogene.* 2010; 29(27): 3990-3996.

Kimata, H. *et al.* Effective treatment of disseminated peritoneal colon cancer with new replication-component herpes simplex viruses. *Hepato-Gastroenterol.* 2003; 50(52): 961-966.

Kinzler, K.W. & Vogelstein, B. Lessons from hereditary colorectal cancer. *Cell.* 1996; 87(2): 159-170.

Knickelbein, J.E. *et al.* Noncytotoxic lytic granule-mediated CD8+ T cell inhibition of HSV-1 reactivation from neuronal latency. *Science.* 2008; 322(5899): 268-271.

Kobelt, D. *et al.* The interaction between dendritic cells and herpes simplex virus-1. *Curr Top Microbiol Immunol.* 2003; 276: 145-161.

Kooby, D.A. *et al.* Oncolytic viral therapy for human colorectal cancer and liver metastases using a multi-mutated herpes simplex virus type-1 (G207). *FASEB.* 1999; 13(11): 1325-1334.

Kucharczuk, J.C. *et al.* Use of a "replication-restricted" herpes virus to treat experimental human malignant mesothelioma. *Cancer Res.* 1997; 57(3): 466-471.

Kurozumi, K. *et al.* Effect of tumor microenvironment modulation on the efficacy of oncolytic virus therapy. *J Natl Cancer Inst.* 2007; 99(23): 1768–1781.

Lambright, E.S. *et al.* Oncolytic therapy using a mutant type-1 herpes simplex virus and the role of the immune system. *Ann Thorac Surg.* 1999; 68(5): 1756-1760.

Lambright, E.S. *et al.* Effect of preexisiting anti-herpes immunity on the efficacy of herpes simplex viral therapy in a murine intraperitoneal tumor model. *Mol Ther.* 2000; 2(4): 387-393.

Lee, C.Y. *et al.* MicroRNA regulation of oncolytic herpes simplex virus-1 for selective killing of prostate cancer cells. *Clin Cancer Res.* 2009; 15(16): 5126-5135.

Leib, D.A. *et al.* Interferons regulate the phenotype of wild-type and mutant herpes simplex viruses in vivo. *J Exp Med.* 1999; 189(4): 663-672.

Leopardi, R. *et al.* The herpes simplex virus 1 protein kinase Us3 is required for protection from apoptosis induced by the virus. *Proc Natl Acad Sci USA.* 1997; 94(15): 7891-7896.

Liang, L. & Roizman B. Expression of gamma interferon-dependent genes is blocked independently by virion host shutoff RNase and by Us3 protein kinase. *J Virol.* 2008; 82(10): 4688-4696.

Lin, R. *et al.* The herpes simplex virus ICP0 RING finger domain inhibits IRF3- and IRF7-mediated activation of interferon-stimulated genes. *J Virol.* 2004; 78(4): 1675-1684.

Liu, T.C. *et al.* Trichostatin A and oncolytic HSV combination therapy shows enhanced antitumoral and antiangiogenic effects. *Mol Ther.* 2008; 16(6):1041–1047.

Lorence, R.M. *et al.* Complete regression of human fibrosarcoma xenografts after local Newcastle disease virus therapy. *Cancer Res.* 1994a; 54(23): 6017-6021.

Lorence, R.M. *et al.* Complete regression of human neuroblastoma xenografts in athymic mice after local Newcastle disease virus therapy. *J Natl Cancer Inst.* 1994b; 86(16): 1228-1233.

Lun, X. *et al.* Myxoma virus is a novel oncolytic virus with significant antitumor activity against experimental human gliomas. *Cancer Res.* 2005; 65(21): 9982-9990.

Luo, S. *et al.* Combination of vesicular stomatitis virus matrix protein gene therapy with low-dose cisplatin improves therapeutic efficacy against murine melanoma. *Cancer Sci.* 2010; 101(5): 1219-1225.

Mace, A. *et al.* Potential for efficacy of the oncolytic herpes simplex virus 1716 in patients with oral squamous cell carcinoma. *Head and Neck.* 2008; 30(8): 1045-1051.

MacKie, R.M. *et al.* Intralesional injection of herpes simplex virus 1716 in metastatic melanoma. *Lancet.* 2001; 357(9255): 525-526.

Maldonado, A.R. *et al.* Molecular engineering and validation of an oncolytic herpes simplex virus type 1 transcriptionally targeted to midkine-positive tumors. *J Gene Med.* 2010; 12(7): 613-623.

Markert, J.M. *et al.* Conditionally replicating herpes simplex virus mutant, G207 for the treatment of malignant glioma: results of a phase I trial. *Gene Ther.* 2000; 7(10): 867-874.

Markert, J.M. *et al.* Phase Ib trial of mutant herpes simplex virus G207 inoculated pre- and post-tumor resection for recurrent GBM. *Molecular Ther.* 2009; 17(1): 199-207.

McAuliffe, P.E. Effective treatment of pancreatic tumors with two multimutated herpes simplex oncolytic viruses. *J Gastrointest Surg.* 2000; 4(6): 580-588.

Melchjorsen, J. *et al.* Induction of cytokine expression by herpes simplex virus in human monocyte-derived macrophages and dendritic cells is dependent on virus replication and is counteracted by ICP27 targeting NK-kappaB and IRF-3. *J Gen Virol.* 2006; 87(Pt 5): 1099-1108.

Melroe, G.T. *et al.* Herpes simplex virus 1 has multiple mechanisms for blocking virus-induced interferon production. *J Virol.* 2004; 78(16): 8411-8420.

Merrill, M.K. *et al.* Poliovirus receptor CD155-targeted oncolysis of glioma. *Neuro Oncol.* 2004; 6(3): 208-217.

Meyers, M.O. *et al.*, Locoregional strategies for colorectal hepatic metastases. *Clin. Colorectal Cancer.* 2003; 3(1): 34–44.

McKee, T.D. *et al.* Degradation of fibrillar collagen in a human melanoma xenograft improves the efficacy of an oncolytic herpes simplex virus vector. *Cancer Res.* 2006; 66(5): 2509-2513.

McKie, E.A. *et al.* Histopathological responses in the CNS following innoculation with a nonneurovirulent mutant (1716) of herpes simplex virus type 1 (HSV1): relevence for gene and cancer therapy. *Neuropath Appl Neurobiol* 1998; 24(5): 367–372.

Mineta, T. *et al.* Treatment of malignant gliomas using ganciclovir-hypersensitive, ribonucleotide reductase-deficient herpes simplex viral mutant. *Cancer Res.* 1994; 54(15): 3963-3966.

Mineta, T. *et al.* Attenuated multi-mutated herpes simplex virus-1 for the treatment of malignant gliomas. *Nature Med.* 1995; 1(9): 938–943.

Miyatake, S.I. *et al.* Hepatoma-specific antitumor activity of an albumin enhancer-promoter regulated herpes simplex virus in vivo. *Gene Ther.* 1999; 6(4): 564-572.

Moriyama, Y. *et al.* Tumor-suppressor effect of interferon regulatory factor-1 in human hepatocellular carcinoma. *Clin Cancer Res.* 2001; 7(5): 1293-1298.

Morris, S.M. A role for p53 in the frequency and mechanism of mutation. *Mutat Res.* 2002; 511(1): 45-62.

Mossman, K.L. *et al.* Herpes simplex virus ICP0 mutants are hypersensitive to interferon. *J Virol.* 2000; 74(4): 2052-2056.

Mulvey, M. *et al.* Regulation of eIF2alpha phosphorylation by different functions that act during discrete phases in the herpes simplex type 1 life cycle. *J Virol.* 2003; 77(20): 10917-10928.

Muñoz-Fontela, C. *et al.* Transcriptional role of p53 in interferon-mediated antiviral immunity. *Journal of Exp Med.* 2008; 205(8): 1929–1938.

Nakamori, M. *et al.* Effective therapy of metastatic ovarian cancer with an oncolytic herpes simplex virus incorporating two membrane fusion mechanisms. *Clin Cancer Res.* 2003; 9(7): 2727-2733.

Nakamura, H. *et al.* Multimodality therapy with a replication-conditional herpes simplex virus 1 mutant that expresses yeast cytosine deaminase for intratumoral conversion of 5-fluorocytosine to 5-fluorouracil. *Cancer Res.* 2001; 61(14): 5447-5552.

Nakao, A. A *et al.* Clinical experiment of mutant herpes simplex virus HF10 therapy for cancer. *Current Cancer Drug Targets.* 2007; 7(2): 169-174.

Nakao, A. *et al.* A phase I dose-escalation clinical trial of intraoperative direct intratumoral injection of HF10 oncolytic virus in non-resectable patients with advanced pancreatic cancer. *Cancer Gene Ther.* 2011; 18(3): 167-178.

Nemunaitis, J. Vaccines in cancer: GVAX, a GM-CSF gene vaccine. *Expert Rev Vaccines.* 2005; 4(3): 259-274.

Norman, K.L. *et al.* Reovirus oncolysis of human breast cancer. *Hum Gene Ther.* 2002; 13(5): 641-652.

Paladino, P. & Mossman, K.L. Mechanisms employed by herpes simplex virus 1 to inhibit the interferon response. *J Intereferon Cytokine Res.* 2009; 29(9): 599-607.

Paladino, P. *et al.* Cellular localization of the herpes simplex virus ICP0 protein dictates its ability to block IRF3-mediated innate immune reponses. *PLoS One.* 2010; 5(4): e10428.

Papanastassiou, V. *et al.* The potential for efficacy of the modified (ICP34.5(-)) herpes simplex virus HSV1716 following intratumoral injection into human malignant glioma: a proof of principle study. *Gene Ther.* 2002; 9(6): 398-406.

Pasieka, T.J. *et al.* Herpes simplex virus virion host shutoff attenuates establishment of the antiviral state. *J Virol.* 2008; 82(11): 5527-5535.

Pawlik, T.M. *et al.* Oncolysis of diffuse hepatocellular carcinoma by intravascular administration of a replication-competent, genetically engineered herpesvirus. *Cancer Res.* 2000; 60(11): 2790-2795.

Pawlik, T.M. *et al.* Prodrug bioactivation and oncolysis of diffuse liver metastases by a herpes simplex virus 1 mutant that expresses the CYP2B1 transgene. *Cancer.* 2002; 95(5): 1171-1181.

Pecora, A.L. *et al.* Phase I trial of intravenous administration of PV701, an oncolytic virus, in patients with advanced solid cancers. *J Clin Oncol.* 2002; 20(9): 2251-2266.

Pende, D. *et al.* Analysis of the receptor-ligand interactions in the natural killer-mediated lysis of freshly isolated myeloid or lymophoblastic leukemias: evidence for the involvement of the Poliovirus receptor (CD155) and Nectin-2 (CD112). *Blood.* 2005; 105(5): 2066-2073.

Peng, K.W. *et al.* Systemic therapy of myeloma xenografts by an attenuated measles virus. *Blood.* 2001; 98(7): 2002-2007.

Peng, K.W. *et al.* Biodistribution of oncolytic measles virus after intraperitoneal administration into Ifnar-CD46Ge transgenic mice. *Hum. Gene Ther.* 2003a; 14(16): 1565–1577.

Peng, K.W. *et al.* Oncolytic measles viruses displaying a single-chain antibody against CD38, a myeloma cell marker. *Blood.* 2003b; 101(7): 2557-2562.

Peri, P. *et al.* Herpes simplex virus type 1 Us3 gene deletion influences toll-like receptor responses in cultured monocytic cells. *Virol J.* 2008; 21(5): 140.

Peters, G.A. *et al.* Inhibition of PACT-mediated activation of PKR by the herpes simplec virus type 1 Us11 protein. *J Virol.* 2002; 76(21): 11054-11064.

Phuangsab, A. *et al.* Newcastle disease virus therapy of human tumor xenografts: antitumor effects of local or systemic administration. *Cancer Lett.* 2001; 172(1): 27-36.

Pitha, P.M. *et al.* Role of the interferon regulatory factors (IRFs) in virus-mediated signalling and regulation of cell growth. *Biochimie.* 1998; 80(8-9): 651-658.

Platanias, L.C. Mechanisms of type-I- and type-II-interferon-mediated signalling. *Nat Rev Immunol.* 2005; 5(5): 375-386.

Poppers, J. *et al.* Inhibition of PKR activation by the proline-rich RNA binding domain of the herpes simplex virus type 1 Us11 protein. *J Virol.* 2000; 74(23): 11215-11221.

Rajan, B. *et al.* Survival in patients with recurrent glioma as a measure of treatment efficacy: prognostic factors following nitrosourea chemotherapy. *Eur J Cancer* 1994; 30A(12): 1809–1815.

Rampling, R. Chemotherapy. Determining the appropriate treatment. In: Hopkins A, Davies EH (eds) *Improving Care for Patients with Malignant Glioma.* Royal College of Physicians: London, 1997; pp 63–74.

Rampling, R. Modern aspects of radiation therapy for glial tumours of the brain. *Forum.* 1998; 8(3): 289–301.

Rampling, R. *et al.* Toxicity evaluation of relication-competent herpes simplex virus (ICP34.5 mull mutant 1716) in patient with recurrent malignant glioma. *Gene Ther.* 2000; 7(10): 859-866.

Randazzo, B.P. *et al.* Treatment of experimental intracranial murine melanoma with neuroattenuated herpes simplex virus type 1 mutant. *Virology* 1995; 211(1): 94–101.

Randazzo, B.P. *et al.* Treatment of experimental subcutaneous human melanoma with a replication-restricted herpes simplex virus mutant. *J Invest Dermatol.* 1997; 108(6): 933-937.

Reichard, K.W. *et al.* Retinoic acid enhances killing of neuroblastoma cells by Newcastle disease virus. *J Pediatr Surg.* 1993; 28(10): 1221-1225.

Ries, S.J. & Brandts, C.H. Oncolytic viruses for the treatment of cancer: current strategies and clinical trials. *Drug Discovery Today.* 2004; 9(17), 759-768.

Rodriguez, R. *et al.* Prostate attenuated replication competent adenovirus (ARCA) CN706: a selective cytotoxic for prostate-specific antigen-positive prostate cancer cells. *Cancer Res.* 1997; 57(13): 2559-2563.

Rodrigues, R. *et al.* Bovine herpesvirus type 1 as a novel oncolytic virus. *Cancer Gene Ther.* 2010; 17(5): 344-55.

Roizman, B. & Sears, A.E. Herpes simplex viruses and their replication. In: Fields, B.N. *et al.* (eds.). *Fundamental Virology, Third Edition* (Lippincott-Raven Publishers, Philadelphia) 1996; pp. 1043-1107.

Rosen, C.B. *et al.* Liver resection for metastatic colonic and rectal carcinoma. In: Cohen, A.M., and Winawer, S.J. (eds.). *Cancer of the Colon, Rectum, and Anus* (McGraw-Hill, New York) 1995; pp. 805–821.

Rosenberg, S.A. *et al.* Cancer immunotherapy: moving beyond current vaccines. *Nat Med.* 2004; 10(9): 909–915.

Sadler, A.J. & Williams, B.R. Interferon-inducible antiviral effectors. *Nat Rev Immunol.* 2008; 8(7): 559-568.

Saira, K. *et al.* The infected cell protein 0 encoded by bovine herpesvirus 1 (bICP0) induces degradation of interferon response factor 3 and, consequently, inhibits beta interferon promoter activity. *J Virol.* 2007; 81(7), 3077-3086.

Salomoni, P. & Pandolfi, P.P. The role of PML in tumor suppression. *Cell.* 2002; 108(2): 165-170.

Sànchez, R. & Mohr, I. Inhibition of cellular 2′-5′ oligoadenylate synthetase by the herpes simplex virus type 1 Us11 protein. *J Virol.* 2007; 81(7): 3455-3464.

Sen, G.C. & Sarkar, S.N. The interferon-stimulated genes: targets of direct signalling by interferons, double-stranded RNA and viruses. *Curr Top Microbiol Immunol.* 2007; 316:233-2350.

Senzer, N. *et al.* Phase II clinical trial of a granulocyte-macrophage colony-stimulating factor-encoding, second-generation oncolytic herpesvirus in patients with unresectable metastatic melanoma. *Journal of Clinical Oncol.* 2009; 27(34): 5763-5771.

Schulze, T. *et al.* Efficiency of adjuvant active specific immunization with Newcastle disease virus modified tumor cells in colorectal cancer patients following resection of liver metastases: results of a prospective randomized trial. *Cancer Immunol Immunother.* 2009; 58(1): 61-69.

Shen, Y., & Nemunaitis, J. Herpes simplex virus 1 (HSV-1) for cancer treatment. *Cancer Gene Ther.* 2006; 13(11), 975-992.

Shinozaki K. *et al.* Oncolysis of multifocal hepatocellular carcinoma in the rat liver by hepatic artery infusion of vesicular stomatitis virus. *Mol Ther.* 2004; 9(3): 368-376.

Sobol, P.T. & Mossman, K.L. ICP0 prevents RNase L-independent rRNA cleavage in herpes simplex virus type 1-infected cells. *J Virol.* 2006; 80(1): 218-225.

Stanford, M.M. & McFadden, G. Myxoma virus and oncolytic virotherapy: a new biologic weapon in the war against cancer. *Expert Opinion Biol Ther.* 2007; 7(9): 1415-1425.

Stanford, M.M. *et al.* Myxoma virus in the European rabbit: interactions between the virus and its susceptible host. *Vet Res.* 2007; 38(2): 299-318.

Stojdl, D.F. *et al.* Exploiting tumor-specific defects in the interferon pathway with a previously unknown oncolytic virus. *Nat Med.* 2000; 6(7): 821-825.

Strong, J.E. & Lee, P.W. The v-erbB oncogene confers enhanced cellular susceptibility to reovirus infection. *J Virol.* 1996; 70(1): 612-616.

Strong, J.E. *et al.* The molecular basis of viral oncolysis: usurpation of the Ras signalling pathway by reovirus. *EMBO.* 1998; 17(12): 3351-3362.

Subach, B.R. *et al.* Morbidity and survival after 1,3-bis(2-chloroethyl)-1-nitrosourea wafer implantation for recurrent glioblastoma: a retrospective case-matched cohort series. *Neurosurgery.* 1999; 45(1): 17–22; discussion 22–23.

Suzutani, T. *et al.* The role of the UL41 gene of herpes simplex virus type 1 in evasion of non-specific host defense mechanisms during primary infection. *J Gen Virol.* 2000; 81(Pt 7): 1763-1771.

Sypula, J. *et al.* Myxoma virus tropism in human tumor cells. *Gene Ther. Mol. Biol.* 2004; 81: 108-114.

Takakuwa, H. *et al.* Oncolytic viral therapy using a spontaneously generated herpes simplex virus type 1 variant for disseminated peritoneal tumor in immunocompetent mice. *Arch Virol.* 2003; 148(4): 813-825.

Tamura, T. *et al.* The IRF family transcription factors in immunity and oncogenesis. *Annu Rev Immunol.* 2008; 26: 535-584.

Taniguchi, T. *et al.* IRF family of transcription factors as regulators of host defense. *Annu Rev Immunol.* 2001; 19: 623-655.

Teshigahara, O. *et al.* Oncolytic viral therapy for breast cancer with Herpes Simplex Virus Type 1 mutant HF10. *J. Surg. Oncol.* 2004; 85(1): 42-47.

Toda, M. *et al.* Treatment of human breast cancer in a brain metastatic model by G207, a replication-competent multimutated herpes simplex virus 1. *Hum Gene Ther.* 1998; 9(15): 2177-2185.

Toda, M. *et al.* Tumor growth inhibition by intratumoral inoculation of defective herpes simplex virus vectors expressing granulocyte-macrophage colony-stimulating factor. *Mol Ther.* 2000; 2(4): 324-329.

Todo, T. *et al.* In situ expression of soluble B7-1 in the context of oncolytic herpes simplex virus induces potent antitumor immunity. *Cancer Res.* 2001a; 61(1): 153-161.

Todo, T. *et al.* Oncolytic herpes simplex virus vector with enhanced MHC class I presentation and tumor cell killing. *Proc Natl Acad Sci USA.* 2001b; 98(11): 6396-6401.

Todo, T. Oncolytic virus therapy using genetically engineered herpes simplex viruses. *Hum Cell.* 2002; 15(3): 151-159.

Turin, L. *et al.* BHV-1: New Molecular Approaches to Control a Common and Widespread Infection. *Molecular Medicine.* 1999; 5(5), 261-284.

Vaha-Koskela, M.J. *et al.* Oncolytic viruses in cancer therapy. *Cancer Letters.* 2007; 254(2), 178-216.

Valyi-Nagy, T. *et al.* A thymidine kinase-negative HSV-1 strain establishes a persistent infection in SCID mice that features uncontrolled peripheral replication but only marginal nervous system involvement. *Virology.* 1994; 199(2): 484-490.

Varghese, S. & Rabkin, S.D. Oncolytic herpes simplex virus vectors for cancer virotherapy. *Cancer Gene Ther.* 2002; 9(12): 967-978.

Verpooten, D. *et al.* Control of TANK-binding kinase 1-mediated signalling by the gamma(1)34.5 protein of herpes simplex virus 1. *J Biol Chem.* 2009; 284(2): 1097-1105.

Vile, R. *et al.* The oncolytic virotherapy treatment platform for cancer: unique biological and biosafety points to consider. *Cancer Gene Ther.* 2002; 9(12): 1062-1067.

Wakimoto, H. *et al.* Effects of innate immunity on herpes simplex virus and its ability to kill cells. *Gene Ther.* 2003; 10(11): 983-990.

Wang, F. *et al.* Disruption of Erk-dependent type I IFN induction breaks the myxoma virus species barrier. *Nat. Immunol.* 2004; 5(12): 1266-1274.

Wang, F. *et al.* RIG-I mediates the co-induction of tumor necrosis factor and type I interferon elicited by myxoma virus in primary human macrophages. *PLoS Pathog.* 2008; 4(7): e1000099.

Wang, G. *et al.* Infection of human cancer cells with myxoma virus requires Akt activation via interaction with a viral ankyrin-repeat host range factor. *Proc. Natl. Acad. Sci. USA.* 2006; 103(12): 4640 -4645.

Wein, L.M. *et al.* Validation and analysis of a mathematical model of a replication-competent oncolytic virus for cancer treatment: implications for virus design and delivery. *Cancer Res.* 2003; 63(6): 1317-1324.

Werden, SJ. *et al.* Pharmacological Manipulation of the Akt Signaling Pathway Regulates Myxoma Virus Replication and Tropism in Human Cancer Cells. *Journal of Virol.* 2010; 84(7): 3287-3302.

Willett, C.G. *et al.* Direct evidence that the VEGF specific antibody bevacizumab has antivascular effects in human rectal cancer. *Nat Med.* 2004; 10(2): 145–147.

Wong, R.J. *et al.* Effective treatment of head and neck squamous cell carcinoma by an oncolytic herpes simplex virus. *J Am Coll Surg.* 2001; 193(1): 12-21.

Wong, R.J. *et al.* Angiogenesis inhibition by an oncolytic herpes virus expressing interleukin 12. *Clin Cancer Res.* 2004; 10(13): 4509-4516.

Yamamura, H. *et al.* Identification of the transcriptional regulatory sequences of human calponin promoter and their use in targeting a conditionally replicating herpes vector to malignant human soft tissue and bone tumors. *Cancer Res.* 2001; 61(10): 3969-3977.

Yoon, S.S. *et al.* An oncolytic herpes simplex virus type 1 selectively destroys diffuse liver metastases from colon carcinoma. *FASEB J.* 2000; 14(2): 310-311.

Zamarin, D. *et al.* Genetically engineered Newcastle disease virus for malignant melanoma therapy. *Gene Ther.* 2009; 16(6): 796-804.

Zhang, Y.Q *et al.* Enhancing the therapeutic effect against ovarian cancer through a combination of viral oncolysis and antigen-specific immunotherapy. *Mol Ther.* 2010; 18(4): 692–699.

Zhao, H. *et al.* Recombinant Newcastle disease virus expressing human interleukin-2 serves as a potential candidate for tumor therapy. *Virus Res.* 2008; 136(1-2): 75-80.
Zhou, G. *et al.* Construction and properties of a herpes simplex virus 1 designed to enter cells solely via the IL-13alpha2 receptor. *Proc Natl Acad Sci USA.* 2006; 103(14): 5508-5513.

19

Gene Therapy of Melanoma Using Inactivated Sendai Virus Envelope Vector (HVJ-E) with Intrinsic Anti-Tumor Activities

Yasufumi Kaneda[1], Eiji Kiyohara[1,2],
Toshimitsu Itai[3] and Toshihiro Nakajima[3]
[1]*Division of Gene Therapy Science,*
[2]*Department of Dermatology, Graduate School of Medicine,*
Osaka University, Suita, Osaka
[3]*GenomIdea, Inc., 1-8-31 Midorigaoka, Ikeda, Osaka,*
Japan

1. Introduction

Despite the development of various cancer treatments, including surgical treatment, radiation, and anti-cancer reagents, cancer cells are not completely eliminated from the body in many cases, which allows the tumors to recur. Disease recurrence is the most difficult problem in cancer treatment. Much attention has been paid to cancer immunotherapy as a strategy to eliminate cancer cells from patients (1). However, numerous failures of cancer immunotherapy have indicated the difficulty of achieving anti-cancer immunity (1, 2). Cancer tissues produce factors that attenuate anti-tumor immunity and eventually induce immunotolerance against cancers in tumor-bearing individuals (3, 4). Therefore, to successfully eradicate cancer, first the tumor mass must be reduced as much as possible through surgery, radiation and chemotherapy; then, immunotherapy should be provided to increase the immune-activation signals and decrease the immune-suppression signals (5-7). Thus, multi-lateral strategies are needed in cancer treatment. Gene therapy has been anticipated to be a new tool for cancer treatment (8). Much attention has been also paid to immuno-gene therapy (9). However, it is still very difficult to achieve long-term remissions in cancer patients (10). Based on the concept of multi-lateral strategies, the control of multiple pathways of cancer growth is also necessary in gene therapy. We have developed a hemagglutinating virus of Japan envelope (HVJ-E) vector by using inactivated Sendai virus as a pseudovirion for gene and drug delivery (11). This vector can deliver siRNA, DNA, proteins, and anti-cancer drugs to cells *in vitro* and *in vivo* (12).

We previously reported that HVJ-E itself has a strong anti-tumor effect against mouse tumors, such as colon carcinoma and renal carcinoma, by the activation of cytotoxic T lymphocytes and natural killer cells and the suppression of regulatory T cells (13, 14). Recently, we also determined the direct tumor-killing activity of HVJ-E through the induction of type I interferon on hormone-resistant human prostate cancer cells and human glioblastoma cells (15, 16). Thus, HVJ-E is a versatile gene and drug delivery vector with intrinsic anti-cancer activities. Therefore, it is expected that synergistic anti-tumor effects can be achieved by HVJ-E vector with incorporated therapeutic molecules.

Melanoma is a one of the most aggressive tumors due to its strong ability to metastasize. In the United States, there were an estimated 62,480 new melanoma cases and 8,420 deaths caused by melanomas in 2008 (17). Although the 5-year survival rate of patients with localized melanoma at the early stage is greater than 90%, the survival rate drops to less than 20% once the melanoma has metastasized to distant sites (17).

Many chemotherapeutic agents have been used alone or in combination to treat melanoma (18). However, these therapies are insufficient for the eradication of melanoma cells, and recurrences are often observed. A recent report indicates that B-RAF inhibitor is a promising treatment for malignant melanoma patients (19). However, after the initial response, melanoma recurrence frequently occurred in the inhibitor-treated patients due to the up-regulation of other signaling molecules, such as RTK or N-RAS (20). Thus, when some signaling pathways are inhibited, cancer cells become resistant to the drug by the up-regulation of other pathways. Another report showed that the resistance to B-RAF inhibition in melanoma could be overcome by targeting both MEK and IGF-1receptor-mediated PI3 kinase (21). However, even when these pathways are inhibited, the elimination of all cancer cells is unlikely. Molecular-targeting drugs are very attractive because of their selectivity. However, this strategy may fall into a vicious cycle because cancers are heterogeneous and become adaptive to the drugs. Thus, a novel strategy is needed for the treatment of melanoma.

In the present study, we tested the possibility of HVJ-E with or without a therapeutic gene for the effective treatment of melanoma in a mouse model. We incorporated the IL12 gene into the HVJ-E vector (IL12/HVJ-E) and compared the tumor regression induced by IL12/HVJ-E and HVJ-E (without IL12 cDNA). We also performed a series of six HVJ-E injections into both mouse and human melanomas in mouse models to compare the suppression of tumor growth and survival time with three injections of HVJ-E.

2. Materials and methods

Cell lines and animals: Mouse melanoma F10 cells were purchased from the American Tissue Culture Collection, and human melanoma Mewo cells were purchased from the Japanese Collection of Research Bioresources. Mouse melanoma B16-BL6 cells expressing the luciferase gene were prepared by GenomIdea Inc. (Ikeda, Osaka, Japan). Cancer cells were grown in DMEM supplemented with 10% fetal bovine serum and 5% penicillin-streptomycin and maintained at 37°C in a humidified atmosphere with 5% CO2. Murine bone marrow-derived DCs were generated as previously described. More than 90% of these DCs were positive for CD11c. Five- to six-week-old male C.B-17/IcrCrj-SCID mice and C57BL/6 mice were purchased from Charles River Inc. (Yokohama, Japan) and maintained in a temperature-controlled, pathogen-free room. All animals were handled according to the approved protocols and guidelines of the Animal Committee of Osaka University.

HVJ-E preparation and siRNA transfection: HVJ (VR-105 parainfluenza 1 Sendai/52, Z strain) propagated in HEK293 cells was collected and inactivated by UV irradiation (99 mJ/cm^2) and β-propiolactone. The inactivated HVJ suspension (HVJ-E) was purified by GenomIdea Inc. by using four different columns. The titer of HVJ-E was examined by neuraminidase activity (mNAU). One mNAU corresponded to approximately 5 x 10^7

particles. Two hundred micrograms of plasmid DNA was mixed with 2000 mNAU HVJ-E in the presence of Tween 80 (final concentration, 0.05%).

Cytokine measurements: Mouse dendritic cells or F10 melanoma cells were seeded at 5 x 10^4 cells/well in 96-well plates. The following day, HVJ-E (MOI: 10^2 - 10^4) was added, and the cells were cultured for another 24 hr. After this, cytokines and chemokines were measured within the supernatant by ELISA performed with commercially available reagents (PBL Biomedical Laboratories, Piscataway, NJ, USA).

TUNEL assay: Twenty-four hours after three injections of HVJ-E or PBS, tissue sections were prepared by using a microtome. The sections were washed twice with PBS and fixed with 4% paraformaldehyde for 15 min at 4°C. The terminal deoxynucleotide transferase-mediated dUTP nick-end labeling (TUNEL) assay was performed according to the protocol of an *in situ* Apoptosis Detection Kit (Takara Bio Inc.).

Quantitative real-time RT-PCR: Isogen (Nippon Gene, Japan) was used to extract total RNA from tumors that had been resected and washed in PBS. A total of 2 μg of total RNA was reverse transcribed into cDNA and analyzed as *in vitro*. Probes and primer pairs specific for murine DX5, CD8, CD11c, and glyceraldehyde-3-phosphate dehydrogenase (GAPDH) were purchased from Applied Biosystems. The concentration of target genes was determined by using the comparative CT method (threshold cycle number at the cross-point between amplification plot and threshold), and values were normalized to an internal GAPDH control.

ELISPOT assay: Mice were sacrificed 7 days after the fifth IP injection. Splenocytes were harvested from the spleen and cultured as previously described (15). A total of 1×10^4 lymphocytes were cultured with 0.2×10^4 mitomycin C-treated F10 cells at 37°C for 24 hr. The assay was performed by using a mouse IFN-gamma ELISPOT kit (R&D Systems). The number of spots was counted under a dissecting microscope (Leica, Cambridge, UK).

Tumor growth *in vivo*: Viable melanoma cells were re-suspended in 100 μl of PBS and intradermally injected into the backs of the mice. When each tumor had grown to approximately 4-6 mm in diameter, the mice were treated with intra-tumor injections of HVJ-E (in a total volume of 100 μl) or 100 μl of PBS. Tumor size was measured in a blinded manner with slide calipers, and tumor volume was calculated with the following formula: tumor volume (mm^3) = length × $(width)^2$ / 2. In a spontaneous lung metastasis model, B16-BL6 cells (10^6 cells) were subcutaneously inoculated into a C57BL/6 mouse. The mice were injected with HVJ-E (300, 1000 and 2000 mNAU) or PBS three times on days 4, 8 and 12. On day 26, the mice were sacrificed. Lungs were isolated and fixed with 10% formalin solution, and the size and number of metastatic foci were examined.

Statistical analysis: *In vitro* results were analyzed with the Student's non-paired *t*-test. Comparisons of *in vivo* results were made by using Kaplan-Meyer's method or Dunnett's test. Differences with P values < 0.05 were considered statistically significant.

3. Results

HVJ envelope (HVJ-E) was constructed by inactivation of HVJ (hemagglutinating virus of Japan; Sendai virus) with ß-propiolactone (0.0075% - 0.001%) or UV irradiation (99 mjoule/cm^2), as described previously, and then purified by ion-exchange column chromatography and gel filtration. The diameter of HVJ-E was 220 nm, and the zeta potential was approximately –5 mV. Exogenous plasmid DNA was incorporated into inactivated HVJ by treatment with mild detergent and centrifugation (10,000 g, 5-10 min). Various detergents, such as Triton X-100, NP-40, deoxycholate and Tween 80, were available for incorporating exogenous DNA into HVJ-E. The exogenous DNA incorporation rate was approximately 15% - 20% and did not vary significantly among the different detergents. However, when detergent-treated HVJ-E was added to dendritic cells or melanoma cells, the cytokine production from those cells was varied. IL-6, which plays a major role in the anti-tumor immunity of HVJ-E, was produced from dendritic cells treatment with Tween 80-treated HVJ-E as well as non-treated HVJ-E while it was dramatically suppressed by HVJ-E treated with other detergents (Fig. 1A). Tween 80-treated HVJ-E maintained the production of interferon-α and RANTES from dendritic cells, but Triton X-100-treated HVJ-E lost this ability (Fig. 1B and C). The optimum concentration of Tween 80 was 0.05%, which also enabled the incorporation of exogenous DNA into HVJ-E (data not shown). Mouse melanoma B16-F10 cells produced a small amount of interferon-β in response to HVJ-E. As shown in Fig. 1D, Tween 80-treated HVJ-E stimulated interferon-β secretion from melanoma cells in a dose-dependent manner. However, the interferon-β production induced by Triton X-100-treated HVJ-E was greatly suppressed. Therefore, we used 0.05% Tween 80-treated HVJ-E for cancer treatment in a mouse model.

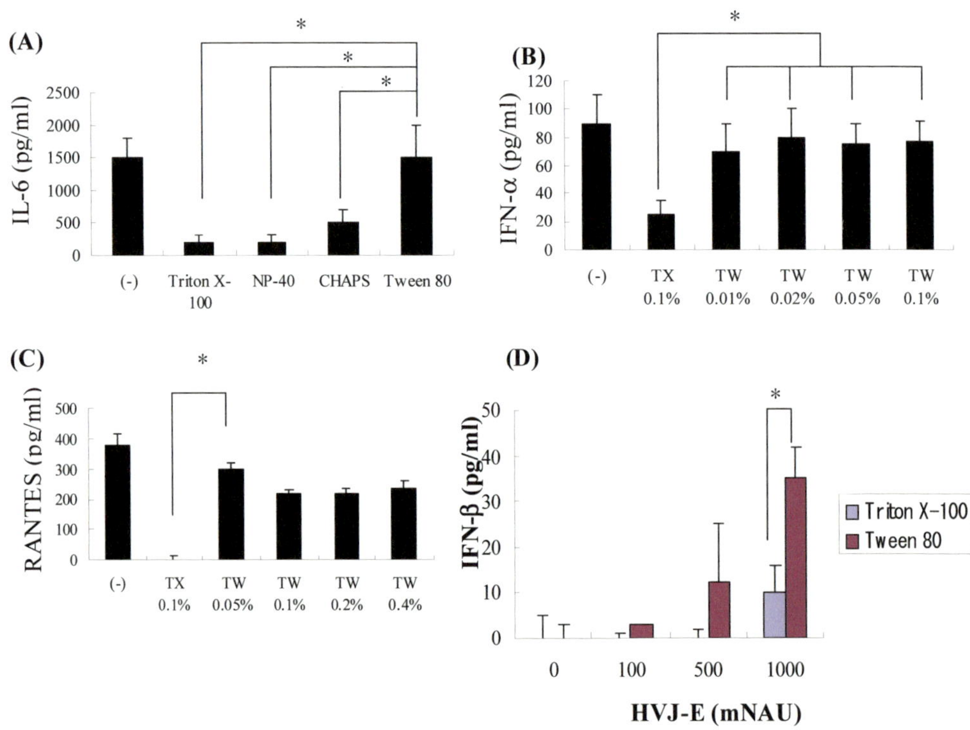

Fig. 1. The effect of detergent on the production of cytokine and chemokine from dendritic cells and tumor cells treated with HVJ-E.

IL-6 (A), IFN-α (B) and RANTES (C) in mouse dendritic cells were assessed by using ELISA kits 24 hours after HVJ-E treatment. In (A), HVJ-E was treated with detergent (0.2% Triton X-100, 0.1% NP-40, 1.25 CHAPS or 0.05% Tween 80). The concentration of each detergent was required for incorporation of plasmid DNA into HVJ-E. In (B) and (C), 0.1% Triton X-100 (TX) and 0.01 - 0.4 % Tween 80 (TW) were used.

To test the anti-tumor effects of Tween 80-treated HVJ-E, mouse melanoma B16-F10 cells were intradermally inoculated into C57BL/6 mice. When the diameter of the tumor was approximately 5 mm, various amounts of HVJ-E were injected into tumors in a series of three injections with 4 days between injections (Fig. 2). Tumor regression was induced by HVJ-E. After three injections of HVJ-E (1000 mNAU), a TUNEL assay was performed on tumor sections to detect apoptosis. As shown in Fig. 3, TUNEL-positive cells were abundantly observed in the tumor tissues treated with HVJ-E but not in normal tissues.

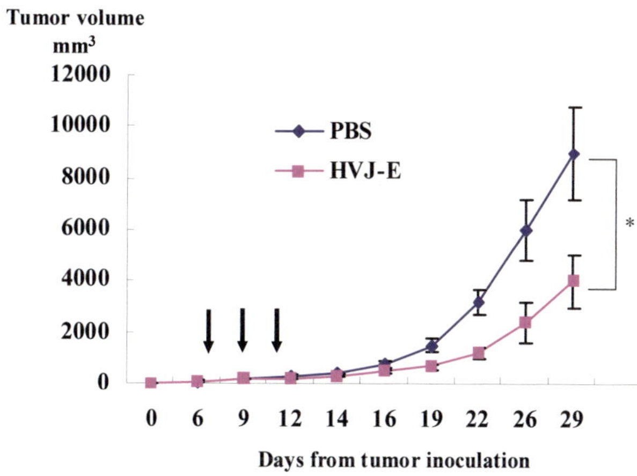

Fig. 2. Mouse melanoma treatment by three-times injection of HVJ-E

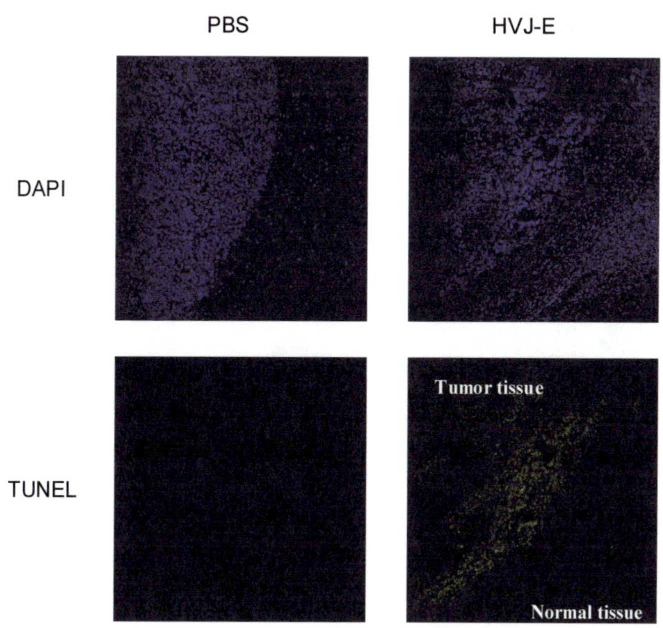

Fig. 3. Apoptotic cells in the tumor tissue by the injection of HVJ-E

C57BL/6 mice (each group; n=5) were challenged with 5×10^5 F10 cells by intradermal injection on the dorsal surface. After tumors reached 4~6 mm in diameter, 1000 mNAU HVJ-E or PBS was injected into the tumors once every other day on days 6, 8 and 10. Tumor diameter was measured to calculate tumor volume. Bars, SD. *P <0.05.
Twenty-four hours after the third injection of HVJ-E (1000 mNAU) or PBS, tissue sections were prepared for a TUNEL assay. Successive sections were stained with DAPI to confirm the position of nuclei. The boundary between tumor and normal tissues was confirmed by H-E staining of successive sections and shown by a white dotted line.
As we have previously reported the generation of multiple anti-tumor immunities by HVJ-E, the infiltration of immune cells into the tumor bed was analyzed by RT-PCR at 48 hours after the last of three injections of HVJ-E (1000 mNAU). CD11c, CD8 and DX5 were highly expressed in melanoma tissues (Fig. 4A), indicating the infiltration of dendritic cells, $CD8^+$ T cells and NK cells. Two weeks later, the cytotoxic T-cell response was evaluated by ELISPOT assay (Fig. 4B). A significant increase in interferon-γ spots was detected in spleen cells from mice injected with HVJ-E.
The subcutaneous mouse melanoma (B16-BL6) cells spontaneously metastasized to the lung. When the subcutaneous tumor mass was treated with HVJ-E, the ratio of mice with more than one melanoma focus in the lungs significantly decreased (Table 1). In particular, the number of large-sized metastatic foci (>0.7 mm in diameter) were dramatically reduced.

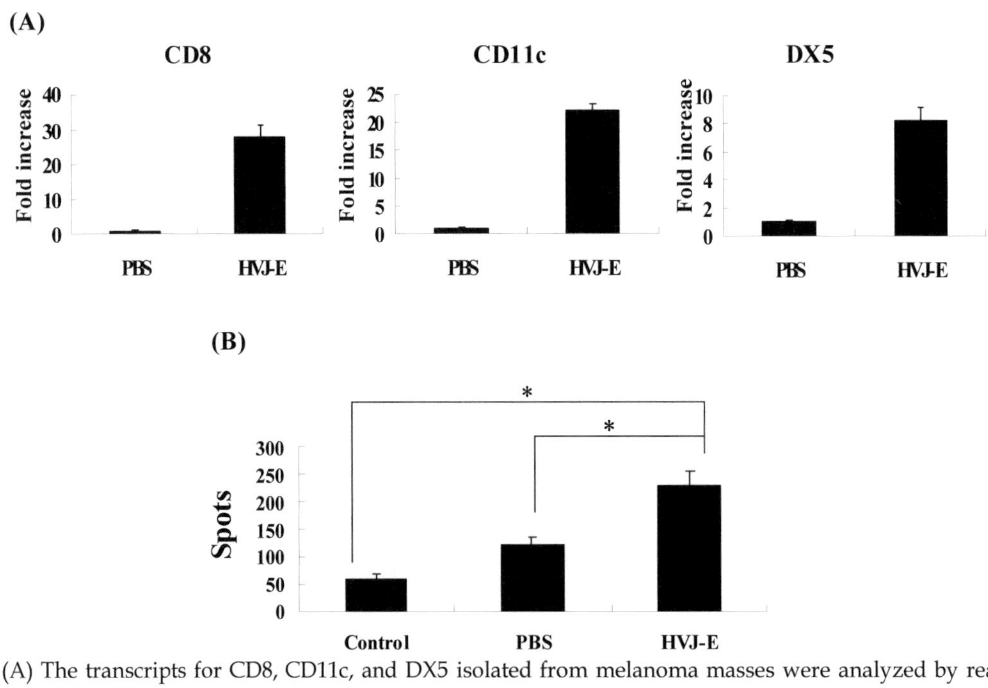

(A) The transcripts for CD8, CD11c, and DX5 isolated from melanoma masses were analyzed by real-time PCR. Values were normalized to an internal GAPDH control. The ratio of each transcript from HVJ-E-treated samples to that from PBS-injected samples is shown as the fold increase. Bars, SD. (B) ELISPOT assay of IFN-γ from lymphocytes collected from the spleen 7 days after the last injection of HVJ-E or PBS. Control samples were prepared from lymphocytes collected from untreated tumor-bearing mice. Bars, SD. *P <0.05.

Fig. 4. Infiltration of immune cells into tumor tissue by intratumoral injection of HVJ-E

Group	n	Lung (%)		
		Total	>0.4 mm in length	>0.7 mm in length
PBS	10	100	80	70
HVJ-E 300 mNAU	11	82	18*	9-
HVJ-E 1000 mNAU	8	38*	13*	0-
HVJ-E 2000 mNAU	9	44*	22*	0-

*Statistical significance vs. PBS at $p<0.05$ by Steel's test
- Impossible for statistical analysis

Table 1. Ratio of mouse with more than one metastatic focus in lung

To increase the anti-tumor effects of HVJ-E, mouse IL-12 cDNA (IL-12/HVJ-E) was incorporated into HVJ-E, and the resulting vector was injected into the intradermal tumor mass of B16-BL6 cells. As shown in Fig. 5A, a series of three injections of IL-12/HVJ-E was more effective for melanoma regression than mock HVJ-E that contained vector plasmid without IL-12 cDNA. The survival and body weight change of tumor-bearing mice were analyzed. Fig 5B shows that 90% of mice injected with three times were alive on day 46, when all the mice injected with either mock HVJ or PBS had died. There was no decrease in the body weight of mice treated with IL-12/HVJ-E. No significant difference was observed in the growth rate of the PBS and IL-12/HVJ-E groups (Fig. 5C).

(A)

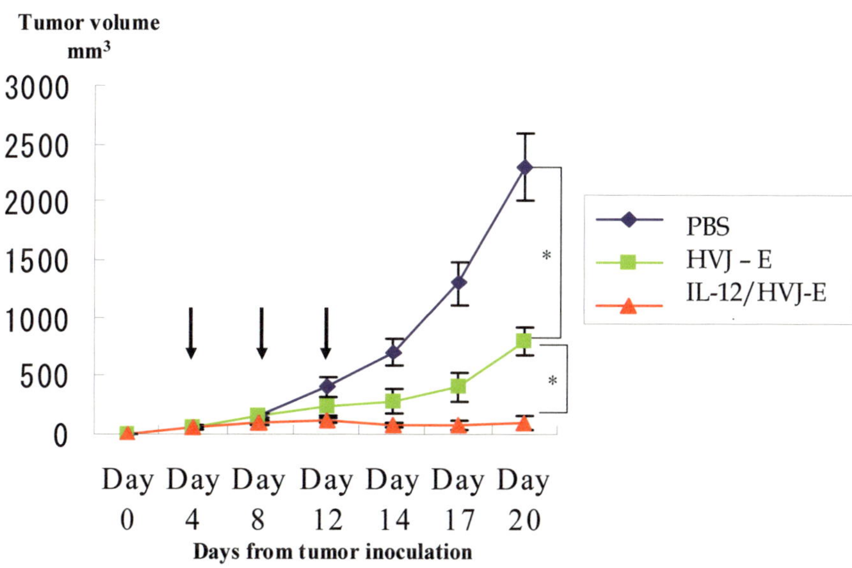

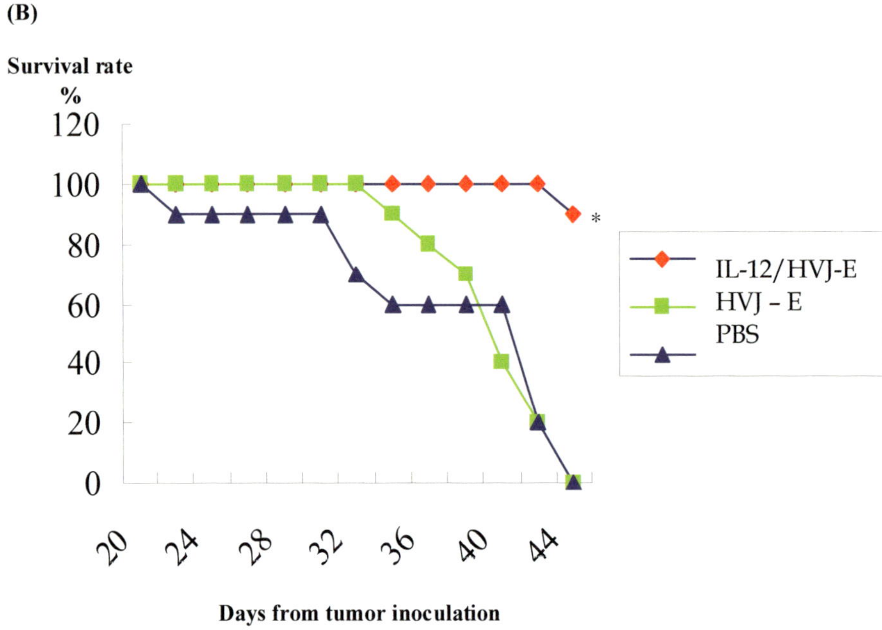

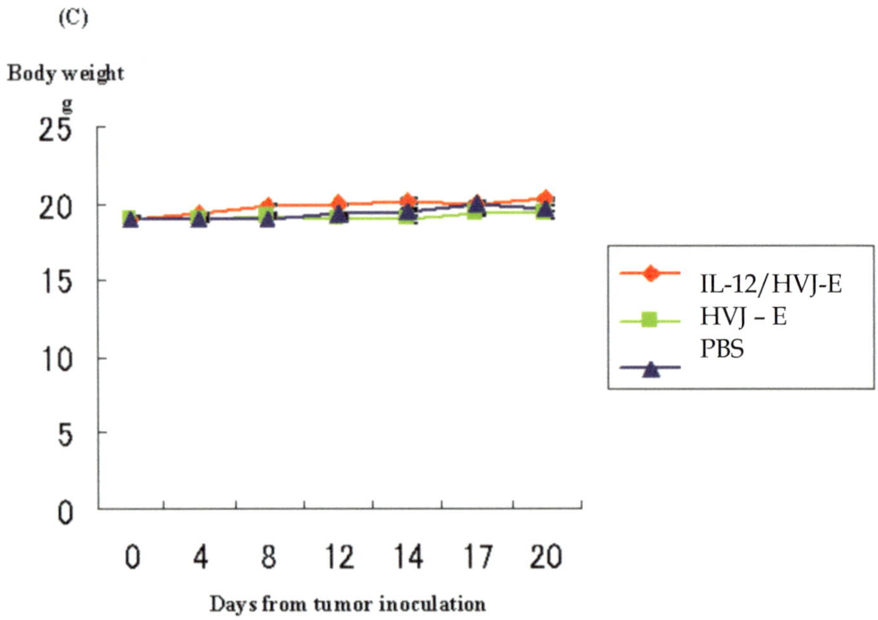

(A) C57BL/6 mice (each group; n=5) were challenged with 10^6 B16-BL6 cells by intradermal injection on the dorsal surface. After tumors reached 4~6 mm in diameter, HVJ-E (1000 mNAU), HVJ-E containing IL-12 cDNA or PBS were injected into the tumors on days 4, 8 and 12. Tumor diameter was measured to calculate tumor volume. Bars, SD. *P <0.05. (B) The survival of mice injected with HVJ-E (1000 mNAU) containing IL-12 cDNA (IL12/HVJ-E) or HVJ-E containing vector plasmid without IL12 (mock HVJ-E) or PBS (each group; n=10) is shown. *P <0.05. (C) Body weight of mice treated with IL12/HVJ-E, mock HVJ-E or PBS is shown (each group; n=10).

Fig. 5. Gene therapy of mouse melanoma by IL-12/HVJ-E

Three injections of HVJ-E without a therapeutic gene resulted in a significant regression of melanoma growth (Fig. 2), but the survival of tumor-bearing mice was not significantly prolonged as compared with the mice injected with PBS. Then, we tested whether a series of six injections of HVJ-E without therapeutic genes could prolong mouse survival. We found that the series of six injections inhibited melanoma (B16-BL6) growth and significantly prolonged the survival (Fig. 6 A and B). A similarly prolonged survival was also observed in B16-F10 melanoma model mice that received six HVJ-E injections (data not shown). Based on these results, we attempted to treat human melanoma (Mewo) in immunodeficient SCID mice. Six injections of HVJ-E suppressed the growth of human melanoma in a dose-dependent manner and significantly prolonged mouse survival (Fig. 7A and B).

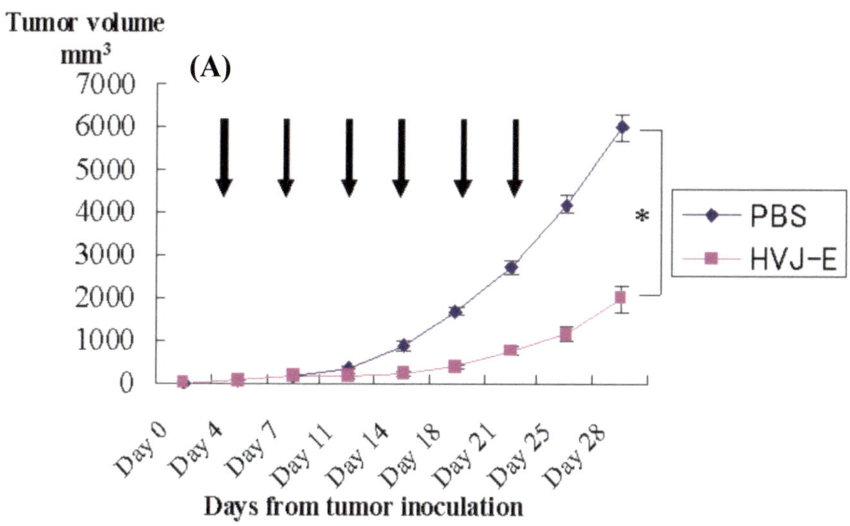

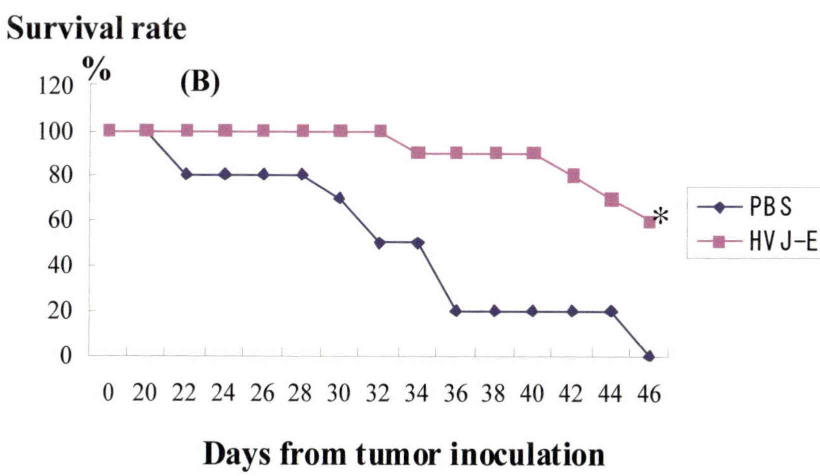

(A) A series of six injections of HVJ-E (1000 mNAU) or PBS was administered to mice with intradermal tumor B16-BL6 melanoma on days 4, 8, 12, 16, 20 and 24 (each group; n=5). Bars, SD. *P <0.05. (B) The survival of mice injected with HVJ-E (1000 mNAU) or PBS (each group; n=10) is shown. *P <0.05.

Fig. 6. Mouse melanoma treatment by six times injection of HVJ-E

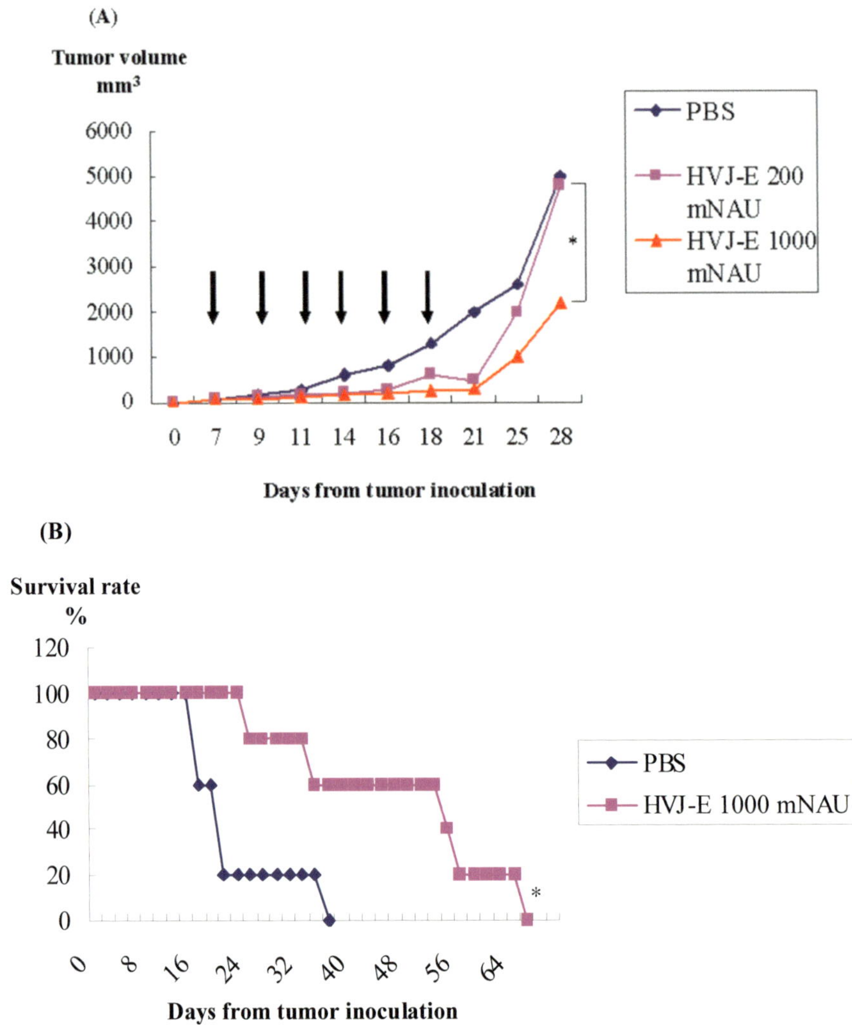

(A) Human melanoma Mewo cells (10^6 cells) were inoculated intradermally into SCID mice. Six injections of HVJ-E (200 mNAU, 1000 mNAU) or PBS were administered to the mice on days 7, 9, 11, 13, 15 and 17 (each group; n=5). Bars, SD. *P <0.05. (B) The survival of mice injected with HVJ-E (1000 mNAU) or PBS (each group; n=10) is shown. *P <0.05.

Fig. 7. Human melanoma treatment by six-times injection of HVJ-E

4. Discussion

HVJ-E was originally developed as a vector for the delivery of drugs and genes (11, 12). Then, it was found that vector itself has anti-tumor activities (13-16). For cancer treatment, a single modality of therapeutic strategy is not sufficient. By using HVJ-E, multi-lateral cancer treatment can be achieved by incorporating therapeutic molecules into HVJ-E with intrinsic anti-tumor activities. Here, we demonstrate that the anti-tumor activities of HVJ-E are enhanced by the incorporation of IL-12 cDNA. Our previous reports showed that HVJ-E induces the production of interferon-α, -β, IL-6 and CXCL10 in mouse dendritic cells

(13, 14). However, interferon-γ was not produced from dendritic cells treated with HVJ-E. Rather, interferon-γ was secreted from NK cells exposed to interferon-β produced from HVJ-E-treated dendritic cells (14). Since interferon-γ plays a key role in anti-tumor immunity (22), we selected IL-12, which induces interferon-γ in immune cells, for incorporation into HVJ-E. Local injection of the IL-12 gene into melanoma by using the canarypox virus or naked plasmid DNA has already been clinically tested and shows promising results (23, 24). In the present study, the IL-12 gene was coupled with HVJ-E, which has intrinsic anti-tumor activities; therefore, synergistic anti-tumor effects were expected. Indeed, in mouse tumor models of melanoma, IL-12/HVJ-E enhanced tumor regression and prolonged mouse survival more effectively as compared to mock HVJ-E without IL-12 cDNA. However, even when the therapeutic gene was not used, more frequent injections of HVJ-E increased the anti-tumor activities and prolonged the mouse survival. This result might be due to the accumulation of the anti-tumor effects of HVJ-E. A similar regression of human melanoma tumors in immunodeficient SCID mice was achieved by six injections of HVJ-E without therapeutic genes. In SCID mice, which lack T-cell immunity, NK cells activated by HVJ-E play a role in tumor suppression, as previously reported (14). Additionally, HVJ-E induces cancer cell killing in some human tumors, such as prostate cancer (15), glioblastoma (16), neuroblastoma and mammary carcinoma (YK; unpublished data). We found that HVJ-E itself induced apoptosis in Mewo cells in a dose-dependent manner, although the efficiency was not as high as the efficiency in glioblastoma and prostate cancers. This activity of HVJ-E also achieved significant regression of human melanoma in SCID mice and prolonged mouse survival. In SCID mice inoculated with Mewo cells, we compared the efficacy of HVJ-E to the efficacy of a clinically used anti-melanoma reagent, dacarbazine (DTIC). Three intratumoral injections of HVJ-E were sufficient for overcoming the tumor suppression effect by six intraperitoneal injections of DTIC.

The anti-tumor immunity induced by HVJ-E was shown to be caused by the production of cytokines and chemokines (14), which are produced in response to the recognition of viral RNA by RIG-I (25-27). HVJ-E contains viral RNA fragments (200 - 300 bases) that also have the potential to be recognized by RIG-I (28). Therefore, it is likely that the production of chemokines and cytokines induced by HVJ-E depends on the amount of viral RNA fragments introduced into the cytoplasm by membrane fusion. As shown in Figure 1, the production is dependent on the treatment of HVJ-E with detergent. We recently found that depletion of cholesterol from HVJ by methyl-β-cyclodextrin attenuated the infectivity of the virus due to the irreversible dysfunction of fusion protein (29). It is speculated that some detergents, such as Triton X-100 and NP-40, may damage fusion activity, while other detergents such as Tween 80 may maintain that activity. The difference might be due to the amount of envelope lipids depleted by the detergent treatment. Although the reason remains to be elucidated, Tween 80-treated HVJ-E is recommended for the treatment of cancer and infectious disease, and Triton X-100-treated HVJ-E is recommended for the treatment of other diseases, such as cardiovascular disease and inflammatory disease, which are exacerbated by cytokines and chemokines.

It has been determined that the selective cancer-killing activity of HVJ-E is mediated through the RIG-I/MAVS signaling pathway, which is activated by viral RNA fragments of HVJ-E (YK; manuscript in preparation). Therefore, Tween 80-treated HVJ-E can be equipped with both anti-tumor immunities and cancer-killing activities.

Recently, we also demonstrated the augmentation of the anti-tumor activities of HVJ-E by incorporating siRNA against motor protein Eg5 in glioblastoma treatment (30). The ability of Eg5 siRNA to induce cell-cycle arrest compensated for HVJ-E in conducting apoptosis. Since the mechanism of apoptosis induced by Eg5 siRNA is different from that induced by HVJ-E, the combination of HVJ-E with Eg5 siRNA creates a synergistic anti-tumor effect. Thus, if a molecule to promote cancer progression after HVJ-E treatment is identified by comprehensive microarray analysis of transcripts in cancer cells, the combination of HVJ-E and siRNA against that molecule will be recommended as an effective cancer treatment.

5. Acknowledgment

This study was supported by the Program for Promotion of Fundamental Studies in Health Sciences of the National Institute of Biomedical Innovation (Project ID:10-03), the Northern Osaka (Saito) Biomedical Knowledge-Based Cluster Creation Project, a grant-in-aid for Promoting Science from the Ministry of Education, Culture, Sports, Science and Technology of Japan, and grants from the Ministry of Health, Labor, and Welfare of Japan.

6. References

[1] Rosenberg S. Progress in human tumour immunology and immunotherapy. Nature 2001; 411, 380-384.

[2] O'Neill D and Bhardwaj N. (2005) Exploiting dendritic cells for active immunotherapy of cancer and chronic infection. Methods Mol Med. 109:1-18.

[3] Gross S, Walde P. Immunosuppressive mechanisms in human tumors; why we still cannot cure cancer. Imunol Lett. 2008; 116, 7-14.

[4] Kim R, Emi M, and Tanabe K. Cancer immunosuppression and autoimmune disease: beyond immunosuppressive network for tumor immunity. Immunology 2006; 119: 254-264.

[5] Kirkwood JM, Tarhini AA, Panelli MC, et al. Next generation of immunotherapy for melanoma. J. Clin. Oncol. 2008;20:3445-3455.

[6] Samuel M, Chow PK, Chan S-Y, et al. Neoadjuvant and adjuvant therapy for surgical resection of hepatocellular carcinoma. Database Syst Rev. 2009, Jan 21;(1):CD001199.

[7] Dudley ME, Yang JC, Sherry R, et al. Adoptive cell therapy for patients with metastatic melanoma: evaluation of intensive myeloablative chemoradiation preparative regimens. J Clin Oncol. 2008;26:5233-5239.

[8] Moon C, Oh Y, and Roth JA. Current status of gene therapy for lung cancer and head and neck cancer. Clin Cancer Res. 2003; 9:5055-5067.

[9] Vera JF, Brenner MK, Dotti G. Immunotherapy of human cancers using gene modified T lymphocytes. Curr Gene Ther. 2009 Oct;9(5):396-408.

[10] Gajewski TF, Louahed J, Brichard VG. Gene signature in melanoma associated with clinical activity: a potential clue to unlock cancer immunotherapy. Cancer J. 2010;16(4):399-403.

[11] Kaneda Y, Nakajima T, Nishikawa T, et al. Hemagglutinating virus of Japan (HVJ) envelope vector as a versatile gene delivery system. Mol Ther. 2002;6(2):219-226.

[12] Kaneda Y. Applications on hemagglutinating virus of Japan in therapeutic delivery system. Expert Opinion Drug Delivery 2008;5:221-33.

[13] Kurooka M and Kaneda Y. Inactivated Sendai virus particles eradicate tumors by inducing immune responses through blocking regulatory T cells. Cancer Res. 2007;67:227-236.
[14] Fujihara A, Kurooka M, Miki T, et al. Intratumoral injection of inactivated Sendai virus particles elicits strong antitumor activity by enhancing local CXCL10 expression and systemic NK cell activation. Cancer Immunology Immunotherapy 2008;57:73-84.
[15] Kawaguchi Y, Miyamoto Y, Inoue T, et al. Efficient eradication of hormone-resistant human prostate cancers by inactivated Sendai virus particle. Int. J. Cancer 2009;124: 2478-87.
[16] Tanaka M, Shimbo T, KikuchiY, Matsuda M, Kaneda Y. Sterile alpha motif containing domain 9 (SAMD9) is involved in death signaling of malignant glioma treated with inactivated Sendai virus particle (HVJ-E) or type I interferon. Int. J. Cancer 2010;126: 1982-1991.
[17] Atkins MB, Buzaid AC, Houghton AN. Systemic chemotherapy and biochemotherapy. In: Cutaneous-Melanoma (Balch CM, et al. eds) 4th ed. Quality Medical Publishing. St. Louis, 2003; 589-604.
[18] Huncharek M, Caubet JF, McGarry R. Single-agent DTIC versus combination chemotherapy with or without immunotherapy in metastatic melanoma: a meta-analysis of 3273 patients from 20 randomized trials. Melanoma Res 2001; 11: 75-81.
[19] Bollag G, Hirth P, Tsai J, et al. Clinical efficacy of a RAF inhibitor needs broad target blockade in BRAF-mutant melanoma. Nature. 2010;467(7315):596-599.
[20] Nazarian R, Shi H, Wang Q, et al. Melanomas acquire resistance to B-RAF (V600E) inhibition by RTK or N-RAS upregulation. Nature. 2010;468(7326):973-977.
[21] Villanueva J, Vultur A, Lee JT, et al. Acquired resistance to BRAF inhibitors mediated by a RAF kinase switch in melanoma can be overcome by cotargeting MEK and IGF-1R/PI3K. Cancer Cell. 2010;18(6):683-695.
[22] Gomes AQ, Martins DS, Silva-Santos B. Targeting gamma delta T lymphocytes for cancer immunotherapy: from novel mechanistic insight to clinical application. Cancer Res. 2010;70(24):10024-10027.
[23] Triozzi PL, Strong TV, Bucy RP, et al. Intratumoral administration of a recombinant canarypox virus expressing interleukin 12 in patients with metastatic melanoma. Hum Gene Ther. 2005; 16(1):91-100.
[24] Heinzerling L, Burg G, Dummer R, et al. Intratumoral injection of DNA encoding human interleukin 12 into patients with metastatic melanoma: clinical efficacy. Hum Gene Ther. 2005 Jan;16(1):35-48.
[25] Takeuchi O, Akira S. Innate immunity to virus infection. Immunol Rev. 2009;227:75-86.
[26] Yoneyama M, Fujita T. Recognition of viral nucleic acids in innate immunity. Rev. Med. Virol. 2010; 20, 4-22.
[27] Kato H, Takeuchi O, Sato S, Yoneyama M, Yamamoto M, Matsui K, Uematsu S, Jung A, Kawai T, Ishii KJ, Yamaguchi O, Otsu K, Tsujimura T, Koh C-S, Sousa CR, Matsuura Y, Fujita, T and Akira S. Differential roles of MDA5 and RIG-I helicases in the recognition of RNA viruses. Nature 2006; 441: 101-105.
[28] Schlee M, Hartmann E, Coch C, et al. Approaching the RNA ligand for RIG-I? Immunolog. Rev. 2009; 227, 66-74.

[29] Fujita H. Tamai K, Kwachi M, et al. Methyl-beta cyclodextrin alters the production and infectivity of Sendai virus. Archiv. Virol. In press.

[30] Matsuda M., Yamamoto T., Matsumura A, et al. Highly efficient eradication of intracranial glioblastoma using Eg5 siRNA combined with HVJ envelope. Gene Therapy 2009; 16, 1465-1476.

20

Pharmacokinetic Study of Viral Vectors for Gene Therapy: Progress and Challenges

Xianxing Xu[1], Jingwen Yang[2] and Yuanguo Cheng[1]
[1]*Department of Pharmacology, State Key Laboratory of Pathogen and Biosecurity, Beijing Institute of Microbiology and Epidemiology,*
[2]*Department of neurobiology, Beijing Institute of Basic Medical Science, PR China*

1. Introduction

Gene therapy may be described as the use of genes as medicines to treat disease, or, more precisely, as the delivery of nucleic acids by means of vectors to patients for some therapeutic purpose (Thanou, M. *et al.*, 2007). The major goal of gene therapy is to introduce a functional gene into a target cell and restore protein production that is absent or deficient due to a genetic disorder (Neeltje, A. *et al.*, 2003). This approach is a potentially powerful method for the treatment of diseases for which classical pharmacotherapy is unavailable or not easily applicable.

Gene therapy is a therapeutic modality with enormous promise, which is also considered to have failed to deliver much of therapeutic significance in spite of all the apparent clinical interest. Clinical trial activity in gene therapy began in 1989, peaked in 1999, and is now currently declining (Thanou, M. *et al.*, 2007). This decline was marked by some clinical trial problems, including a death from toxic liver shock during an adenovirus-based clinical trial in 1999 (Marshall, E., 2000), the anomalous appearance of a transgene in the gonads during adeno-associated virus-based preclinical trials in 2001 (Arruda, V. R. *et al.*, 2001), signs of hypertension in lipofection clinical trials in 2005 (Pro-1) (MacLachlan, I. *et al.*, 1999), and the development of leukemia in retrovirus-based clinical trials for ex vivo treatment of X-linked severe combined immunedeficiency (X-linked SCID) (Cavazzana-Calvo, M. *et al.*, 2004; Gaspar, H. B., & Thrasher, A. J., 2005).

Lessons from those frustrated results suggest that more basic research is required in gene therapy study, including mechanism of diseases and features of viral vectors. In order to modify a specific cell type or tissue, the therapeutic gene must be efficiently delivered to the cell, so that it will express at the appropriate level for a sufficient duration. Thus, identifying the ideal means of carriage for viral gene therapy is the key rate-limiting step in the development of most promising gene therapy strategies. In spite of long-term and extensive efforts to develop *in vivo* gene delivery systems, little achievements have been reported, especially as far as clinical applications are concerned. Apparently, the development of gene delivery systems will be one of the most critical issues for the success of *in vivo* gene therapy.

Over the years, two broad approaches have been used to deliver therapeutic genes to cells, viral vectors and non-viral vectors. These two kinds of vectors are different as regard to efficiency, ease of production and safety. Preclinical and current clinical trial data suggest that non-viral vector systems are much less affected by immunogenicity, toxicity, and oncogenicity. However, the lack of delivery efficacy and short-term expression in *in vivo* also pose their greatest drawback.

By contrast, viral-based vectors are feasible for modification and long-term gene expression, meanwhile, they are characterized by their infectivity and satisfactory targeting, all of which make them even more attractive as gene delivery systems. Nowadays, many viral vectors have been developed and frequently used in the present gene therapy studies, such as Adenovirus, Adeno-associated virus, retroviruses, herpes simplex virus type 1 and vaccinia virus. The real success has been reported with a serotype 5 adenovirus vector delivering the p53 tumor suppressor gene (Gendicine, the World's first commercial gene therapy product, licensed for use in China) (Pearson S. *et al.*, 2004). Viral vectors have also been applied in the treatment of monogenic diseases. In 2000, the World's first curative gene therapy trial was reported after bone marrow cells were isolated from patients with X-linked SCID (Cavazzana-Calvo, M. *et al*, 2000). In a word, gene therapy with viral vectors has been proven effective in a variety of model systems.

However, studies have also shown that even if some common characteristics exist, an important variability is introduced by the administration route, the promoter and other key components of the construct (targeting modifications, etc) (Dani, S.U., 1999). The variability results in a variety of challenges, including circumvention of immune responses against viral vectors and difficulty in transferring the genes to a sufficient number of cells to change the phenotype, and in controlling the expression of the gene (Worgall, S. & Crystal, R.G., 2007). Thus, it is currently admitted that pharmacokinetic studies should be carried out prior to any clinical trial for a promising viral gene therapy. Additionally, preexisting knowledge about the viral vectors, including the viral vector titration standardization issues, specific formulation and purification process, also prompts for dedicated pharmacokinetic studies.

Therefore, this chapter reviews the general strategies of the pharmacokinetic studies in viral gene therapy, provides an overview of the pharmacokinetic characteristics of viral vectors and the methods used in pharmacokinetic analysis of viral gene therapy, details the challenges and discusses the strategies being used to improve the analytical modality in viral gene therapy.

2. Pharmacokinetic characteristics of viral vectors

Viral vectors currently available for gene therapy can roughly be categorized into integrating and non-integrating vectors. Vectors based on adeno-associated virus and retroviruses (including lentivirus and foamy virus) are classified as integrating vectors as they have the ability to integrate their viral genome into the chromosomal DNA of the host cells, which will possibly achieve lifelong gene expression. Vectors based on adenovirus (Ad), modified vaccinia virus of Ankara (MVA) and herpes simplex virus type 1 (HSV-1) represent the non-integrating vectors (Pfeifer, A. & Verma, I.M., 2001). These vectors deliver their genomes into the nucleus of the target cells, where they remain episomal. The different behavior between these two kinds of viruses will frequently determine their difference in the availability at the target cells and also the undesirable sites following *in vivo* administration.

Accordingly, principles of pharmacokinetic study are equally applicable to conventional small-molecule drugs and biotech drugs (Meibohm, B., 2006), including viral vectors.

However, viral vectors often exhibit unique pharmacokinetic properties that are different from others.

As described previously, replication-deficient viral vectors remain *in vivo* for a temporal period due to rapidly elimination through degradation as well as by the clearance (Senoo, M., *et al*, 2000; Hackett, N.R., *et al*, 2000). Usually, the elimination of viral vectors within tissues or within the blood compartment results from the action of both endonucleases and exonucleases (Goncalves, MA. *et al.*, 2002). Hence, viral nucleic acids must be extracted and detected as soon as possible when performing a pharmacokinetic study with PCR method in case of rapid degradation. However, the suitability or yield of nucleic acid from extraction procedures can vary depending on the nucleic acid and the biological material (Kok, T. *et al.*, 2000). Great differences were found on the recoveries of viral DNA between tissues and blood as shown in Table 1, most experiments produced recovery of greater than 50%, while some were relative low but stable. Interestingly, the lowest recovery was found in blood (Lovatt, A., 2002). Therefore, efficient extraction of target nucleic acid should be evaluated for the particular target and biological material to be used.

Animal tissue	Recovery (%)
Brain	60-90
Kidney	70-95
Spleen	68-80
Lung	50-75
Gonads	60-90
Muscle	10-40
Blood	10-20
Heart	70-100
Lymph node	30-90
Liver	65-100

Table 1. Recovery of 10~100 copies of viral nucleic acid target per 100 microgram of animal tissue extracted with the Qiagen DNA mini kit (tissue and blood protocol)Additionally, it is very important to determine the optimal blood compartment for quantitative measurement of virus in peripheral blood specimens. Perlman, J. *et al.* compared the use of whole blood (WB), plasma, and peripheral blood mononuclear cells (PBMC) for the detection of adenovirus in peripheral blood specimens from a pediatric HSCT recipient population, and higher viral loads were in WB and plasma than in PBMC (Perlman, J. *et al.*, 2007).

In viral gene therapy, gene expression and duration is an important criterion and controlled by the choice of promoter, CpG content, topological form of DNA etc. Although viral vectors are structurally similar to the wild-type progenitor virus, they generally lack some or all of the viral genes, so that their ability to replicate is frequently impeded or obliterated (Worgall, S. & Crystal, R.G., 2007). Hence, the lack of sustained transgene expression may be another important characteristic of viral vectors, and must be taken into account when setting up treatment regiments and investigating their pharmacokinetics. What's more, controlling the gene expression is a challenge that needs to be addressed.

Ideally, each delivery problem should be assessed in the round from the site of administration to target cells of interest. And viral vectors probably present a much greater risk of oncogenicity, particularly retroviral vectors that mediate insertion into actively

expressing gene loci, thereby creating a high risk of oncogenesis (Pfeifer, A. & Verma, I.M., 2001). This condition must be considered during pharmacokinetic studies.
In short, gene therapy should be seen as a somatic medicine that seeks to treat disease at a more fundamental level than most other therapeutic modalities are capable of. In this field, viral vectors have been extremely attractive as delivery system. An understanding of the pharmacokinetic behavior of these vectors will be utmost important when designing an effective therapeutic regimen, also will provide a comprehensive review of viral vectors and stimulate novel approaches to improve their pharmacokinetics.

3. Methods used in pharmacokinetic evaluation of viral vectors

As for pharmacokinetic study of viral vectors in gene therapy, the appropriate methods are of vital importance. With the development of science and technology, there have been many advances in the field of pharmacokinetic study in viral gene therapy. Many approaches have been developed over the past decades, especially in the utilization of molecular strategies for the detection and quantification of viral vectors.

3.1 Radioactive tracers

Radioactive tracers are compounds containing one or more radioactive atoms that allow for easy detection and measurement. Tracers are frequently used to track the localization of a specific compound or to trace the path of a compound through a series of chemical reactions. A number of different radioactive forms of hydrogen, carbon, phosphorus, sulfur, and iodine are commonly used in biochemical assays, metabolism studies, and medical diagnostics (Rennie M., 1999).
A radioactive tracer is identical in chemical composition to the compound of interest and is administered in minute amounts that do not perturb the experimental system. The tracer behaves in exactly the same way as an unlabeled molecule, but the tracer molecule continually gives off radiation that can be detected with a Geiger counter, scintillation counter or other type of radiation detection instrument. Zinn K.R. *et al.* labeled recombinant adenovirus serotype 5 knob with the gamma emitter ^{99m}Tc (Zinn, K.R. *et al.*, 1998). Maarten ter Horst *et al.* also used ^{99m}Tc to track the distribution of adenoviral vector (Maarten ter Horst *et al.*, 2006). Studies suggest that this technology is sensitive and the radiolabeling process had no effect on receptor binding. However, it is not available in clinic research because the tracers will give off radiation and labs specific for isotope detection are required, which limits its application in research.

3.2 Polymerase Chain Reaction (PCR)

The polymerase chain reaction (PCR), developed in 1983 by Kary Mullis, is a scientific technique to amplify a single or a few copies of a piece of DNA across several orders of magnitude, generating thousands to millions of copies of a particular DNA sequence (Bartlett & Stirling, 2003). It is now a common and usually indispensable technique used in medical and biological research for a variety of applications, including DNA cloning for sequencing, DNA-based phylogeny, functional analysis of genes, identification of genetic fingerprints, and diagnosis of diseases (Saiki, RK. *et al.*, 1988; Glorioso J.C. *et al.*, 1995). A few years ago, the main approach was defining generic biodistribution properties of viral vectors by designing studies often relying on transgene expression and mostly nonvalidated PCR techniques.

This method has greatly advanced the development of viral gene therapy and progressively helped defining important features of these vectors. But it is just a semi-quantification technology with critical problems, including the number of replicates, the necessity of an internal control, the specificity and the carryover contamination during sample treatment. Besides, the limit of quantification is not as sensitive as expected. In our study, the detection limit of Ad DNA was 10,000 copies per microliter (Figure.1, data unpublished), which greatly hampers the utility of PCR technology in DNA detection when the concentration of DNA in the sample is less than the level mentioned above.

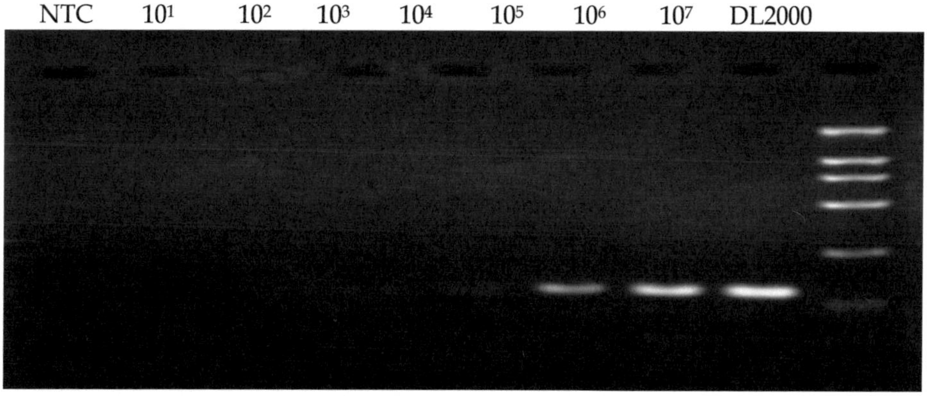

Fig. 1. Validation of the limit of detection of PCR.
Concentrations of DNA in reactions range from 10^7~10^1 copies per microliter.

3.3 Southern blotting

Southern blot, developed by Edwin Southern at Edinburgh University in the 1975, allows investigators to determine the molecular weight of a restriction fragment, to measure relative amounts in different samples and to locate a particular DNA sequence within a complex mixture. In this method, DNA (genomic or other source) is digested with a restriction enzyme, separated by gel electrophoresis and transferred from the agarose gel onto a membrane. The membrane is then incubated with a probe, a single-strand DNA labeled either radioactively or enzymatically (e.g. alkaline phosphatase or horseradish peroxidase), which will form a double-strand DNA with its complementary DNA sequence. Finally, the location of the probe is detected by directly exposing the membrane to X-ray film or chemiluminescent methods. Southern blotting had ever played an important role in viral gene therapy. Henderson Y.C. *et al* developed a method for detecting adenovirus in serum and urine with Southern Blot. Ponnazhagan S. *et al* used it to evaluate Ad2 in nonpermissive human cells (Ponnazhagan S. *et al.*, 1995). Cichon G *et al.* and Bernt KM *et al.* also applied it to investigate gene therapy with adenovirus vectors (Cichon G. *et al.*, 1999; and Bernt K.M. *et al.*, 2003). Those studies suggest its high sensitivity, reproducibility and specificity. However, this method requires a long time and careful manipulation to avoid contamination.

3.4 Western blot

Western blot, developed by W. Neal Burnette from the laboratory of George Stark at Stanford, is an effective and useful method to detect and characterize proteins in small amounts. In this protocol, gel electrophoresis is used to separate proteins by length of the polypeptide (denaturing conditions) or by the 3-D structure of the protein (native/ non-denaturing conditions). The proteins are then transferred to a membrane (typically nitrocellulose or PVDF), where they are probed using antibodies specific to the target protein. This technique is usually used to evaluate the distribution of vectors by detecting expression of target genes in tissues and demonstrates high specificity and sensitivity, therefore, has been widely used in viral gene therapy. Fanxia Shen *et al.* applied it to evaluate hypoxia-inducible vascular endothelial growth factor gene expression mediated by adeno-associated viral vector- in mice (Shen FX, *et al.*, 2006).

3.5 Immunohistochemistry

Immunohistochemistry (IHC) refers to the process of detecting antigens (e.g., proteins) in cells of a tissue section by exploiting the principle of antibodies binding specifically to antigens in biological tissues (RAMOS-VARA J. A., 2005). ICH staining is widely used in the diagnosis of abnormal cells such as those found in cancerous tumors. Specific molecular markers are characteristic of particular cellular events such as proliferation or cell death (apoptosis). IHC is also widely used in basic research to understand the distribution and localization of biomarkers and differentially expressed proteins in different parts of a biological tissue. Visualising an antibody-antigen interaction can be accomplished in a number of ways. In the most common instance, an antibody is conjugated to an enzyme such as peroxidase that can catalyse a colour-producing reaction. Alternatively, the antibody can also be tagged to a fluorophore, such as fluorescein or rhodamine (Elias J.M., 2003).

This method could provide precise information about the distribution of target proteins. However, there are several potential problems that will affect the outcome of the procedure. Although antibodies show preferential avidity for specific epitopes, endogenous biotin or reporter enzymes or primary/secondary antibody cross-reactivity are common causes of strong background staining that can mask the detection of the target antigen, while weak staining may be caused by poor enzyme activity or primary antibody potency. Furthermore, autofluorescence may be due to the nature of the tissue or the fixation method (Grizzle W.E. *et al.*, 2001).

3.6 Real-time quantitative polymerase chain reaction (Q-PCR)

The idea to monitor the PCR reaction in the thermal cycler as it progresses was first realized by Higuchi and colleagues in 1992 (Higuchi R. *et al.*, 1992). And the first commercial platform was the Applied Biosystems ABI Prism 7700 Sequence Detection System, followed by the Idaho Technology LightCycler (Wittwer C.T. *et al.*, 1997). The principle of Q-PCR is based on monitoring of a fluorescent signal arising during the amplification process. In this technique two methods are used to obtain fluorescent signals from the PCR products (Fig. 2). One method involves the use of DNA- specific intercalating dyes such as SYBR Green I and the other is to use fluorescent resonance energy transfer (FRET) such as TaqMan® probes (Didenko V.V., 2001).

Q-PCR has revolutionised the detection and quantification of nucleic acid due to its improved rapidity, sensitivity, reproducibility, reduced risk of carry-over contamination, and ability to quantify viral nucleic acid directly from samples (Morris T. *et al.*, 1996; Lovatt A. *et al.*, 1999; Nitsche A. *et al.*, 1999). As a result, real-time PCR assays, as an attractive tool for precise evaluation of nucleic acid, have received wider acceptance than conventional PCR assays in the field of gene therapy.

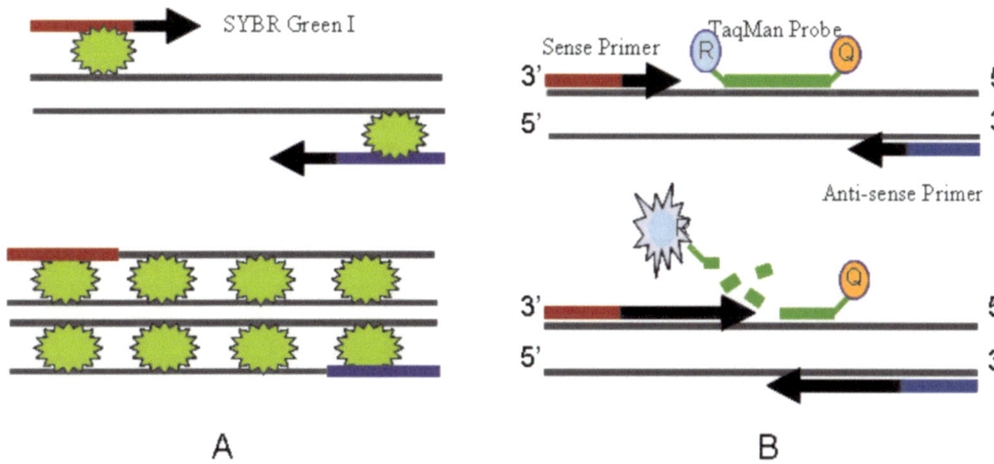

Fig. 2. Two methods used to obtain fluorescent signals from the PCR products.
(A) SYBR Green I; (B) TaqMan® probes.

Quantification of viral vectors by a TaqMan real-time PCR assay has been previously reported. Our team employed TaqMan real-time PCR system to investigate the dynamics of Ad5-LFA-3/IgG1 by measuring its concentration in the blood of rhesus macaques and organs of rats (Xu XX *et al.*, 2009). Miyazawa N. *et al.* examined the kinetics of adenovirus genomic DNA delivery to the nucleus by measuring viral DNA with TaqMan-PCR (Miyazawa N. *et al.*, 1999). Senoo M. *et al.* assessed the tissue distribution of recombinant adenovirus in mice and guinea pigs via TaqMan-PCR (Senoo M., *et al*, 2000). Hackett *et al.* also used TaqMan-PCR to track the time-dependent distribution of vectors *in vivo* (Hackett N.R. *et al*, 2000). These studies support the feasibility of utilizing Q-PCR to track viral vectors.

3.7 *In vivo* imaging system (IVIS)

In conventional experimental strategies, temporal information about biological processes is often obtained through repeated, time-stacked animal sacrifice. If fine temporal analysis is sought during the observation of key biological stages in normal development or disease, the number of animals required per experiment can be quite large (Christopher H.C. & Michael H.B., 2002). Noninvasive imaging methods enable gene expression assays to be conducted in living animals, and they comprise the emerging field of *in vivo* imaging in which a variety of imaging modalities are used for real-time visual monitoring and assessment of biological processes in living animals (Ntziachristos V., 2006). As shown in Fig.3, this technology greatly reduces the number of animals sacrificed per experiment because they allow the comprehensive assessment of each animal over the entire duration of the process (Contag P.R. *et al.*, 1998; Rocchetta H.L. *et al.*, 2001).
Despite obvious progress in gene therapy, the recent failure of trials using adenoviral vectors reminds us that the use of viral vectors has risks that should be carefully assessed. What's more, great the progress in viral vector production, and a better understanding of molecular aspects of vector delivery and targeting issues, has created the need for imaging techniques that could address the problems and opportunities inherent to gene therapy development. As noted previously, *in vivo* imaging could play a unique role in preclinical and clinical

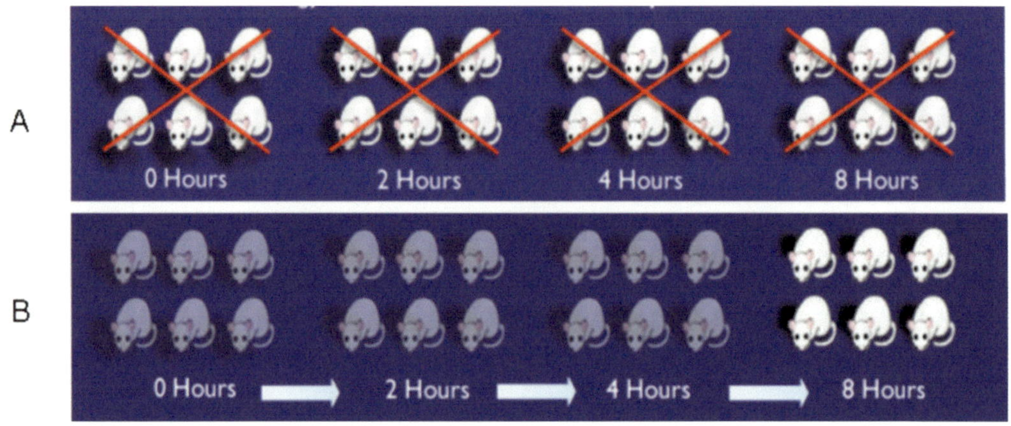

Fig. 3. Comparison of conventional experimental strategies and Noninvasive imaging methods. (A) conventional experimental strategies; (B) Noninvasive imaging methods

gene therapy research and answer the following fundamental questions asked by gene therapists:

- How long would the vector reach its target after *in vivo* administration?
- How many of the vectors are in the target?
- When the expression would take place?
- How long would the expression last?
- Did gene transfer take place?

There have been many recent advances in imaging research to provide answers to these questions mentioned above, and particularly in the utilization of such strategies for the distribution studies of viral vectors. The imaging technology alone, however, can only yield limited information, and pharmacokinetics parameters remain unclear. In this regard, more efforts are required to develop multi-modality imaging strategies allowing for co-registration of high resolution anatomical data together with high sensitive molecular information.

4. Challenges and prospects

As noted previously, viral gene therapy research has evolved considerably since the first clinical trials of this technology. The range of therapeutic targets has also expanded from the treatment of monogenetic disorders to the prevention and treatment of acquired diseases, and so has the number and range of possible therapeutic nucleic acids. This therapeutic modality represents one of the most important developments to occur in medicine. On the other hand, certain technical problems arising from pharmacokinetic studies of viral gene therapy remain to be overcome.

Design and development of ideal gene delivery vectors (Table. 2) are among the main challenges in the evolution of experimental gene therapy into a clinically acceptable mainstream therapy (Rubanyi, G.M., 2001). In spite of the relatively undemanding nature of the selected viral vectors in clinical trials, results from many early stage clinical trials have been frequently disappointing due to the inadequacy of the vectors. The main hurdle for successful viral gene therapy has been the host response to the gene therapy vector, the lack of long-term gene expression, and problems related to the viral property of integration (Neeltje A. K. & Inder M. V. 2003), all of which represent the general aim of pharmacokinetic studies in viral gene therapies. Together, the choice of vector, the design of the expression cassette, and the coding sequence of the genes determine the pharmacokinetics of vectors. Additionally, innovations in vector design will require a better understanding of delivery problems, both at the level of intracellular trafficking of viral DNA to the nucleus and at the level of biological fluid stability and tissue penetration. Hence, much more basic research is needed to interpret the mechanism of viral gene therapy.

Insert size	capacity for one or more genes
Targeting	delivery to specific cell types or gene expression limited to target cells
Regulation	controllable expression levels of transgenes
Safety and stability	safe for the patient and the environment- devoid of the risk of insertional mutagenesis
Immune response	appropriate
Titles	high concentrations and stable final product
Manufacture	easy, reproducible, possible for scale-up and standardization

Table 2. The ideal vector for gene transfer in gene therapy protocols (Dani, S.U., 1999).

Over the past decades, the process and validation of bioanalytical methods have been well developed to generate pharmacokinetic data and provide ADME (absorption, distribution, metabolism, and elimination) information on biotech drugs. However, pharmacokinetic principles of viral gene therapy are far away from sufficiency in spite of long-term and extensive efforts, which requires more considerations when developing bioanalytical approaches in gene therapy with viral vectors, including validation and assay implementation.

Despite recent advances in analytical techniques, further improvements in current analysis modalities are still at the center stage. As mentioned above, all of the technologies mentioned in the review have played important roles during the development of viral gene therapy and provided us important information. But only limited material can be obtained when these methods are used alone.

Challenges including pharmacokinetic studies and analytical methods were shortly described above. It is evident that overcoming these barriers will contribute greatly to the development of viral gene therapy.

In recent years, more attention has been paid on new viral vectors and modifying the existing ones to make them have less toxicity and immunity, besides, with ideal pharmacokinetic features. A number of strategies have evolved to enhance the targeting of gene transfer vectors by genetic or chemical modification on the surface of the vector. Gene expression directed by the transferred gene can be regulated by inducible promoters, tissue-specific promoters, and *trans*-splicing. And many hybird or chinmeric vectors have emerged. Mizuguchi H. *et al.* developed adenovirus vectors containing chimeric type 5 and type 35 fiber proteins, which exhibit altered and expanded tropism and increase the size limit of foreign genes (Mizuguchi H. & Hayakawa T., 2002). Lars Mullera *et al.* developed hybrid vectors HSV–EBV (hepies-simplex-virus-epstein-barrvirus hybrid amplicons) to transfer genes into hepatocytes (Mullera L. *et al.*, 2005). Goncalves MA *et al.* developed

AAV-Ad hybrid vectors, improving the transfer efficiency and expression duration (Goncalves M.A. *et al.*, 2002). These approaches will, consequently, provide more vectors practicable in clinical gene therapies.

Besides, on the basis of what mentioned above, no single modality is ideal for all possible applications and, thus, new protocols for pharmacokinetic studies have been developed in viral gene therapy. Wood M. *et al.* investigated the biodistribution of Ad vector following systemic administration with a PCR and luciferase assay (Mark Wood *et al.*, 1999), which provided semi-quantitative and qualitative analyses of vector distribution. Pan D. *et al.* applied real-time PCR method and flow-cytometric analysis to measure the distribution of lentiviral Vector and expression of target gene in various organs (Dao Pan *et al.*, 2002). And our team used TaqMan real-time PCR and *in vivo* imaging system to track the time-dependent distribution of rAd5/35 *in vivo* post intramuscular injection. The vector was found to remain primarily at the injection site for about eight weeks, at which point it became undetectable (Fig. 4). This result was also shown by *in vivo* imaging of rAd5/35-luc in Balb/c mice (Fig. 5). What's more, as shown in Fig. 6, the whole process of luciferase expression could be monitored in Balb/c mice post-injection with rAd5/35-luc. Quantitative and qualitative results could be attained through the utility of real-time PCR and IVIS technology in biodistribution study of viral gene therapy. In general, the combination of these two approaches provides a rapid, simple approach for a precise, visible result and will ultimately accelerate the progress of gene therapy studies.

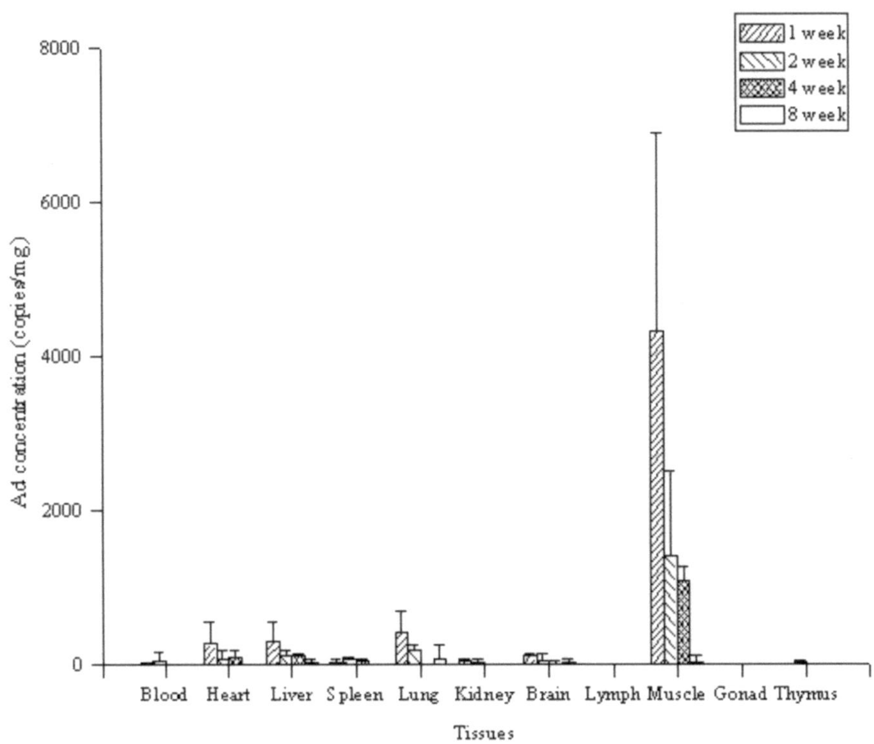

Fig. 4. Biodistribution of rAd5/35-HGEC in tissues of Balb/c mice post-injection with 1.6×10^{9}vp

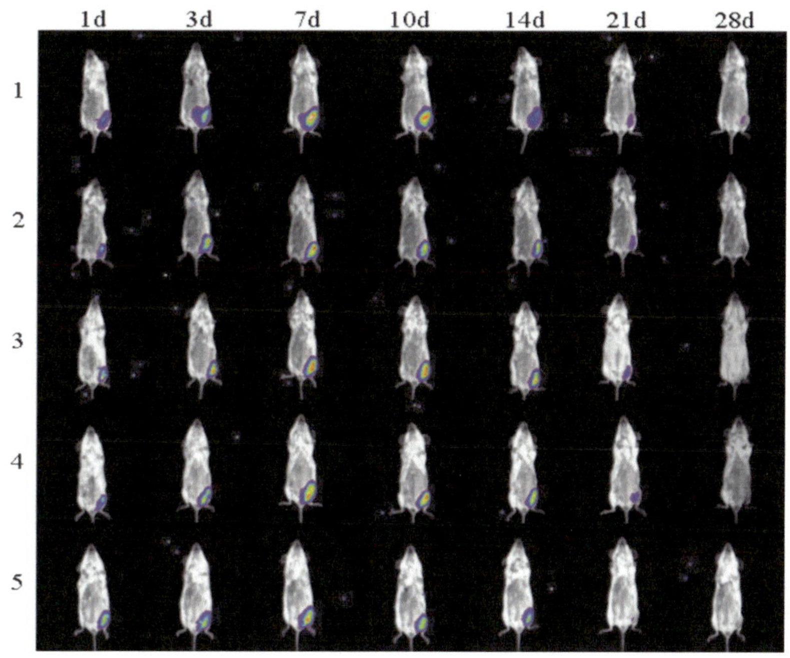

Fig. 5. Luciferase expression in Balb/c mice post-injection with rAd5/35-luc (2×10^{10}vp) (n=5)

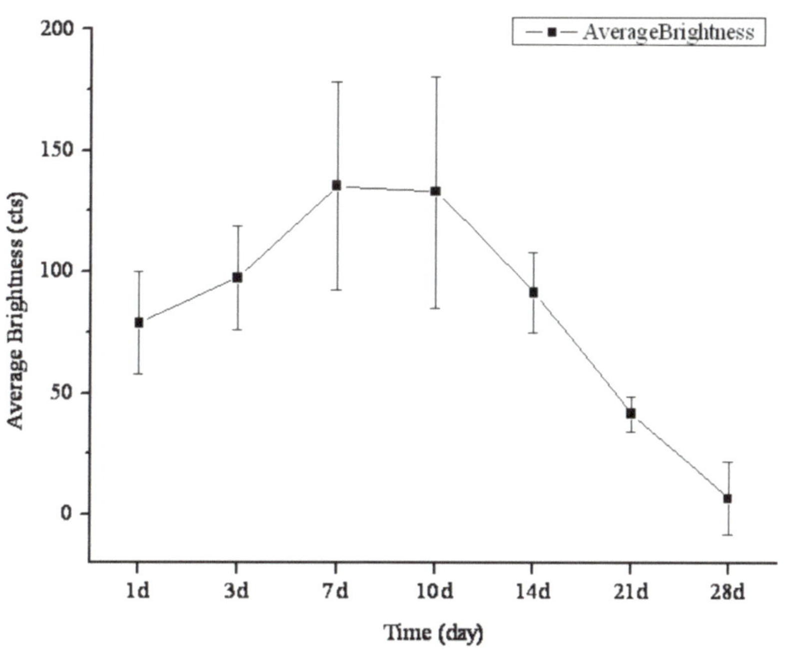

Fig. 6. Duration of luciferase expression in Balb/c mice post-injection with rAd5/35-luc (2×10^{10}vp) (n=5) .

The young field of viral gene therapy promises major medical progress toward the cure of a broad spectrum of human diseases, and has generated great hopes. To achieve this goal, scientists from many different disciplines should participate and pull together as a team. Geneticists must identify target genes while the task for the virologists is to develop efficient and safe vectors. Finally, clinicians carry out clinical trials with vectors optimized for the disease and the medical requirements of the patients (Pfeifer, A. & Verma, I.M., 2001).
On the whole, progress has been made in addressing many of these challenges over the past decades. Based on the continued focus on solving these issues, the knowledge gained from the successes and the setbacks will prove beneficial in viral gene therapy, and there is no doubt that prodigious work will result in innovative technology for pharmacokinetic studies.

5. Conclusion

Gene therapy with viral vectors has been proven very effective in a variety of model systems. And great progress has been made in pharmacokinetic studies of viral gene therapy. However, there are still many challenges, including the host response to the viral vectors, the lack of long-term gene expression, and the risks related to integration into the host genome. Thus, understanding of the pharmacokinetic behavior of viral vectors and developing ideal methods for pharmacokinetic studies will greatly accelerate the development of gene therapy. It's believed that gene therapy has the power to become a dominant therapeutic modality in the future - but all in good time.

6. References

Pfeifer, A. & Verma, I.M., (2001) Gene Therapy: Promises and Problems. *Annual Review of Genomics and Human Genetics*. 2: 177–211.

Arruda VR, Fields PA, Milner R, Wainwright L, De Miguel MP, Donovan PJ, Herzog RW, Nichols TC, Biegel JA, Razavi M, Dake M, Huff D, Flake AW, Couto L, Kay MA & High KA. (2001) Lack of germline transmission of vector sequences following systemic administration of recombinant AAV-2 vector in males. Molecular Therapy. 4: 586–592.

Lovatt A. (2002) Applications of quantitative PCR in the biosafety and genetic stability assessment of biotechnology products. Reviews in Molecular Biotechnology. 82: 279-300

Bartlett & Stirling, (2003) A Short History of the Polymerase Chain Reaction. In: Methods Mol Biol. 226:3-6.

Meibohm, B. (2006) The role of Pharmacokinetics and Pharmacodynamics in the Development of Biotech Drugs, In: Pharmacokinetics and Pharmacodynamics of Biotech Drugs: Principles and case studies, Bernd Meibohm, pp, 3-13, WILEY-VCH Verlag GambH & Co. KGaA, ISBN-13: 978-3-527-31408-9, Germany.

Bernt, K.M., Ni, S., Li, Z.L., Shayakhmetov D.M. & Lieber A. (2003) The effect of sequestration by nontarget tissues on anti-tumor efficacy of systemically applied, conditionally replicating adenovirus vectors. Molecular Therapy. 8: 746–755.

Cichon G., Hartmut H. Schmidt, Tahar Benhidjeb, Peter Löser, Sabine Ziemer, Regina Haas, Nicole Grewe, Frank Schnieders, Jörg Heeren, Michael P. Manns, Peter M. Schlag & Michael Strauss. (1999) Intravenous administration of recombinant adenoviruses causes thrombocytopenia, anemia and erythroblastosis in rabbits. *Journal of Gene Medicine*. 1: 360–371.

Cavazzana-Calvo, M., Hacein-Bey, S., de Saint Basile, G., Gross, F., Yvon, E., Nusbaum, P., Selz, F.; Hue, C., Certain, S., & Casanova, J. L., (2000). Gene therapy of human severe combined immunodeficiency (SCID)-X1 disease[J]. Science, 288(5466): 669~672

Cavazzana-Calvo, M., Thrasher, A., & Mavilio, F. (2004) The future of gene therapy. Nature. 427: 779–781.

Christopher H. Contag & Michael H. Bachmann. (2002) Advances In In Vivo Bioluminescence Imaging Of Gene Expression. Annu. Rev. Biomed. Eng. 4:235–260.

Contag PR, Olomu IN, Stevenson DK & Contag CH. 1998. Bioluminescent indicators in living mammals. Nat. Med. 4:245–247.

Pan D., Gunther R., Duan W., Wendell S., Kaemmerer W., Kafri T., Verma I.M. & Whitley C.B. (2002) Biodistribution and Toxicity Studies of VSVG-Pseudotyped Lentiviral Vector after Intravenous Administration in Mice with the Observation of in Vivo Transduction of Bone Marrow. Melocular Therapy, 6: 19-29.

Dani, S.U., (1999) The challenge of vector development in gene therapy. Brazilian Journal of Med ical and Biological Research. 32: 133-214.

Didenko, V.V., (2001) DNA probes using fluorescence resonance energy transfer (FRET): designs and applications. Biotechniques .31: 1106-1121.

Elias JM (2003) Immunohistochemical methods. In: Immunohistopathology. A Practical Approach to Diagnosis, ed. Elias JM, 2nd ed., pp. 1–110. ASCP Press, Chicago, IL.

Shen FX, Su H, Fan Y, Chen Y, Zhu Y, Liu W, Young WL & Yang GY. (2006) Adeno-Associated Viral Vector-Mediated Hypoxia-Inducible Vascular Endothelial Growth Factor Gene Expression Attenuates Ischemic Brain Injury After Focal Cerebral Ischemia in Mice. Stroke, 37: 2601-2606

Gaspar, H. B., & Thrasher, A. J. (2005) Expert Opinion on Biological Therapy. 5: 1175–1182.

Glorioso JC, DeLuca NA & Fink DJ. (1995) Development and application of herpes simplex virus vectors for human gene therapy. Annu Rev Microbiol. 49:675-710.

Gonçalves MA, van der Velde I, Janssen JM, Maassen BT, Heemskerk EH, Opstelten DJ, Knaän-Shanzer S, Valerio D & de Vries AA. (2002) Efficient gene ration and amplification of high - capacity adeno - associated virus Padenovirus hybrid vectors. Journal of Virology. 76(21) :10734 - 10744.

Grizzle WE, Stockard CR, Billings PE. (2001) The effects of tissue processing variables other than fixation on histochemical staining and immunohistochemical detection of antigens. J Histotechnol. 24: 213–219.

Hackett, N. R., El Sawy, T., Lee, L. Y., Silva, I., O'Leary, J., Rosengart, T. K., Crystal R.G., (2000) Use of quantitative TaqMan Real-Time PCR to track the time-dependent distribution of gene transfer vectors in vivo. Molecular Therapy, 2: 649–656.

Henderson Y.C., Liu T.J., Clayman G.L., (1998) A simple and sensitive method for detecting adenovirus in serum and urine. Journal of Virological Methods. 71: 51–56.

Higuchi, R., Dollinger, G., Walsh, P.S. & Griffith, R., (1992) Simultaneous amplification and detection of specific DNA sequences. Biotechnology (NY). 10: 413-417.

Mizuguchi H. & Hayakawa T. (2002)Adenovirus vectors containing chimeric type 5 and type 35 fiber proteins exhibit altered and expanded tropism and increase the size limit of foreign genes. Gene. 285:69–77.

Kok, T., Wati, S., Bayly, B., Devonshire-Gill, D. & Higgins, G., (2000) Comparison of six nucleic acid extraction methods for the detection of viral DNA or RNA sequences in four different non-serum specimen types. Journal of Clinical Virology. 16: 59-63.

Lovatt A, Black J, Galbraith D, Doherty I, Moran MW, Shepherd AJ, Griffen A, Bailey A, Wilson N& Smith KT. (1999) High throughput detection of retrovirus- associated reverse transcriptase using an improved Fluorescent Product Enhanced Reverse Transcriptase Assay(F-PERT) and its comparison to conventional detection methods. Journal of Virology Methods. 82: 185-200.

ter Horst M., Verwijnen S.M., Brouwer E, Hoeben R.C., de Jong M., de Leeuw B.H., Sillevis Smitt P.A. (2006) Locoregional Delivery of Adenoviral Vectors. Journal of Nuclear Medicine. 47: 1483-1489

Marshall, E. (2000) Gene Therapy on Trial. Science. 288 (5468): 951-957.

Wood M., Perrotte P., Onishi E., Harper M.E., Dinney C., Pagliaro L. & Wilson D.R. (1999) Biodistribution of an adenoviral vector carrying the luciferase reporter gene following intravesical or intravenous administration to a mouse. Cancer Gene Therapy.6: 367–372.

MacLachlan, I., Cullis, P., & Graham, R. W., (1999) Curr. Opin. Molecular Therapy. 1: 252–259.

Miyazawa, N., Leopold, P. L., Hackett, N. R., Ferris, B., Worgall, S. & Falck-Pedersen, E., (1999) Fiber swap between adenovirus subgroups B and C alters intracellular trafficking of adenovirus gene transfer vectors. Journal of Virology, 73: 6056–6065.

Morris, T., Robertson, B. & Gallagher, M., 1996. Rapid reverse transcription-PCR detection of hepatitis C virus RNA in serum using TaqMan fluorogenic detection system. Journal of Clinical Microbiology. 34: 2933-2936.

Müller L, Saydam O, Saeki Y, Heid I & Fraefel C. (2005) Gene transfer into hepatocytes mediated by hepies simplex-virus-epstein-barrvirus hybrid amplicons. Journal of Virological Methods. 123: 65- 72.

Kootstra N.A. & Verma I.M. (2003) Gene Therapy With Viral Vector. Annu. Rev. Pharmacol. Toxicol. 43: 413–439.

Hackett N.R., Sawy T.E., Lee L.Y., Silva I., O'Leary J., Rosengart T.K. & Crystal R.G. (2000) Use of Quantitative TaqMan Real-Time PCR to Track the Time-Dependent Distribution of Gene Transfer Vectors in Vivo. Molecular Therapy. 2: 649-656.

Nitsche, A., Steuer, N., Schmidt, C.A., Landt, O. & Siegert, W., (1999) Different real-time PCR formats compared for the quantitative detection of human cytomegalovirus DNA. Clinical Chemistry. 45: 1932-1937.

Perlman, J., Gibson, C., Pounds, S.B., Gub, Z., Bankowski, M.J., & Haydenb, R.T. (2007) Quantitative real-time PCR detection of adenovirus in clinical blood specimens: A comparison of plasma, whole blood and peripheral blood mononuclear cells. Journal of Clinical Virology. 40: 295-300.

Pearson, S., Jia H & Kandachi, K., (2004) China approves first gene therapy[J]. Nature Biotechnology, 22(1): 3~4.

Ponnazhagan S., Woody M.J., Wang XS, Zhou SZ & Srivastava A. (1995) Transcriptional transactivation of parvovirus B19 promoters in nonpermissive human cells by adenovirus type 2. Journal of Virology. 69: 8096-8101.

RAMOS-VARA J. A. (2005) Technical Aspects of Immunohistochemistry. Vet Pathol. 42:405-426.

Rennie M., (1999) An introduction to the use of tracers in nutrition and metabolism . *Proceedings of the Nutrition Society*. 58 (4): 935-944.

Rocchetta HL, Boylan CJ, Foley JW, Iversen PW, LeTourneau DL, McMillian CL, Contag PR, Jenkins DE & Parr TR Jr. (2001) Validation of a noninvasive, real-time imaging technology using bioluminescent Escherichia coli in the neutropenic mouse thigh model of infection. Antimicrob. Agents Chemother. 45:129-137

Rubanyi, G.M. (2001) The future of human gene therapy. Mol.Aspects Med. 22, 113-142.

Saiki, RK; Gelfand DH, Stoffel S, Scharf SJ, Higuchi R, Horn GT, Mullis KB & Erlich HA (1988). Primer-directed enzymatic amplification of DNA with a thermostable DNA polymerase. Science. 239 (4839): 487-491.

Senoo, M., Matsubara, Y., Fujii, K., Nagasaki, Y., Hiratsuka, M. & Kure, S., (2000). Adenovirus-mediated in utero gene transfer in mice and guinea pigs: Tissue distribution of recombinant adenovirus determined by quantitative TaqMan-polymerase chain reaction assay. Molecular Genetics and Metabolism. 69: 269-276.

Worgall S. & Crystal R.G. (2007) Gene Therapy, In: Principles of Tissue Engineering, 3rd Edition, ed. by Lanza, Langer, and Vacanti, Copyright © 2007, Elsevier, Inc.

Thanou, M., Waddington, S., & Miller, A D., (2007) Gene Therapy. Comprehensive Medicinal Chemistry II, 297-319, Elsevier Ltd. ISBN (set): 0-08-044513-6, ISBN (Volume 1) 0-08-044514-4, USA.

Ntziachristos V. (2006) Fluorescence Molecular Imaging. *Annual Review of Biomedical Engineering*. 8:1-33.

Wittwer, C.T., Ririe, K.M., Andrew, R.V., David, D.A., Gundry, R.A. & Balis, U.J. (1997) The LightCycler: a microvolume multisample fluorimeter with rapid temperature control. Biotechniques. 22: 176-181.

Xu XX, Shui X, Chen ZH, Shan CQ, Hou YN & Cheng YG (2009) Development and Application of a Real-time PCR Method for Pharmacokinetic and Biodistribution Studies of Recombinant Adenovirus. Molecular Biotechnology. 43:130-137.

Zinn KR, Douglas JT, Smyth CA, Liu HG, Wu Q, Krasnykh VN, Mountz JD, Curiel DT & Mountz JM. (1998) Imaging and tissue biodistribution of 99mTc-labeled adenovirus knob (serotype 5). Gene Therapy. 5: 798–808.